Radiographic
Image
Analysis

second edition

Radiographic Image Analysis

Kathy McQuillen Martensen, MA, RT(R)

Director, Radiologic Technology Education
University of Iowa Hospitals and Clinics
Iowa City, Iowa

ELSEVIER
SAUNDERS

ELSEVIER
SAUNDERS

11830 Westline Industrial Drive
St. Louis, Missouri 63146

Notice

Neither the Publisher nor the Author assume any responsibility for any loss or injury and/or
damage to persons or property arising out of or related to any use of the material contained in this
book. It is the responsibility of the treating practitioner, relying on independent expertise and
knowledge of the patient, to determine the best treatment and method of application for the patient.

The Publisher

International Standard Book Number 13: 978-0-7216-3925-3
International Standard Book Number 10: 0-7216-3925-9

Publisher: Andrew Allen
Acquisitions Editor: Jeanne Wilke
Senior Developmental Editor: Linda Woodard
Publishing Services Manager: Patricia Tannian
Project Manager: Sarah Wunderly
Designer: Kathi Gosche

Printed in United States

Last digit is the print number: 9 8 7 6 5 4 3 2 1

To my parents, Pat and Dolores McQuillen
and to my husband, Van
and to my children, Nicole, Zachary, and Adam

Deanna Butcher, MA, RT(R)
Program Director
St. Luke's College
Sioux City, Iowa

Charles Frances, MEd, RT(R), (QM)
Department Chair and Associate Professor
Idaho State University
Pocatello, Idaho

Mari P. King, EdD, RT(R), CDT
Health Sciences Division Chair
Associate Professor, Medical Imaging
College Misericordia
Dallas, Pennsylvania

Beckey J. Miller, MS, RT(R)
Program Director/Chairperson
Horry-Georgetown Technical College
Conway, South Carolina

Barbara Peacock, BS, RT(R), (CT)
Radiography Clinical Coordinator
Cumberland County College
Vineland, New Jersey

Kenneth A. Roszel, MS, RT(R)
Program Director
Geisinger Health System
Danville, Pennsylvania

Loraine D. Zelna, MS, RT(R), (MR)
Associate Professor
College Misericordia
Dallas, Pennsylvania

The purpose of this book is to supply educators, students, and radiographers with the information needed to analyze radiographic images for accuracy and to know how to adjust mispositioning or technical equipment to obtain an optimal image when a less than optimal one has been obtained, to prepare for the certification examination by the ARRT, and to develop a high degree of problem-solving ability, as well as provide a practical image analysis reference for working technologists. For each of the most commonly performed radiographic positions/projections, this book provides an accurately positioned image with labeled anatomy, many examples of poorly positioned images, photographs of a model demonstrating accurate patient positioning and demonstrating examples of patient mispositioning, and an image analysis criteria list. For each criterion listed, a discussion is provided that correlates the analysis criteria with the corresponding patient or central ray set-up procedure that defines how the resulting image will appear if the correct patient or central ray set-up procedure is not followed, and that explains radiographic principles as they relate to the criterion. The images for each procedure that demonstrate poor patient and central ray positioning are grouped together. Next to each of these images is a synopsis discussing the mispositioning, and how the patient or central ray should be repositioned to obtain an optimal image.

Since the publication of the first edition of *Radiographic Critique*, many advances in imaging technology have occurred, the ASRT has revised the suggested radiography curriculum and included a more inclusive outline for the image analysis course with a strong emphasis on critical thinking, the cost of health care has continued to rise, demanding a need for more proficient technologists, and my image analysis knowledge has expanded.

NEW CONTENT

In the second edition the reader will notice a new chapter covering the digestive system, the addition of digital and pediatric imaging throughout the chapters, as well as new discussions on mobile and trauma imaging, image distortion, technical adjustments for poor image visibility, and equipment-related artifacts. Approximately 80% of the radiographic images have been replaced with higher quality digital images, the format has been streamlined and tables added for easier reference, and 34 new position/projections have been included.

The ability to accurately produce and analyze images and provide the best possible patient care is the goal of every technologist. It is hoped that this text will contribute substantially to that goal.

ALSO AVAILABLE

Workbook for Radiographic Image Analysis, edition 2, is available for separate purchase and provides the learner with ample opportunities to practice and apply the information presented in the text. The workbook includes extra images beyond those in the text for analysis, so the student can hone imaging and evaluation skills. It also includes learning objectives and many exercises.

FOR THE INSTRUCTOR

An Instructor's Resource Manual accompanies the text. This resource consists of:
- Instructor's Manual, which includes in-depth chapter outlines, Learning Activities, and Laboratory Activities
- Test Bank, which includes over 350 questions in Examview format.
- Electronic Image Collection, which includes all the images from the text in PowerPoint and jpeg format.

The ICR is also posted on Evolve, which also includes a Course Management System for instructors and Websites for students.

EVOLVE ONLINE COURSE MANAGEMENT

Evolve is an interactive learning environment designed to work in coordination with *Radiographic Image Analysis*. Instructors may use Evolve to provide an Internet-based course component that reinforces and expands on the concepts delivered in class. Evolve may be used to publish the class syllabus, outlines, and lecture notes; set up "virtual office hours" and email communication; share important dates and information through the online class Calendar; and encourage student participation through Chat Rooms and Discussion Boards. Evolve allows instructors to post exams and manage their grade books online. An online version of the Instructor's Resource Manual is also available on Evolve. For more information, visit http://www.evolve.elsevier.com/Martensen/imageanalysis/ or contact an Elsevier sales representative.

ACKNOWLEDGMENTS

I would like to express my gratitude to the following individuals who have helped shape this edition and provided the support required to accomplish the work.

Stephanie Harris, Zanetta Hoehle, Brandi Huber, Stephanie Ellingson, and Shelley Matzen, for the willingness to help me locate interesting images, review sections of the book, and listen, test, and question my analysis concepts. Thank you also for your support and friendship.

The University of Iowa Hospitals and Clinics' Radiologic Technology Classes of 1988 to 2005, who have been my best teachers, as they have challenged me with their questions and insights.

Adam Martensen, Angie Rausch, Cade Rausch, Kendrick Harris, Jeff Stellinga, and Stephanie Harris for helping with the photography and working as models.

Jeanne Wilke, Linda Woodard, Jennifer Moorhead, Sarah Wunderly, and the entire Elsevier Saunders team for their support, assistance, and expertise in planning and developing this project.

To the professional colleagues, book reviewers, educators, and technologists that have evaluated, sent me compliments and suggestions, and questioned concepts in the first edition. Please continue to do so.

My husband, Van, for picking up where I left off, allowing me the time needed to complete this work.

KMM

CONTENTS

Radiographic
Image
Analysis

Guidelines for Image Analysis

In radiographic positioning and diagnostic imaging classes, one learns the skills needed to obtain optimal images of all body structures. An optimal image is one that demonstrates all the most desired features. It would demonstrate maximum recorded detail; perfect patient positioning; excellent penetration, contrast, and density; and no motion or removable artifacts.

Unfortunately, because of patient condition, equipment malfunction, or technologist error, such perfection is not obtained for every image that is produced. A less-than-optimal image should be thoroughly evaluated to determine the reason for error so the problem can be corrected before the examination is repeated. An image should never have to be taken a third time because the error was not accurately identified from the first mispositioned image.

This book cannot begin to identify the standards of acceptability within all the different imaging facilities. What might be an acceptable standard in one facility may not be in another. Even if an image is not optimal but is still passable according to your facility's standards, it should be carefully studied to determine whether your skills could be improved before the next similar examination. Study the technical factors, such as placement of radiation protection, name identification plate (ID plate) and markers, and degree of collimation, to determine whether you can improve the locations or can increase collimation for your next patient. Closely studying the patient's positioning can reveal habits in positioning that can be corrected to improve imaging. For example, if you believe you are positioning the femoral epicondyles perpendicular to the image receptor (IR) for a lateral knee image but the images you take consistently demonstrate the lateral condyle anterior to the medial condyle, you may learn to alter your positioning technique by increasing the anterior rotation of the patient by the distance usually demonstrated between the two condyles on

your images. This rotation should compensate for your error and should yield an image with perpendicular alignment of the condyles.

As you study the images in this book, you may find that many of them are acceptable within your facility, even though they do not meet optimal standards. The goal of this work is not to dictate to your facility what should be acceptable and unacceptable images. It is to help you focus on improving your image analysis and positioning skills and to provide a guideline on how the patient or central ray was mispositioned for an image containing an error.

TERMINOLOGY
Positioning and Anatomical Placement Terminology

Many terms are used in radiography to describe the path of the x-ray beam; the patient's position; the precise location of an anatomical structure; the position of one anatomical structure in relation to another; and the way a certain structure will change its position as the patient moves in a predetermined direction. These terms can be used singly or in combinations. Familiarity with radiography terminology will help you to understand statements made throughout this text and to converse competently with other professionals in the medical field. The combining form of each term is shown in parentheses.

Anatomical position: Refers to positioning the patient with the arms and legs extended and the face, arms, hands, legs, and feet placed in an anteroposterior (AP) projection. This is the starting point from which imaging procedures are referenced.

Anterior (antero-): Refers to the front surface of the patient; used to express something that is situated at or directed toward the front: *The sternum is anterior to the vertebral column.* Includes the palms and tops of the feet as in anatomical position.

Decubitus position: Refers to the patient lying down on a table or cart while a horizontally directed central ray is used. Also stated with the term *decubitus* is the surface (lateral, dorsal, or ventral) that is placed adjacent to the table or cart: *The patient is in a left lateral decubitus position.*

Distal (disto-): Refers to a structure that is situated away from the source or beginning: *The foot is distal to the ankle.* Or, *The splenic flexure is distal to the hepatic flexure.*

Dorsal (dorso-): See *posterior.*

Inferior (infero-): Refers to a structure within the patient's torso that is situated closer to the feet; used when comparing the locations of two structures: *The symphysis pubis is inferior to the iliac crest.*

Lateral (latero-): Refers to the patient's sides; used to express something that is directed or situated away from the patient's median plane or to express the outer side of an extremity: *The kidneys are lateral to the vertebral column.* Or, *Place the IR against the lateral surface of the knee.*

Lateral position: Refers to positioning of the patient so that the side of the torso or extremity being imaged is placed adjacent to the IR. When a lateral position of the torso, vertebrae, or cranium is defined, the term *right* or *left* is also included to state which side of the patient is placed closer to the IR: *The patient was in a left lateral position when the chest image was taken.*

Medial (medio-): Refers to the patient's median plane; used to express something that is directed or situated toward the patient's median plane or to express the inner side of an extremity: *The sacroiliac joints are medial to the anterior superior iliac spines (ASISs).* Or, *Place the IR against the medial surface of the knee.*

Oblique position: Refers to rotation of a structure away from an AP or posteroanterior (PA) projection. When obliquity of the torso, vertebrae, or cranium is defined, the terms *right* or *left* and *anterior* or *posterior* are used with the term *oblique,* to indicate which side of the patient is placed closer to the IR. In a right anterior oblique (RAO) position the patient is rotated so that the right, anterior surface is placed closer to the IR. When obliquity of an extremity is defined, the term *medial* (internal) or *lateral* (external) is used with the term *oblique* to indicate which way the extremity is rotated from anatomical position and which side of the extremity is positioned closer to the IR. For a medial oblique position of the wrist, the medial side of the arm is placed closer to the IR.

Posterior (postero-): Refers to the back of the patient; used to express something that is situated at or directed toward the back: *The knee joint is posterior to the patella.* Includes the backs of the hands and bottoms of the feet as in anatomical position.

Proximal (proximo-): Refers to a structure that is closest to the source or beginning: *The shoulder joint is proximal to the elbow joint.* Or, *The hepatic flexure is proximal to the splenic flexure.*

Superior (supero-): Refers to a structure within the patient's torso that is situated closer to the head; used when comparing the locations of two torso structures: *The thoracic cavity is superior to the peritoneal cavity.*

Ventral (ventro-): See *anterior.*

The following list contains frequently used combinations of the preceding terms. You might recognize some of them as *projections,* a term used to describe the entrance and exit points of the x-ray beam as it passes through the body when an image is taken. The projections have been starred (*). In a projection the path from the first location to the second must be straight.

anteroinferior	inferolateral	posterolateral
anterolateral	inferosuperior*	posteromedian
anteromedian	lateromedial*	posterosuperior
anteroposterior*	mediolateral*	superoinferior*
anterosuperior	posteroanterior*	superolateral
	posteroinferior	

Body Plane Terminology

Following are body planes that are used throughout this textbook. Becoming familiar with them will help you to better understand how the patient and central ray or IR are positioned.

Coronal plane: An imaginary plane that passes through the body from side to side and divides it into two (not necessarily equal) sections, one anterior and one posterior.

Midcoronal plane: An imaginary plane that passes through the body from side to side and divides it into equal anterior and posterior sections or halves.

Midsagittal or median plane: An imaginary plane that passes through the body anteroposteriorly or posteroanteriorly and divides it into equal right and left sections or halves.

Sagittal plane: An imaginary plane that passes through the body anteroposteriorly or posteroanteriorly and divides it into right and left sections that are not necessarily equal.

General Terminology

Following are definitions of terms relating to patient or central ray positioning, anatomical alignment and identity, and technical procedures used throughout this book.

Abduct: To move an extremity outward, away from the torso. The humerus is abducted when it is elevated laterally.

Adduct: To move an extremity toward the torso. The humerus is adducted when it is positioned closer to the torso after being abducted.

Align: To bring into line or alignment: *The lower leg and foot are aligned at a 90-degree angle with each other for a lateral foot image.*

Articulation: A joint or place where two bones meet.

Caudal: The foot end of the patient: *A caudally angled central ray is directed toward the patient's feet.*

Central ray: The center of the x-ray beam. It is used to center the anatomical structure and IR.

Cephalic: The head end of the patient. A cephalically angled central ray is directed toward the patient's head.

Concave: Curved or rounded inward: *The anterior surface of the metacarpals is concave.*

Condyle: Rounded projection on a bone that often articulates with another bone.

Convex: Curved or rounded outward: *The posterior surface of the metacarpals is convex.*

Cortical outline: The outer layer of a bone that is demonstrated on an image as the white outline of an anatomical structure.

Depress: To lower or sink down, positioning at a lower level.

Detail: A part of the whole structure: *The trabeculae are details in the femoral bone.*

Deviate: To move away from the normal or routine.

Distortion: The misrepresentation of the size or shape of the structure being examined.

Dorsiflexion: The act of moving the toes and forefoot upward.

Elevate: To lift up or raise, positioning at a higher level.

Elongate: To make one axis of an anatomical structure appear to be disproportionately longer on the image than the opposite axis. Angling the central ray while the part and IR remain parallel with each other will elongate the axis toward which the central ray is angled.

Eversion: The act of turning the plantar foot surface as far laterally as the ankle will allow.

Extension: A movement that results in straightening of a joint. With extension of the elbow, the arm is straightened. Extension of the cervical vertebrae shifts the patient's head posteriorly in an attempt to separate the vertebral bodies.

External (lateral) rotation: The act of turning the anterior surface of an extremity outward or away from the patient's torso midline.

Flexion: A movement that bends a joint. With flexion of the elbow, the arm is bent. Flexion of the cervical vertebrae shifts the patient's head forward in an attempt to bring the vertebral bodies closer.

Foreshorten: To make one axis of an anatomical structure appear to be disproportionately shorter on the image than the opposite axis. Positioning the long axis of the lower leg at a 45-degree angle with the IR while the central ray is perpendicular to the IR foreshortens the image of the lower leg on the image.

Internal (medial) rotation: The act of turning the anterior surface of an extremity inward or toward the patient's torso midline.

Inversion: The act of turning the plantar foot surface as far medially as the ankle will allow.

Longitudinal or lengthwise (LW): Refers to the long axis of the anatomical structure or object being discussed.

A longitudinal axis on a 14- × 17-inch (35- × 43-cm) IR would parallel the IR's longer (17-inch or 43-cm) length. The longitudinal axis of a patient's thorax would parallel the midsagittal plane. To position the IR LW with the patient means to align the IR's longitudinal axis with the patient's longitudinal axis.

Magnification: Proportionately increasing or enlarging both axes of a structure. The gonadal contact shield is magnified on the image if it is placed on top of the patient.

Object–image receptor distance (OID): Distance from the object being imaged to the IR.

Palpate: Act of touching or feeling a structure through the skin.

Plantar flexion: The act of moving the toes and forefoot downward.

Profile: The outline of an anatomical structure: *The glenoid fossa is demonstrated in profile on a Grashey method image.*

Project: The act of throwing the image of an anatomical structure forward: *An angled central ray projects the anatomical part situated farther away from the IR farther than the anatomical part situated closer to the IR.*

Pronate: To rotate or turn the upper extremity medially until the hand's palmar surface is facing downward or posteriorly.

Protract: To move a structure forward or anteriorly: *The shoulder is protracted when it is drawn forward.*

Radial deviation: While maintaining a PA projection, move the distal hand toward the radial side as much as the wrist will allow.

Recorded detail: The sharpness of structures that have been included on the image.

Retract: To move a structure backward or posteriorly: *The shoulder is retracted when it is drawn backwards.*

Source–image receptor distance (SID): The distance from the anode's focal spot to the IR.

Superimpose: To lie over or above an anatomical structure or object.

Supination: Rotating or turning the upper extremity laterally until the hand's palmar surface is facing upwardly or anteriorly.

Symmetrical: Structures on opposite sides demonstrating the same size, shape, and position.

Trabecular pattern: The supporting material within cancellous bone. It is demonstrated on an image as thin white lines throughout a bony structure.

Transverse, horizontal, or crosswise (CW): Refers to a plane that is at a 90-degree angle from the longitudinal axis of the anatomical structure or object being discussed. The transverse axis of a 14- × 17-inch (35- × 43-cm) IR would parallel the shorter (14-inch or 35-cm) length. The transverse axis on a patient's thorax would be perpendicular to the midsagittal plane.

Ulnar deviation: While maintaining a PA projection, turn the distal hand toward the ulnar side as much as the wrist will allow.

Technical Terminology

Following are definitions of technical terms.

Artifact: An undesirable structure or substance recorded on the image. It may or may not be covering information.

Cathode ray tube (CRT) monitor: Electronic monitor used for display and/or manipulation of the resulting digital image.

Compensating filter: An absorbing substance added in the path of the x-ray beam that will remove photons from the beam. The filter is used to even out the density of structures that are imaged at the same time and vary in part thickness, such as the femur or lower leg.

Computed radiography: Projection radiography that uses photostimulable phosphor plates (imaging plates) as the IR.

Contrast: The number of shades of gray that represent the different structures on the image.

Density: The degree of darkness on an image.

Diagnostic specifier: In computed radiography, the examination indicator chosen by the technologist before the plate is processed; tells the reader the anatomical structure, position, and projection under which the image plate is to be processed.

Digital radiography: The use of detectors that convert x-ray energy to electrical energy that is delivered directly to a computer, where the anatomical image is digitally processed and displayed.

Grid: A device consisting of lead strips that is placed between the patient and IR for the purpose of reducing the amount of scatter radiation reaching the receptor.

ID plate: The area on the resulting image that indicates the patient and facility's identification information, procedure completed, and date and time the procedure was completed.

Imaging plate: The plate used in computed radiography that is coated with a photostimulable phosphor material that absorbs the photons exiting the patient, resulting in the formation of a latent image that is released and digitized before being sent to a computer.

Imaging receptor (IR): A device that receives the radiation leaving the patient. Conventional radiography uses a screen-film system, and computed radiography uses an imaging plate.

Normalization (automatic scaling): A process by which the computed radiography system automatically corrects for manually set and automatic exposure errors to produce consistently optimal images.

Quantum mottle: A mottled or grainy appearance of an image when insufficient milliampere-seconds (mAs) have been used.

Radiolucent: Allowing the passage of x-radiation. A radiolucent object appears dark on an image.

Radiopaque: Preventing the passage of x-radiation. A radiopaque object appears white on an image.

Resolution: The differentiation of individual structures or details from one another on an image.

Scatter radiation: Radiation that has changed in direction from the primary beam because of an interaction with the patient or other structure. Because it is emitted in random directions it carries no useful signal or subject contrast.

Windowing: In digital radiography, postprocessing manipulation feature by which the technologist adjusts image contrast and density.

DISPLAYING IMAGES

Before an image is evaluated for accuracy, it is displayed on a CRT monitor or made available in the form of a hard-copy radiograph and displayed on a view box. This section describes the proper procedure for displaying images on the CRT monitor or hanging hard-copy radiographs on the view box. For any image presented in the book but not listed here, the proper hanging procedure is described in the discussion of the image, in the section on marker placement.

The following are global guidelines for displaying images on a CRT monitor or hanging hard-copy radiographs of different parts, positions, and projections:

- Torso, vertebral, cranial, shoulder, and hip images: as if the patient were standing in an upright position
- Finger, wrist, and forearm images: as if the patient were hanging from the fingertips
- Elbow and humerus images: as if they were hanging from the patient's shoulder
- Toe and AP and oblique foot images: as if the patient were hanging from the toes
- Lateral foot, ankle, lower leg, knee, and femur images: as if they were hanging from the patient's hip
- Decubitus chest and abdominal images: generally displayed so that the side of the patient that was positioned upward when the image was taken is upward on the displayed image
- Axiolateral positions of the shoulder and hip: with the patient's anterior surface up and posterior surface down

Whether the front or back of the image is placed against the view box or displayed as if on a view box is determined by the projection or position presented, as described in the following section.

Anteroposterior and Posteroanterior Projections and Oblique Positions of the Torso, Vertebrae, and Cranium

- Images taken in an AP or PA projection or oblique position should be displayed as if the viewer and the patient are facing one another. The right side of the patient's image is on the viewer's left, and the left side of the patient's image is on the viewer's right.
- Whenever AP projections or posterior oblique positions are taken, the R (right) or L (left) marker appears correct when the image is accurately displayed, as long as the

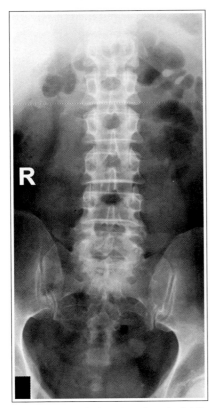

Figure 1-1. Accurately displayed and marked AP projection.

Lateral Positions of the Torso, Vertebrae, and Cranium

- The marker placed on a lateral image of the torso, vertebrae, or cranium represents the side of the patient positioned closer to the IR. If the patient is positioned with the left side against the imaging table for a lateral lumbar vertebrae image, a left marker should be placed on the IR.

- If this marker is placed anteriorly (in front of the lumbar vertebrae), the image can be displayed in the same manner as an AP/PA projection, with the left marker placed on the viewer's right side or the right marker placed on the viewer's left side (Figure 1-3). In general, accurately displayed laterally positioned images demonstrate a correct marker as long as the marker was placed on the IR face-up before the image was taken. One exception to this guideline may be when left lateral chest images are displayed; often, reviewers prefer left lateral chest images to be displayed as if they had been taken in the right lateral position.

Extremities

- Extremity images are displayed as if the viewer's eyes were the x-ray beam going through the image in the same manner in which the photons went through the extremity when it was imaged. If a PA right-hand image is viewed, it should be displayed so the thumb is positioned

marker was placed on the IR face-up before the image was taken (Figure 1-1).

- When PA projections or anterior oblique positions are taken, the R or L marker appears reversed if placed face-up when the image is accurately displayed (Figure 1-2).

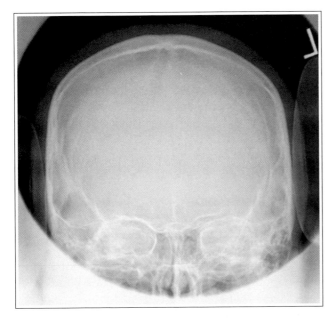

Figure 1-2. Accurately displayed PA projection.

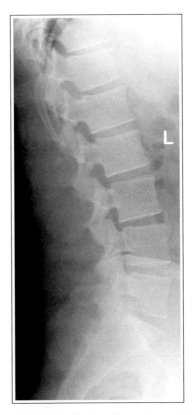

Figure 1-3. Accurately displayed laterally positioned image.

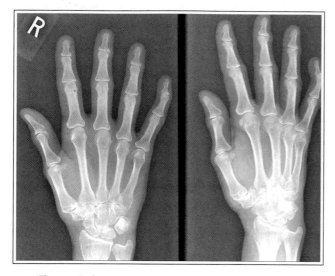

Figure 1-4. Accurately displayed extremity image.

toward the viewer's left side (Figure 1-4). If the viewer places his or her right hand against an accurately displayed image of a hand in a PA projection, it should be aligned as the image is (i.e., the thumb and fingers should appear in the same order). For a lateral right-hand image, the palmar side of the hand should be directed toward the viewer's left side. This indicates that the medial (ulnar) side of the hand was positioned closer to the IR and that the x-ray beam went from the lateral side of the patient's hand to the medial side.

- As long as the R or L marker is placed on the IR face-up before the image is taken, it will be demonstrated accurately when the image is correctly displayed.

IMAGE ANALYSIS FORM

Once a hard-copy radiograph is correctly displayed or is presented on the CRT monitor, it should be evaluated for positioning and technical accuracy. The analysis should follow some consistent system or method, to ensure that all aspects of the image are considered. The image analysis form shown in Figure 1-5 contains a checklist that covers all the aspects of image analysis. For each item, several questions should be asked regarding an image; these questions are presented and discussed in the remainder of this section. The answers to all the questions, taken together, will determine whether the image is acceptable. The checklist can be used whenever you evaluate an image.

The approach to image analysis outlined in Figure 1-5 is the approach taken in the image analysis sections of this book. Each item listed on the image analysis form represents a particular aspect of image analysis. The following discussion explores in depth each of these aspects. Every item on the image analysis form is presented below in **boldface** and followed by a series of questions, shown in *italics*, that will help you determine whether the item may be checked as satisfactorily completed.

Facility's identification requirements—facility name, patient name and age, and examination time and date—are visualized on the image.

1. Is the facility's name visible on the image?

Each hard-copy radiograph should have the facility's name permanently imprinted on the film's emulsion. This is accomplished by photoflashing the ID plate when using a screen-film system. When digital radiography is used, the facility's name is automatically added to the image during the printing process. This information identifies ownership.

2. Are the patient's name and age or birth date visible on the image, and are they accurate?

The correct patient's name and age or birth date should be permanently photoflashed to the ID plate or displayed on the CRT monitor. This information should be typed and legible. Evaluate all the images within a routine series to ensure that the correct name is imprinted or displayed on each image. Never assume that an image has been correctly photoflashed or assigned to the correct patient. Always double-check. Flash cards can be easily switched or forgotten, or the examination assigned to the wrong patient.

If the wrong name or age has been photoflashed onto the ID plate when using a screen-film system, the correct information should be attached over the incorrect patient information before the radiographs are sent to be interpreted. If incorrect patient information was assigned to an image when digital radiography was used, the examination should be reattributed to the correct patient before the image is sent to the archiving system. If a radiograph is sent to the archiving system with the wrong patient associated with it, the image may be seen or evaluated by a physician before the change is made, resulting in an inaccurate diagnosis and unnecessary or inaccurate treatment of the wrong patient.

3. Are the examination time and date visible on the image?

The accuracy of examination time and date are necessary to distinguish the images in a timed series and to match images with their accompanying requisition and report.

4. Is the ID plate positioned so it does not obscure any anatomy of interest?

ID plate placement is evaluated on every image for optimal location. Has it obscured any anatomy of interest, or was it positioned in a place that is acceptable? By evaluating where the ID plate is positioned on all images taken using the screen-film system, one can locate the best place to position the ID plate for future reference. When the IR is positioned LW, the ID plate is placed in the upper right or lower left corner. When the IR is positioned CW, the ID plate is placed in the lower right or upper left corner.

Image Analysis Form

Exam _____

_____ Facility's identification requirements — facility name, patient name and age, and examination time and date — are visualized on the image.

_____ Correct marker (eg., R/L, arrow) is visualized on image and demonstrates accurate placement.

_____ Required anatomy is present on image.

_____ The relationships between the anatomical structures are accurate for the projection/position demonstrated.

_____ Image is demonstrated without unwanted distortion.

_____ Bony cortical outlines and/or soft tissue structures are sharply defined.

_____ Maximum collimation efforts are evident on image.

_____ Radiation protection is present on image when indicated, and good radiation protection practices were used during procedure.

_____ Smallest possible IR size has been used, and the IR and anatomical structures have been accurately aligned to include the required anatomy with tight collimation.

_____ Correct image receptor system was used.

_____ Density and penetration are optimal, visualizing the required bony and soft tissue structures.

_____ Image contrast optimally visualizes the bony and soft tissue structures of interest.

_____ No preventable artifacts are present on the image

_____ The ordered procedure and the indication for the exam have been fulfilled.

_____ The requisition and other post-procedure requirements have been completed, and the repeat/reject analysis information has been provided as indicated by your facility.

Image is: _____ acceptable _____ unacceptable

If image is unacceptable, describe what measures should be taken to produce an acceptable image. If image is acceptable, but not optimal, describe any factors that could be adjusted to obtain an optimal image.

Figure 1-5. Image analysis form.

Guidelines for determining the best location to position the ID plate are as follows:

- Place the ID plate outside the collimated field whenever possible.
- Position the ID plate away from the direction in which the central ray is angled.
- Position the ID plate next to the narrowest anatomical structure.

Digital imaging systems vary with regard to how the patient information is displayed. Regardless of the system used, the ID plate placement for digital radiography is not as sensitive as it is for a screen-film system because the information is displayed outside the collimated area. After the image is displayed, the blocker location can be adjusted to move it away from anatomy of interest.

Marking Images

Correct markers (R, L, arrow, etc.) are visible on the image and demonstrate accurate placement.

Lead markers are used to identify the patient's right and left sides, to indicate variations in the standard procedure, or to show the amount of time that has elapsed in timed procedures such as intravenous urography and small bowel studies. The markers are constructed of lead so as to be radiopaque (unable to be penetrated with radiation). Whenever a marker is placed on the IR within the collimated light field, radiation will be unable to penetrate it, resulting in an unexposed, white area on the image where the marker was located.

1. Is the marker visualized within the collimated field and so it does not obscure areas of interest?

Proper marker placement ensures that the marker will be present on the image: The marker must be positioned within the collimated light field so radiation will strike it. Place the markers on the IR instead of on the imaging table or patient. This placement avoids marker distortion and magnification and prevents scatter radiation from crossing beneath the marker, fogging the area on the IR where the marker would be visualized. It also ensures that the marker will not be projected off of the IR. Figure 1-6 shows a

marker that is undistorted and can be clearly seen, as well as two examples of marker fogging, magnification, and distortion that resulted from placement of the marker on the patient or imaging table instead of directly on the IR.

When collimating less than the size of the IR used, it can be difficult to determine exactly where to place the marker on the IR so it will remain within the collimated field and not obscure anatomical areas of interest. The best way of accomplishing this is to first collimate the desired amount and then use the collimator guide (Figure 1-7) to determine how far from the IR's midline to place the marker. Although different models of x-ray equipment have different collimator guides, the information displayed by all is similar. Each guide explains the IR coverage for the SID and amount of longitudinal and transverse collimation being used. If a 14- × 17-inch (35- × 43-cm) IR is placed in the Bucky tray at a set SID, and the collimator guide indicates that the operator has collimated to an 8- × 17-inch (20- × 43-cm) field size, the marker should be placed 3½ to 4 inches (10 cm) from the IR's longitudinal midline in order to be included in the collimated field (Figure 1-8). If the field was also longitudinally collimated, the marker would have to be positioned within this dimension, as well. In the preceding example, if the collimator guide indicates that the longitudinal field is collimated to a 15-inch (38-cm) field size, the marker would have to be placed 7½ inches (19 cm) from the IR's transverse midline (see Figure 1-8).

Usually, an IR provides many areas in which to place the marker so it does not obscure needed information. Before taking an image, imagine where the areas of interest will be located, and then situate the marker on the IR where it is least likely to obscure anatomy of interest. Because the area of interest is most often located in the center of the collimated field, it is best to position markers as far away from the center of the IR as possible.

2. Is the marker positioned in the best possible location for the projection and position being presented?

This question is best considered separately for each projection and position.

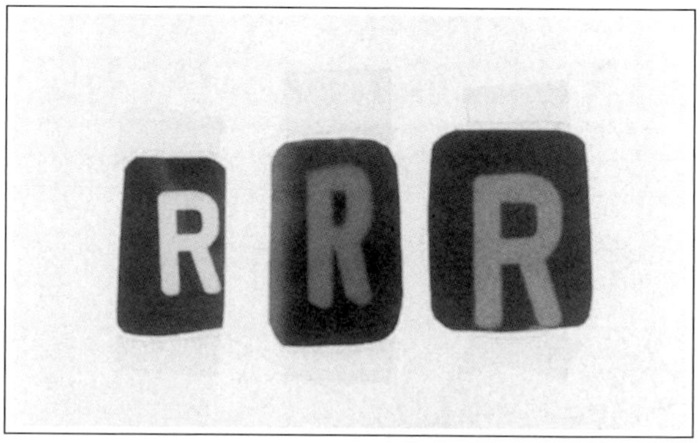

Figure 1-6. Marker magnification and distortion.

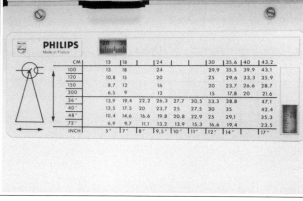

Figure 1-7. Collimator guide.

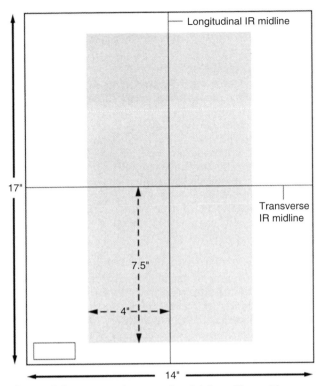

Figure 1-8. Marker placement for tightly collimated image.

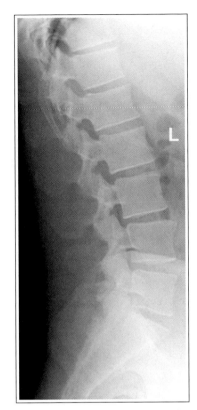

Figure 1-9. Marker placement for lateral position.

Anteroposterior and Posteroanterior Projections of the Torso, Vertebrae, and Cranium: For AP and PA projections, a right or left marker should be placed laterally within the collimated field on the side being marked. The patient's vertebral column is the dividing plane for the right and left sides. If marking the right side, position the R marker to the right of the vertebral column; if marking the left side, position the L marker to the left of the vertebral column (see Figure 1-1).

Lateral Positions of the Torso, Vertebrae, and Cranium: When a patient is placed in a lateral position, the right or left marker placed on the IR should indicate the side of the patient positioned closer to the IR. If the patient's left side is positioned closer to the IR for a lateral lumbar vertebrae, place an L marker on the IR (Figure 1-9). Whether the marker is placed anteriorly or posteriorly to the lumbar vertebrae does not affect the accuracy of the image's marking, although the images of markers placed posteriorly are often overexposed (Figure 1-10).

Oblique Positions of the Torso, Vertebrae, and Cranium: In the oblique position, one side of the patient's body is situated closer to the IR than the other side. The marker placed on the IR for the oblique position should identify the side of the patient that is positioned closer to the IR and should be placed on the correct side of the patient. In an RAO position, place an R marker on the IR; for a left posterior oblique (LPO) position, place an L marker on the IR (Figure 1-11). As with the AP/PA projections, the vertebral column is the plane used to divide the right and left sides of the body. For the right posterior oblique (RPO) position,

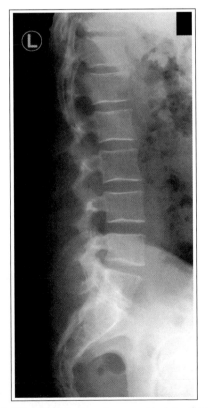

Figure 1-10. Poor marker placement in lateral position.

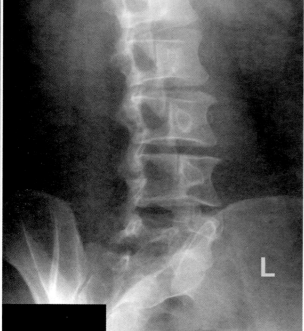

Figure 1-11. Marker placement for oblique position.

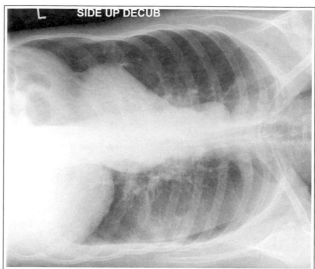

Figure 1-12. Marker placement for decubitus position.

place the R marker to the right of the vertebral column; for the left anterior oblique (LAO) position, place the L marker to the left of the vertebral column.

Lateral Decubitus Position of the Torso: Marking for the lateral decubitus position is identical to that for the AP/PA projection. Place an R marker to the right of the vertebral column when the right side is being identified and an L marker to the left of the vertebral column when the left side is being identified. In this position it is easier to place the marker on the IR, and the marker will be better

visualized if the side of the patient that is positioned up, away from the cart or imaging table on which the patient is lying, is the side marked. Along with the right or left marker, use an arrow marker pointing up toward the ceiling or lead lettering to indicate which side of the patient is positioned away from the cart or imaging table (Figure 1-12).

Projections and Positions of the Extremities: The marker placed on the IR should identify the side of the patient being imaged, an R marker to indicate the right side and an L marker to indicate the left side. When routine series of projections and positions for the fingers, hands, wrists, forearms, elbows, toes, feet, ankles, and lower legs are taken, more than one position is often placed on the same IR. For such examinations, it is necessary to mark only one of the positions placed on the IR as long as they are all images of the same anatomical structure (Figure 1-13). If positions of a right anatomical structure and its corresponding left are placed on the same IR, mark both images

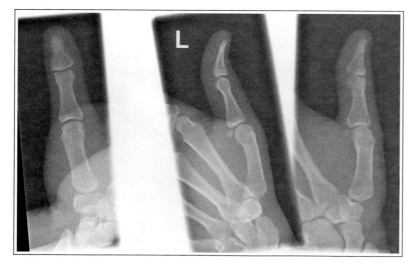

Figure 1-13. Marker placement for unilateral extremity image on one receptor.

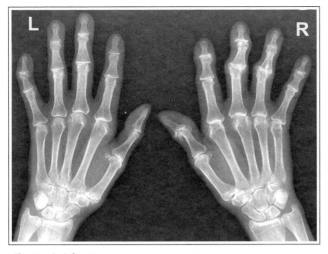

Figure 1-14. Marker placement for bilateral extremity images.

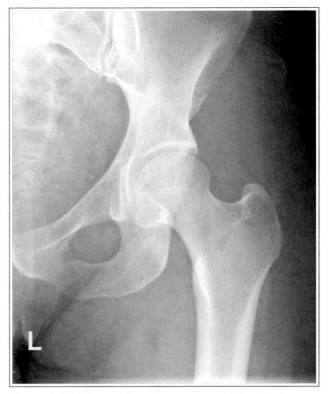

Figure 1-16. Poor marker placement on an AP projection of hip.

with the correct R or L marker (Figure 1-14). The only way to ensure that a marker will be demonstrated on the image is to place it within the collimated light field and corresponding radiation field.

Projections and Positions of the Shoulder and Hips: The marker placed on the IR for these images should indicate the side of the patient being imaged, an R marker for the patient's right side and an L marker for the patient's left side (Figure 1-15). It is best to place the marker laterally on AP/PA projections and oblique positions to prevent it from obscuring medial anatomical structures and to eliminate possible confusion about which side of the patient is being imaged. Figure 1-16 demonstrates an AP hip image with the marker placed medially. Because the marker is placed at the patient's midsagittal plane, the reviewer might conclude that the technologist was marking the other hip.

Lateral Cross-Table Images: When an examination is taken cross-table, as for a lateral shoulder or hip image or to evaluate trauma to the vertebral column, position the marker anteriorly to prevent it from obscuring structures situated along the posterior edge of the IR. The marker used should indicate the right or left side of the patient when the extremities, shoulder, or hip is imaged (Figure 1-17) and

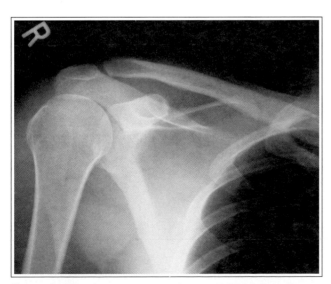

Figure 1-15. Marker placement for an AP projection of shoulder.

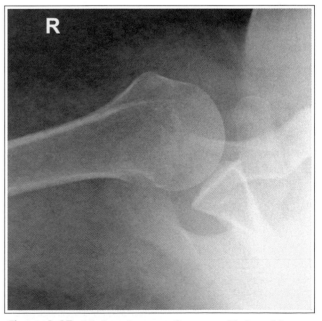

Figure 1-17. Marker placement for cross-table lateral image.

the side of the patient positioned closer to the IR when the torso, vertebrae, or cranium is imaged (see Figure 1-9).

3. Double-check the marker for accuracy. Does the R or L marker correspond to the correct side of the patient?

Mismarking an image can have many serious implications, including treatment of the incorrect anatomical structure. After an image has been produced, evaluate it to determine whether the correct marker has been placed on the image. An R marker is shown on the image if the right side of the body was imaged, and an L marker is shown if the left side of the body was imaged. This same analysis should be done for the lateral position; is an R marker visible if the right side of the patient was positioned closer to the IR, or is an L marker visible if the left side of the patient was placed closer to the IR?

Screen-Film System: If both sides of the body are demonstrated on the same radiograph, as with an AP projection of the pelvis or abdomen, evaluate it to ensure that an R marker is placed to the right of the vertebral column or an L marker is placed to the left of the vertebral column. When the screen-film system is used, this analysis can be accomplished by using the patient ID plate. Begin by hanging the image on the view box in the same manner as it was placed in the Bucky diaphragm. (For PA projections, hang the image as if the patient's back were facing you. This is not the proper way to hang such an image but is a method for determining marker accuracy.) The ID plate is in the lower right corner or the upper left corner on the image. Then, position yourself as the patient was positioned with respect to the IR. If the patient was in an AP projection, turn your back to the image; if the patient was in a PA projection, face the image. The marker on the image should correspond to your right or left side: an R marker on your right side or an L marker on your left side.

When a marker on an image is only faintly visible, circle it and rewrite the information it displays next to it. *Do not write the information over it* (Figure 1-18).

Digital Radiography: Digital imaging systems allow the technologist to add an R or L marker during postprocessing if it was partially positioned outside the collimated light field during the exposure (Figure 1-19). Do not cover up the original marker.

If the R or L marker does not appear on the image or the image has been mismarked, it is best to repeat the image. Do not guess or rely on what you may believe to be a "sure" sign. The heart shadow, which is normally located on the left side of the thorax, may be shifted toward the right because of a disease process (Figure 1-20) or because the patient has situs inversus (total or partial reversal of the body organs).

When the images presented in the analysis sections of this book were photographed, the areas of importance were enlarged to better show the anatomy so positioning could be evaluated. Unfortunately, the enlargement often eliminated the markers that were placed on the images. To prevent redundancy, I have not evaluated marker

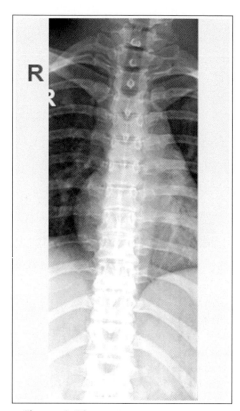

Figure 1-18. Partially visible marker.

existence or placement on any of these images, although this omission in no way is meant to decrease the importance of proper image marking. Use the guidelines presented in this section to evaluate marker placement on images you analyze.

Required anatomy is present on image.

1. Is the anatomy required for this projection and position demonstrated on the image?

For each projection and position a technologist images, not only is the area of interest required on the image, but a certain amount of the surrounding anatomy is also necessary.

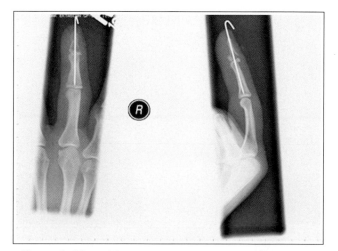

Figure 1-19. Adding marker with computed radiography.

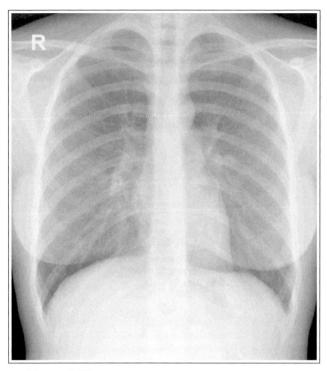

Figure 1-20. AP chest image with accurate marking.

For example, because radiating wrist pain may be a result of a distal forearm fracture, all wrist positions require that one fourth of the distal forearm be included with the wrist examination. A lateral ankle image should include 1 inch (2.5 cm) of the fifth metatarsal base to rule out a Jones fracture. Become familiar with the anatomy to be included on each image, as indicated in the critique section of this book, to avoid overcollimation or undercollimation and unnecessary repeats.

Patient Obliquity and Extremity Flexion

The relationships among the anatomical structures are accurate for the projection and position demonstrated.

1. Are the anatomical structures accurately displayed on the image for the projection and position demonstrated, as indicated in the analysis section of this book or defined by your imaging facility?

Evaluate each image for proper anatomical alignment as defined in the image analysis sections of this book. Each projection and position that is described demonstrates a specific bony relationship, allowing a specific area of interest to be demonstrated. For example, an AP ankle image demonstrates an open talotibial joint space (medial mortise), whereas the oblique image demonstrates an open talofibular joint space (lateral mortise), and the lateral image demonstrates the talar domes and soft-tissue fat pads. Patient positioning and the alignment of the central ray, body part, and IR affect how the anatomical structures are visualized on an image.

Pediatric Bone Development

The images of pediatric patients are very different from those of adults and one another during the various stages of bone growth and development (Figure 1-21). Bones throughout the body enlarge through the deposits of bone at cartilaginous growth regions, and long bones lengthen by the addition of bone material at the epiphyseal plate. Cartilaginous spaces and epiphyseal plates exist throughout the skeletal structure. They appear as dark spaces and lines on images and may look similar to an irregular fracture or joint space to those unfamiliar with pediatric imaging. The appearance of these spaces and lines reduces as the child develops, until early adulthood when they are replaced by bone and no longer are visible on the image. Round bones, such as the carpal and tarsal bones, are rarely formed at birth and therefore are not demonstrated on images of neonatal and very young pediatric patients. Because of this continual state of development, some anatomical relationships described in the imaging analysis sections may not be useful for determining accurate positioning for the pediatric patient. It is beyond the scope of this textbook to explain all the differences that could be demonstrated at different growth stages for each position and projection included in this text. When evaluating pediatric images for proper anatomical alignment, use only the analysis criteria that describe bony structures that are developed enough to use. For example, the PA wrist image analysis describes the

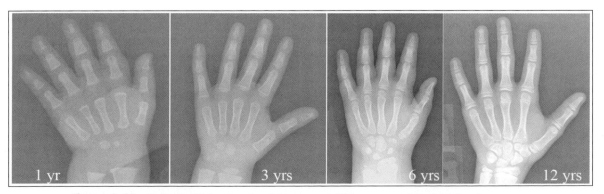

Figure 1-21. Pediatric PA hand and wrist images at different ages of skeletal development.

alignment of the carpal bones and metacarpals to determine accurate positioning. The carpal bone alignment cannot be used to evaluate young pediatric wrists, because all of the carpal bones are not formed, but the metacarpals can be used to determine the accuracy.

Determining the Degree of Patient Obliquity

To align the anatomical structures correctly, it is necessary to demonstrate precise patient positioning and central ray alignment. How accurately the patient is placed in a true AP/PA, lateral, or oblique projection or position, whether the structure is properly flexed or extended, and how accurately the central ray is directed and centered in relation to the structure determines how properly the anatomy is aligned. Because few technologists carry protractors, there must be a method for them to determine whether the patient is in a true AP/PA projection, lateral position, or specific degree of obliquity. For every projection or position described, an imaginary line (e.g., for the midsagittal or midcoronal plane, line connecting the humeral or femoral epicondyles) is given that can be used to align the patient with the IR or imaging table. When the patient is in an AP/PA projection, the reference line should be aligned parallel (0-degree angle) with the IR (Figure 1-22, *A*), and when the patient is in a lateral position, the reference line should be aligned perpendicular (90-degree angle) to the IR (Figure 1-22, *B*). For a 45-degree oblique position, place the reference line halfway between the AP/PA projection and the lateral position (Figure 1-22, *C*). For a 68-degree oblique position, place the reference line halfway between the 45-degree and 90-degree angles (Figure 1-22, *D*). For a 23-degree oblique position, place the reference line halfway

between the 0-degree and 45-degree angles (Figure 1-22, *E*). Even though these five angles are not the only angles used when a patient is positioned for images, they are easy to locate and can be used to estimate almost any other angle. For example, if a 60-degree oblique position is required, rotate the patient until the reference line is positioned at an angle slightly less than the 68-degree mark. I have used the torso to demonstrate this obliquity principle, but it can also be used for extremities. When an oblique position is required, always use the reference line to determine the amount of obliquity. Do not assume that a sponge will give you the correct angle. A 45-degree sponge may actually turn the patient more than 45 degrees if it is placed too far under the patient or if the patient's posterior or anterior soft tissue is thick.

Determining the Degree of Extremity Flexion

For many examinations a precise degree of structure flexion or extension is required to adequately demonstrate the desired information. Technologists need to estimate the degree to which an extremity is flexed or extended when positioning the patient and when critiquing images. When an extremity is in full extension, the degree of flexion is 0 (Figure 1-23, *A*), and when the two adjoining bones are aligned perpendicular to each other, the degree of flexion is 90 degrees (Figure 1-23, *B*). As described in the preceding discussion, the angle found halfway between full extension and 90 degrees is 45 degrees (Figure 1-23, *C*). The angle found halfway between the 45-degree and 90-degree angles is 68 degrees (Figure 1-23, *D*), and the angle found halfway between full extension and a 45-degree angle is 23 degrees (Figure 1-23, *E*). Because most flexible extremities flex

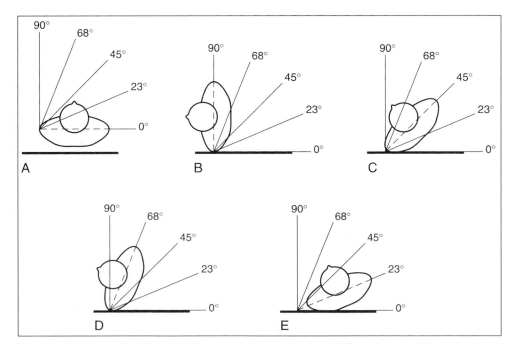

Figure 1-22. Estimating the degree of patient obliquity, viewing the patient's body from the top of the patient's head. See text for explanation.

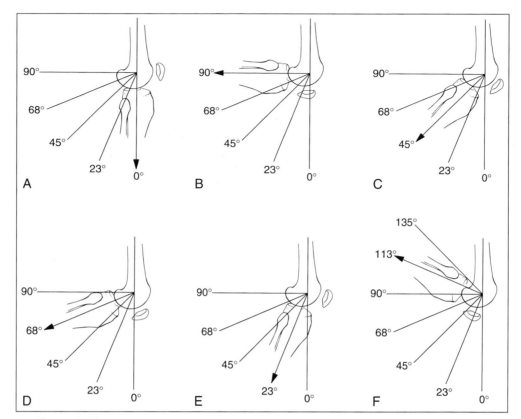

Figure 1-23. Estimating the degree of joint or extremity flexion. See text for explanation.

beyond 90 degrees, the angles 113 and 135 degrees, as demonstrated in Figure 1-23, *F*, should also be known.

Shape Distortion

2. Does your image demonstrate unwanted shape distortion?

Understanding how **the x-ray beam**, and **the alignment of the x-ray beam, part, and IR** shape the image is valuable knowledge that can be used to explain the causes of most of the resulting relationships among the anatomical structures. X-rays used to create an image are emitted from the x-ray tube's focal spot in the form of a fan-shaped beam. The *central ray* is the center of this beam and is used to center the anatomical structure and IR. It is here that the x-ray beam has the least divergence and the image of an anatomical structure demonstrates the least amount of distortion. As one moves away from the center of the beam, the x-rays that are used to record the image diverge and expose the IR at an angle (Figure 1-24). The farther one moves away from the central ray, the larger is the angle of divergence.

Poor beam-part-IR alignment results in shape distortion. To minimize shape distortion on the image, keep the part parallel to the IR and the central ray perpendicular to both the part and the IR (Figure 1-25, *A*). When an object is *shape distorted,* it is either elongated or foreshortened. *Elongation* is the most common shape distortion and occurs when one of the structure's axes appears disproportionately longer on the image than the opposite axis.

Elongation occurs in the following situations:

- The part is not centered to the central ray (referred to as *off-centered*). The central ray is perpendicular to the part, and the IR is parallel with the part (Figure 1-25, *B*).
- The central ray is angled and is not aligned perpendicular to the part, but the IR and the part are parallel with each other (Figure 1-25, *C*).
- The central ray and part are aligned perpendicular to each other, but the IR is not aligned parallel with the part (Figure 1-25, *D*).

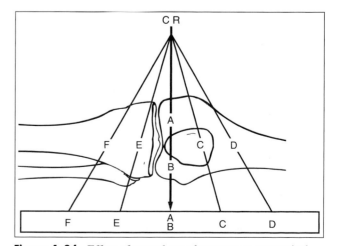

Figure 1-24. Effect of central ray placement on anatomical alignment.

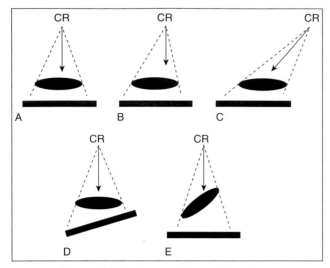

Figure 1-25. Causes of image distortion.

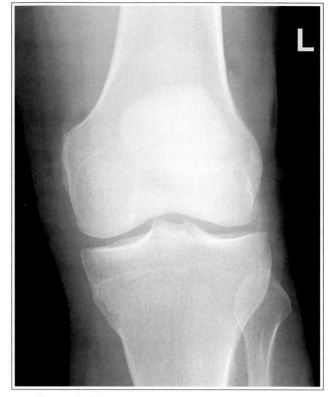

Figure 1-27. AP knee image with open knee joint.

Foreshortening of a structure is demonstrated when one of the structure's axes appears disproportionately shorter on the image than the opposite axis. Foreshortening occurs when the central ray and IR are perpendicular to each other, but the part is angled (Figure 1-25, *E*).

Whether a distorted or nondistorted image is desired depends on what particular anatomical structure is being evaluated and how this structure is aligned with the surrounding structures. For example, to demonstrate the scaphoid bone without foreshortening, you must angle the central ray, thereby distorting the carpal bones that surround the scaphoid bone. To demonstrate the foramen magnum, dorsum sellae, and occipital bone in the AP axial projection of the cranium, the rest of the cranial and facial bones must be distorted. Yet the acromioclavicular joints must not be distorted by positioning the central ray differently in the "with weights" and "without weights" images, or a false diagnosis about separation may result. Refer to the analysis sections of this book to determine whether your image has demonstrated the desired anatomical structures properly.

3. Are the joints of interest open or fracture lines well demonstrated?

Demonstrating Joint Spaces and Fracture Lines: For an open joint space or fracture line to be demonstrated, the central ray must be aligned parallel with the joint or fracture line of interest (Figures 1-26 and 1-27). Failure to accomplish this alignment will result in a closed joint or poor fracture visualization as the surrounding structures are projected into the space or over the fracture line (Figures 1-28 and 1-29).

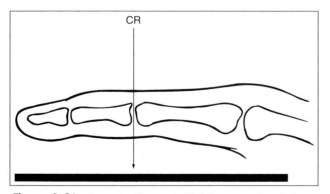

Figure 1-26. Accurate alignment of joint space and central ray.

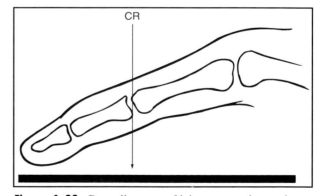

Figure 1-28. Poor alignment of joint space and central ray.

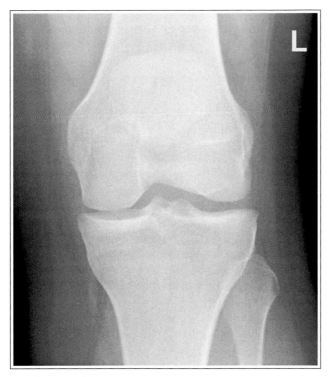

Figure 1-29. AP knee image with closed knee joint.

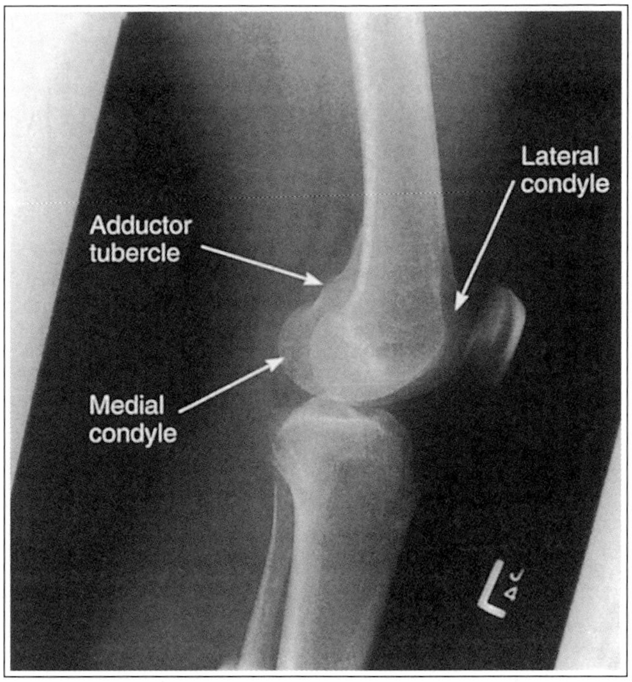

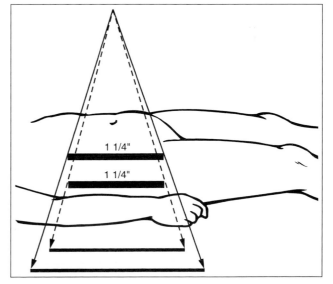

Adductor tubercle

Lateral condyle

Medial condyle

Figure 1-30. Poorly positioned lateral knee image with the medial condyle posterior.

Adjusting for Poor Positioning

4. How should the patient's positioning or central ray be adjusted before the image is obtained again? How much adjustment should be made?

After it is determined that the relationships between the anatomical structures of the projection and position being evaluated are inaccurate, you must decide how the patient or central ray was mispositioned for such an image to result and how they should be readjusted to reflect accurate anatomical relationships. The guidelines and images presented in the analysis sections of this book for the projection and position being evaluated will help you make this decision. The most difficult structures to identify are those that are identical in shape and size, such as the femoral condyles or talar domes. For these structures, three methods may be used to distinguish the structures from one another.

- Use the structures that surround the area of interest. For example, if a poorly positioned lateral ankle image demonstrates inaccurate AP talar dome alignment and a closed tibiotalar joint space, one cannot view the joint space to determine which talar dome is anterior, but the relationship of the tibia and fibula can easily be used to deduce this information.
- Use bony projections such as tubercles to identify one of the similar structures. For example, the medial femoral condyle can be distinguished from the lateral condyle on a lateral knee image by locating the adductor tubercle that is situated on the medial condyle (Figure 1-30).

- Identify the more magnified of the two structures. The anatomical structure situated farthest from the IR is magnified the most (Figure 1-31). On a left lateral chest image, the right side posterior ribs are situated posterior to the left because they are positioned farther from the IR and are more magnified.

1 1/4"

1 1/4"

Figure 1-31. The part farthest from the IR will be magnified the most.

Steps for Repositioning the Patient for Repeat Images

1. Identify the two structures that are mispositioned. For example, the medial and lateral femoral condyles for a lateral knee image or the petrous ridges and supra-orbital rims for a PA Caldwell cranial image.

2. Determine the number of inches or centimeters that the two mispositioned structures are "off." For example, the anterior surfaces of the medial and lateral femoral condyles should be superimposed on an accurately positioned lateral knee image, but a ½-inch (1.25-cm) gap is present between them on the produced image (see Figure 1-30). Or consider how the supraorbital margins should be demonstrated 1 inch (2.5 cm) superior to the petrous ridges on an accurately positioned PA Caldwell cranial image, but they are superimposed on the produced image (Figure 1-32).

3. Determine if the two structures will move toward or away from each other when the main structure is adjusted. For example, when the medial femoral condyle is moved anteriorly, the lateral condyle moves in the opposite direction (posteriorly). Also, when the patient's chin is elevated away from the chest, the supraorbital margins move superiorly, whereas the petrous ridges, being located at the center, pivoting point in the cranium, do not move.

4. Begin the repositioning process by first positioning the patient as he or she was positioned for the poorly positioned image. From this position move the patient as needed for proper positioning.

5. If the structures move in opposite directions from each other when the patient is repositioned, adjust the patient half the distance that the structures are off. For example, if the anterior surface of the lateral femoral condyle is situated ½ inch (1.25 cm) anterior to the anterior surface of the medial femoral condyle on a poorly positioned lateral knee image (see Figure 1-30), the medial condyle should be rotated anteriorly ¼ inch (0.6 cm).

6. If only one structure moves when the patient is repositioned, adjust the patient so the structure that moves is adjusted the full amount. For example, if the petrous ridges should be located 1 inch (2.5 cm) inferior to the supraorbital margins on an accurately positioned PA Caldwell cranial image but they are superimposed (see Figure 1-32), then adjust the patient's chin 1 inch (2.5 cm) away from the chest, moving the supraorbital margins superiorly and 1 inch (2.5 cm) above the petrous ridges.

Steps for Repositioning the Central Ray for Repeat Images

1. Identify the two structures that are mispositioned—for example, the medial and lateral femoral condyles for a lateral knee image.

2. Determine which of the identified structures is positioned farthest from the IR. This is the structure that will move the most when the central ray angle is adjusted. For example, the medial femoral condyle is positioned farthest from the IR for a lateral knee image.

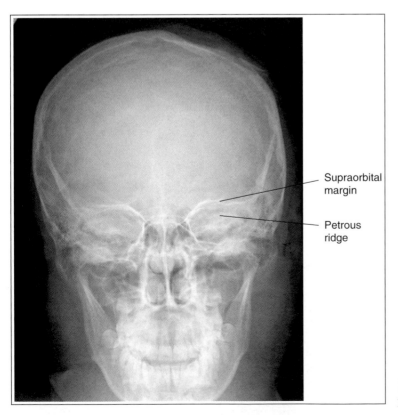

Supraorbital margin

Petrous ridge

Figure 1-32. AP Caldwell cranial image showing poor positioning.

3. Determine the direction in which the structure situated farthest from the IR must move to be positioned accurately with respect to the other structure. For example, in Figure 1-30 the medial femoral condyle must be moved anteriorly toward the lateral condyle to obtain accurate positioning.

4. Determine the number of inches or centimeters the two mispositioned structures are off on the image. For example, the anterior surfaces of the medial and lateral femoral condyles should be superimposed on an accurately positioned lateral knee image, but a ½-inch (1.25-cm) gap is present between them on the produced image (see Figure 1-30).

5. Estimate how much the structure situated farthest from the image will move per 5 degrees of angle adjustment placed on the central ray. How much the central ray angulation will project two structures away from each other depends on the difference in the actual distance of the structures from each other and the IR. Note that in Figure 1-33 point A is farther away from the IR than point B is. Even though point A is horizontally aligned with point B, an angled central ray used to record these two images would project point A farther inferiorly than point B. If these two structures were closer together (points A and C on Figure 1-33), the amount of separation on the image would be less. If these two structures were farther apart (points A and D on Figure 1-33), the separation on the image would be greater.

   Box 1-1 lists guidelines that can be used to determine the degree of central ray adjustment required when dealing with different anatomical structures. For example, the physical space between femoral condyles

> ## BOX 1-1 Central Ray Adjustment Guidelines for Structures Situated at the Central Ray*
>
> - If the identified physical structures (actual bone, not as seen on radiographic image) are separated by ½-1¼ inches, a 5-degree central ray (CR) angle adjustment will move the structure situated farthest from IR approximately ⅛ inch (0.3 cm).
> - If the identified physical structures are separated by 1½-2¼ inches, a 5-degree CR angle adjustment will move the structure situated farthest from the IR approximately ¼ inch (0.6 cm).
> - If the identified physical structures are separated by 2½-3¼ inches, a 5-degree CR angle adjustment will move the structure situated farthest from the IR approximately ½ inch (1.25 cm).
> - If the identified physical structures are separated by 3-4½ inches, a 5-degree CR angle adjustment will move the structure situated farthest from the IR approximately ¾ inch (1.9 cm).

*Structures situated away from the CR will also be affected by divergence of the x-ray beam and amount of source-image distance used and may require less adjustment than indicated above.

of the knee is approximately 2 inches (5 cm). Using the *central ray adjustment guidelines* in Box 1-1, we find that structures that are 2 inches apart will require a 5-degree central ray angle adjustment to move the part situated farthest from the IR 0.25 inch (0.6 cm) more than the structure situated closer to the IR.

6. Place the needed angulation on the central ray, as determined by steps 4 and 5 above, and direct the central ray in the direction indicated in step 3 above. For example, if a lateral knee image demonstrates a separation between the medial and lateral femoral condyle of ½ inch (1.25 cm), then the central ray would need to be adjusted 10 degrees and directed toward the part farthest from the IR that needs to be moved in order to superimpose the condyles on the image. To obtain an optimal lateral knee image for Figure 1-30 using the central ray only to improve positioning, it should be angled 10 degrees and directed anteriorly. This will move the medial condyle ½ inch (1.25 cm) anteriorly. To obtain an optimal PA Caldwell image for Figure 1-32 using the central ray, it should be angled 20 degrees in a cephalic direction, moving the petrous ridges, which are situated furthest from the IR, 1 inch (2.5 cm) superiorly toward the supraorbital margins.

Performing Mobile and Trauma Imaging

The goal of mobile and trauma imaging is the same as that of routine imaging: to demonstrate accurate relationships among the anatomical structures for the projection and position imaged, without causing further patient injury and with minimal discomfort. The following are general guidelines for obtaining this goal.

1. Based on the requisition or request form, determine the images that will be needed and the order in which they will be completed. First obtain the images that will give information about the most life-threatening

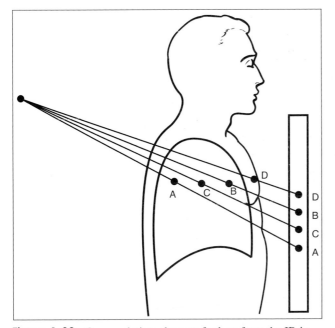

Figure 1-33. On angulation, the part farthest from the IR is projected the most.

condition (cross-table lateral cervical spine if cervical fracture is questioned or when obtaining an AP chest image for a patient having difficulty breathing). Speed is of the essence in many mobile and trauma situations, because the patient can be quite ill. Having a thought-out plan of action before starting allows the technologist to work in an organized and speedy manner. As a general rule, after the initial images associated with life-threatening conditions have been exposed and checked by the radiologist or physician, the remaining images are exposed in an order that will require the least amount of central ray adjustment. All AP images are exposed, then the central ray is moved horizontally for the lateral images.

2. Gather and organize the supplies (IRs, IR holders, positioning aides, disposable gloves, radiation protection supplies, etc) that will be needed, and determine the starting technical factors (kilovolt peak [kVp], mAs, automatic exposure control [AEC]) for the needed images. Cover the positioning aides and IRs to protect them from contamination.

3. Determine the degree of patient mobility, alertness, and ability to follow requests. Can the patient be placed in a seated position or be rotated to one side? Can the arm or leg fully extend or flex? When the patient is asked to breathe deeply, can he or she follow the request? Can the patient control movement?

4. Assess the site of interest for physical signs of injury (swelling, bruising, deformity, pain). Understanding the degree of injury will help the technologist prevent further injury during the positioning process.

5. Determine whether positioning devices (such as slings, backboards, and casts) and artifacts (such as heart leads, clothing, and jewelry) may be removed and, if not, whether they will obscure the area of interest on the ordered images. If positioning devices or artifacts will obscure the area, consult with the radiologist or ordering physician about possible alternatives (e.g., taking a slight oblique instead of a true lateral). Technical adjustments may also be needed as a result of the increase in absorption that may occur because of the positioning device or artifact. Either increase (+) or decrease (−) the kVp or mAs from the routine amount for the patient thickness measurement as indicated in Table 1-1.

6. Obtain the requested images. The technologist should use the routine positioning guidelines for patient positioning, central ray centering, IR size, collimation, and so on when obtaining mobile and trauma images. For patients who are unable to perform the routine positioning requirements, adaptations to this setup are to be made. Never force the patient into a position. Instead, adjust the central ray and IR. As long as the central ray, part, and IR form the same alignments, identical images will result. The word *part* with regard to alignment refers to the specific plane, imaginary line, or anatomical structure used to position the patient with the central ray and IR in routine positioning.

- Routine lateral foot positioning requires that the foot's lateral surface be aligned parallel to the IR and the central ray be aligned perpendicular to the part and the IR. In this situation the lateral foot surface is the part, because it is what is used to position the foot in relation to the central ray and IR.

- If the lateral foot image is taken on the imaging table, the patient will externally rotate the leg until the lateral foot surface is parallel to the IR, and the central ray will be aligned perpendicular to the IR and part (Figure 1-34).

- If the lateral foot image is taken in a standing position, the IR will be positioned vertically and the central ray horizontally. Even though the setup appears different, the central ray–part-IR alignments are the same as in the previous setup. The lateral foot surface is positioned parallel to the IR, and the central ray is perpendicular to the IR and lateral foot surface. Many times when a cross-table image is created the projection taken is opposite. For a routine tabletop lateral foot image a mediolateral projection is performed, whereas a lateromedial projection is used for cross-table images. To obtain identical images for both projections the technologist must maintain the same central ray–part-IR alignment. This mean that the lateral surface of the foot must still be positioned parallel to the IR for a lateromedial projection, even if this surface is not placed directly adjacent to the IR. On a lateral foot image, this will require the medial aspect of the heel to be positioned slightly away from the IR (Figure 1-35).

- If a patient arrives in the radiology department in a wheelchair and is unable to easily move to the imaging table for the lateral foot image, the

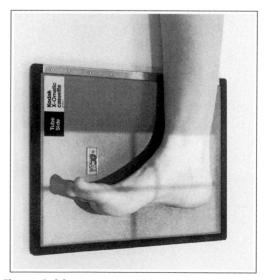

Figure 1-34. Tabletop mediolateral foot positioning.

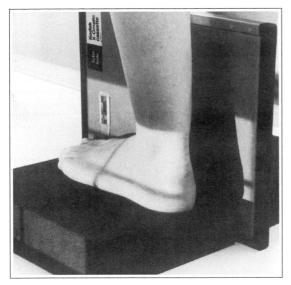

Figure 1-35. Standing lateromedial foot positioning.

image can be obtained with the patient remaining in the wheelchair. First, align the lateral foot surface with the IR, and then align the central ray perpendicular to the IR and lateral foot surface. Again, because the relationships among the central ray, IR, and part are the same as in the two previous setups, the resulting image will be identical (Figure 1-36).

- For oblique images, begin by aligning the central ray with the plane, line, or anatomical structure that is used for an AP projection of the part being imaged. Next, adjust the central ray in the direction needed to set up the correct alignment between the central ray and structure. Because the degree of angulation in which patients are rotated for oblique images is always referenced from the AP/PA projection, the amount of angle adjustment would be the same as the required degree of obliquity. For a routine internal oblique elbow image the central ray is aligned at a 45-degree angle with an imaginary line connecting the humeral epicondyles (the medial epicondyle is placed farther from the tube than the lateral). To obtain the same image in a patient who is unable to rotate the arm, the technologist first positions the central ray perpendicular to the line connecting the epicondyles and then adjusts the angle 45 degrees medially, positioning the medial epicondyle farther from the x-ray tube than the lateral. The IR would then be angled so it is perpendicular to the central ray (Figure 1-37).

- Aligning the IR with the central ray should be done whenever possible to obtain a true image. At times this cannot be accomplished, as with an oblique examination of the torso where the patient is unable to move from a supine position. When this is the case, the IR may have to remain "as is" or be positioned as close to perpendicular with the central ray as possible. The resulting image will demonstrate elongation, but the anatomical alignment of the structures, the required joint space visibility, and so on should be demonstrated as required for the image. The more acute the central ray and IR angle, the greater will be the elongation.

7. Use a grid if the patient part thickness is over 5 inches (13 cm) and over 70 kVp is used. Evaluate the alignment of the central ray and grid. Is the central ray aligned accurately with the center of the grid? If a central ray angle is used, is it angled with the grid lines? Is the grid level? Is the SID within the grid's focusing range? Is the correct side of the grid facing the central ray?

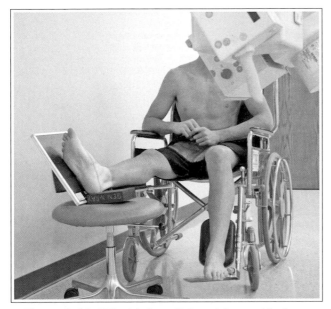

Figure 1-36. Wheelchair mediolateral foot positioning.

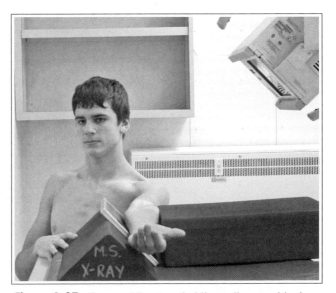

Figure 1-37. Trauma AP external oblique elbow positioning.

8. Set an optimal kVp and mAs or AEC for the anatomical structure and position and projection being imaged. Adjust the kVp or mAs as needed for patient conditions (see Table 1-1).

9. Use good radiation protection practices. Ask female patients if there is any chance they could be pregnant. Never assume that other staff members have asked. Use gonadal shielding whenever possible, collimate tightly, and provide those assisting with patient holding during the exposure with aprons and lead gloves. Images of the extremity should not be taken by placing the IR and part on the patient's torso unless it is the only means of obtaining accurate positioning. If this is the case, always place a lead apron between the IR and torso. Not all of the radiation directed toward the IR is absorbed; high-energy beams will exit the back of the IR, exposing structures beneath.

10. Never leave a confused patient or a trauma patient unattended in the imaging room.

11. Process the images and evaluate them for positioning and technical accuracy. Determine if repeated images are needed and how much adjustment will be required.

12. Repeat any necessary images.

13. Return the patient to the emergency room or, if the images were taken with the mobile unit, replace the bed, monitoring devices, and personal items to the positions they occupied when you entered the room or to positions that make the patient most comfortable.

14. Disinfect all equipment, IRs, and positioning devices used during the procedures.

Image is demonstrated without unwanted size distortion.

1. Does your image demonstrate the least possible amount of magnification?

Because (1) no image is taken with the part situated directly on the IR, (2) no anatomical structure imaged is flat, and (3) not all structures are imaged with a perpendicular beam, all images demonstrate some type of distortion. The amount of **size distortion**, or **magnification**, depends on how far each structure is from the IR. The farther away the part is situated, the more magnified the structure will be (see Figure 1-31). *Size distortion* is present when all axes of a structure have been equally magnified. Size distortion also results when the same structure, situated at the same OID, is imaged at a different SID.

Detail Sharpness

Bony cortical outlines and/or soft-tissue structures are sharply defined.

1. Was a small focal spot used when indicated?

A detail smaller than the focal spot used to produce the image will not be visible. This is why a small focal spot is recommended when fine detail demonstration is important, such as images of the extremities. Compare the trabecular patterns on the ankle images in Figures 1-38 and 1-39.

TABLE 1-1	Technical Adjustments for Trauma Patients	
Immobilizing Device or Patient Condition	**kVp Adjustment**	**mAs Adjustment**
Small to medium plaster cast	+5-7 kVp	+50%-60%
Large plaster cast	+8-10 kVp	+100%
Fiberglass cast	+3-4 kVp	+25%-30%
Inflated air splint	No adjustment	No adjustment
Wood backboard	+5 kVp	+25%-30%
Ascites (accumulation of fluid in abdomen or swelled joint)		+50%-75%
Pleural effusion (fluid in pleural cavity)		+35%
Pneumothorax (fluid within lungs)	−8% kVp	
Postmortem imaging of head, thorax, and abdomen (because of pooling of blood and fluid)		+35%-50%
Soft tissue injury (used for foreign objects, such as slivers of wood, glass, or metal, embedded in the soft tissue and to demonstrate the upper airway)	−15%-20% kVp	

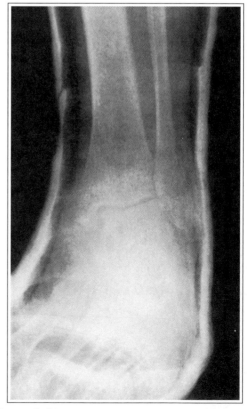

Figure 1-38. Recorded detail using large focal spot.

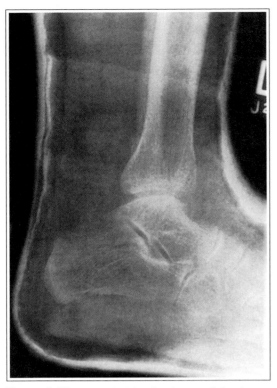

Figure 1-39. Recorded detail using small focal spot.

Figure 1-38 was taken using a large focal spot, and Figure 1-39 was taken using a small focal spot. Notice how use of a small focal spot increases the visibility of the bony trabeculae.

Today's imaging equipment allows a small focal spot to be chosen for many high-radiation exposures. On an AEC examination the milliamperage selected by the equipment is low when a small focal spot is chosen, resulting in the need for a long exposure time to obtain the density required to adequately visualize the torso structures. Long exposure times often result in the demonstration of patient motion on the image. Weigh the expected exposure time and the possibility of motion against the advantages gained by choosing a small focal spot. If the patient's thickness measurement is large or the patient's ability to hold still is not reliable, a large focal spot and high milliamperage might be chosen.

2. Does the image demonstrate signs of unwanted patient motion or unhalted respiration?

The term *motion unsharpness* refers to lack of sharpness in an image that is most often caused by patient movement during the exposure. This movement can be voluntary or involuntary. *Voluntary motion* refers to the patient's breathing or otherwise moving during the exposure. It can be controlled by explaining to the patient the importance of holding still, making the patient as comfortable as possible on the imaging table, using the shortest possible exposure time, and employing positioning devices. Voluntary motion can be identified on an image by blurred bony cortical outlines (Figure 1-40). *Involuntary motion* is movement the patient cannot control. Its effects will appear the same as those of voluntary motion in most situations, with the exception of within the abdomen. In the abdomen, peristaltic activity of the stomach and small or large intestine can be identified on an image by sharp bony cortices and blurry gastric and intestinal gases (Figure 1-41). The only means of decreasing the blur caused by involuntary motion is to use the shortest possible exposure time, which in some cases is not good enough. At times, normal voluntary motions such as breathing or shaking can become involuntary motions. For example, an unconscious patient is unable to control breathing, and a patient with severe trauma may be unable to control shivering.

A double-exposed image may also appear blurry and can easily be mistaken for an image affected by patient motion (Figure 1-42). When evaluating a blurry image, look at the cortical outlines of bony structures that are lying longitudinally and transversely. Is there only one cortical outline to represent each bony structure, or are there two? Is one outline lying slightly above or to the side of the other? If one outline is demonstrated, the patient moved during the exposure, but if two are demonstrated, the image was exposed twice, and the patient was in a slightly different position for the second exposure.

3. Does the anatomy of interest demonstrate the least possible amount of magnification?

Magnification of an anatomical structure reduces its recognizability and blurs the recorded details. For magnification

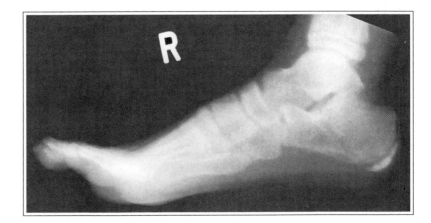

Figure 1-40. Voluntary patient motion.

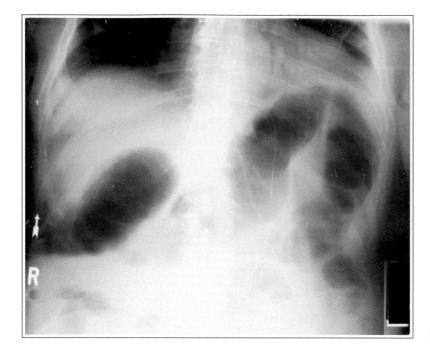

Figure 1-41. Involuntary patient motion.

to be prevented, the anatomical structure of interest should always be positioned as close to the IR as possible.

4. Was a detail screen used when indicated?

Departments often have more than one receptor system to choose from. A detail screen system increases the recognizability of the image's recorded details and is often used for extremity images. Compare the trabecular patterns on the hand images in Figure 1-43. Figure 1-43 demonstrates a hand image exposed using a low-speed, detail screen and using a faster-speed, nondetail screen. Notice how use of a detail screen increases the visibility of the bony trabeculae.

5. Does evidence suggest poor screen-film contact?

Poor screen-film contact results when a screen-film system is used and a foreign object is wedged between

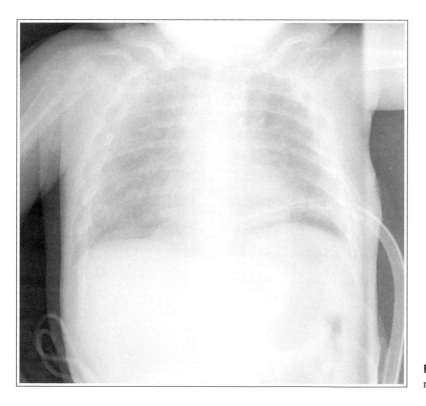

Figure 1-42. Double exposed computed radiography chest image.

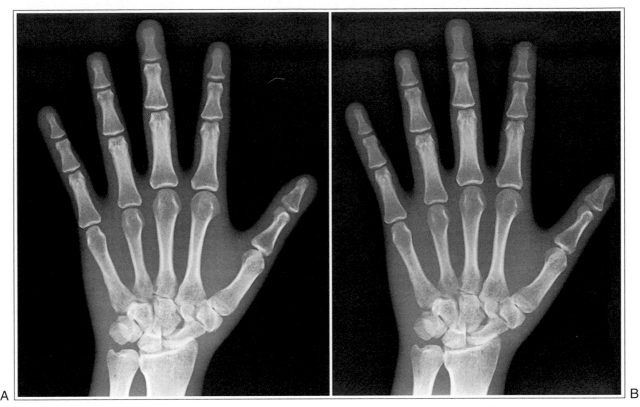

Figure 1-43. Comparing recorded detail between low-speed (**A**) and high-speed (**B**) screens.

the IR and the screen or the cassette is damaged or warped. Radiographically, poor screen-film contact is demonstrated by a blurred image only in the area in which the screen and film are not making direct contact. Figure 1-44 demonstrates an oblique hand image. Note how the hand image is sharp everywhere except at the second and third digits. Because it would be impossible for these two fingers to move without causing the rest of the hand to also move, it can be concluded that this blurring is a result not of patient motion but of poor screen-film contact. The screen should be thoroughly cleaned and tested on a phantom. If the test radiograph does not demonstrate improved screen-film contact, the cassette should be replaced.

6. If using a computed radiography imaging system, was the smallest possible IR used?

The smallest possible IR should be employed when using a **computed radiography imaging system**. The quality of image resolution in computed radiography is partly determined by the size of the image matrix. The *image matrix* refers to the layout of pixels (cells) in rows and columns (Figure 1-45). The image is formed when each pixel in the matrix is given a brightness value that will represent an area on the object being imaged. The larger the matrix, the higher the pixel numbers and the better the spatial resolution will be. The size of the matrix is determined both by the equipment and the computer

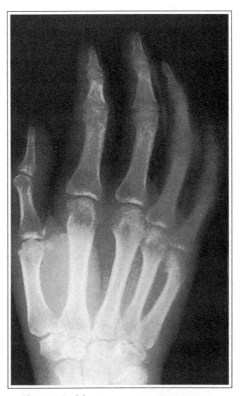

Figure 1-44. Poor screen-film contact.

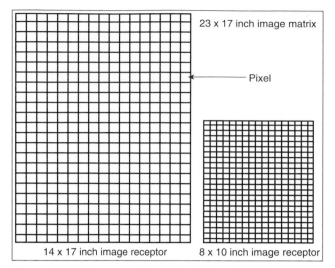

Figure 1-45. Image matrix and pixel sizes with different IR sizes.

capacity used and is the same for a system no matter which size IR is used. Even though the size of the matrix is the same whether an 8- × 10-inch or 14- × 17-inch IR is used, the 8- × 10-inch IR will contain pixels of smaller size, providing an image with better spatial resolution (Figure 1-46).

Collimation

Maximum collimation efforts are evident on image.

1. Is a collimated border present on all four sides of the image?

Good collimation practices are necessary to decrease the radiation dosage by limiting the amount of patient tissue exposed and to improve the visibility of recorded details and the image contrast by reducing the amount of scatter radiation that reaches the IR. As a general rule, each image should demonstrate a small collimated border around the entire image of interest. This is particularly helpful in computed radiography, because during the image-acquisition process the reader distinguishes the useful regions of the image by locating the edges of the collimation (a process known as *exposure field recognition*), so information beyond the collimation borders is not used during the analysis. The only time this rule does not apply is when the entire IR must be used to prevent clipping of needed anatomy, as in chest and abdominal imaging. This collimated border not only demonstrates good collimation practices but also can be used to determine the exact location of central ray placement. Make an imaginary X on the image by diagonally connecting the corners of the collimated border (Figure 1-47). The center of the X indicates the central ray placement for the image.

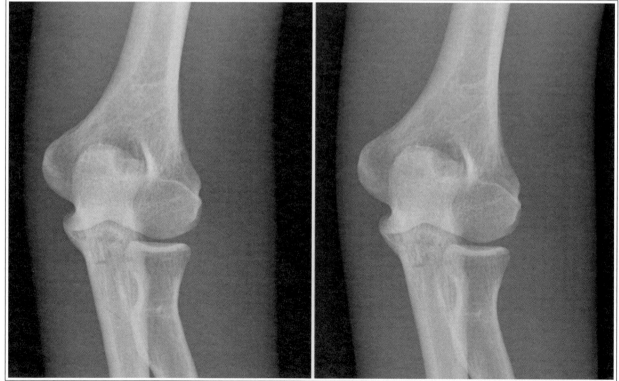

Figure 1-46. Comparing spatial resolution between large and small IR sizes using computed radiography. **A,** 8- × 10-inch IR. **B,** 14- × 17-inch IR.

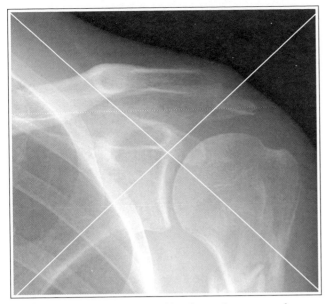

Figure 1-47. Using collimated borders to locate central ray placement.

Accurate placement of the central ray and alignment of the long axis of the part with the collimator's longitudinal light line are two positioning practices that will aid in obtaining tight collimation. When collimating, do not allow the collimator's light field to mislead you into believing you have collimated more tightly than you actually have. When the collimator's central ray indicator is positioned on the patient's torso and the collimator is set to a predetermined width and length, the light field demonstrated on the patient's torso does not represent the true width and length of the field set on the collimator. This is because x-rays (and the collimator light if the patient was not in the way) continue to diverge as they move through the torso to the IR, increasing the field size as they do so (Figure 1-48).

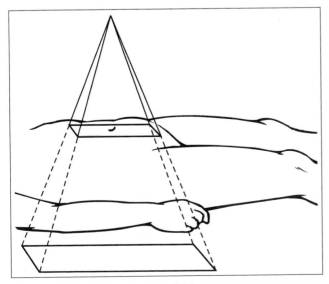

Figure 1-48. Collimator light field versus receptor coverage.

The thicker the part being imaged, the smaller the collimator's light field that appears on the patient's skin surface. On a very thick patient, it is often difficult to collimate the needed amount when the light field appears so small, but on these patients, tight collimation demonstrates the largest improvement in the visibility of the recorded details.

Learn to use the collimator guide (see Figure 1-7) to determine the actual IR coverage. For example, when an AP lumbar vertebrae image is taken, the transversely collimated field should be reduced to an 8-inch (20-cm) field size. Because greater soft-tissue thickness has nothing to do with an increase in the size of the skeletal structure, the transverse field should still be reduced when one is imaging a thick patient part. Accurately center the patient by using the centering light field, then set the transverse collimation length to 8 inches by using the collimator guide. Be confident that the IR coverage will be sufficient even though the light field appears small.

2. Have you collimated to within ¹/₂ inch (1.25 cm) of the patient's skinline on all extremity, chest, and abdominal images?

All extremity images should demonstrate the collimated borders positioned next to the skinline of the thickest area of interest. Figure 1-49 shows an AP forearm image. Note that the transversely collimated borders are adjacent to the elbow, the thickest area of the forearm.

Often, chest and abdominal images show very little collimation because the entire IR is needed to demonstrate the required anatomy. Whenever a small patient is imaged,

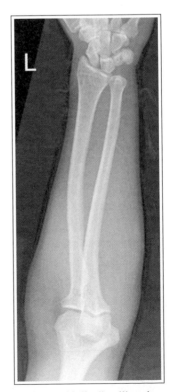

Figure 1-49. Proper "to skinline" collimation on an AP forearm image.

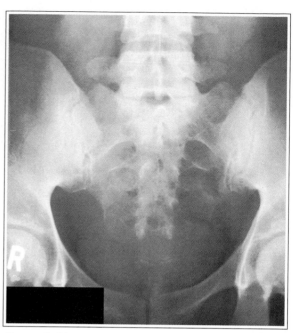

Figure 1-51. Proper collimation on an AP sacral image.

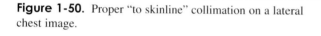

Figure 1-50. Proper "to skinline" collimation on a lateral chest image.

however, collimated borders should be demonstrated within ½ inch (1.25 cm) of the patient's skinline (Figure 1-50).

On some x-ray equipment the collimator head can be rotated without rotating the entire tube column. This capability allows the technologist to increase collimation on anatomical structures such as the humerus and clavicle, which are not aligned directly with the longitudinal or transverse axes of the light field. Rotating just the collimator head does not affect the alignment of the beam with the grid; this alignment is affected only when the tube column is rotated. Severe rotation of the collimator head should be avoided when using computed radiography, as it may affect the exposure field recognition process.

3. Have you collimated to the specific anatomy desired on images involving structures within the torso?

When imaging a specific body structure within the torso, bring the collimated borders as close to the structure as possible. Use palpable anatomical structures around the area of interest to determine how close the borders are to the structure of interest. For the AP sacral image shown in Figure 1-51, for example, the longitudinally collimated field was closed to the palpable symphysis pubis because the sacrum is located superior to the symphysis pubis on an accurately positioned sacral image, and the transversely collimated field was closed to the palpable ASISs because the sacrum is located medial to them.

4. Are all required anatomical structures visible on the image?

Evaluate all images to determine whether the required anatomical structures have been included. Poor centering

or overcollimation can result in the clipping of required anatomy (Figure 1-52).

Clipping of required anatomy can also result from overcollimation on a structure that is not placed in direct contact with the IR, such as for a lateral third or fourth finger or

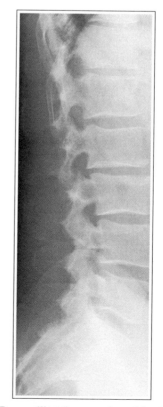

Figure 1-52. Poor collimation on a lateral lumbar vertebral image.

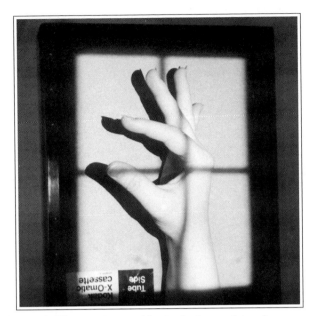

Figure 1-53. Viewing an object's shadow to determine proper collimation.

lateral hand image. Clipping occurs because the divergence of the x-ray beam has not been taken into consideration during collimation. To prevent clipping, view the shadow of the object projected onto the IR by the collimator light (Figure 1-53). It will be magnified. This magnification is similar to the magnification the x-ray beam undergoes when the image is created. Allow the collimated field to remain open enough to include the shadow of the object, ensuring that the object will be shown in its entirety on the image.

When the images presented in the critique sections of this book were photographed, the areas of importance were enlarged to better demonstrate the anatomy so positioning could be evaluated. Unfortunately, this has eliminated the collimated borders. To prevent redundancy, I have not evaluated the collimation on any of these images, but this decision in no way is meant to decrease the importance of proper collimation. Use the guidelines presented in this section to judge the adequacy of collimation on images you evaluate.

Radiation Protection

Radiation protection is present on the image when indicated, and good radiation protection practices were used during the procedure.

Proper gonadal shielding practices have been proved to reduce radiation exposure of the female gonads by approximately 50% and of the male gonads by approximately 90% to 95%.[1] Gonadal shielding is recommended in the following situations:

- When the gonads are within 2 inches (5 cm) of the primary x-ray beam
- If the patient is of reproductive age

- If the gonadal shield does not cover information of interest

Professional technologists must always strive to improve skills and to develop better ways to ensure good patient care while obtaining optimal images. All images should be evaluated for the accuracy of gonadal shielding. It is by studying our shielding habits that we learn to improve and perfect them.

1. Is gonadal shielding evident and accurately positioned on male and female patients when the gonads are within the primary beam and shielding is therefore indicated?

Gonadal Shielding in the AP Projection for Female Patients: Shielding the gonads of the female patient for an AP image of the pelvis, hip, or lumbar vertebrae requires more precise positioning of the shield to prevent the obscuring of pertinent information. The first step in understanding how to properly shield an adult female is to know which organs should be shielded and their location. These organs are the ovaries, uterine (fallopian) tubes, and uterus. The uterus is found at the patient's midline, superior to the bladder. It is approximately 3 inches (7.5 cm) in length; its inferior aspect begins at the level of the symphysis pubis, and it extends anterosuperiorly. The uterine tubes are bilateral, beginning at the superolateral angles of the uterus and extending to the lateral sides of the pelvis. Tucked between the lateral side of the pelvis and the uterus and inferior to the uterine tubes are the ovaries. The exact level at which the uterus, uterine tubes, and ovaries are found varies from patient to patient. Figures 1-54 and 1-55 show images from two different hysterosalpingograms. Notice the variation in the location of the uterus, uterine tubes, and ovaries in these two patients. Because the location of these organs within the inlet pelvis cannot be determined with certainty, the entire

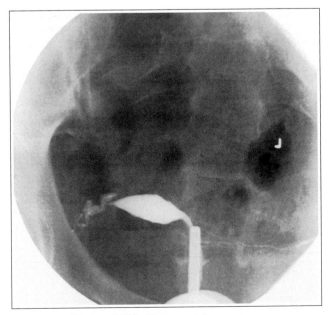

Figure 1-54. Hysterosalpingogram.

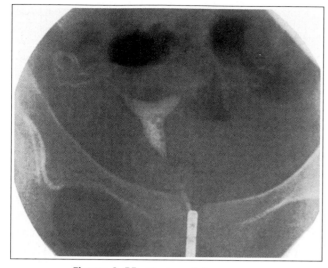

Figure 1-55. Hysterosalpingogram.

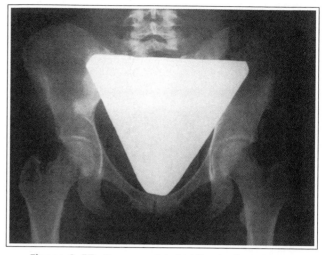

Figure 1-57. Poor gonadal shielding in the female.

inlet pelvis should be shielded to ensure that all the reproductive organs have been protected.

To properly shield the female gonad, use a flat contact shield made from at least 1 mm of lead and cut to the shape of the inlet pelvis (Figure 1-56). Oddly shaped and male (triangular) shields do not effectively protect the female patient (Figure 1-57). The dimensions of the shield used should be varied according to the amount of magnification the shield will demonstrate, which is determined by the OID, as well as the size of the patient's pelvis, which increases from infancy to adulthood. Each department should have different-sized contact or shadow shields for variations in female pelvic sizes for infants, toddlers, adolescents, and young adults.

To position the shield on the patient, place the narrower end of the shield just superior to the symphysis pubis and allow the wider end of the shield to lie superiorly over the reproductive organs. Side-to-side centering can be evaluated by placing an index finger just medial to each ASIS. The sides of the shield should be placed at equal distances from the index fingers. It may be wise to tape the shield to

the patient. Patient motion such as breathing may cause the shield to shift to one side, inferiorly, or superiorly.

Gonadal Shielding in the AP Projection for Male Patients: The reproductive organs that are to be shielded on the male are the testes, which are found within the scrotal pouch. The testes are located along the midsagittal plane inferior to the symphysis pubis. Shielding the testes of a male patient for an AP image of the pelvis or hip requires more specific placement of the lead shield to avoid obscuring areas of interest. For these examinations a flat contact shield made from vinyl and 1 mm of lead should be cut out in the shape of a right triangle (one angle being 90 degrees). Round the 90-degree corner on this triangle. Place the shield on the adult patient with the rounded corner beginning approximately 1 to 1½ inches (2.5 to 4 cm) inferior to the palpable superior symphysis pubis. When accurately positioned, the shield frames the inferior outlines of the symphysis pubis and inferior ramus and extends inferiorly until the entire scrotum is covered (Figure 1-58). Each department should have different-sized male contact

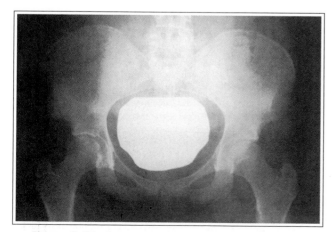

Figure 1-56. Proper gonadal shielding in the female.

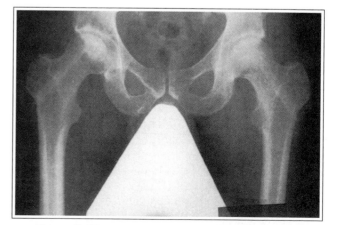

Figure 1-58. Proper gonadal shielding in the male.

shields for the variations in male pelvic sizes for infants, youths, adolescents, and young adults.

Gonadal Shielding in the Lateral Position for Male and Female Patients: When male and female patients are imaged in the lateral position, use gonadal shielding whenever (1) the gonads are within the primary radiation field and (2) shielding will not cover pertinent information. In the lateral position, male and female patients can be similarly shielded with a large flat contact shield or the straight edge of a lead apron. Begin by palpating the patient's coccyx and elevated ASIS. Next, draw an imaginary line connecting the coccyx with a point 1 inch posterior to the ASIS, and position the longitudinal edge of a large flat contact shield or half-lead apron anteriorly against this imaginary line (Figure 1-59). This shielding method can be safely used on patients being imaged for lateral vertebral, sacral, or coccygeal images without fear of obscuring areas of interest (Figure 1-60).

2. Were radiation protection measures used for patients whose radiosensitive cells were positioned within 2 inches (5 cm) of the primary beam?

Shielding of radiosensitive cells should be done whenever they lie within 2 inches (5 cm) of the primary beam. *Radiosensitive cells* are the eyes, thyroid, breasts, and gonads. To protect these areas, place a flat contact shield constructed of vinyl and 1 mm of lead or the straight edge of a lead apron over the area to be protected. Because the atomic number of lead is so high, radiation used in the diagnostic range will be readily absorbed within the shield.

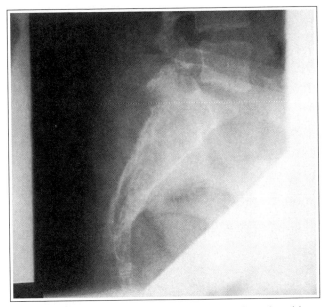

Figure 1-60. *Proper gonadal shielding in the lateral position.*

3. Was tight collimation used?

Tight collimation reduces the radiation exposure of anatomical structures that are not required on the image. Its use on chest images will reduce exposure of the patient's thyroid; on a cervical vertebral image, it will reduce exposure of the eyes; on a thoracic vertebrae image, it will reduce exposure of the breasts; and on a hip image, it will reduce exposure of the gonads. Even when radiation protection efforts are not demonstrated on the image, good patient care standards dictate their use.

4. Are any anatomical artifacts demonstrated on the image?

Anatomical artifacts are anatomical structures of the patient or x-ray personnel that are demonstrated on the image but should not be there. An example of such an artifact is shown in Figure 1-61. Notice how the patient's other hand was used to help maintain the position. This is not an acceptable practice. Many sponges and other positioning tools are available to adequately position and immobilize the patient. Whenever the hands of the patient or x-ray personnel must be within the radiation field, they must be properly attired with lead gloves.

5. Were personnel who remained in the room during the exposure given protective clothing?

All personnel and family members should be asked to leave the room before the x-ray exposure is made. If the patient cannot be left alone in the room during the exposure, lead-protection clothing such as aprons, thyroid shields, glasses, and gloves should be worn by the personnel during any x-ray exposure. Anyone remaining in the room should also stand as far from the primary beam as possible.

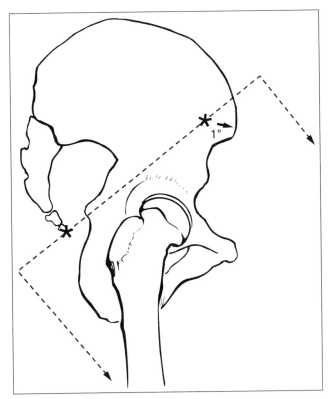

Figure 1-59. Gonadal shielding for the lateral position in both male and female.

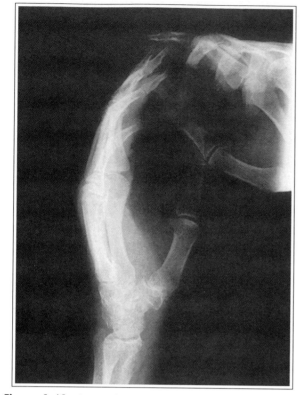

Figure 1-61. Anatomical artifact. Poor radiation protection.

The smallest possible IR size has been used, and the IR and anatomical structures have been accurately aligned to include the required anatomy with tight collimation.

1. Was the IR positioned CW or LW correctly to accommodate required anatomy?

Evaluate the image to determine whether all the required anatomy has been included. Deciding whether to place the IR CW or LW is a simple matter of positioning it so that all the required anatomy can easily be demonstrated on the image. If the IR is placed CW for an adult forearm image, the IR will not be long enough to accommodate the wrist and elbow joints on the same IR. This is why adult forearm images are taken with the IR aligned LW.

Body Habitus

2. Was the IR positioned CW or LW correctly to accommodate the patient's body habitus?

Be aware of the three basic body types when positioning a patient for a PA/AP chest or AP abdominal image: hypersthenic, sthenic, and asthenic. The *hypersthenic* patient has a wide, short thorax and a broad peritoneal cavity with a high diaphragm (Figure 1-62). This body type requires the IR to be placed CW for PA/AP chest images in order to include the entire lung field and requires two CW IRs to be used for an AP abdominal image in order to demonstrate the entire peritoneal cavity. The *asthenic* patient has a long,

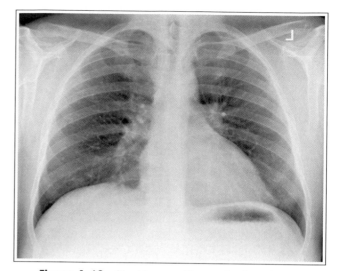

Figure 1-62. Chest image of hypersthenic patient.

narrow thoracic cavity and a narrow peritoneal cavity with a lower diaphragm (Figure 1-63). The *sthenic* body type is between the hypersthenic and asthenic body types (Figure 1-64). Both the asthenic and sthenic body types require the IR to be placed LW for the PA/AP chest and AP abdominal images in order to include the entire lung field and peritoneal cavity, respectively.

3. Was the smallest possible IR used, and were as many projections and positions as possible placed on the same IR without collimation field overlap?

Screen-Film System: With the rising cost of health care, we must do whatever we can to reduce the cost of

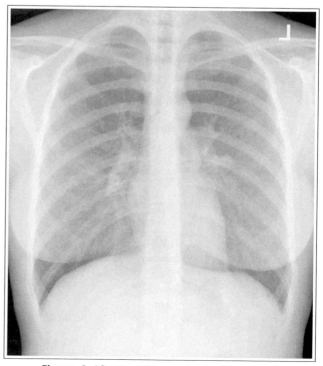

Figure 1-63. Chest image of asthenic patient.

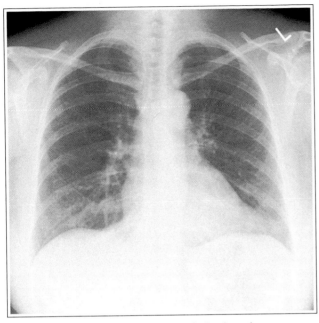

Figure 1-64. Chest image of sthenic patient.

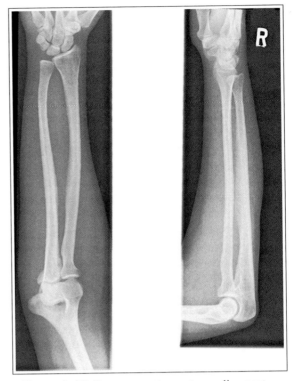

Figure 1-65. Proper receptor-anatomy alignment.

imaging procedures. When using a screen-film system, choosing the correct IR size for an examination and, when possible, exposing more than one image on the same IR is part of cost efficiency. How the IR is placed (LW or CW) often dictates how many images can be placed on the IR. For example, a 10- × 12-inch (24- × 30-cm) IR placed CW can accommodate three images of the wrist, but the same size IR placed LW has space available for only two images.

Computed Radiography: The smallest possible IR should be employed when using a computed radiography imaging system, to provide optimal spatial resolution. Because the same imaging plate can be used over and over again, the same cost-reduction argument cannot be used as with screen-film systems.

When positioning more than one image on the IR for computed radiography, the images should be evenly distributed on the IR without overlapping the collimation fields. Such overlapping will result in poor exposure field recognition during the image-acquisition process and may result in poor image normalization (rescaling).

Also consider the similarity in the thickness of the parts being imaged when deciding whether or not to place the images on the same receptor. When the image plate is read, only one diagnostic specifier can be chosen for the receptor, resulting in the same normalization process occurring for all the images placed on the receptor. The thickness difference may result in one of the images being inadequately normalized and consequently too light or dark.

4. If more than one projection or position is placed on the same IR, were they all aligned in the same direction?

When an extremity is imaged and more than one projection or position is exposed on the same IR, similar anatomical structures should be located at the same end of

the IR. For example, when the AP and lateral images of the forearm are placed on the same 14- × 17-inch (35- × 43-cm) IR, the elbows in the two images are to be demonstrated at the same end of the IR (Figure 1-65). Failure to keep this alignment makes displaying and viewing of the image difficult (Figure 1-66).

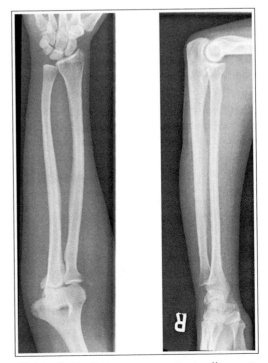

Figure 1-66. Poor receptor-anatomy alignment.

Correct IR system was used.

1. Have you chosen the correct IR system for the body part being imaged?

Receptor systems are chosen for their ability to demonstrate fine recorded details or for their speed. The more details a system can demonstrate, the less speed the system has, and consequently the more radiation exposure is needed to obtain adequate density.

Use low-speed, detail screen for most extremity examinations. This system is for tabletop work only and should not be used when a grid is employed or when a thick body part is being imaged. Use a medium-speed system when the detail capability provides little benefit. For example, hands and feet can have hairline fractures that may be visualized only on a detail screen; because a fracture of the femoral bone is very obvious, however, we do not need to see small details to identify it. Use a high-speed system for examinations such as those performed for scoliosis, in which the bony cortical outlines are all that need to be demonstrated for measurements to be taken. Such a system should not be used when information about the structure itself is desired.

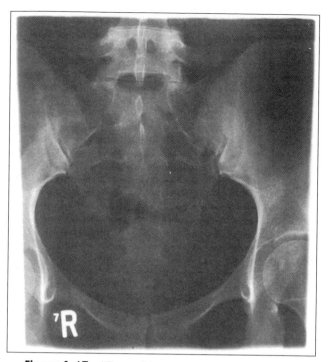

Figure 1-67. AP sacral image overexposed by 100%.

Density and Penetration

Density and penetration are optimal, demonstrating the required bony and soft-tissue structures.

1. Does the image have optimal density to demonstrate the bony trabeculae and soft-tissue structures of interest?

Study the area of interest on each image to determine whether it demonstrates adequate density to visualize the bony trabeculae and soft-tissue structures of interest. However, many factors affect image density; the factor to use when controlling density is milliampere per second (mAs).

Screen-Film Systems: When an image is *overexposed* (too much mAs used), it demonstrates density that is so dark the bony and soft-tissue structures of interest are not well visualized. On such an image the contrast is acceptable. Even though the overall image will be dark, the cortical outlines of the bone should remain high in contrast. Figure 1-67 demonstrates an overexposed AP sacral image.

An *underexposed* image (not enough mAs used) demonstrates density so light that the bony trabecular patterns cannot be evaluated. Usually on light images, unless underexposure is extreme, the demonstration of the soft-tissue structures is better. Because underexposed and underpenetrated images demonstrate low density, it is necessary to learn to identify each technical error. One way to distinguish whether an image has been underexposed rather than underpenetrated is to study the bony cortical outlines of the structures of interest. On an image that has been underexposed, the cortical outlines are visible, even though their density is light, whereas an underpenetrated image will not demonstrate areas of the cortical outlines that were not penetrated. Figure 1-68 shows an underexposed AP image of the thoracic vertebrae.

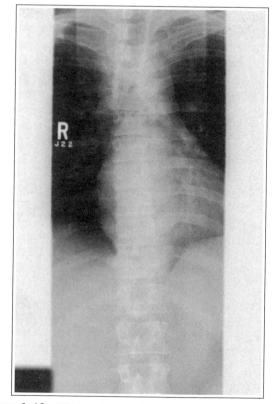

Figure 1-68. AP thoracic vertebrae image underexposed by 100%.

Computed Radiography: Computed radiography systems automatically make adjustments in density to produce consistently optimal images over a wide range of exposure values. If the exposure value is very low, the computed radiography processing system is unable to produce an image that is adequate. Patient dosage and spatial resolution are the issues of concern when deciding if the exposure was adequate. Each of the several computed radiography manufacturers uses a different method to indicate the amount of exposure reaching the phosphor plate. For example, the Fuji system uses a sensitivity number. This number is inversely proportional to the exposure, meaning that as the exposure is increased the sensitivity number decreases. The acceptable exposure range for the Fuji system is a sensitivity number between 75 and 500. The Kodak system uses an index number to indicate exposure. This number is directly proportional to the exposure, meaning that as the exposure is increased the index number also increases. The acceptable index number range is between 1700 and 2200.

An overexposed computed radiography image will have an exposure indicator number outside the acceptable range (a sensitivity number below 75 or an index number above 2200), and the image density and contrast will be adequate, because it will be normalized (scaled) by the reader acquisition system before being displayed on the CRT monitor. The patient would have received more radiation than would have been needed to produce the image.

An underexposed computed radiography image will have an exposure indicator number outside the acceptable range (a sensitivity number above 500 or an index number below 1700); the image will have a noisy, mottled appearance (**quantum mottle**) (Figure 1-69); and the image density and contrast will be adequate, because the reader acquisition system will have normalized the digital information before displaying it on the CRT monitor.

When an exposure indicator number outside the acceptable range has been obtained, the amount of adjustment in exposure needed to bring the number within the range varies with system manufacturers. Technologists should refer to the system's operator manual to determine the correct adjustment required. For example, the Kodak system recommends a 100% increase or 50% decrease in exposure to increase or decrease the exposure index number by 300, respectively.

2. What adjustments should be made for inadequate density or when the computed radiography exposure indicator number is outside the acceptable range?

Density Changes with Manually Set Examinations (Screen-Film Systems): Before changing the technique and repeating an examination because the image is too dark or light, evaluate all other factors that affect image density. Was the SID set correctly? Did you read the technique chart correctly and set the kVp and mAs as stated on the technique chart? Was the patient measured correctly? Did you use the correct receptor system, and was the correct IR placed in that system? Was a grid used if required? Only if these additional technical preparations were correct can one conclude that the image was dark or light because the mAs or kVp was inaccurately set.

When image density is inadequate, mAs is the controlling factor of choice. How much adjustment in mAs should be made to obtain an optimal image is directly proportional to the amount of increase or decrease in density that is needed. Typically three adjustments can be made when making density changes. It takes much practice to be able

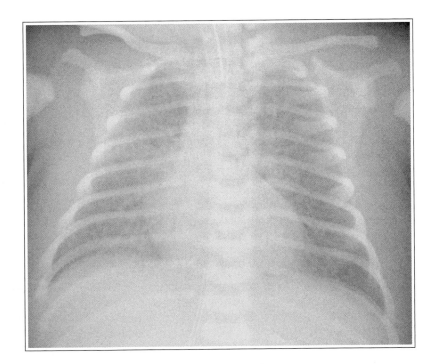

Figure 1-69. Computed radiography image demonstrating quantum mottle caused by underexposure.

to visually distinguish the difference in density each of these adjustments would make. One way to describe how much density adjustment each of these represents is to study some hypothetical conversations that might occur in a radiology department about an image that is inadequately exposed. The adjustment that would provoke such statements is also noted in the following list.

- *Hypothetical conversation:* "We have to repeat this image because of motion. The density is okay, but it could be just a little lighter (or darker)." A 30% change in mAs adjusts the image density just enough for the eyes to be able to visualize that a change has been made. This amount of adjustment should never be used when an image needs to be repeated because the density is too light or dark. However, it is an ideal adjustment to make when the image demonstrates acceptable but not optimal density and needs to be repeated because of a factor other than density, such as an artifact, patient motion, or mispositioning. To calculate a 30% change, multiply the original mAs value by 0.3; then, add the result to the original mAs value to increase density or subtract the result from the original mAs value to decrease the density.

- *Hypothetical conversation:* "This image is too light (dark). Maybe we could pass it depending on what radiologist is working today, but I'd feel better if it was repeated." (See Figures 1-67 and 1-68.) When an image is light or dark enough for you to question whether it should be repeated or whether it is close enough for the radiologist to accept, don't immediately say it definitely needs to be repeated. If it does need to be repeated, a 100% change should be made if it is too light and a 50% change made if it is too dark. To calculate a 100% increase in density, multiply the original mAs by 2: If the original mAs was 20, the new mAs would be 40. To calculate a 50% decrease in density, divide the original mAs by 2 so that if the original mAs was 20, the new mAs would be 10.

- *Hypothetical conversation:* "This image is way too light (dark). We definitely have to repeat it." (See Figures 1-70 and 1-71.) When an image is so light or dark that you immediately know without question that it needs to be repeated, a 300% or 400% change should be made if it is too light, and a 33% or 25% change if it is too dark. To calculate a 300% or 400% increase in density, multiply the original mAs by 3 or 4, respectively. To calculate a 33% or 25% decrease in density, multiply the original mAs by 0.33 or 0.25, respectively, and subtract the result from the original mAs.

Density Changes with Automatic Exposure or Phototimed Examinations (Screen-Film Systems): Overexposed or underexposed images obtained using the AEC are primarily a result of poor patient and ionizing chamber alignment. An overexposed image results when the ionization chamber chosen is located beneath a structure that has a higher atomic number or is thicker or

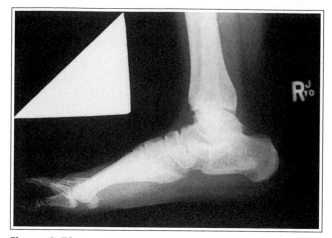

Figure 1-70. Lateral foot image underexposed by 300% to 400%.

denser than the structure of interest. For example, when an AP abdomen image is taken, the outside ionization chambers should be chosen and situated within the soft tissue, away from the lumbar vertebrae, to yield the desired abdominal soft-tissue density. If the chamber situated under the lumbar vertebrae is used instead, the capacitor (device that stores energy) requires a longer exposure time to reach its maximum filling level and terminate the exposure. This occurs because of the high atomic number of bone and the higher number of photons that bone absorbs compared with soft tissue. The result will be an image with adequate bone density but overexposed soft tissue. Similar results occur when the AEC is used on patients with metal prostheses. Because the metal's atomic number is so much higher than that of bone and soft tissue and because the AEC attempts to adequately expose the metal structure, these structures will be overexposed on the resulting image.

An underexposed image results, however, when the ionization chamber chosen is located beneath a structure that has a lower atomic number or is thinner or less dense than the structure of interest. When an AP lumbar vertebrae

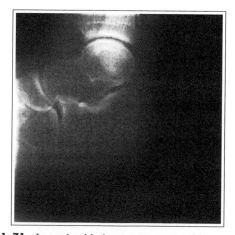

Figure 1-71. Lateral ankle image overexposed by 300% to 400%.

image is taken, the center ionization chamber is chosen and centered directly beneath the lumbar vertebrae. If one or both of the outside chambers are used or the center ionization chamber is off center, the image is underexposed, because soft tissue, which has a lower atomic number than bone, is above the activated chamber.

An underexposed image also results if a portion of the activated chamber has not been covered with body tissue, such as can happen when shoulder structures are imaged. The part of the chamber not covered with tissue collects radiation so quickly that it will charge the capacitor to its maximum level, terminating the exposure before proper density of the shoulder structures has been reached. Premature termination of the exposure can also be avoided with tight collimation practices, because table and body scatter radiation will charge the capacitor.

An overexposed image may result when the structure of interest is in close proximity to thicker structures and both are situated above the activated ionization chamber. For example, it is best not to use the AEC on an AP "open-mouth" projection of the dens. With this examination the upper incisors, occipital cranial base, and mandible add thickness to the areas superior and inferior to the dens and atlantoaxial joint. This added thickness causes the area of interest to be overexposed, because more time is needed for the capacitor to reach its maximum level as photons are absorbed in the thicker areas.

In most facilities, the automatic exposure thyristor (a device used to set the maximum capacitor charge) is set to accommodate the most frequently used film-screen combination. If a higher-speed screen-film combination is used with this thyristor setting, the resulting image is overexposed; if a lower-speed screen-film combination is used, the resulting image is underexposed. The AEC will not adjust for the receptor system speed.

Density Changes with Manually Set and Automatic Exposure or Phototimed Examinations (Digital and Computed Radiography): To produce consistently optimal images, computed radiography systems automatically correct for manually set or automatic exposure errors through a process called *normalization.* Such corrections can be made without image degradation with overexposures as high as 120% and underexposures as low as 60% from the ideal range.[2] Ideally, this process should be kept to a minimum to ensure the highest image quality and reasonable patient dosage. The amount of normalization to an image can be estimated through the exposure indicator number. The more this value is outside the ideal range for the system used, the more normalization occurred to result in the image presented. Exposure indicator numbers that specify higher-than-ideal exposure values typically do not require repeating because of image quality, although the reason for this high value should be investigated, as excessive patient dosage was rendered to produce them. Exposure indicator numbers that specify lower-than-ideal exposure values may necessitate repeating the procedure because of the mottled image appearance (see Figure 1-69).

Digital radiography also allows for postprocessing manipulation of the image's contrast and density to better demonstrate an area of interest. This process, called *windowing,* occurs after the image is displayed on the CRT monitor. Adjusting the window level allows the viewer to increase or decrease the density of the overall image, and adjusting the window width allows the viewer to increase or decrease the contrast of the overall image.

Before an image is processed the radiographer chooses a **diagnostic specifier** that indicates the anatomical structure that is being processed and its position and projection. Unless the correct diagnostic specifier is chosen the resulting image may not display optimal density values.

During image processing the digital data is evaluated and manipulated before being displayed. First, the digital data are used to construct a histogram (graphic display of the distribution of pixel values). The histogram graphs the pixel value (density) with the frequency of occurrence, defining areas of bone, soft tissue, contrast media, metal, and unattenuated areas. The results of the histogram analysis are correlated with a "look-up table" (characteristic curve) that best displays the anatomical part being imaged. The look-up table that is used for this correlation is determined when the radiographer chooses the diagnostic specifier (anatomical structure, position and projection) before the image plate is scanned. If the correlation between the histogram and look-up table suggests a low or high exposure, the electrical signal will be adjusted accordingly to compensate for the error. This process is called *normalization.* If the incorrect diagnostic specifier is used, the image quality may be inadequate for the intended purpose, because the raw data will not be normalized correctly for the examination. This error is easily detected, because the study name is noted in the data field underneath each digital image and may be corrected by reprocessing it under the correct diagnostic specifier as long as it has not yet been sent to the archiving system.

Patient positioning, pathological condition, internal artifact, and missing or additional anatomy can affect the created histogram because these factors affect pixel value distribution in the histogram, resulting in incorrect normalization even when the correct diagnostic specifier was chosen. Poor patient positioning—such as not centering the part to the center of the IR, having the collimation edges overlap when more than one image is placed on the IR, or using poor collimation that results in poor normalization—can be corrected by improving the centering, spacing the images evenly, and collimating tightly. The different computed radiography manufacturers have different methods of obtaining optimal images under the other circumstances. For example, the image may be processed under a different scanning mode (Fuji) or processed under a different anatomical specifier (Kodak).

Guidelines for obtaining the most accurate normalization of a digital image are as follows:
- Choose the correct diagnostic specifier for the anatomical structure imaged and the position and projection.

- For nonroutine positioning situations, pathological conditions, internal artifacts, and missing or added anatomy, follow the manufacturer's guidelines for choosing the most appropriate diagnostic specifier or processing mode.
- Center the structure being imaged in the center of the IR.
- Do not overlap collimation edges when more than one image is placed on an IR.
- Collimate tightly.

3. Does the image have adequate penetration to demonstrate the cortical outlines of the structures of interest?

Penetration of the primary beam's photons is controlled by the kilovoltage that is used. An image that has been adequately penetrated demonstrates the cortical outlines of the thinnest and thickest bony structures of interest. If the anatomical structure of interest has not been *penetrated* (not enough kVp used), the image demonstrates too little density, but in comparison with an underexposed image, the cortical outlines of the thickest parts of the structure are not visible. Figure 1-72 demonstrates an underpenetrated AP hip image, and Figure 1-73 demonstrates an underexposed image. Note that if a transparency were laid over the images and an outline of the bony structures drawn on the transparency with lines made only where the cortical outlines of the bone were clearly visible, many of the hip structures around the acetabulum would not be drawn.

If the cortical outlines of the structure of interest can be seen even though the image density is light, it can be concluded that the mAs needs adjusting; if the cortical outlines of the structure cannot be seen and the image density is light, a kVp adjustment is required.

4. How much adjustment in technique should be made for inadequate penetration?

Changing Penetration: An underpenetrated image may also demonstrate inadequate density. The amount of density adjustment that is needed must also be considered when deciding how much kVp adjustment is to be made.

- If an image has to be repeated because it was underpenetrated and the density (refer to the density discussion earlier in this chapter for explanation) was 100% too light, increase the kVp by at least 15%. (If 50 kVp was the level used on the original image, the new kVp level is calculated by taking 50×0.15 and adding the result [7.5] to the original 50 kVp; the new kVp value would be 57.5.) The mAs should remain the same as that used on the original image, because a 15% kVp change will also increase density by 100% (see Figure 1-72).
- If an image is underpenetrated and light enough to require a 300% or 400% density adjustment, a combination kVp and mAs change is indicated. Figure 1-73 demonstrates an underpenetrated AP shoulder image. How much of the adjustment should be with kVp in this situation depends on your departmental standard for contrast and can be determined by using the optimal kVp level for the structure being imaged as a guideline. As a general rule the kVp should be kept relatively close to the optimal level. First, calculate a 15% increase in the kVp. Is this new kVp reasonably

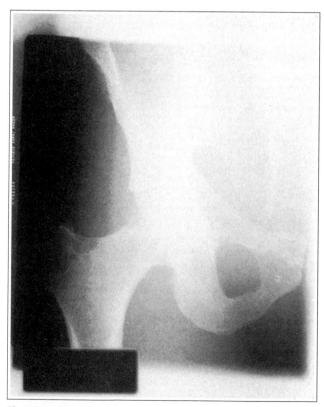

Figure 1-72. Underpenetrated AP hip image needing a 100% density change.

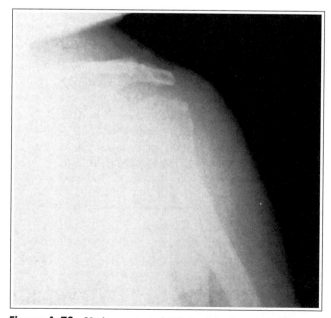

Figure 1-73. Underpenetrated AP shoulder image needing a 400% density change.

close to the optimal level for the structure being imaged? If so, you know there will be a significant penetration change, and any additional density adjustment could be made with mAs without negatively affecting image contrast. (Because a 15% increase in kVp is equivalent to a 100% density change, increase the mAs by 50% to 100% to obtain a total of a 300% or 400% change, respectively.) Increasing the kVp too far above optimum results in an increase in scatter radiation being directed toward the *IR* and a decrease in image contrast.

Compensating Filters and Anode-Heel Effect

5. Has a compensating filter been used when indicated and has the thinnest end of a long bone or vertebral column been positioned at the anode end of the tube when a 17-inch (43-cm) length IR is used to obtain homogeneous density across the structure?

With some examinations, when an exposure is set that will adequately demonstrate one structure of interest, other structures of interest are overexposed. This occurs because of the differences in thickness among the structures being imaged. AP projections of the shoulder, feet, and thoracic vertebrae are three examples that demonstrate this problem. To offset this thickness difference and obtain homogeneous density, place a compensating filter over or under the thinnest structures (Figure 1-74). A **compensating filter** absorbs x-ray photons before they reach the IR. The thicker part of the filter absorbs more photons than the thinner part. Set a technique that will adequately expose the thickest part being examined. If the filter has been accurately positioned, it will absorb the excessive radiation directed toward the thinnest structures, resulting in uniform image density throughout the image. Figures 1-75 and 1-76 show AP foot images. The image in

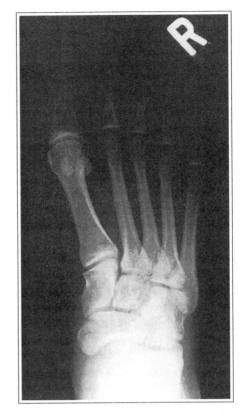

Figure 1-75. Compensating filter was not used on toes.

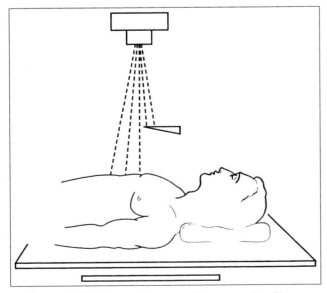

Figure 1-74. Proper placement of compensating filter.

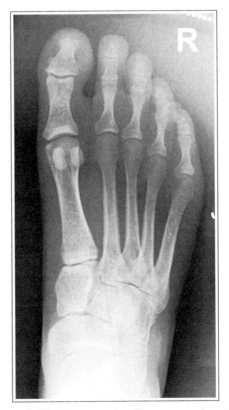

Figure 1-76. Compensating filter was used on toes.

Figure 1-75 was taken without using a compensating filter, whereas the image in Figure 1-76 was taken with a compensating filter positioned over the distal metatarsals and phalangeal regions. Notice the increased visibility of anatomical structures covered by the compensating filter.

If the compensating filter is inaccurately positioned, there will be a density variation defining where the filter was and was not placed over the structures (Figure 1-77). Having too much of the filter positioned over or under a structure that does not need it will result in too many of the photons being absorbed and too little image density in the area.

Because of the superior contrast resolution demonstrated on digital radiography over conventional screen-film, compensating filters are often not needed to demonstrate structures with differing thickness.

Another exposure factor that should be considered when positioning long bones and the vertebral column where a long 17-inch (43-cm) field length is used to accommodate the structure is the **anode-heel effect**. When a long (17-inch [43-cm]) field length is used, a noticeable density variation occurs across the entire field size that is significant enough between the ends of the field that when they are compared it can be seen. This density variation is a result of greater photon absorption that occurs at the thicker "heel" portion of the anode compared with the thinner "toe" portion when a long field is used. Consequently, image density at the anode end of the tube is less because fewer photons emerge from that end of the tube than that at the cathode end.

Using this knowledge to our advantage can help us produce images of long bones and the vertebral column that

TABLE 1-2	Guidelines for Positioning to Incorporate the Anode-Heel Effect	
Projection(s)	Placement of Anode	Placement of Cathode
AP and lateral forearm	Wrist	Elbow
AP and lateral humerus	Elbow	Shoulder
AP and lateral lower leg	Ankle	Knee
AP and lateral femur	Knee	Hip
AP thoracic vertebrae	Cephalic	Caudal
AP lumbar vertebrae	Cephalic	Caudal

demonstrate uniform density at both ends. Position the thinner side of the structure at the anode end of the tube and the thicker side of the structure at the cathode end. Set an exposure (mAs) that will adequately demonstrate the midpoint of the structure (where the central ray is centered). Because the anode will absorb some of the photons aimed at the anode end of the IR and the thinnest structure, but not as many of the photons aimed at the cathode end and the thickest structure, a more uniform density across the part will be demonstrated. Table 1-2 provides guidelines for positioning structures to take advantage of the anode-heel effect. Because the density variation between the ends of the IR is only approximately 30%, the anode-heel effect will not adequately adjust for large thickness differences but will help to improve images of the structures listed in Table 1-2.

Image Contrast

The image contrast optimally visualizes the bony and soft-tissue structures of interest.

1. Does the image contrast optimally demonstrate the bony and soft-tissue structures of interest?

Kilovoltage is the primary exposure factor used to manipulate image contrast in digital and conventional radiography. The kilovoltage should be selected based on the penetration needed for the part being imaged, but more importantly, it should be selected to produce the level of contrast (high or low) necessary to best visualize the anatomic structures of interest. Digital radiography has a contrast resolution that is superior to that of conventional radiography because it has the capability of displaying a much greater range of densities (gray shades) for a given exposure than conventional radiography does. A system that can display a greater number of shades of gray (dynamic range) provides an image with superior contrast resolution.

Image contrast is affected by the kilovoltage employed when the image is made. For every structure within the body there exists an optimum kVp level that provides sufficient penetration and optimal contrast for that body structure. However, situations and different patient conditions occur in which this optimum kVp level does not provide the

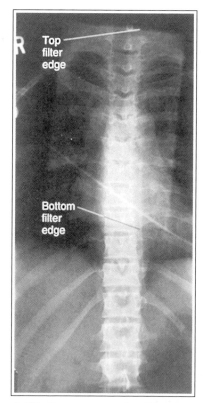

Figure 1-77. Poor compensating filter placement.

best contrast. In these cases the kVp must be adjusted from the routinely used optimal level to obtain a scale of contrast that will better demonstrate the structures of interest.

Adjusting Image Contrast: If the contrast on an image is very low (Figure 1-78), very little difference is demonstrated between the shades of gray and the image lacks a bright white shade. A low-contrast image results when the kVp level is too high. If the contrast on the image is too high (Figure 1-79), the anatomical structures are demonstrated with black and white shades and very few gray shades. A high-contrast image results when the kVp level is set too low for the structure being imaged.

When the density on the image is adequate but the contrast level is not sufficient to adequately visualize all the anatomical structures, the contrast level can be adjusted by varying kVp, and the density can be maintained by counteracting the kVp adjustment with a comparable mAs adjustment. If higher contrast is desired, decrease the original kVp used by 15% and increase the mAs value used by 100%. For example, if the original settings were 80 kVp at 10 mAs, the new settings are 68 kVp at 20 mAs. If you wish lower contrast, increase the original kVp used by 15% and decrease the mAs value used by 50%. For example, if the original technique was 80 kVp at 10 mAs, the new technique would be 92 kVp at 5 mAs. In both of these situations the image density has remained the same as in the original image, because the density adjustment made with kVp is offset by an equal mAs adjustment. The amount of kVp adjustment depends on how dramatic a

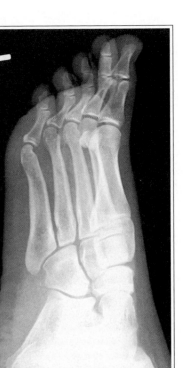

Figure 1-79. High-contrast image.

contrast change is desired. As a general rule you should stay relatively close to the optimal kVp level for the structure being imaged to prevent insufficient penetration.

Contrast on Pediatric Images: Pediatric images are taken to demonstrate fractures, dislocations, congenital anomalies, and pathologies. The bones of infants and children are less dense and more porous than adult bones, resulting in less image contrast being demonstrated between the bone and soft tissue in children than on adult images.

2. Has the amount of scatter radiation produced been effectively controlled?

The contrast that an image displays also depends on how much **scatter radiation** was allowed to reach the IR. An increase in scatter radiation causes a decrease in image contrast and a decrease in the visibility of details. Tight collimation and the use of a grid whenever the kVp is above 70 controls the amount of scatter radiation that reaches the IR.

Flat contact shields can also be used to control the amount of scatter radiation that reaches the IR. When the anatomical structures being examined demonstrate an excessive amount of scatter fogging along the outside of the collimated borders (such as the lateral lumbar vertebrae), place a large flat contact shield or the straight edge of a lead apron along the appropriate border. Doing this greatly improves the visibility of the recorded details. Compare the lateral lumbar vertebral images in Figure 1-80 and Figure 1-81. Figure 1-80 was taken with a lead contact

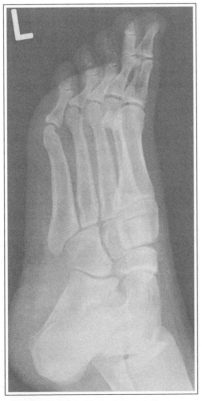

Figure 1-78. Low-contrast image.

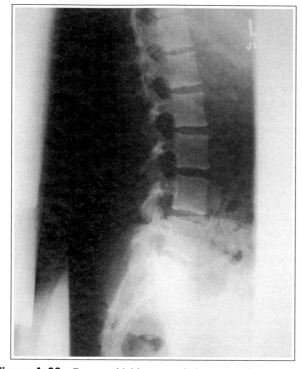

Figure 1-80. Contact shield was used along posterior collimated border.

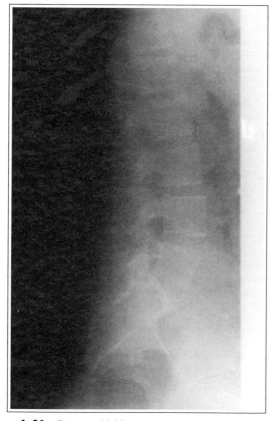

Figure 1-81. Contact shield was not used along posterior collimated border.

shield placed against the posterior edge of the collimator's light field. A contact shield was not used for Figure 1-80. Note the improvement in visualization of the lumbar spinous processes with use of the contact shield.

Controlling scatter radiation is very important when using digital imaging. The phosphor makeup of the IRs used in digital imaging makes them more sensitive to scatter radiation, so techniques such as collimation and grid usage should be increased to reduce the amount of scatter radiation reaching the IR.

Artifacts

No preventable artifacts are present on the image.

1. Are any artifacts visible on the image?

An *artifact* is any undesirable structure or substance recorded on an image. They may be grouped into the following categories: (1) anatomical structures that obscure the area of interest or have no purpose for being there and can be removed from the image; (2) externally removable objects such as patient or hospital possessions; (3) internal objects such as prostheses or monitoring lines; and (4) appearances that result from improper use of equipment.

Before an image is taken, it may be wise to have the patient change into a hospital gown and to ask whether any patient possessions are located in or around the area being imaged. Patients are often nervous and may forget to remove articles of clothing, or for sentimental reasons they may not remove jewelry pieces, so you should recheck the area of interest even after the patient has changed into a gown. Once the patient is positioned and the IR is ready to be exposed, take a last look to make sure all hospital possessions that can be moved out of the imaging field have been moved. Check that those things that must remain in the field, such as heart monitoring leads, have been shifted so that they will superimpose the least amount of information.

2. Can you identify the artifact demonstrated on the image?

It would be impossible to demonstrate in this book all the possible artifacts that can appear on an image, but it is important for technologists to familiarize themselves with as many artifacts as possible. The more aware we are of what causes artifacts on the image, the more careful patient and technical preparation procedures we learn to follow. It might be wise for your department to keep an envelope of images that had to be repeated because of artifacts. From time to time these can be studied to help keep all technologists current on the possibilities for facility-related artifacts.

Most possession-related artifacts are demonstrated on the image as lighter densities than the anatomical structures that surround them. Artifacts that are related to poor film or phosphor plate handling, such as film creases, static, and light leaks, most often exhibit greater density. The following discussion concerns different categories of image artifacts and common examples of each.

Anatomical Artifacts

Anatomical Structures. An anatomical artifact is any anatomical structure that is within the image that could have been removed. This includes those that are superimposed over an area of interest, as well as those that are not superimposed over an area of interest but are still located within the collimated field and could easily have been excluded. A common anatomical artifact is the patient's own hand or arm. Figure 1-82 shows a supine abdominal image in which the patient's hands are superimposed over the upper abdominal region. More than likely the patient was not positioned in this manner when the technologist left the room. Between when the technologist positioned the patient and when the exposure was taken, however, the patient found a more comfortable position. This example stresses the importance of explaining examinations to patients so that they understand how important it is that they remain in the position in which the technologist places them. This example also shows the importance of rechecking each patient's position before the exposure is taken if much time has elapsed between positioning the patient and exposing the image. It is also not uncommon for a patient who is experiencing hip or lower back pain from lying on the imaging table to place a hand beneath an affected hip. This will result in superimposition of the hip and hand on the image. Remember that the patient does not know that repositioning because of discomfort is not acceptable. Figure 1-83 shows a chest image, produced with a mobile x-ray machine, which was taken with the patient's

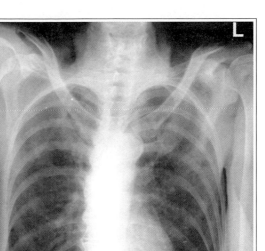

Figure 1-83. Anatomical artifact; patient's arms included in chest image.

arms positioned tightly against the sides. Because humeri are not evaluated on a chest image, there is no reason for them to be included, and they could easily have been shifted out of the imaging field.

Double-Exposure Artifacts: A double-exposed image occurs when two exposures are taken on the same IR without processing having been done between them. The images exposed on the IR can be totally different and easy to identify, such as an AP and lateral lumbar vertebrae images (Figure 1-84), or they may be the same image with almost identical overlap. Double-exposures of images of the same procedure typically appear blurry and can easily be mistaken for patient motion (Figure 1-85). When evaluating a blurry image, look at the cortical outlines of bony structures that are lying longitudinally and transversely. Is there only one cortical outline to represent each bony structure, or are there two? Is one outline lying slightly above or to the side of the other? If one outline is demonstrated, the patient moved during the exposure, but if two are demonstrated, the image was exposed twice and the patient was in a slightly different position for the second exposure. Another indication of a double-exposed image in conventional radiography is its density (Figure 1-86). When the screen-film system is used, a double-exposed image will result in high image density because the film was exposed to radiation twice. When digital radiography is used, a double-exposed image will not demonstrate high density, because the image will be normalized during processing (see Figure 1-42). In this process the density obtained from overexposure will automatically be decreased to the normal or average amount for the examination indicated.

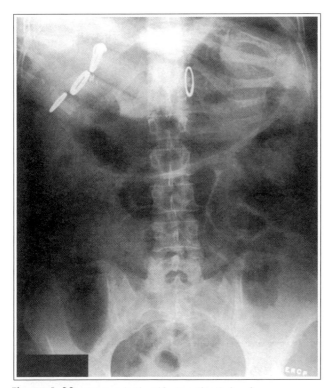

Figure 1-82. Anatomical artifact; patient's hands superimposed on supine abdominal image.

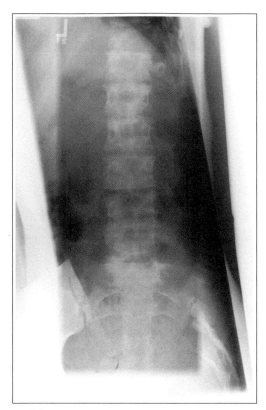

Figure 1-84. Screen-film double exposure. AP and lateral vertebral images.

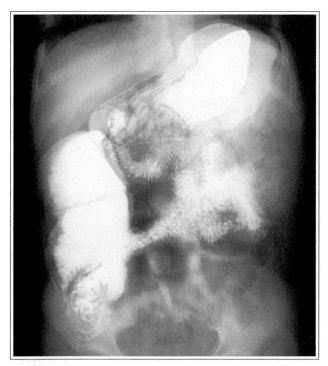

Figure 1-85. Screen-film double exposure. Two abdominal images with barium in stomach and intestines.

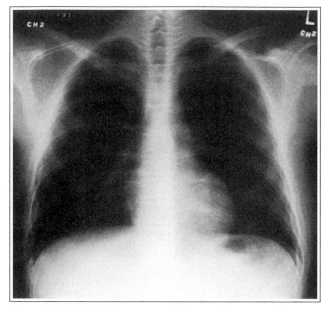

Figure 1-86. Double exposure of chest using screen-film system.

External Artifacts

An external artifact is found outside the patient's body, such as a patient's possession that remained in a pocket or a hospital possession (e.g., needle cap, ice bag) that was lying on top of or beneath the patient. Common external artifacts include earrings, rings, necklaces, bra hooks, dental structures, hairpins, heart-monitoring lines, and gown snaps (Figure 1-87). Two external artifacts that

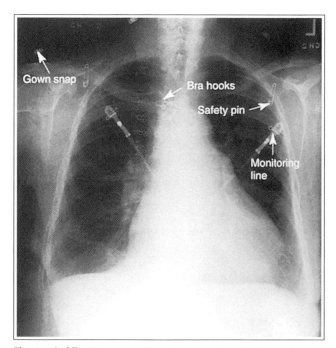

Figure 1-87. External artifacts from patient clothing and hospital monitoring equipment.

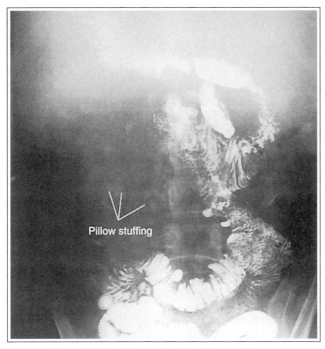

Figure 1-88. External artifact from a pillow.

that can create artifacts on the image is the best way of preventing them.

Internal Artifacts

Internal artifacts are found within the patient. They cannot be removed and must be accepted. Examples of commonly seen internal artifacts are prostheses (Figures 1-89 and 1-90) and pins, pacemakers (see Critique Image 17, Chapter 2), central venous pressure line or chest tube (Figure 1-91), and nasogastric tubes.

If an artifact that is normally not found within the body is identified on an image, it is the technologist's duty to discretely search and interview the patient or to consult the ordering physician to determine whether the artifact is locatable outside the patient's body. If it is not found, it may have been introduced into the patient through one of the body orifices. Your search and interview discoveries should be recorded on the patient's requisition. Figure 1-92 shows a pelvic image of a patient who had swallowed several batteries.

Equipment-Related Artifacts

Equipment-related artifacts are caused by improper use of the imaging equipment.

Grid Alignment Artifact. Grid alignment artifacts are grid lines that result from the use of stationary grids and the improper use of all grid types. They occur because the grid's lead strips absorb primary radiation and are visible as small white lines on the image. Grid line artifacts caused

are not as common but do occasionally appear are caused by pillows (Figure 1-88) and by the imprinted designs on shirts and pants (Figure 1-89). Most of these artifacts can easily be avoided with proper patient preparation and positioning. Being aware of as many objects as possible

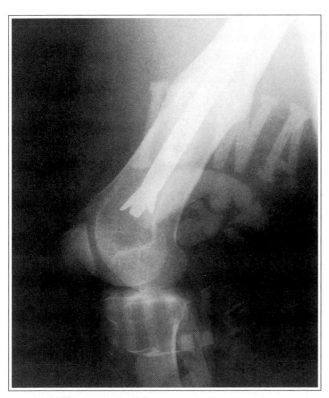

Figure 1-89. External and internal artifacts caused by imprint of patient clothing and leg prosthesis.

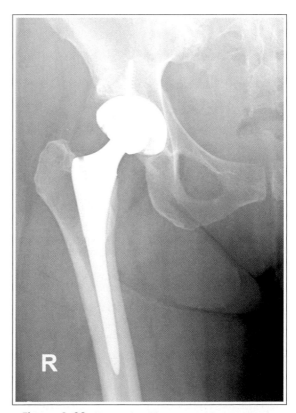

Figure 1-90. Internal artifact caused by prosthesis.

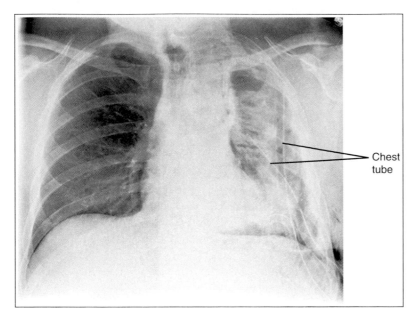

Figure 1-91. Internal artifact: two chest tubes.

by improper grid use are more noticeable when higher-ratio grids are used and can be avoided by choosing a moving grid whenever possible and by properly aligning the central ray and grid.

Causes of grid cut-off include the following:

- If a parallel grid was tilted (off level) or the central ray was angled toward the grid's lead strips, the image demonstrates grid lines on the side toward which the central ray was angled (Figures 1-93, *A*, and 1-94).
- If a parallel or focused grid was off focus (taken at source-image distance outside focusing range), the image demonstrates grid lines on each side of the image (Figures 1-93, *B*, and 1-95).
- If a focused grid was tilted (off level) or the central ray was angled toward the grid's lead strips, the image demonstrates grid lines across the entire image (Figures 1-93, *C*, and 1-96).

- If a focused grid was inverted, the image demonstrates grid lines on each side of the image (Figures 1-93, *D*, and 1-97).
- If a focused grid was off center (central ray not centered on the center of the grid), the image demonstrates grid lines across the entire image (Figures 1-93, *E*, and 1-98). If the image was taken with the table Bucky, the image will not be in the center of the IR but will be demonstrated to one side.

When conventional screen-film radiography is used, an image taken with a grid alignment artifact demonstrates a loss in density where the grid lines are shown. The degree of

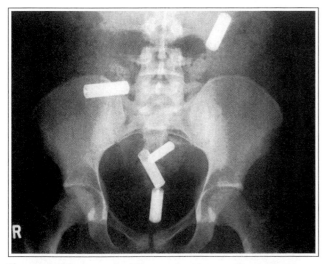

Figure 1-92. Internal artifact; patient has swallowed five batteries.

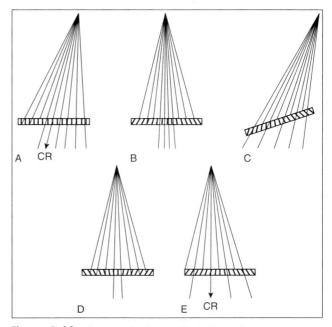

Figure 1-93. Causes of grid cutoff. **A,** Central ray angled against grid's lead lines. **B,** Off focused. **C,** Off level. **D,** Inverted. **E,** Off center.

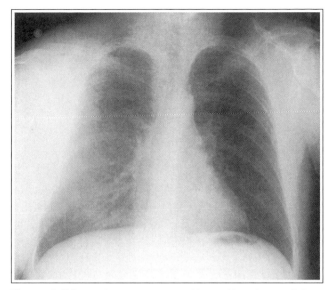

Figure 1-94. Equipment-related artifact. Either the parallel grid was tilted or the central ray was angled toward the grid's lead strips.

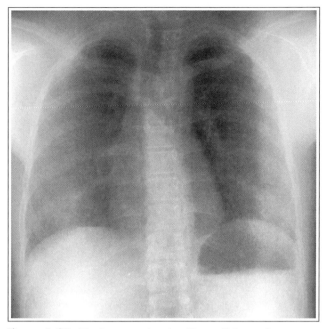

Figure 1-95. Equipment-related artifact: off-focused grid cutoff.

density loss will be greater on the side toward which the central ray is angled and will increase with increased severity of misalignment. Density loss will also be greater when higher grid ratios are used. This density decrease may not be demonstrated in digital radiography, and if it is it may not be as noticeable because the image will be normalized during processing. In this process the density will automatically be increased to the normal or average amount for the examination indicated.

Moiré Grid Artifact. The computed radiography moiré grid artifact occurs when a stationary grid is used and the imaging plate is placed in the plate reader so that the grid's lead strips are aligned parallel with the scanning direction, resulting in a wavy line pattern on the image (Figure 1-99). It is more common with grids that have a frequency below 60 lines/cm. The moiré grid artifact can be eliminated by using a moving grid to blur lines and a grid frequency of

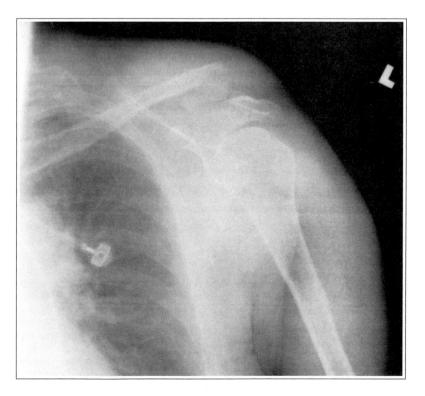

Figure 1-96. Equipment-related artifact. The focused grid was tilted or the central ray was angled toward the grid's lead strips.

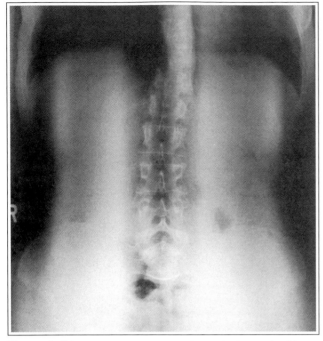

Figure 1-97. Equipment-related artifact. The focused grid was inverted.

60 lines/cm or above and by processing the image so that the grid's lead strips are aligned perpendicular to the plate reader's laser scanning direction. When the reader scans a 10- × 12-inch or 14- × 17-inch imaging plate it is scanned across its short axis. To position the grid's lead strips perpendicular to the scanning direction the grid's lead strips should be placed with the long axis of the imaging plate. An 8- × 10-inch imaging plate is scanned across its long axis. To position the grid's lead strips perpendicular to the scanning direction the grid's lead strips should be aligned with the short axis of the imaging plate.

Phantom Image Artifact. Phantom images are artifacts in computed radiography that occur when the IR is not adequately erased before the next image is exposed on it.

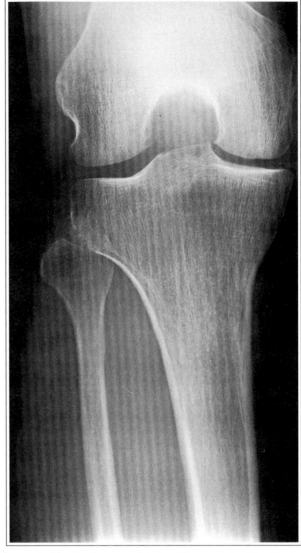

Figure 1-99. Equipment-related artifact: moiré grid artifact. (Courtesy Cesar LJ, Schueler BA, Zink FE, Daly TR, Taubel JP, Jorgensen LL. Artefacts found in computed radiography, *Br J Radiol* 74:195-202, 2001.)

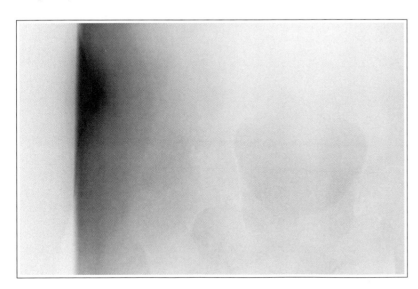

Figure 1-98. Equipment-related artifact: off-centered grid cutoff.

The resulting image is a light shadow of the image that was previously exposed onto the phosphors on the plate. After the exposure the imaging plate is placed into the reader for processing. Information stored on the plate is released when it is exposed to a red laser light. After the image-acquisition process is complete, the plate goes to the erasing block, where it is exposed to a high intensity light to release any remaining stored energy. The erasure block system is capable of erasing a phosphor plate that has received up to five times the normal exposure. If an exposure is greater than this, stored energy in the form of a phantom image will remain on the plate and when re-exposed and read may be seen on the new image, appearing similar to a double-exposed image. For this artifact to be prevented, the phosphor plate should be sent back to the erasure block for a second erasing when the exposure indicator number indicates an excessive exposure was used to create the image.

Phantom images may also be produced when the IR is accidentally exposed to scatter radiation when left in the room during other exposures or has not been used for 24 hours and has collected a sufficient exposure from natural background radiation. Avoid storing IRs in radiation areas. Completion of a secondary erasure before using a phosphor plate that has not been used for some time will prevent this artifact.

Film Handling and Processing Artifacts. Improper film handling and processing can cause artifacts such as film creases, static (Figure 1-100), fog, stains, scratches (Figure 1-101), and hesitation marks (Figure 1-102). They can be avoided by following a good quality control program for the darkroom, film storage, and processor.

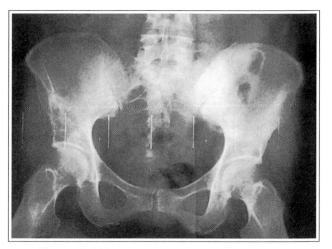

Figure 1-101. Film-handling artifact: scratches.

Phosphor Plate Handling Artifacts. Dust or dirt particles and scratches on the surface of the phosphor plate produce small white dots or curved white lines, respectively (Figure 1-103). Dust or dirt artifacts can be corrected by cleaning the screen. Scratches are permanent, and replacement of the plate is required to eliminate them.

3. What is the location of the artifact with respect to a palpable anatomical structure?

Whenever an external or an unidentifiable internal artifact is demonstrated on an image, discretely examine and interview the patient to determine the artifact's location. To pinpoint where to look for the artifact, study the image

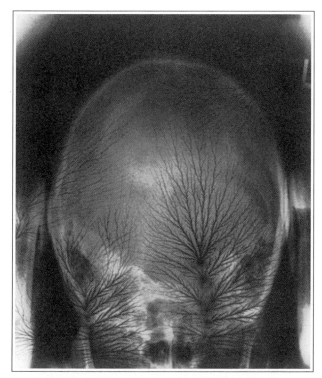

Figure 1-100. Film-handling artifact: static.

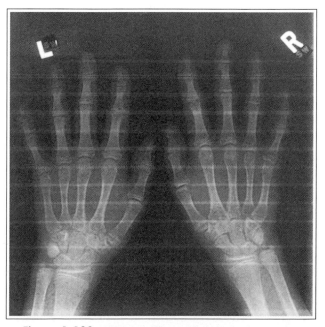

Figure 1-102. Film-handling artifact: hesitation marks.

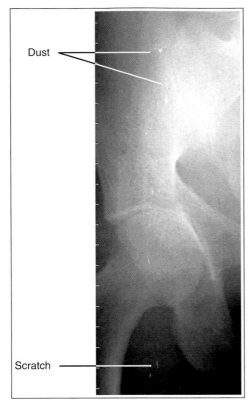

Figure 1-103. Equipment-handling artifact: phosphor plate scratches and dust on AP hip image.

to locate a palpable anatomical structure situated close to the artifact. This is the area where the search should begin.

4. Does the image have to be repeated because of the artifact?

If an artifact that can be eliminated obscures any portion of the area of interest, the image needs to be repeated. A gown snap superimposed on an area of the lungs on a chest image can easily obscure a small lesion. A ring can easily obscure a hairline finger fracture.

If the artifact is located outside the field of interest, the image does not need to be repeated, although the patient should be discretely examined and interviewed to determine whether the artifact is located externally or internally.

The ordered procedure and the indication for examination have been fulfilled.

1. Has the routine series for the body structure ordered been completed as determined by your facility?

One of the last steps to take before deciding whether an image is acceptable is to make sure that you have taken all the images that are recommended by your facility for the body part being imaged. For example, many facilities require that both an AP projection and a lateral position be taken whenever images of the knee are requested.

This series of images provides the reviewer with the needed positions to accurately evaluate the patient's knee.

2. Do the images in the routine series fulfill the indication for the examination, or must additional images be taken?

Not only should the entire series be taken, but you should also determine whether the indication for the examination has been fulfilled. If an elbow examination is ordered and the indication for the examination was to evaluate or rule out a radial head fracture, an additional external oblique or radial head–capitulum position of the elbow may be needed to effectively rule out this fracture. Consult with the reviewer before allowing the patient to leave the imaging department.

POSTPROCEDURE REQUIREMENTS

The requisition and other postprocedure requirements have been completed, and the repeat or reject analysis information has been provided as indicated by your facility.

1. Has the requisition been completed?

These are the sections of the requisition that should be completed by the technologist: (1) the number and sizes of films that were used during conventional screen-film radiography; (2) the number of images obtained during digital imaging; (3) the mAs, kVp, and distance used; (4) the room number where the images were taken; (5) the technologist's name; (6) the date and time of the procedure; and (7) any additional patient history obtained from the patient-technologist interview (Figure 1-104).

Recording the number and sizes of films or images obtained on the requisition tells the reviewer how many images are to be evaluated. The name(s) of the technologist(s) involved in the examination is valuable information if a question arises about the image or patient or if the patient is found to have a contagious disease and measures need to be taken to protect the technologist(s). Recording the same date and time of the procedure on the requisition as are shown on the image, as well as double-checking that the name of the patient is correct, provides a means of verifying that the requisition goes with a certain set of images.

The patient's history should be completed by the ordering physician before the requisition arrives in the imaging facility; any information the technologist has learned from interviewing and observing the patient that might assist the reviewer in the diagnosis should be added, however. This area of the form may also be used to note any situation necessitating departure from the routine examination procedure. For example, if a hand image was taken with the patient's ring still on the finger because the ring could not be removed, the technologist should record this fact in the patient history or notes section of the requisition so that the reviewer understands why the ring appears on the image.

**PHYSICIAN ORDER FOR
RADIOLOGIC/NUCLEAR MEDICINE
Consultation/Request for Procedure**

Department of Radiology

DATE

HOSP. NO.

NAME

BIRTHDATE

ADDRESS

IF NOT IMPRINTED, PLEASE PRINT DATE, HOSP. NO., NAME AND LOCATION

**Procedure
Scheduled for**   Date _____   Time _____

Known Allergies _____

Female of Child-Bearing Age   ☐ Yes   ☐ No

**Patient
Transport**   ☐ Walk   ☐ Cart   ☐ Chair   ☐ Isolette

Oxygen   ☐ Yes   ☐ No   **Diabetic**   ☐ Yes   ☐ No

Pregnant   ☐ Yes   ☐ No   **Lactating**   ☐ Yes   ☐ No

Isolation   ☐ Strict   ☐ Respiratory   ☐ Protective
☐ Wound/Skin   ☐ Enteric   ☐ Blood   ☐ Secretion/Excretion

☐ **Routine**   ☐ **ASAP**   ☐ **STAT**   ☐ **Portable**
STAT Report   ☐ Yes   ☐ No
Phone _____   Pager No. _____

Imaging Specialty   ☐ Ultrasound   ☐ Magnetic Resonance Imaging   ☐ Computed Tomography   ☐ Nuclear Medicine

Procedure _____
_____

Patient diagnosis _____

REASON FOR EXAM/CLINICAL FINDINGS _____
_____

**Physician's
Signature** _____   CLP No. _____   Date _____   **Return
Report To** _____   Phone _____

Radiology use only

14 x 17		KV	MAS	DIST
11 x 14	PA			
10 x 12	LAT			
8 x 10				
9 x 9				
6 x 12				

Fluoro Time (min) _____   Actual Date of Proc. _____

Room _____   Actual Time of Proc. _____

Procedure _____

Physician _____   Technologist/
Sonographer _____

Notes _____
_____
_____

Contrast _____   Date _____

PHARMACEUTICALS AND AGENTS
Radiopharmaceuticals Administered _____   Amount _____   Time _____   By _____
Route of Administration   ☐ I.V.   ☐ Oral   Other _____   Lot No. _____
Radiopharmaceuticals Administered _____   Amount _____   Time _____   By _____
Route of Administration   ☐ I.V.   ☐ Oral   Other _____   Lot No. _____

IMAGING INSTRUCTIONS _____
_____
_____
_____

**PHYSICIAN'S RADIOPHARMACEUTICAL/
ADJUNCT DRUG PRESCRIPTIONS**
_____
_____
_____

☐ **Outpatient**   ☐ **Inpatient**

**Technologist's
Signature** _____

Figure 1-104. The requisition form. The areas to be filled out by the technologist are shaded. *(Courtesy of the University of Iowa Hospital and Clinics.)*

# OF EXAM FILMS	OVE	UNE	POS	PRO	ART	FOG	MOT	EQF	OTH
04 X 05 [ ]	[ ]	[ ]	[ ]	[ ]	[ ]	[ ]	[ ]	[ ]	[ ]
06 X 12 [ ]	[ ]	[ ]	[ ]	[ ]	[ ]	[ ]	[ ]	[ ]	[ ]
08 X 10 [ ]	[ ]	[ ]	[ ]	[ ]	[ ]	[ ]	[ ]	[ ]	[ ]
09 X 09 [ ]	[ ]	[ ]	[ ]	[ ]	[ ]	[ ]	[ ]	[ ]	[ ]
10 X 12 [ ]	[ ]	[ ]	[ ]	[ ]	[ ]	[ ]	[ ]	[ ]	[ ]
11 X 14 [ ]	[ ]	[ ]	[ ]	[ ]	[ ]	[ ]	[ ]	[ ]	[ ]
14 X 14 [ ]	[ ]	[ ]	[ ]	[ ]	[ ]	[ ]	[ ]	[ ]	[ ]
14 X 17 [ ]	[ ]	[ ]	[ ]	[ ]	[ ]	[ ]	[ ]	[ ]	[ ]
14 X 36 [ ]	[ ]	[ ]	[ ]	[ ]	[ ]	[ ]	[ ]	[ ]	[ ]
14 X 51 [ ]	[ ]	[ ]	[ ]	[ ]	[ ]	[ ]	[ ]	[ ]	[ ]
OTHER [ ]	[ ]	[ ]	[ ]	[ ]	[ ]	[ ]	[ ]	[ ]	[ ]

Figure 1-105. Example of a repeat or reject analysis card. *ART,* Artifact; *EQF,* equipment failure; *FOG,* film fog; *MOT,* patient motion; *OTH,* other; *OVE,* overexposure; *POS,* error in patient positioning; *UNE,* underexposure. (Courtesy of the University of Iowa Hospital and Clinics.)

2. Has the repeat or reject analysis information been supplied?

The facility's repeat or reject analysis card, an example of which is shown in Figure 1-105, should be filled out to indicate any positioning or technical errors that occurred during the procedure. This information provides your facility with a means of distinguishing areas where patient service can be improved through in-service personnel training or equipment repair.

Image is acceptable or unacceptable. If image is unacceptable, describe what measures should be taken to produce an acceptable image. If image is acceptable but not optimal, describe factors that could be adjusted to obtain an optimal image.

When an image meets all the necessary requirements, it is considered an optimal image and it should not be repeated. When an image is not optimal but may be acceptable, the question arises whether it is poor enough to repeat or whether the information needed can be obtained without exposing the patient to further radiation. Here are the factors that should be considered when making this decision:

- Your facility's standards
- The age and condition of the patient
- The conditions under which the patient was imaged
- Whether obvious pathology is evident
- Whether the indications for the examination have been fulfilled

Each facility has its own standards that will determine whether an image should be repeated. If standards are low, improving imaging skills can raise them, thereby increasing the accuracy of diagnosis. The age and condition of the patient as well as the situation under which the

patient was imaged carry the largest weight in the decision to repeat an image. Sometimes a less-than-optimal image must be accepted because repeating the image is impossible, as in a surgery case; at other times the patient cannot or will not cooperate. Whenever an examination is accepted that does not meet optimal standards, record on the requisition any information about the patient's condition or setup situation that resulted in acceptance of such an examination. A less-than-optimal image may also be passed when the indication for the examination is clearly fulfilled by the images obtained. For example, a lower leg examination is taken without the required knee joint when the patient history states that the patient has a distal fibular fracture and the indication for the examination is to evaluate the healing of the distal fibular fracture. In this case it is obvious that the patient's knee is not being evaluated. As long as the distal fibula is included in its entirety on the original image, the image should not be repeated.

It is important that all unacceptable images and those less-than-optimal images that have been accepted are studied carefully to determine whether the situation(s) that caused them could be eliminated on future examinations. When an image is repeated, the overall radiation dose to the patient increases and the cost of patient care rises because reimaging requires more technologist time, supplies, and equipment use.

REFERENCES

1. Fauber TL. *Radiographic imaging and exposure,* St Louis, 2004, Mosby.
2. Carroll QB. *Fuchs's radiographic exposure, processing and quality control,* ed 7, Springfield, Ill, 2003, Charles C Thomas.

Image Analysis of the Chest and Abdomen

CHEST

The following image analysis criteria are used for all chest images and should be considered when completing the analysis. Position- or projection-specific criteria relating to these topics are discussed, along with the other criteria for each position or projection.

The facility's identification requirements are visible on the image as identified in Chapter 1.

A right or left marker identifying the correct side of the patient is present on the image and is not superimposed over anatomy of interest.

- Specific placement of the marker is as described in Chapter 1.

Radiation protection practices, as defined in Chapter 1, have been followed.

No evidence of preventable artifacts, such as undergarments, necklaces, and gown snaps, is present.

- It is recommended that the patient be instructed to remove all clothing above the waist and to change into a snapless hospital gown before the procedure. The most common chest image artifacts are necklaces and bra hooks.

The lung markings, diaphragm, heart borders, hilum, greater vessels, and bony cortical outlines are sharply defined.

- Sharply defined recorded details are obtained when patient respiration and body movements are halted and when the least amount of object–image receptor distance (OID) is maintained. A 72-inch (183-cm) source–image receptor distance (SID) is used to decrease the magnification of the heart and lung details.

Beam penetration is sufficient on chest images when the thoracic vertebrae and mediastinal structures are demonstrated. Contrast and density are adequate when the vascular lung markings are visible throughout the lung field.

- An optimal kilovolt-peak (kVp) technique, as shown in Table 2-1, sufficiently penetrates the chest structures and provides the contrast scale necessary to visualize the lung details. A grid should be used to absorb the scatter radiation produced by the thorax, increasing detail visibility, unless otherwise indicated. To obtain optimal density, set a manual milliampere-seconds (mAs) based on the patient's thorax thickness or choose the appropriate automatic exposure control (AEC) chamber when recommended (Table 2-1).

TABLE 2-1	Chest Technical Data			
Position or Projection	**kVp**	**Grid**	**AEC Chamber(s)**	**SID**
PA projection	110	Grid	Both outside	72 inch (183 cm)
Lateral position	125	Grid	Center	72 inch (183 cm)
AP projection	70-80	Nongrid		48-50 inch (120-125 cm)
AP projection	80-100	Grid	Both outside	48-50 inch (120-125 cm)
Lateral decubitus position	125	Grid	Center	72 inch (183 cm)
AP axial (lordotic) projection	125	Grid	Both outside	72 inch (183 cm)
Oblique position	125	Grid	Over lung of interest	72 inch (183 cm)

AEC, Automatic exposure control; *AP,* anteroposterior; *kVp,* kilovolt peak; *PA,* posteroanterior; *SID,* source–image receptor distance.

CHEST: POSTEROANTERIOR PROJECTION

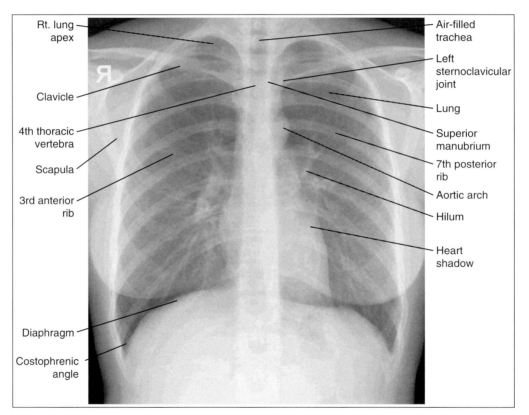

Figure 2-1. Posteroanterior chest image with accurate positioning.

Image Analysis

Beam penetration is adequate on a posteroanterior (PA) chest image when the thoracic vertebrae and posterior ribs are seen through the heart and mediastinal structures. Contrast and density are adequate when the vascular lung markings and fluid levels or air within the pleural cavity, when present, are demonstrated.

- Vascular lung markings are scattered throughout the lungs and are evaluated for changes that may indicate pathology. A pneumothorax (presence of air in

pleural cavity) (Figure 2-2) or pneumectomy (removal of lung) (Figure 2-3) may be indicated if no lung markings are present, whereas excessive lung markings may suggest lesions such as fibrosis, interstitial or alveolar edema, or compression of the lung tissue. To demonstrate precise fluid levels when a pleural effusion is suspected, chest images should be taken with the patient upright and the x-ray beam horizontal. With this position the air rises and the fluid gravitates to the lowest position, creating an air-fluid line or separation. This separation can be identified as a decrease in density on the image

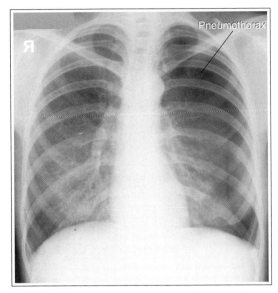

Figure 2-2. Posteroanterior chest image demonstrating a pneumothorax.

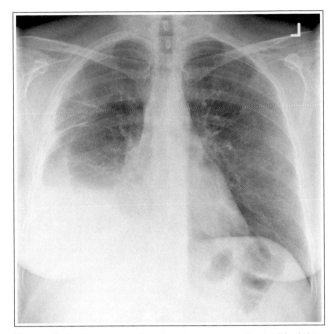

Figure 2-4. Posteroanterior chest image on patient with right side pleural effusion.

wherever the denser fluid is present in the lung field (Figure 2-4 and Figure 2-5). The erect PA chest image is also an excellent method of discerning the presence of free intraperitoneal (within abdominal cavity) air beneath the diaphragm (Figure 2-6).

The seventh thoracic vertebra is at the center of the collimated field. Both lungs from apices to costophrenic angles are included within the field.

- Centering a perpendicular central ray to the midsagittal plane, at a level approximately 7½ inches (18 cm)

inferior to the vertebra prominens (seventh cervical spinous process), places the seventh thoracic vertebra in the center of the image. The seventh thoracic vertebra is identified on the image by counting down the vertebral column from the first thoracic vertebra, which is located just superior to the lung field and is

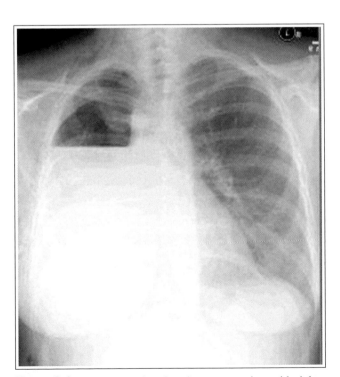

Figure 2-3. Posteroanterior chest image on patient with right side pneumectomy.

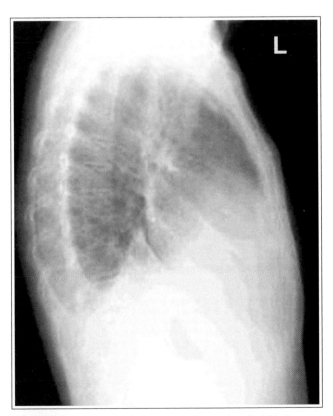

Figure 2-5. Lateral chest image demonstrating fluid in lower lung field.

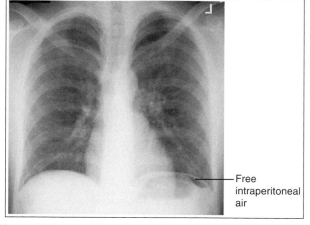

Figure 2-6. Posteroanterior chest image demonstrating free intraperitoneal air.

the first vertebra that demonstrates rib attachment. This central ray placement also centers the lung field on the image. Center the image receptor (IR) to the central ray. Open the transversely collimated field to within ½ inch (2.5 cm) of the patient's lateral skinline. For most adult PA chest images, the full IR length is needed, although you should collimate longitudinally on small patients.

- *IR size and direction:* A 14- × 17-inch (35- × 43-cm) IR should be large enough to include all the required anatomical structures. The direction of IR placement (crosswise versus lengthwise) must also be considered to ensure full lung coverage. For the average sthenic patient and the asthenic patient, whose lung fields are long and narrow, position the IR lengthwise. For the hypersthenic patient, whose lung fields are short and wide, position the IR crosswise.

- *Change in lung dimensions on inspiration:* Along with body type, consider how the lung expands on deep inspiration when choosing IR size and placement. On inspiration the lungs expand in three dimensions: transversely, anteroposteriorly, and vertically. Evaluate the transverse and vertical dimensions to determine how the IR should be placed. When a patient takes a deep breath, will the costophrenic angles still be included on the image? Determine this by placing a hand along the patient's side at the level of the costophrenic angles, then asking the patient to inhale. If your hands remain within the IR's boundaries on inspiration, the IR is wide enough to accommodate the patient. If your hands move outside the IR's boundaries on inspiration, consider using a larger IR or placing the IR crosswise. It is the vertical dimension that will demonstrate the greatest expansion. During high levels of breathing, as when we coax a patient into deep inspiration for a chest image, the vertical dimension can increase by as much as 4 inches (10 cm). This full vertical lung expansion is necessary to

demonstrate the entire lung field. Imaging the patient in an upright position and encouraging a deep inspiration by taking the exposure at the end of the second full inspiration allow demonstration of the greatest amount of vertical lung field. Circumstances that may prevent full lung expansion include disease processes, advanced pregnancy, excessive obesity, being seated in a slouching position, and confining abdominal clothing.

A PA projection is demonstrated. The distances from the vertebral column to the sternal (medial) ends of the clavicles are equal, and the lengths of the right and left corresponding posterior ribs are equal.

- To avoid chest rotation, position the patient's shoulders and arms at equal distances from the IR and instruct the patient to distribute body weight evenly on both feet and to face forward (Figure 2-7). Special attention should be given to female patients who have had one breast removed. The side of the patient on which the breast was removed may need to be placed at a greater OID than the opposite side to prevent rotation. A rotated chest image demonstrates distorted mediastinal structures and may create an uneven density between the lateral borders of the chest. This density difference occurs because the x-ray beam traveled through less tissue on the chest side positioned away from the IR than on the side positioned closer to the IR. It may be detected when the chest has been rotated as little as 2 or 3 degrees. Because any variation in structural relationships or density may represent a pathological condition, the importance of providing nonrotated PA chest images cannot be overemphasized.

- *Detecting rotation:* Rotation is readily detected on a PA chest image by evaluating the distances between

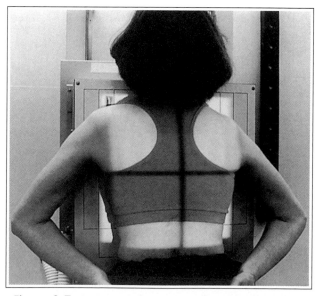

Figure 2-7. Proper patient positioning for PA chest image.

the vertebral column and the sternal ends of the clavicles and by comparing the lengths of the posterior ribs. On a nonrotated PA chest image these distances and lengths should be equal, respectively. On a rotated PA projection the sternal clavicular end that demonstrates the least vertebral column superimposition and the side of the chest with the greatest posterior rib length represents the side of the chest positioned farthest from the IR (see Image 1).

- *Distinguishing scoliosis from rotation:* Scoliosis is a condition of the spine that results in the vertebral column's curving laterally instead of remaining straight. Scoliosis can be distinguished from rotation by comparing the distance from the vertebral column to the lateral lung edges down the length of the lungs. On images of a rotated patient the distances are uniform down the length of the lung field, although when both lungs are compared the distance is shorter on one side. If the patient has scoliosis, the vertebral column to lateral lung edge distances vary down the length of each lung and between each lung (see Image 2). The amount of distance variation increases with the severity of the scoliosis.

Clavicles are positioned on the same horizontal plane.

- The lateral ends of the clavicles are positioned on the same horizontal plane as the medial clavicle ends by depressing the patient's shoulders. Accurate clavicle positioning lowers the lateral clavicles, positioning the middle and lateral clavicles away from the apical chest region and providing better visualization of the apical lung field. When a PA chest image is taken without depression of the shoulders, the lateral ends of the clavicles are elevated, causing the middle and lateral clavicles to be demonstrated within the apical chest region (see Image 3).

The humeri are abducted away from the chest, and the scapulae are located outside the lung field.

- Placing the back of the patient's hands on the hips draws the humeri away from the chest. This positioning also allows the patient to easily rotate the elbows and shoulders anteriorly in order to place the scapulae outside the lung field. When the scapulae are accurately positioned, the superolateral portion of the lungs is better visualized. If a chest image is taken without anterior rotation of the elbows and shoulders, the scapulae are seen superimposing the superolateral lung field (see Image 4). Many dedicated chest units provide holding bars for the patient's arms. When using these units, make certain the shoulders are protracted. If the patient is unable to protract the shoulders while using the bars, position the patient's arms as described previously.

The manubrium is superimposed by the fourth thoracic vertebra, with approximately 1 inch (2.5 cm) of the apical lung field visible above the clavicles,

and the lungs and heart are demonstrated without foreshortening.

- The tilt of the midcoronal plane determines the relationship of the manubrium to the thoracic vertebrae, the amount of apical lung field seen above the clavicles, and the degree of lung and heart foreshortening. When the midcoronal plane is vertical, the manubrium is projected at the level of the fourth thoracic vertebra, approximately 1 inch (2.5 cm) of the apices is visible above the clavicles, and the lungs and heart are demonstrated without foreshortening. If the superior midcoronal plane is tilted anteriorly (forward), however, as demonstrated in Figure 2-8, the lungs and heart are foreshortened, the manubrium is situated at the level of the fifth thoracic vertebra or lower, and more than 1 inch (2.5 cm) of the apices is demonstrated above the clavicles (see Image 5). This positioning error most often occurs during imaging of women with pendulous breasts and patients with protruding abdomens. Conversely, if the superior midcoronal plane is tilted posteriorly (backward), as demonstrated in Figure 2-9, the lungs and heart are foreshortened, the manubrium is situated at a level between the first and third thoracic vertebrae, and less than 1 inch (2.5 cm) of the apices is demonstrated above the clavicles (see Image 6).

- *Poor midcoronal plane versus poor shoulder positioning:* When a PA chest image is taken with the patient's upper midcoronal plane tilted toward the IR, the clavicles are not always demonstrated

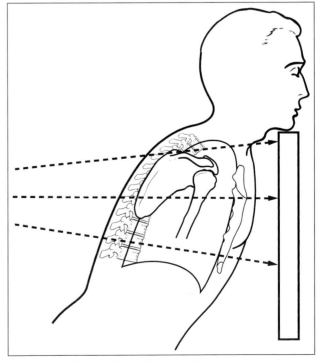

Figure 2-8. Chest foreshortening.

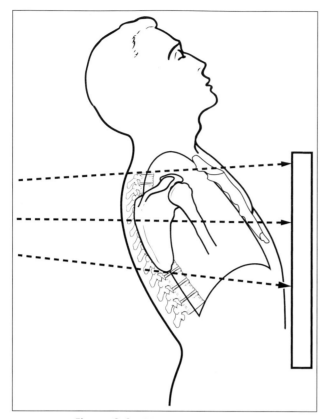

Figure 2-9. Chest foreshortening.

horizontally but may be seen vertically (see Image 5). Distinguish poor shoulder positioning from poor mid-coronal plane positioning by measuring the amount of lung field visualized superior to the clavicles and determining which vertebrae are superimposed over the manubrium. An image with poor shoulder positioning demonstrates decreased lung field superior to the clavicles and the manubrium at the level of the fourth vertebra. An image with the upper midcoronal plane tilting anteriorly demonstrates increased lung field superior to the clavicles and the manubrium at a level inferior to the fourth vertebra.

Ten or 11 posterior ribs are demonstrated above the diaphragm, indicating full lung aeration.

- To obtain maximum lung aeration, take the exposure with the patient in an upright position and after the second full inspiration. When the patient is positioned upright, the abdominal organs and diaphragm shift inferiorly, providing more space for maximum vertical lung expansion.
- Total lung capacity is best obtained when the patient is coaxed into a deep inspiration. In practice this is accomplished by taking the image after the patient's *second* full inspiration. If fewer than 10 posterior ribs are demonstrated, the lungs were not fully inflated. Before repeating the procedure,

attempt to obtain a deeper inspiration and determine whether a patient condition might have caused the poor inhalation. Chest images that are taken on expiration may also demonstrate a decrease in image density, because a decrease in air volume increases the concentration of pulmonary tissues.

- ***Expiration chest image:*** Abnormalities such as a pneumothorax or foreign body may indicate the need for an expiration chest image. For such an image, all evaluation requirements listed for a PA chest image should be met except the number of ribs demonstrated above the diaphragm. On an expiration chest image, as few as nine posterior ribs may be demonstrated, the lungs are denser, and the heart shadow is broader and shorter (see Image 7). When manually setting technique, it may be necessary to increase the exposure (mAs) when a PA chest projection is taken on expiration and lung details are of interest.

Posteroanterior Chest Image Analysis

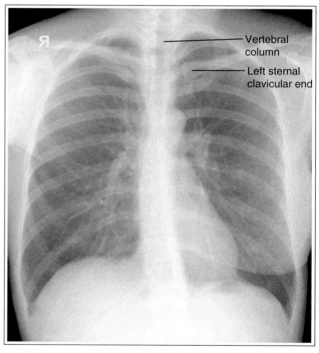

Vertebral column

Left sternal clavicular end

Image 1.

Analysis. The left sternal clavicular end is visualized without vertebral column superimposition, and the left posterior ribs demonstrate greater length than the right posterior ribs. The patient was slightly rotated, with the right side of the chest positioned closer to the IR than the left. (This is a right anterior oblique [RAO] position.)

Correction. To offset chest rotation, position the left shoulder closer to the IR. The shoulders should be at equal distances from the IR.

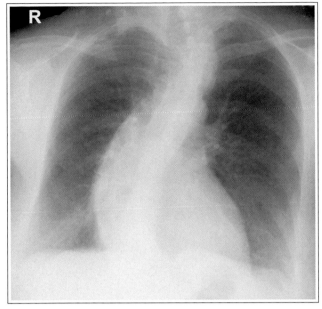

Image 2.

Analysis. The distances from the vertebral column to the lateral rib edges down the length of lungs varies, indicating the patient has scoliosis.

Correction. No correction movement is required.

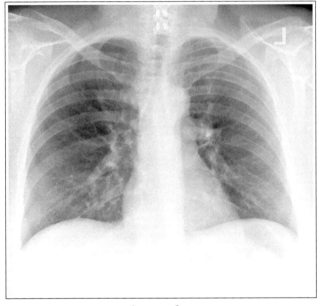

Image 3.

Analysis. The clavicles are not horizontal, and the lateral ends of the clavicles are elevated, obscuring the apices. The manubrium is situated at the level of the fourth thoracic vertebra, and approximately 1 inch (2.5 cm) of the apices is demonstrated superior to the clavicles, indicating that the midcoronal plane was adequately positioned. The patient's shoulders were not depressed.

Correction. Depress the patient's shoulders.

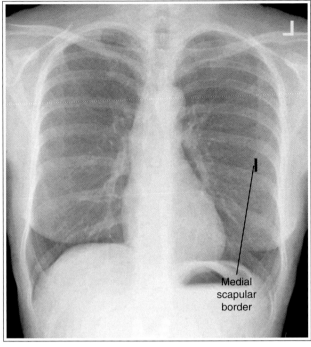

Image 4.

Analysis. The medial borders of the scapulae are demonstrated within the superolateral lung field; the shoulders and elbows were not anteriorly rotated.

Correction. Rotate the elbows and shoulders anteriorly, to draw the scapulae out of the lung field.

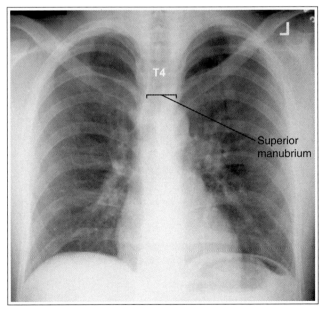

Image 5.

Analysis. The manubrium is situated at the level of the fifth thoracic vertebra, and more than 1 inch (2.5 cm) of the apices is demonstrated superior to the clavicles. The upper midcoronal plane was tilted anteriorly (see Figure 2-8).

Correction. Move the patient's upper thorax posteriorly until the midcoronal plane is vertical.

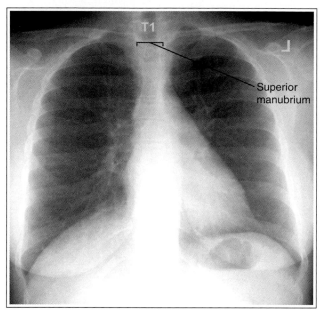

Image 6.

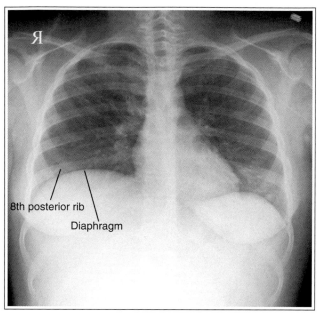

Image 7.

Analysis. The manubrium is situated at the level of the second thoracic vertebra, and less than 1 inch (2.5 cm) of the apices is demonstrated superior to the clavicles. The upper midcoronal plane was tilted away from the IR (see Figure 2-9).

Correction. Move the patient's upper thorax toward the IR until the midcoronal plane is vertical.

Analysis. Only the first through eighth posterior ribs are demonstrated above the diaphragm; the image was taken at the end of expiration.

Correction. If an expiration PA chest image is desired, no change in respiration is required. If an inspiration PA chest image is desired, repeat the image, making the exposure after the second full inspiration.

CHEST: LEFT LATERAL POSITION

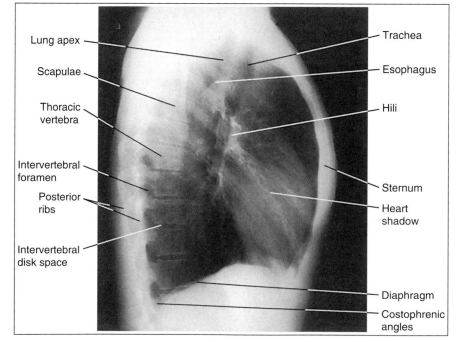

Figure 2-10. Lateral chest image with accurate positioning.

Image Analysis

The midcoronal plane, at the level of the eighth thoracic vertebra, is at the center of the collimated field. The entire lung field, including apices, costophrenic angles, and posterior ribs, is included within the field.

- Centering a perpendicular central ray to the midcoronal plane, at a level approximately 8½ inches (21.25 cm) inferior to the vertebra prominens, places the central ray at the level of the eighth thoracic vertebra. This lower centering, compared with that for the PA chest image, is needed to include the right costophrenic angle on the image. Because the right costophrenic angle is positioned at a long OID and the central ray is centered superior to it, the costophrenic angle is projected inferiorly. Center the IR to the central ray.

- Positioning the midcoronal plane vertically prevents forward or backward leaning, which may result in clipping of the sternum or posterior ribs. Open the transversely collimated field to within ½ inch (1.25 cm) of the lateral skinline. For most adult lateral chest images, the full IR length is needed, although you should collimate longitudinally on small patients.

- A 14- × 17-inch (35- × 43-cm) lengthwise IR should be adequate to include all the required anatomical structures.

A lateral chest position is demonstrated. The posterior and the anterior ribs are nearly superimposed, demonstrating no more than a ½-inch (1-cm) space between them; the sternum is in profile; and the intervertebral foramina of the thoracic vertebrae are open.

- To avoid chest rotation align the shoulders, the posterior ribs, and the posterior pelvic wings perpendicular to the IR (Figure 2-11). This alignment,

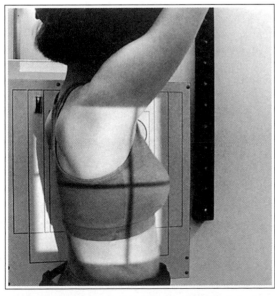

Figure 2-11. Proper patient positioning for lateral chest image.

which nearly superimposes each pair, is accomplished by resting an extended flat hand against each, respectively, then adjusting the patient's rotation until the hand is positioned perpendicularly to the IR. Because the right lung field and ribs are positioned at a greater OID than the left lung field and ribs, the right lung field and ribs are more magnified. This magnification prevents the posterior and anterior ribs from being directly superimposed. Routinely, approximately a ½-inch (1-cm) separation is demonstrated between the right and left posterior ribs, with the right posterior ribs projecting behind the left. When the posterior ribs are directly superimposed, this separation is demonstrated between the anterior ribs (see Image 8).

- **Detecting chest rotation:** Chest rotation is effectively detected on a lateral chest image by evaluating the degree of superimposition of the posterior ribs and anterior ribs. When more than ½ inch (1.25 cm) of space exists between the right and left anterior ribs or between the right and left posterior ribs, the chest was rotated for the image. A rotated lateral chest image obscures portions of the lung field and distorts the heart and hilum shadows.

- **Distinguishing the right and left lungs:** When a rotated lateral chest image has been obtained, determine how to reposition the patient by identifying the hemidiaphragms and therefore the lungs. The first and easiest method of discerning the hemidiaphragm is to identify the *gastric air bubble.* On an upright patient, gas in the stomach rises to the fundus (superior section of stomach), which is located just beneath the left hemidiaphragm (see Images 8 and 10). If this gastric bubble is visible on the image, you know that the left hemidiaphragm is located directly above it. The second method of distinguishing one lung from the other uses the heart shadow. Because the heart shadow is located in the left chest cavity and extends anteroinferiorly to the left hemidiaphragm, outlining the *superior heart shadow* enables you to recognize the left lung. As demonstrated in Figure 2-12, if the left lung is positioned anteriorly, the outline of the superior heart shadow continues beyond the sternum and into the anterior lung (see Image 9). Figure 2-13 demonstrates the opposite rotation; the right lung is positioned anteriorly. Note how the superior heart shadow does not extend into the anterior situated lung but ends at the sternum (see Image 10). It is most common on rotated lateral chest images for the left lung to be rotated anteriorly and the right lung rotated posteriorly.

- **Repositioning the rotated patient:** Once the lungs have been identified, reposition the patient by rotating the thorax. When the left lung was anteriorly positioned on the original image, rotate the left thorax posteriorly, and when the right lung was anteriorly positioned, rotate the right thorax posteriorly. Because both lungs move simultaneously, the amount of adjustment

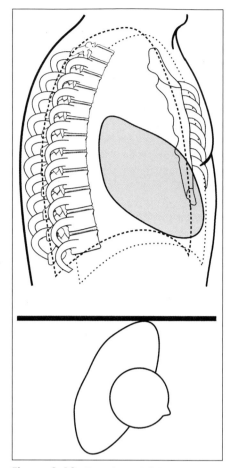

Figure 2-12. Rotation—left lung anterior.

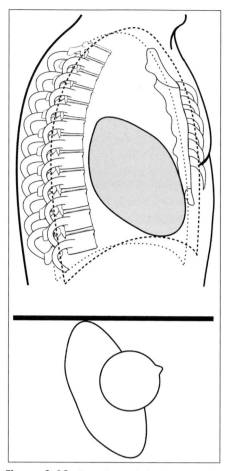

Figure 2-13. Rotation—right lung anterior.

should be only half of the distance demonstrated between the posterior ribs.

- ***Distinguishing scoliosis from rotation:*** On images of patients with spinal scoliosis, the lung field may appear rotated because of the lateral deviation of the vertebral column (see Image 11). The anterior ribs are superimposed, but the posterior ribs demonstrate differing degrees of separation, depending on the severity of scoliosis. View the accompanying PA chest image to confirm this patient condition. Although the separation between the posterior ribs is not acceptable beyond 1/2 inch (1.25 cm) on a patient without scoliosis, it is acceptable on a patient with the condition.

The lungs are demonstrated without foreshortening, with nearly superimposed hemidiaphragms.

- ***Lung foreshortening:*** To obtain a lateral chest image without lung foreshortening, position the midsagittal plane parallel with the IR. When imaging a patient with broad shoulders and narrow hips, it is essential to place the hips away from the IR to maintain a parallel midsagittal plane. In 90% of persons the right lung and diaphragm are situated at a slightly higher elevation than the left lung and diaphragm. This elevation is caused by the liver, which is situated

directly below the right diaphragm. Because the right diaphragm is elevated, one might expect it to be demonstrated above the left diaphragm when the patient is imaged from the side, but this is not true when the midsagittal plane is correctly positioned. Because the anatomical part positioned farthest from the IR diverges and magnifies the most, the right lung will be projected and magnified more than the left lung. The resulting image demonstrates near superimposition of the two hemidiaphragms. When the midsagittal plane has not been positioned parallel with the IR, lung foreshortening and poor hemidiaphragm positioning occur.

- ***Poor midsagittal plane positioning:*** Figure 2-14 demonstrates lateral chest positioning in which the patient's shoulders and hips were both resting against the IR, causing the inferior midsagittal plane to tilt toward the IR. This positioning projects the right hemidiaphragm inferior to the left on the image (see Image 12). When such an image has been obtained, determine how the patient was mispositioned by using one of the methods described previously to distinguish the right lung from the left lung. Before retaking a lateral chest image because of foreshortening, scrutinize the patient's accompanying

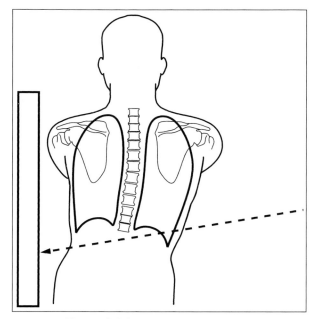

Figure 2-14. Chest foreshortening.

PA projection image to determine whether the patient is one of the 10% of persons whose hemidiaphragms are at the same height or whether a pathological condition is causing the left hemidiaphragm to be projected above the right (Figure 2-15).

- ***Right versus left lateral chest image:*** A left lateral chest image and a right lateral chest image have two distinct differences: the size of the heart shadow and the superimposition of the hemidiaphragms. Both differences are a result of a change in OID and magnification. For a right lateral chest image, the right thorax is positioned closer to the IR. In this position, any anatomical

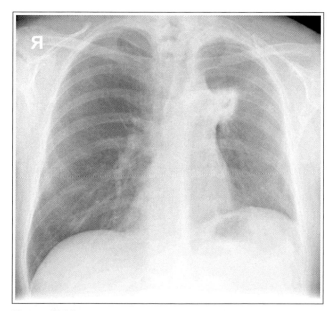

Figure 2-15. Posteroanterior chest image demonstrating an elevated left hemidiaphragm.

structures located in the right thorax are magnified less than structures located in the left thorax, because of the difference in OID. Radiographically the heart shadow is more magnified and the left hemidiaphragm projects lower than the right hemidiaphragm (see Image 13). One advantage of obtaining a right rather than a left lateral chest image is the increase in right lung radiographic detail that results from positioning of the right lung closer to the IR.

No superimposition of humeral soft tissue over the anterior lung apices is present.

- ***Humeral positioning:*** Placing the humeri in an upright vertical position and instructing the patient to cross the forearms above the head prevent superimposition of the humeral soft tissue over the anterior lung apices (see Image 14). Many dedicated chest units provide holding bars for the patient's arms. When they are used, make sure the humeri are placed high enough to prevent this soft-tissue overlap. If the holding bars cannot be raised high enough and the patient is able to prevent motion, position the patient's arms as just described.
- ***Pacemaker:*** The pacemaker is used to regulate the heart rate by supplying electrical stimulation to the heart. This electrical signal stimulates the heart the needed amount to maintain an effective rate and rhythm. The internal pacemaker is surgically implanted in the patient's chest. Care should be taken when positioning a patient whose pacemaker was inserted within 24 hours of the examination. Elevation of the left arm should be avoided to prevent dislodging of the pacemaker and catheter.[1]

The anteroinferior lung and the heart shadow are well defined.

- This area is most clearly defined when the patient is imaged in a standing position. If the patient is seated and leaning forward, the anterior abdominal tissue is compressed, obscuring the anteroinferior lung and the heart shadow; this is especially true in an obese patient (see Image 15). Consideration of patient condition dictates how the image will be taken. To best demonstrate this region on the seated patient, have the patient lean back slightly, allowing the anterior abdominal tissue to relax. Do not lean the patient so far back, however, that the posterior lungs are not on the image.

The hemidiaphragms demonstrate a gentle, cephalically bowed contour, and the eleventh thoracic vertebra is entirely superimposed by the lung field, with the hemidiaphragms visible inferior to it, indicating full lung aeration.

- ***Maximum lung aeration:*** To obtain maximum lung aeration, take the exposure after the second full inspiration with the patient in an upright position. When a lateral chest image demonstrates the hemidiaphragms with an exaggerated cephalic bow, in addition to a

portion of the eleventh thoracic vertebra inferior to
the hemidiaphragms in a patient with no condition to
have caused such an image, full lung aeration has not
been accomplished (see Image 16). Repeat the procedure with a deeper patient inspiration. The lungs
must be inflated for lung markings to be evaluated.
Chest images that are taken on expiration may also
demonstrate a decrease in image density, because a
decrease in air volume increases the concentration
of pulmonary tissues.

When the patient is in an upright position and fluid
is present in the inferior lungs, the hemidiaphragms
are not clearly identifiable (see Figure 2-5).

- **Identifying the eleventh thoracic vertebra:** The
  eleventh thoracic vertebra can be identified by locating the twelfth thoracic vertebra—which has the last
  rib attached to it—and counting up one. To confirm
  this finding, evaluate the curvature of the posterior
  aspect of the thoracic and lumbar bodies. The thoracic
  curvature is kyphotic (forward curvature), and the
  lumbar curvature is lordotic (backward curvature).
  Follow the posterior vertebral bodies of the lower
  thoracic and upper lumbar vertebrae, watching for the
  subtle change in curvature from kyphotic to lordotic.
  The twelfth thoracic vertebra is located just above this
  change (Figure 2-16). On most fully aerated adult lateral chest images the diaphragms are demonstrated
  dividing the body of the twelfth thoracic vertebra.

Lateral Chest Image Analysis

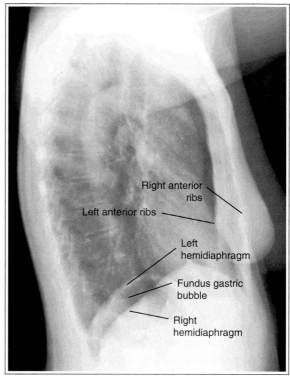

Image 8.

Analysis. Posterior ribs are directly superimposed, and
approximately ½ inch (1.25 cm) of space is present
between the right and left anterior ribs.

Correction. No correction movement is required. The
superimposition is a result of the increased magnification of
the right lung over the left lung as a result of the greater OID.

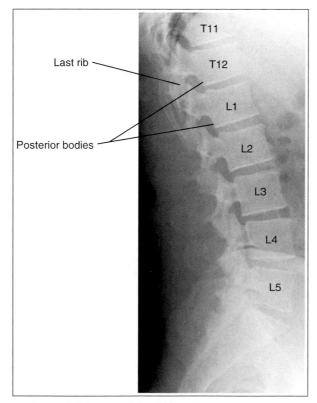

Figure 2-16. Identifying the twelfth thoracic vertebra.

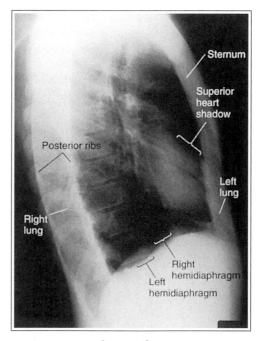

Image 9.

Analysis. The right and left posterior ribs are separated by more than ¹/₂ inch (1.25 cm), indicating that the chest was rotated. The gastric bubble has not been demonstrated, but the superior heart shadow is seen extending beyond the sternum and into the anteriorly situated lung, verifying that it is the left lung. The patient was positioned with the left thorax rotated anteriorly and the right thorax rotated posteriorly.

Correction. Position the right thorax slightly anteriorly. The amount of movement should be only half the distance between the posterior ribs. For this patient the movement should be approximately 1 inch (2.5 cm).

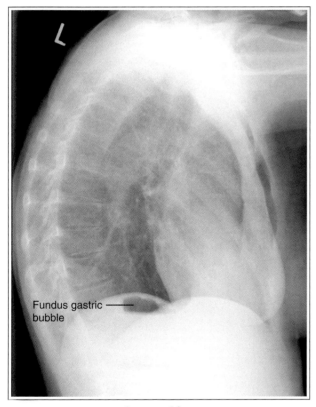

Image 10.

Analysis. The right and left posterior ribs are separated by more than ¹/₂ inch (1.25 cm), indicating that the chest was rotated. The superior heart shadow does not extend beyond the sternum and the gastric air bubble is demonstrated adjacent to the posteriorly situated lung, verifying that the right lung is situated anterior to the sternum, and the left lung posteriorly. The patient was positioned with the right thorax rotated anteriorly and the left thorax rotated posteriorly.

Correction. Position the right thorax posteriorly.

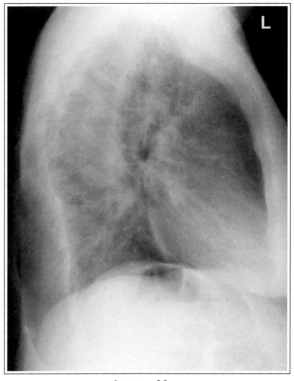

Image 11.

Analysis. The right and left posterior ribs demonstrate differing degrees of separation. The patient has scoliosis. Evaluate the patient's accompanying PA projection image to confirm this finding.

Correction. No correction movement is required. A lateral chest image of a patient with scoliosis demonstrates uneven posterior rib separation.

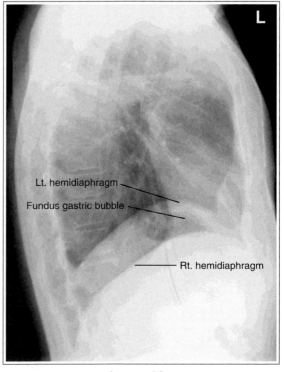

Image 12.

Analysis. The left hemidiaphragm is superior to the right hemidiaphragm. This is verified by the visualization of the gastric bubble below the left hemidiaphragm. The patient's lower thorax was situated closer to the IR than the upper thorax (see Figure 2-14).

Correction. Before repeating the image, scrutinize the patient's accompanying PA projection image carefully. Determine whether the hemidiaphragms are at the same height or whether a pathological condition might have caused the left diaphragm to be projected above the right (see Figure 2-15). If no such condition is evident, repeat the procedure; shift the patient's hips away from the IR until the midsagittal plane is parallel with the IR.

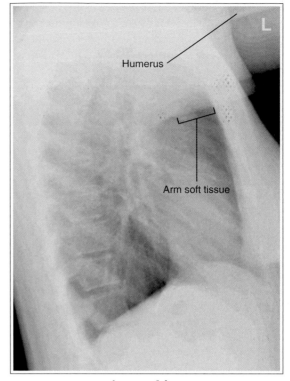

Image 14.

Analysis. The humeral soft-tissue shadows are obscuring the anterior lung apices.

Correction. Have the patient raise the arms until the humeri are vertical, removing them from the field.

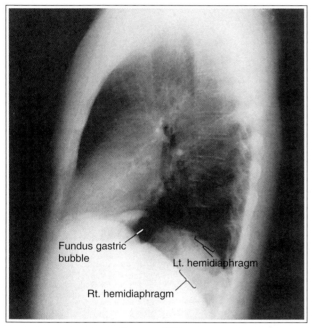

Image 13.

Analysis. This is a right lateral chest image. The right hemidiaphragm is situated superior to the left hemidiaphragm, and the heart shadow is enlarged.

Correction. If a right lateral chest image is desired, no correction is needed. Otherwise, a left lateral chest image should be obtained.

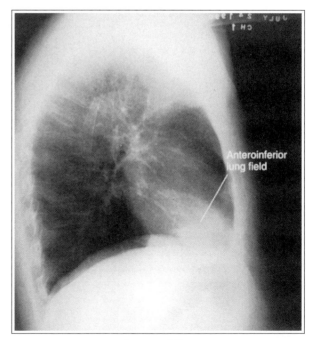

Image 15.

Analysis. The anterior abdominal tissue is pressing against the anteroinferior lung and heart shadows, preventing their clear visualization. The patient was leaning forward in a seated position.

Correction. Allow patient to lean back slightly, relaxing the abdominal tissue. Do not lean the patient so far back, however, that the posterior lungs are not on the image.

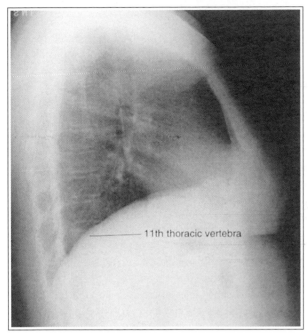

Image 16.

Analysis. A portion of the eleventh thoracic vertebra is demonstrated inferior to the hemidiaphragms. The image was not taken after full inspiration.

Correction. Coax the patient into taking a deeper inspiration.

CHEST: ANTEROPOSTERIOR PROJECTION (SUPINE OR WITH MOBILE X-RAY UNIT)

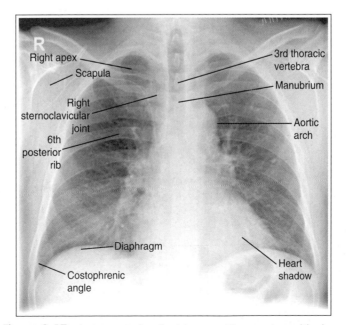

Figure 2-17. Anteroposterior chest image with accurate positioning.

Image Analysis

The time of examination and degree of patient elevation are demonstrated when indicated.

- Indicating the time of day on the image is especially important if the patient's progress is being followed and multiple chest images are to be taken on the same day. Knowledge of the degree of elevation helps the reviewer determine the exact amount of fluid in the patient's lungs.

- *Air-fluid levels:* To demonstrate precise air-fluid levels when pleural effusion is suspected, chest images should be taken with the patient upright and the x-ray beam horizontal. With this position, the air rises and the fluid gravitates to the lowest position, creating an air-fluid separation. This separation is identified as a decrease in density on the image wherever the dense fluid is present in the lung field (Figure 2-18). If the patient is positioned only partially upright, the fluid line will slant, like water in a tilted jar. The true amount of fluid cannot be discerned on an image unless the fluid is level; in the slanted position the chest may appear to have more fluid than it actually does. When the patient is supine, the fluid is evenly spread throughout the lung field, preventing visualization of fluid levels.

No evidence of removable monitoring lines is present.

- All patient monitoring lines that can be removed or shifted out of the lung field should be. When patient monitoring lines remain within the lung field, they may obscure lung details (see Image 17).

Contrast, density, and penetration are adequate to demonstrate the internal tubes and lines when present. Soft-tissue outlines of the air-filled trachea, the heart shadow, and the cortical outline of posterior and anterior ribs are visualized.

- A grid is not always employed in portable imaging, because it is difficult to ensure that the grid and central ray are aligned accurately, preventing grid cutoff. When no grid is used, a lower kVp technique is needed to prevent excessive scatter radiation from reaching the IR and hindering contrast. Although the lower kVp will sufficiently penetrate the lung field, it seldom provides enough penetration to allow visualization of structures within and behind the heart shadow.

- *Heart penetration on mobile chest images:* When a chest image is used to evaluate the placement of apparatus positioned within the mediastinal region, such as a pulmonary arterial line (also known as a *Swan-Ganz catheter*) or central venous (CV) pressure line, the heart shadow should be penetrated. The accurate placement of these lines cannot be evaluated without heart penetration. Accomplish this penetration by increasing the kVp. The resulting image will demonstrate a penetrated heart shadow with the thoracic vertebrae, posterior ribs, and chest lines, such as pulmonary arterial line or CV pressure lines, clearly demonstrated through it. The amount of scatter radiation reaching the IR will also increase, resulting in overall lower image contrast.

Endotracheal tube (ET): The ET is a stiff, thick-walled tube that is used to inflate the lungs. The distal tip of the ET should be positioned 1 to 2 inches (3 to 5 cm) superior to the tracheal bifurcation (carina) when the neck is in a neutral position (Figure 2-19). With neck flexion and

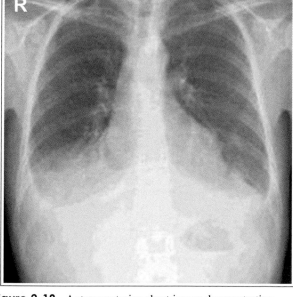

Figure 2-18. Anteroposterior chest image demonstrating fluid in lower lung region.

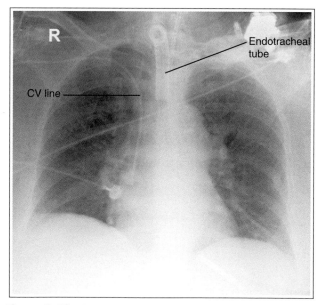

Figure 2-19. Anteroposterior chest image demonstrating an endotracheal tube and central venous line.

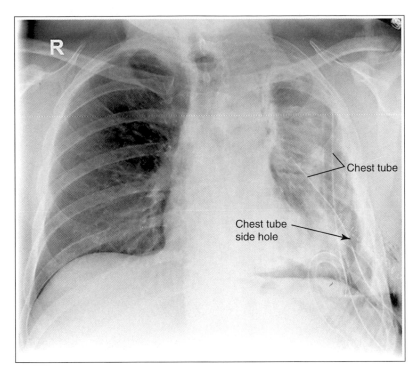

Figure 2-20. Anteroposterior chest image demonstrating two chest tubes.

extension, the tip can move 1 inch (2 cm) superiorly and inferiorly, respectively. The most common mispositioning of this device is placement of the ET into the right main bronchus, causing hyperinflation of the right lung and collapse of the left lung. Images taken for ET placement should demonstrate adequate penetration and density to visualize the upper mediastinal region.

Thoracostomy tube (chest tube): The thoracostomy tube is a 1.25-cm diameter, thick-walled tube that is used to remove fluid or air from the pleural space when it is preventing negative pressure in the intrapleural space from aiding in lung expansion. Failure to remove the fluid or air may result in collapse of the lung. For drainage of air the tube is placed anterosuperiorly within the pleural space, typically at the level of the second or third intercostal space at the midclavicular line (Figure 2-20). For drainage of fluid the tube is typically placed within the pleural space laterally at the midaxillary line at the level of the fifth or six intercostal space. The side hole of the thoracostomy tube, which is marked by an interruption of the radiopaque identification line, should be placed within the thoracic cavity, medial to the inner ribs. Images taken for thoracostomy tube placement should demonstrate adequate density and penetration to visualize the radiopaque identification line interruptions at the side hole.

CV line: The CV line is a small (2 to 3 mm), radiopaque catheter that is used to allow infusion of substances that are too toxic for peripheral infusion, such as for chemotherapy, total parenteral nutrition, dialysis, or blood transfusions. The CV line is commonly inserted into the subclavian or jugular vein and extends to the superior vena cava, approximately 2 to 3 cm above the right atrial junction (Figure 2-21). Images taken for CV line placement should demonstrate

adequate density and penetration to visualize the line and lung conditions that may result if tissue perforation occurs during line insertion, such as pneumothorax or hemothorax.

Pulmonary arterial line (Swan-Ganz catheter): The pulmonary arterial line is similar to the CV line but is longer. It is used to measure atrial pressures, pulmonary artery pressure, and cardiac output. The measurements obtained are used to diagnose ventricular failure and monitor the effects of specific medication, exercise, and stress on heart function. The pulmonary arterial line is inserted in the subclavian, internal or external jugular, or femoral vein and is advanced through the right atrium into the pulmonary artery (Figure 2-22). Images taken for pulmonary arterial line placement should demonstrate adequate density and penetration to visualize the line and mediastinal structures to determine adequate placement.

Pacemaker: The pacemaker is used to regulate the heart rate by supplying electrical stimulation to the heart. This electrical signal will stimulate the heart the needed amount to maintain an effective rate and rhythm. The internal pacemaker is surgically implanted in the patient's chest. On a PA or anteroposterior (AP) chest image the pacemaker catheter tip should be seen at the apex of the right ventricle (see Image 17). Care should be taken when positioning a patient whose pacemaker was inserted within 24 hours of the examination. Elevation of the left arm should be avoided to prevent dislodging of the pacemaker and catheter.

Because the radiographer is the first to see images, it is within his or her scope of practice to inform the radiologist or attending physician when a mispositioned line is suspected. Familiarizing yourself with the accurate placement of these lines will provide the knowledge needed

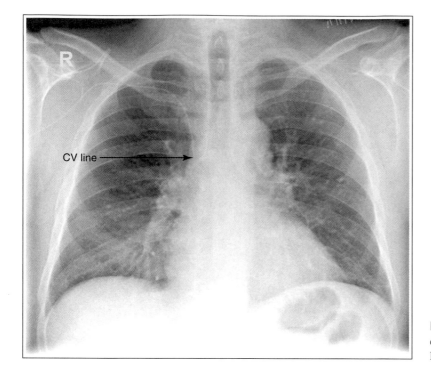
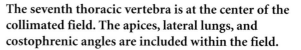

Figure 2-21. Anteroposterior chest demonstrating accurate central venous *(CV)* line placement.

to identify when a mispositioning of a line is suspected (see Image 18).

The heart demonstrates increased magnification when the images are compared with routine chest images.

- A 40- to 48-inch (102- to 120-cm) SID is used. This SID is lower than that used for routine chest images and demonstrates greater heart magnification because of the increase in x-ray divergence.

The seventh thoracic vertebra is at the center of the collimated field. The apices, lateral lungs, and costophrenic angles are included within the field.

- Centering the central ray to the midsagittal plane at a level approximately 4 inches (10 cm) inferior to the jugular notch places the seventh thoracic vertebra in the center of the image. This central ray placement also centers the lung field on the image. Center the IR to the central ray. Open the longitudinally collimated field to within ½ inch (2.5 cm) of the

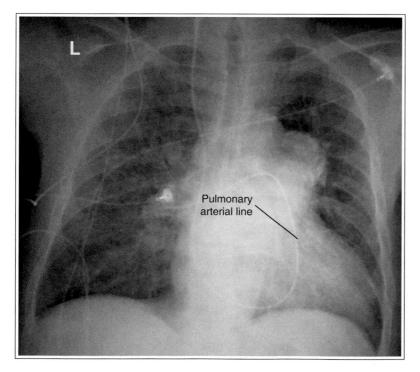

Figure 2-22. Anteroposterior chest image demonstrating accurate pulmonary arterial *(PA)* line placement.

lateral skinline. For most adult AP chest images, the full 14-inch (35-cm) length is needed. A 14- × 17-inch (35- × 43-cm) IR should be adequate to include all the required anatomical structures.

- **IR size and direction for mobile chest image:** The direction of IR placement (crosswise versus lengthwise) must also be considered to ensure full lung coverage. For the asthenic and hypersthenic patient, position the IR crosswise. For the sthenic patient whose lung field is long and narrow, position the IR lengthwise. On inspiration the lungs expand in three dimensions: transversely, anteroposteriorly, and vertically. Evaluate the transverse dimension to determine the direction in which the IR should be placed. View the lateral sides of the chest during the patient's deep inspiration to determine whether the lateral margins of the chest will remain within the IR boundaries. If the lateral chest margins move outside the IR boundaries during inspiration, consider placing the IR crosswise. It is safe to position the IR crosswise on most patients for portable chest imaging because the vertical dimension does not fully expand in a recumbent or seated patient.

The chest demonstrates an AP projection when the distances from the vertebral column to the sternal ends of the clavicles and the lengths of the right and left corresponding posterior ribs are equal.

- The patient, IR, and central ray must be accurately aligned to avoid chest rotation. To align the patient and IR, place the patient's shoulders and pelvis on a straight plane and position the IR parallel with the bed (Figure 2-23). On beds with special padding, it may be necessary to place a sponge beneath one side of the IR to keep it level and parallel. Because the patient's chest and IR move simultaneously, if the IR is not level, the chest is rotated. To align the central

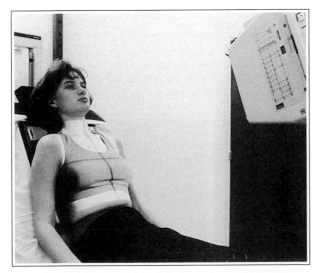

Figure 2-23. Proper patient positioning for anteroposterior chest image.

ray with the patient and IR, adjust the central ray position until it is perpendicular to the midcoronal plane and IR. If the central ray is angled to the right or left side of the patient instead of being perpendicular, the anatomical structures farthest from the IR (manubrium and clavicles) will be projected in the direction toward which the central ray is angled.

- **Detecting chest rotation on a mobile image:** You can detect poor IR balance or poor central ray alignment and, consequently, chest rotation by evaluating the distances between the vertebral column and the sternal ends of the clavicles and by comparing the lengths of the posterior ribs. When the right sternal clavicular end demonstrates less superimposition of the vertebral column and the right posterior ribs demonstrate greater length than the left, the patient's right side was placed closer to the bed (see Image 17). When the left sternal clavicular end is seen without superimposition of the vertebral column and the left side demonstrates greater posterior rib length than the right, the patient's left side was placed closer to the bed (see Image 19). If the cause of this rotation was poor central ray alignment with the patient and IR, the sternal clavicular end that is superimposed over the least amount of the vertebral column and the posterior ribs that demonstrate the greatest length represent the side of the chest toward which the central ray angle was directed. Angling the central ray toward the right side of the chest will result in the right sternal clavicular end being seen at a greater distance from the vertebral column and greater right side posterior rib length (see Image 17), whereas angling the central ray toward the left side of the chest will result in the left sternal clavicular end being seen at a greater distance from the vertebral column and greater left side posterior rib length (see Image 19). It will be necessary to carefully evaluate the positioning setup on rotated AP chest images to determine whether rotation was caused by poor alignment of the patient and IR with the central ray.

The clavicles are positioned on the same horizontal plane.

- When the patient's condition allows, position the lateral ends of the clavicles on the same horizontal plane as the medial ends by depressing the patient's shoulders. Accurate positioning of the clavicles lowers the lateral ends of the clavicles, positioning the middle and lateral clavicles away from the apical chest region and improving visualization of the apical lung field. If the patient is unable to depress the shoulders, the middle and lateral ends of the clavicles will be seen in the apical chest region.

The scapulae are demonstrated within the lung field. The distal humeri have been abducted out of the imaging field.

- To position most of the scapulae outside the lung field, place the back of the patient's hands on the hips and rotate the elbows and shoulders anteriorly. Most patients who require mobile or supine chest images are incapable of positioning their arms in this manner, resulting in an image with the scapulae positioned in the lung field. In such a situation abduct the patient's arms until they are placed outside the imaging field. Failure to do so will result in unnecessary exposure to the patient's arms (see Image 20).

The manubrium is superimposed over the fourth thoracic vertebra with approximately 1 inch (2.5 cm) of the apices demonstrated above the clavicles, and the posterior ribs demonstrate a gentle cephalically bowed contour.

- The alignment of the central ray with respect to the patient determines the relationship of the manubrium to the thoracic vertebrae, the amount of apical lung field seen above the clavicles, and the contour of the posterior ribs. For accurate alignment of this anatomy, position the central ray perpendicular to the IR and the patient's midcoronal plane. Inaccurate central ray angulation misaligns this anatomy and elongates or foreshortens the heart and lung structures. The anatomical structures that are positioned farthest from the IR will move the greatest distance when the central ray is angled; angling the central ray caudally for a PA chest image projects the manubrium inferior to the fourth thoracic vertebra, demonstrating more than 1 inch (2.5 cm) of lung apices superior to the clavicles, and changes the posterior rib contour to vertical. A caudal angle also elongates the heart and lung structures (see Image 21). Angling the central ray cephalically projects the manubrium superior to the fourth thoracic vertebra, demonstrating less than 1 inch (2.5 cm) of lung apices superior to the clavicles, and changes the posterior rib contour to horizontal. A cephalic angle also foreshortens the heart and lung structures (see Image 22). The more the angulation is mispositioned, either caudally or cephalically, the more distorted the anatomy.
- ***Patient with spinal kyphosis:*** On the supine or mobile chest image of a patient with spinal kyphosis (excess posterior convexity of the thoracic vertebrae), the position of the manubrium and clavicles and the contour of the posterior ribs may appear similar to those on a chest image for which the central ray was angled caudally. Also, if the patient is unable to elevate the chin, it may be superimposed over the apical chest region (Figure 2-24); compensate for this patient condition by using a *slight* (5- to 10-degree) cephalic angulation.
- ***Supine patient:*** For the supine AP chest image the patient's kyphotic upper vertebral column is forced to straighten because of the gravitational pull on it. This straightening causes the manubrium and clavicles to move superiorly and results in the image demonstrating less than 1 inch (2.5 cm) of apical lung field superior to the clavicles. Placing a 5-degree caudal angle on the central ray can offset this.

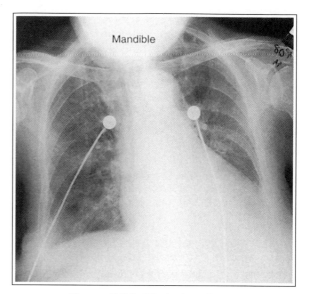

Figure 2-24. Kyphotic patient.

Nine or 10 posterior ribs are demonstrated above the diaphragm, indicating full lung aeration for the nonerect chest image.

- In a supine or seated patient the diaphragm is unable to shift to its lowest position because the abdominal organs are compressed and push against the diaphragm. As a result the lungs are not fully aerated, and only 9 or 10 posterior ribs are demonstrated above the diaphragm. To obtain maximum lung aeration in a patient who is able to follow instructions, take the exposure after the second full inspiration. If less than nine posterior ribs are demonstrated, then full lung expansion has not been obtained (see Image 23).
- ***Unconscious or ventilated patient:*** For the unconscious patient observe chest movement and expose after the patient takes a deep breath. For patient who is being ventilated with a conventional ventilator, observe the ventilator's pressure manometer (Figure 2-25, *A*). The exposure should be taken when the manometer digital bar or analog needle moves to its highest position. If a high-frequency ventilator is being used, the exposure may be made at any time, because this ventilator maintains the lung expansion at a steady mean pressure without the bulk gas exchange of the conventional type (Figure 2-25, *B*).

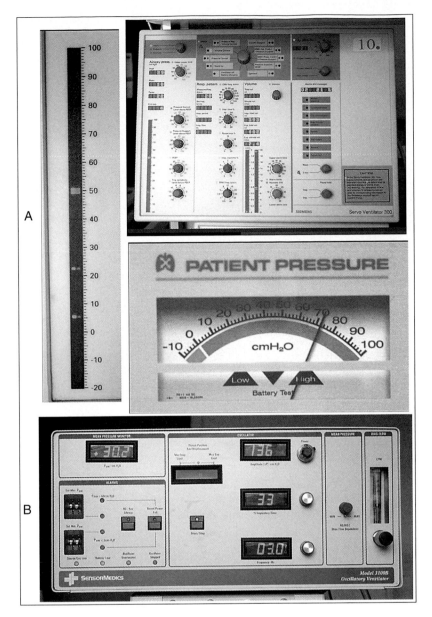

Figure 2-25. **A,** Conventional and **B,** high-frequency ventilators.

Anteroposterior Chest Image Analysis

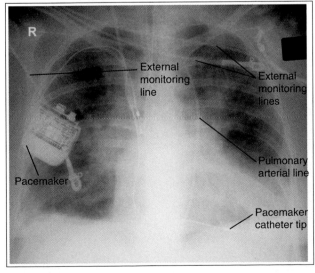

Image 17.

Analysis. Several external patient monitoring lines are superimposed over the lung field. An internal heart pacemaker and pulmonary arterial line are demonstrated. The right sternal clavicular end is visualized away from the vertebral column, whereas the left sternal clavicular end is superimposed over the vertebral column, and the right posterior ribs demonstrate greater length than the left. The IR was not positioned parallel with the bed but was positioned with the right side placed closer to the bed than the left, or the central ray was not aligned perpendicular to the IR but was angled toward the right side.

Correction. If the external monitoring lines can be removed, do so. If the lines cannot be removed, shift them to overlie the least amount of lung field. Place a sponge beneath the right IR border to position the IR parallel with the bed or angle the central ray toward the left side of the patient until it is aligned perpendicular to the IR.

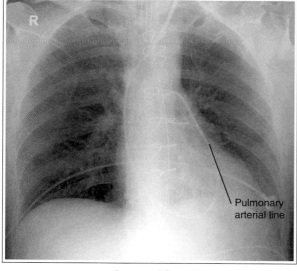

Image 18.

Analysis. The pulmonary arterial line demonstrates poor placement, as it was not advanced to the pulmonary artery.

Correction. When a chest image is being taken to determine the accuracy of line placement, the technologist should alert the radiologist or attending physician immediately if poor line placement is suspected.

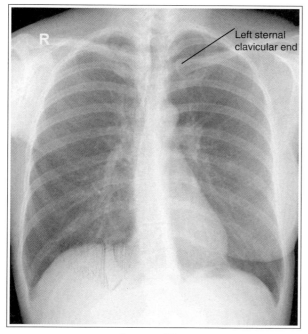

Image 19.

Analysis. The left sternal clavicular end is visualized away from the vertebral column, whereas the right sternal clavicular end is superimposed over the vertebral column, and the left posterior ribs demonstrate greater length than the right posterior ribs. The IR was not positioned parallel with the bed but was positioned with the left side placed closer to the bed than the right, or the central ray was not aligned perpendicular to the IR but was angled toward the left side.

Correction. Place an elevating device beneath the left IR border to position the IR parallel with the bed, or angle the central ray toward the right side of the patient until it is aligned perpendicular to the IR.

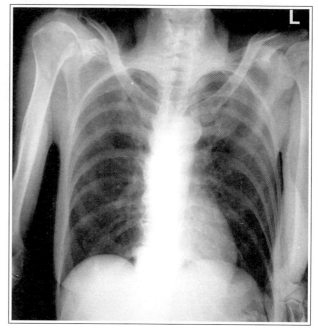

Image 20.

Analysis. The patient's arms were not abducted away from the chest region, unnecessarily exposing them.

Correction. Abduct the patient's arms until they are placed outside the collimated field. Increase the transverse collimation to within ½ inch (1.25 cm) of the patient's skinline.

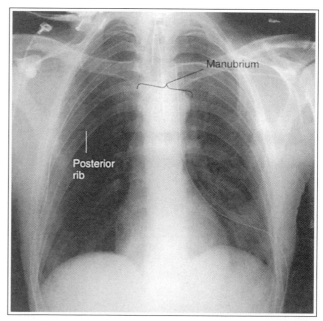

Image 21.

Analysis. The manubrium is superimposed over the fifth thoracic vertebra, more than 1 inch (2.5 cm) of apical lung field is visible above the clavicles, and the lateral clavicular ends are elevated. The posterior ribs demonstrate a vertical contour. All are indications that a caudal angulation was used.

Correction. For this image to be improved, the central ray needs to be adjusted in a cephalad direction until it is aligned perpendicular to the IR.

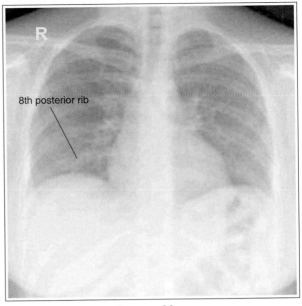

Image 23.

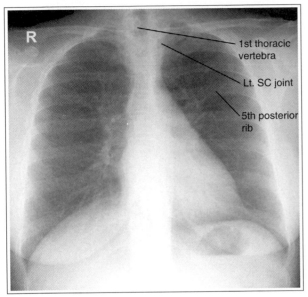

Image 22.

Analysis. The manubrium is superimposed over the second thoracic vertebra, and less than 1 inch (2.5 cm) of apical lung field is visible above the clavicles. The posterior ribs demonstrate a horizontal contour. The central ray was angled cephalically.

Correction. For this image to be improved, the central ray needs to be adjusted caudally until it is aligned perpendicular to the IR.

Analysis. Eight posterior ribs are demonstrated above the diaphragm, indicating that the image was taken with maximum lung aeration.

Correction. If the patient's condition allows, take the exposure after coaxing the patient into a deeper inspiration or at the point at which the ventilator indicates the greatest lung expansion.

CHEST: LATERAL DECUBITUS POSITION (ANTEROPOSTERIOR OR POSTEROANTERIOR PROJECTION)

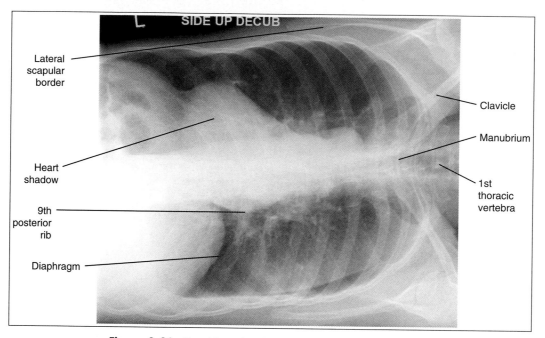

Lateral scapular border

Heart shadow

9th posterior rib

Diaphragm

Clavicle

Manubrium

1st thoracic vertebra

Figure 2-26. Decubitus chest image with accurate positioning.

Image Analysis

An arrow or "word" marker identifying the side of the patient positioned up and away from the imaging table or cart is present on image.

- Place an arrow or "word" marker, indicating side of patient that is positioned away from the imaging table or cart, within collimated light field.

Beam penetration is sufficient to faintly demonstrate the thoracic vertebrae and posterior ribs through the heart and mediastinal structures. Contrast and density are adequate to visualize fluid levels or the presence of air within the pleural cavity.

- *Positioning to demonstrate pleural air or fluid:* The lateral decubitus position is primarily used to confirm the presence of air (pneumothorax) or fluid (pleural effusion) in the pleural cavity. To best demonstrate the presence of air, position the affected side of the thorax away from the tabletop or cart so that the air rises to the highest level in the pleural cavity. If the affected side were placed against the tabletop or cart, the air might be obscured by the mediastinal structures. To best demonstrate fluid in the pleural cavity, position the affected side against the tabletop or cart. This positioning allows the fluid to gravitate to the lowest level of the pleural cavity, away from the mediastinal structures (Figure 2-27).
- *Techniques to demonstrate pleural air or fluid:* Along with positioning efforts, the technique factors

chosen are also very important in identifying a pneumothorax or pleural effusion on a chest image. When a pneumothorax is suspected, demonstration of lung markings is necessary, whereas the absence of such markings indicates a pneumothorax. The lung markings are best demonstrated when the image is neither overexposed nor overpenetrated. A darker density image is acceptable, however, when pleural

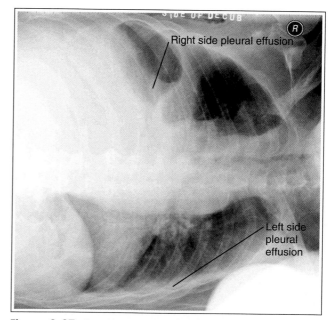

Right side pleural effusion

Left side pleural effusion

Figure 2-27. Decubitus chest image with large right side and small left side pleural effusions.

effusion is suspected. Because fluid is denser than lung tissue, it presents a distinct underexposed, level area on a darker image. When selecting the exposure (mAs) and kVp to be used for a decubitus chest image, evaluate the patient's records carefully to determine whether the technique factors should be set to demonstrate the presence of air or fluid. If a pneumothorax is suspected, decrease the kVp 8% from the routinely used setting. If pleural effusion is suspected, increase the mAs by 35% over the routinely used setting.

The seventh thoracic vertebra is centered within the collimated field. The entire lung field, showing the apices, lateral lungs, and costophrenic angles, is included within the field.

- Centering a perpendicular central ray to the midsagittal plane at a level approximately 7½ inches (18 cm) inferior to the vertebra prominens for the PA projection and 4 inches (10 cm) inferior to the jugular notch for the AP projection places the seventh thoracic vertebra in the center of the image. This central ray placement also centers the lung field on the image. Center the IR to the central ray. Open the longitudinally collimated field to within ½ inch (2.5 cm) of the lateral skinline. For most adult AP chest images, the full 14-inch (35-cm) length is needed. A 14- × 17-inch (35- × 43-cm) IR should be adequate to include all the required anatomical structures. For most patients it is acceptable to use the dedicated chest unit, which will position the IR crosswise to the patient and still include the entire lung field on the image. In a recumbent patient the diaphragm is unable to move to its lowest position on inspiration, preventing full vertical lung expansion. Because the lungs are unable to expand fully, a crosswise IR will provide adequate lung coverage. To be certain the lateral borders are included on the image, center the IR and the central ray to the midsagittal plane.

The chest demonstrates an AP or PA projection. The distance from the lateral edges of the vertebral column to the sternal ends of the clavicles and the lengths of the right and left corresponding posterior ribs are equal.

- The decubitus chest image can be taken in either an AP or a PA projection. In the AP projection it is easier for the patient to maintain a true projection, without rotation, because the knees can be flexed. It is also easier for the patient to move closer to the IR and raise the arms when in an AP position. To avoid chest rotation, align the shoulders, the posterior ribs, and the posterior pelvic wings perpendicular to the cart on which the patient is lying (Figure 2-28). This alignment positions the patient's shoulders and lungs at equal distances from the IR. Accomplish posterior rib and pelvic wing alignment by resting your extended flat hand against each, respectively, then adjusting the patient's rotation until your hand is positioned perpendicularly to

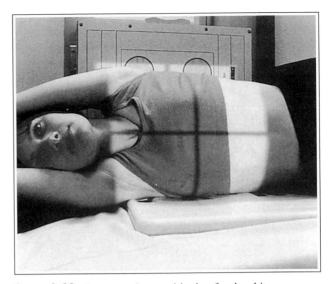

Figure 2-28. Proper patient positioning for decubitus chest image.

the cart. It is most common for a patient to lean the elevated shoulder, lung, and pelvic wing anteriorly when rotated. A pillow or other support placed between the patient's knees may help to eliminate this forward rotation.

- *Detecting chest rotation:* Rotation is readily detected on an AP or PA decubitus chest image by evaluating the distances between the vertebral column and the sternal ends of the clavicles and by comparing the lengths of the posterior ribs. On a nonrotated decubitus chest image, the distances and lengths, respectively, on each side of the patient should be equal. On a rotated AP projection the sternal clavicular end that is superimposed over the lesser amount of the vertebral column, and the side on which the posterior ribs demonstrate the greatest length, is the side of the chest positioned closer to the IR (see Image 24). The opposite is true for a PA projection. For this projection the sternal clavicular end that is superimposed over the least amount of the vertebral column and the posterior ribs that demonstrate the greatest length represent the side of the chest positioned farther from the IR.

- *AP versus PA chest images:* Determine whether a chest image was taken in an AP or a PA projection by analyzing the appearance of the sixth and seventh cervical vertebrae and the first thoracic vertebra. In the AP projection these vertebral bodies and their intervertebral disk spaces are demonstrated without distortion (Figure 2-29). In the PA projection the vertebral bodies are distorted, the intervertebral disk spaces are closed, and the spinous processes and laminae of these three vertebrae are well demonstrated (Figure 2-30). The reason for these variations is related to the divergence of the x-ray beam used to image these three vertebrae and the anterior convexity of the cervical and upper thoracic vertebrae.

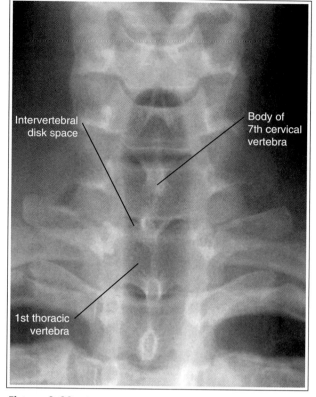

Figure 2-29. Anteroposterior projection of cervical vertebrae.

The arms, mandible, and lateral borders of the scapulae are situated outside the lung field, and the lateral aspects of the clavicles are projected upward.

- The lateral borders of the scapulae are drawn away from the lung field when the patient's arms are

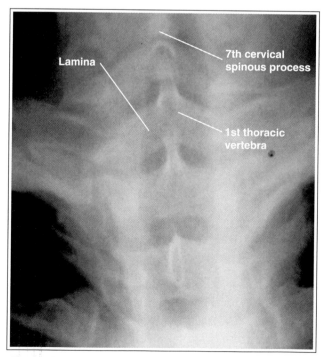

Figure 2-30. Posteroanterior projection of cervical vertebrae.

positioned above the head. This positioning also draws the lateral ends of the clavicles superiorly. If the arms are not positioned in this manner, the arms and the lateral borders of the scapulae are demonstrated within the upper lung field (see Image 24).

- To prevent the chin from being superimposed over the lung apices on the image, position the patient with the chin elevated.

The manubrium and the fourth thoracic vertebra are superimposed, and the lungs and heart are demonstrated without foreshortening.

- The tilt of the midcoronal plane determines the degree of lung and heart foreshortening and the transverse level at which the manubrium is in comparison to the fourth thoracic vertebra. When the midcoronal plane is positioned parallel with the IR, the lungs and heart are demonstrated without foreshortening and the manubrium and fourth thoracic vertebra are superimposed over each other. If the image is taken in an AP projection and the superior midcoronal plane is tilted anteriorly (forward), the manubrium will move inferior to the fourth thoracic vertebra (see Image 25). Conversely, if the superior midcoronal plane is tilted posteriorly (backward), the manubrium will move superior to the fourth thoracic vertebra (see Image 26). If the image is taken in a PA projection and the superior midcoronal plane is tilted anteriorly, the manubrium will move inferior to the fourth thoracic vertebra. Conversely, if the superior midcoronal plane is tilted posteriorly, the manubrium will move superior to the fourth thoracic vertebra.

Nine or 10 posterior ribs are demonstrated above the diaphragm.

- In a recumbent position, the diaphragm is unable to shift to its lowest position owing to pressure from the peritoneal cavity. As a result, the lungs are not fully aerated, and only 9 or 10 posterior ribs are demonstrated above the diaphragm. To obtain maximum lung aeration, the exposure should be taken after the second full inspiration.

The lung field positioned against the cart is demonstrated without superimposition of the cart pad.

- Elevating the patient on a radiolucent sponge or on a hard surface such as a cardiac board prevents the chest from sinking into the cart pad. When the patient's body is allowed to sink into the cart pad, artifact lines are seen superimposed over the lateral lung field of the side placed against the cart. Because fluid in the pleural cavity gravitates to the lowest level, it is in this area that the fluid will be demonstrated, and superimposition of the cart pad and the lower lung field may obscure fluid that has settled in the lowest level.

Decubitus Chest Image Analysis

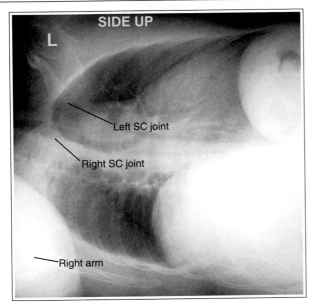

Image 24. AP projection.

Analysis. The right sternal clavicular end is superimposed over the vertebral column, the posterior ribs on the left side demonstrate the greater length, and the arms are superimposed over the right lung apex. The patient's left side was rotated toward the IR, and the arm was positioned at a 90-degree angle to the body.

Correction. Rotate the patient's left side away from the IR until the patient's shoulders, posterior ribs, and posterior pelvic wing are aligned perpendicular to the cart. Elevate the patient's right arm until it is positioned above the lung field.

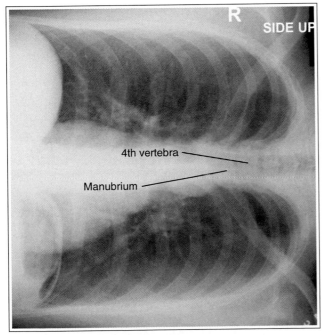

Image 25. AP projection.

Analysis. The manubrium is superimposed over the fifth thoracic vertebra, indicating that the superior midcoronal plane was tilted anteriorly.

Correction. Move the superior midcoronal plane posteriorly until the midcoronal plane is parallel with the IR.

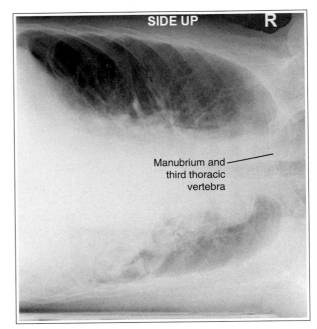

Image 26. AP projection.

Analysis. The manubrium is superimposed over the third thoracic vertebra, indicating that the superior midcoronal plane was tilted posteriorly.

Correction. Move the superior midcoronal plane anteriorly until the midcoronal plane is parallel with the IR.

CHEST: ANTEROPOSTERIOR LORDOTIC PROJECTION

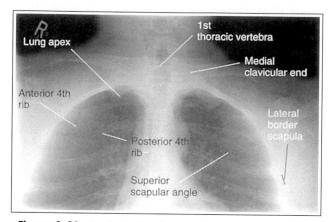

Figure 2-31. Lordotic chest image with accurate positioning.

Image Analysis

Contrast, density, and penetration are adequate to demonstrate the cortical outlines of clavicle, superior thoracic vertebrae, and posterior and anterior ribs.

- Overlying soft tissues, clavicles, and upper ribs often obscure the apical lung markings on a PA projection of the chest. The anterior ends of the first ribs may also project a suspicious-looking shadow in the apices. The lordotic examination is taken to demonstrate areas of the apical lungs obscured on the PA projection and to provide a different anatomical perspective that can be used to evaluate suspicious areas.

The superior lung field is centered within the collimated field. The clavicles, apices, and two thirds of the lung field are included within the field.

- Centering the central ray to the midsagittal plane halfway between the manubrium and the xiphoid positions the superior lung field at the center of the image. Because the lung fields are foreshortened, this centering will include most of the lung fields on the image. A higher centering is required if only the lung apices are desired. Lung foreshortening also creates the need for tight vertical collimation to prevent unnecessary exposure of abdominal and cervical vertebral tissue. Center the IR to the central ray.
- A 14- × 17-inch (35- × 43-cm), lengthwise IR should be adequate to include all the required anatomical structures. Longitudinally collimate to within ½ inch (1.25 cm) of shoulders and transversely collimate to ½ inch (1.25 cm) of lateral skinline.

The medial ends of the clavicles are projected superior to the lung apices at the level of the first thoracic vertebra. The heart shadow can be outlined, although it is foreshortened and wider than on a corresponding PA chest image. The posterior and anterior portions of

the first through fourth ribs lie horizontally and are nearly superimposed.

- The clavicles are projected above the apices, and the upper ribs are superimposed by positioning the patient using one of three methods. First, the patient's back can be arched, leaning the upper thorax and shoulders toward the IR, as demonstrated in Figure 2-32. The correct amount of arching is accomplished when the patient's feet are placed approximately 12 inches (30 cm) away from the IR before the back is arched. The angle formed between the midcoronal body plane and IR should be approximately 45 degrees. Second, the patient remains completely upright, and a 45-degree cephalic central ray angulation is used to shift the clavicles (Figure 2-33). Third, the patient's back is arched as much a possible and the central ray

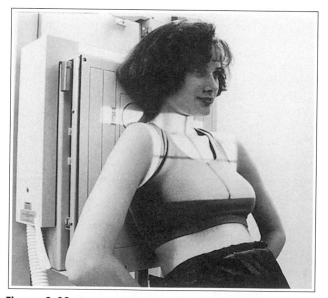

Figure 2-32. Proper patient positioning for lordotic chest image—no central ray angle.

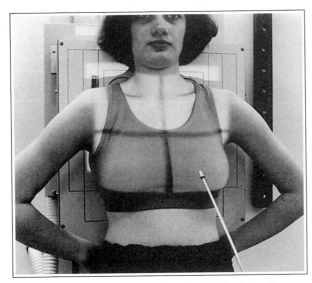

Figure 2-33. Proper patient positioning for lordotic chest image—central ray angled.

is angled cephalically the amount necessary to equal a 45-degree angle. For example, if the patient is able to arch until the midcoronal plane is placed at a 30-degree angle to the IR, the needed central ray angle would be 15 degrees. With each of these methods the clavicles are projected above the apices onto the first thoracic vertebra, and the anterior ribs are projected onto their corresponding posterior ribs.

- *Poor patient or central ray positioning:* Inadequate back extension or central ray angulation is identified on an image when the clavicles are not projected superior to the lung apices and when the anterior and posterior ribs are not superimposed. When the patient's back is not arched enough or when more cephalic angulation is needed, the clavicles superimpose the lung apices, and the anterior ribs are demonstrated inferior to their corresponding posterior rib (see Image 27). If an image is obtained in which lung fields have been so foreshortened that the apices are obscured and the posterior ribs are superimposed and cannot be distinguished, the patient's back was arched too much or the cephalic angle was too extreme (see Image 28).

The lateral borders of the scapulae are drawn away from the lung field, and the superior angles of the scapulae are demonstrated away from lung apices.

- The lateral borders and the superior angles of the scapulae are drawn away from the lung fields by placing the back of the patient's hands on the hips and rotating the elbows and shoulders anteriorly. This position allows visualization of the lung apices without scapular obstruction.

   When the elbows and shoulders are not rotated anteriorly, the lateral borders of the scapulae are demonstrated in the lung fields, and the superior scapular angles are projected into the lung apices (see Image 29).

The chest demonstrates no signs of rotation when the distances from the vertebral column to the sternal ends of the clavicles are equal.

- The patient's shoulders should be equal distances from the IR to prevent rotation. Chest rotation can be identified on an AP lordotic image by evaluating the distance between the vertebral column and the sternal ends of the clavicles or the sternoclavicular (SC) joints. When the distances between the sternal clavicles and the vertebral column are unequal, the SC joint that is superimposed over the smaller amount of the vertebral column is the side of the chest that was positioned closer to the IR.

Anteroposterior Lordotic Chest Image Analysis

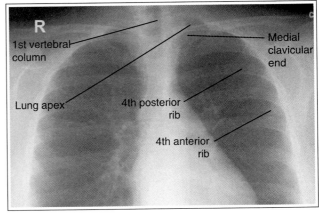

Image 27.

Analysis. The clavicles are superimposed over the lung apices, and the anterior ribs are demonstrated inferior to their corresponding posterior rib. Either the patient's back was not arched enough or the central ray was not angled cephalically enough to obtain a 45-degree angle between the midcoronal plane and central ray.

Correction. If the patient's back was arched to obtain this image, increase the amount of arch or add a cephalic angulation until the midcoronal plane and central ray form a 45-degree angle.

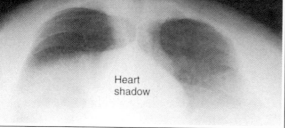

Image 28.

Analysis. The lung fields demonstrate excessive foreshortening, and the individual ribs cannot be identified. Either the patient's back was arched too much or the central ray was angled too cephalically.

Correction. If the patient's back was arched to obtain this image, decrease the amount of arch. If this examination was obtained by using a cephalic angulation, decrease the degree of central ray angulation until the midcoronal plane and central ray form a 45-degree angle.

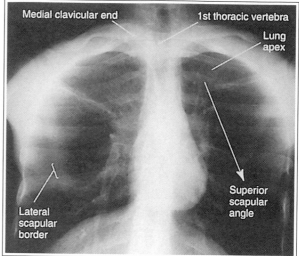

Image 29.

Analysis. The lateral borders of the scapulae are demonstrated within the lung fields, and the superior scapular angles are demonstrated within the apical region. The patient's elbows and shoulders were not rotated anteriorly.

Correction. Place the backs of the patient's hands on the hips, and rotate the elbows and shoulders anteriorly.

CHEST: POSTEROANTERIOR OBLIQUE PROJECTION (RIGHT ANTERIOR OBLIQUE AND LEFT ANTERIOR OBLIQUE POSITIONS)

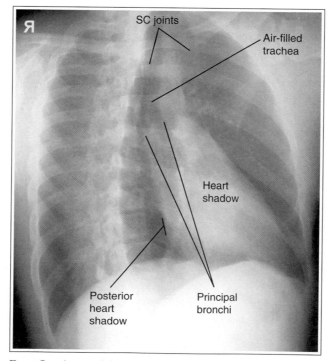

Figure 2-34. Forty-five-degree right anterior oblique chest image with accurate positioning.

Image Analysis

Contrast, density, and penetration are adequate to visualize the soft-tissue outlines of the air-filled trachea and heart shadow and the cortical outlines of posterior and anterior ribs and thoracic vertebrae.

- On the anterior oblique chest image, the lung positioned farther from the IR should demonstrate clear vascular markings. The air-filled trachea should also be demonstrated in the lung field positioned farther from the IR.

The right and left principal bronchi are at the center of the collimated field. The apices, costophrenic angles, and lateral chest walls are included within the field.

- Centering a perpendicular central ray at a level approximately 7½ inches (18 cm) inferior to the vertebra prominens places the central ray at the level of the bronchi. Accurate transverse positioning is obtained when the same amount of IR distance is present on both sides of the patient. A 14- × 17-inch (35- × 43-cm) IR should be adequate to include all the required anatomical structures. Center the IR to the central ray. Open the transversely collimated field to within ½ inch (2.5 cm) of the lateral skinline. For most adult AP chest images, the full 17-inch (43-cm) length is needed, although you should collimate on smaller patients.

Approximately twice as much lung field is demonstrated on one side of the thoracic vertebrae as on the other side, and the SC joints are demonstrated without spinal superimposition, indicating that a 45-degree obliquity has been obtained.

- Rotating the patient until the midcoronal plane is aligned 45 degrees to the IR (Figure 2-35) provides

the reviewer with an additional perspective of the lungs, which will assist in the detection of pulmonary diseases or artifacts. The lung field better demonstrated on an anterior oblique image is the one positioned farther from the IR. An RAO position demonstrates the left lung, whereas a left anterior oblique (LAO) position demonstrates the right lung.

- *Verifying accuracy of obliquity:* When evaluating an image, you can be certain that a 45-degree obliquity has been obtained if (1) twice as much lung field is demonstrated on one side of the thoracic vertebrae as on the other side, and (2) the SC joints, air-filled trachea, and principal bronchi are demonstrated without spinal superimposition. The heart shadow is also demonstrated without spinal superimposition on an RAO chest image, whereas a portion of the heart shadow is superimposed over the thoracic vertebrae on an LAO chest image. Because the heart is located more to the left of the thoracic vertebrae, a 60-degree patient obliquity is necessary to demonstrate the heart shadow without spinal superimposition on the LAO. Figure 2-36 demonstrates a 45-degree LAO chest image. Note that the lung field on one side is twice as large as on the other and that slight superimposition of the thoracic vertebrae and heart shadow is present. Compare this image with the 60-degree LAO chest image shown in Figure 2-37. Note that more than twice as much lung field is present on one side of the thoracic vertebrae as on the other in

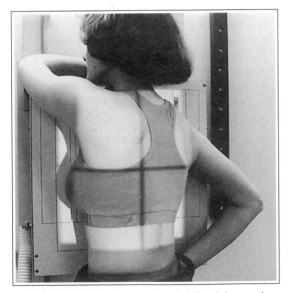

Figure 2-35. Proper patient positioning for right anterior oblique chest image.

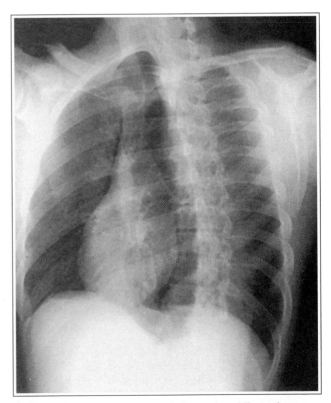

Figure 2-36. Forty-five-degree left anterior oblique chest image with proper positioning.

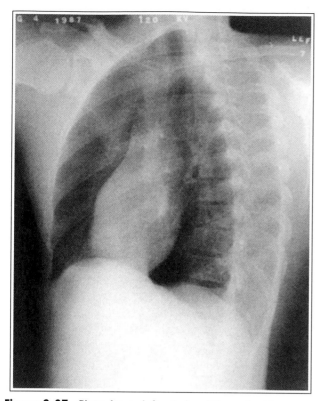

Figure 2-37. Sixty-degree left anterior oblique chest image with proper positioning.

Figure 2-37, and that the heart shadow and thoracic vertebrae are not superimposed. How much obliquity should be obtained depends on the examination indications. When the examination is being performed to evaluate the lung field, a 45-degree oblique image is required; when the outline of the heart is of interest, a 60-degree oblique image is required.

- *Repositioning the inaccurately rotated patient:* If the desired 45-degree obliquity is not obtained on a chest image, compare the amount of lung field demonstrated on both sides of the thoracic vertebrae. If the image demonstrates more than twice the lung field on one side of the thoracic vertebrae as on the other side, the patient was rotated more than 45 degrees. If less than twice the lung field is demonstrated on one side of the thoracic vertebrae as on the opposite side, the patient was not rotated enough (see Image 30). To determine repositioning movements for the 60-degree LAO image, evaluate the heart shadow and thoracic vertebrae superimposition. With adequate obliquity the heart shadow is positioned just to the right of the thoracic vertebrae. If the oblique position is less than 60 degrees, the heart shadow is superimposed over the thoracic vertebrae, as on a 45-degree LAO chest image. Excess obliquity produces an image similar to a rotated lateral chest image.
- *Posterior oblique chest images:* Routinely, anterior oblique images are performed for oblique chest images

because they position the heart closer to the IR. When posterior oblique (right posterior oblique [RPO] and left posterior oblique [LPO]) chest images are taken, however, the preceding evaluation corresponds in the following way. The LPO position demonstrates the lung situated closer to the IR, which is the left lung. To review this position, use the RAO evaluation previously described. For the RPO position, the right lung is of interest and the LAO evaluation should be followed. A 45-degree obliquity is required in the LPO image to rotate the heart away from the thoracic vertebrae, but a 60-degree obliquity is needed for the RPO position.

The manubrium is situated at the same level as the fourth thoracic vertebra with approximately 1 inch (2.5 cm) of the apical lung field visible above the clavicles, and the lungs and heart are demonstrated without foreshortening.

- The tilt of the midcoronal plane determines the relationship of the manubrium to the thoracic vertebrae, the amount of apical lung field seen superior to the clavicles, and the degree of lung and heart foreshortening. When the midcoronal plane is vertical, the manubrium is projected at the level of the fourth thoracic vertebra, approximately 1 inch (2.5 cm) of the apices are visible above the clavicles, and the lungs and heart are demonstrated without foreshortening. In an anterior oblique image, if the superior midcoronal plane is tilted anteriorly (forward), as demonstrated in Figure 2-7, the lungs and heart are foreshortened, the manubrium is situated at a transverse level inferior to the fourth thoracic vertebra or lower, and more than 1 inch (2.5 cm) of apices is demonstrated above the clavicles (see Image 5). Conversely, if the superior midcoronal plane is tilted posteriorly (backward), as demonstrated in Figure 2-8, the lungs and heart are foreshortened, the manubrium is situated at a transverse level above the fourth thoracic vertebra, and less than 1 inch (2.5 cm) of apices is demonstrated superior to the clavicles (see Image 6). The opposite is true for a posterior oblique position. Anterior tilt of the superior midcoronal plane will result in the manubrium projecting inferior to the fourth thoracic vertebra, and posterior tilt of the superior midcoronal plane will result in the manubrium projecting superior to the fourth thoracic vertebra.

Ten or 11 posterior ribs are demonstrated above the hemidiaphragms, indicating full lung aeration.

- To obtain maximum lung aeration, take the exposure after the second full inspiration. If fewer than 10 posterior ribs are demonstrated, the lungs were not fully inflated. Determine whether a patient condition hindered full aeration. If not, repeat the image after full inspiration.

Oblique Chest Image Analysis

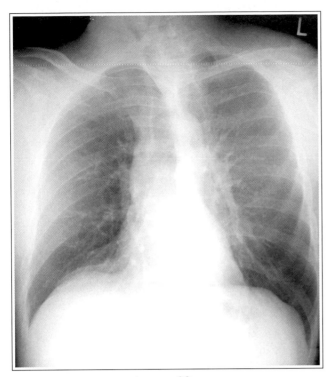

Image 30.

Analysis. This image was taken with the patient in an LAO position. Less than twice the lung field is demonstrated on the left side of the thoracic vertebrae as on the right side. The thoracic vertebrae are superimposed over a portion of the heart shadow and the air-filled trachea. The obliquity was less than 45 degrees.

Correction. Increase the degree of patient obliquity until the midcoronal plane is placed at a 45-degree angle with the IR.

ABDOMEN

The following image analysis criteria are used for all abdominal images and should be considered when the analysis is completed. Position- and projection-specific criteria relating to these topics are discussed along with the other criteria for that position or projection.

Facility's identification requirements are visible on image as identified in Chapter 1.

A right or left marker, identifying the correct side of patient, is present on image and is not superimposed over anatomy of interest. Specific placement of marker is as described in Chapter 1.

Radiation protection practices, as defined in Chapter 1, have been followed.

No evidence of preventable artifacts, such as buttons, zippers, and undergarments, is present (see Figure 2-45).

- The patient should be instructed to remove outer clothing and any underclothes containing artifacts, then to change into a snapless hospital gown before the procedure.

The cortical outlines of the posterior ribs, lumbar vertebrae, and pelvis and the gases within the stomach and intestines are sharply defined.

- Sharply defined recorded details are obtained when patient motion is controlled, respiration is halted, a short exposure time is used, and a short OID is maintained.
- *Voluntary versus involuntary motion:* Two kinds of motion may be evident on an abdominal image: voluntary and involuntary. Voluntary motion is caused by breathing or moving during the exposure. It can be controlled by explaining to the patient the importance of holding still, making the patient as comfortable as possible on the imaging table, and using the shortest possible exposure time. On an image, voluntary motion can be identified as blurred bony cortices and gastric and intestinal gases (see Image 31). Involuntary motion is caused by the peristaltic activity of the stomach or small or large intestine. This movement is considered involuntary because the patient cannot control this movement as with breathing.

TABLE 2-2 **Abdomen Technical Data**				
Position or Projection	**kVp**	**Grid**	**AEC Chamber(s)**	**SID**
AP projection	70-80	Grid	All	40-48 inches (100-120 cm)
Lateral decubitus position	70-80	Grid	Center	40-48 inches (100-120 cm)

AEC, Automatic exposure control; *AP,* anteroposterior; *kVp,* kilovolt peak; *SID,* source–image receptor distance.

The only means of decreasing the blur caused by involuntary motion is to use the shortest possible exposure time, and in some cases this is not good enough. Involuntary motion can be identified on abdominal images as sharp bony cortices and blurry gastric and intestinal gases (see Image 32).

Contrast, density, and penetration are adequate to demonstrate the collections of fat that outline the psoas major muscles and kidneys as well as the bony structures of the inferior ribs and transverse processes of the lumbar vertebrae.

- An optimal kVp technique, as shown in Table 2-2, sufficiently penetrates the soft tissue and bony structures of the abdomen. This kVp setting enhances the subtle radiation absorption differences among the fat, gas, muscles, and solid organs, which mainly consist of water. Because soft-tissue abdominal structures are similar in atomic number and density, whether two soft-tissue structures that border each other are visible or not depends on their arrangement with respect to the gas and fat collections that lie next to them, around them, or within them. These same gas and fat collections are used to identify diseases and masses within the abdomen. The presence or absence of gas, as well as its amount and location within the intestinal system, may indicate a functional, metabolic, or mechanical disease, whereas routinely seen collections of fat may be displaced or obscured with organ enlargement or mass invasion. Use a high-ratio grid to reduce the scatter radiation that reaches the IR, thereby reducing fog and increasing the visibility of the recorded details and providing a higher-contrast image. To obtain optimal density, set a manual mAs based on the patient's abdominal thickness or choose all three AEC chambers.
- *Abdominal anatomy:* The soft-tissue structures that can be outlined if appropriate image density and contrast have been obtained on an abdominal image are the psoas major muscles and kidneys. The psoas major muscles are located lateral to the lumbar vertebrae. They originate at the first lumbar vertebra on each side and extend to the corresponding lesser trochanter. On an AP abdominal image, the psoas major muscles are visible as long triangular soft-tissue shadows on each side of the vertebral bodies.

The kidneys are found in the posterior abdomen and are identified on the image as bean-shaped densities located on each side of the vertebral column 3 inches (7.5 cm) from the midline. The upper poles of the kidney lie on the same transverse level as the spinous process of the eleventh thoracic vertebra, and the lower poles lie on the same transverse level as the spinous process of the third lumbar vertebra. The right kidney is usually demonstrated approximately 1 inch (2.5 cm) inferior to the left kidney because of its location beneath the liver. Occasionally a kidney may be displaced inferior (nephroptosis) to this location, because it is not held in place by adjacent organs or its fat covering; this condition is most often seen in thin patients.

- *Techniques to compensate for specific patient conditions:* The routine manually set exposure factors obtained from the AP body measurement of patients with suspected large amounts of *bowel gas* may overexpose areas of the abdomen that are overlaid with gas (see Image 33). (The patient measures the same whether gas or dense soft tissue causes the thickness.) This increased image density results from the low density (number of atoms per given area) characteristic of gas. As the radiation passes through the patient's body, fewer photons are absorbed where gas is located than where dense soft tissue is present. To compensate for this situation, decrease the exposure (mAs) 30% to 50% or the kVp 5% to 8% from the routinely used manual technique before the image is taken.

An underexposed image may result when patients have *ascites* (invasion of fluid into the peritoneal cavity), *obesity, bowel obstructions, or soft-tissue masses.* This is because sections of the abdomen that normally contain gas or fat do not, resulting in an increase in the density of the soft tissue. To compensate for this situation, increase the exposure (mAs) 30% to 50% or the kVp 5% to 8% from the routinely used technique before the image is taken.

ABDOMEN: ANTEROPOSTERIOR PROJECTION (SUPINE AND UPRIGHT)

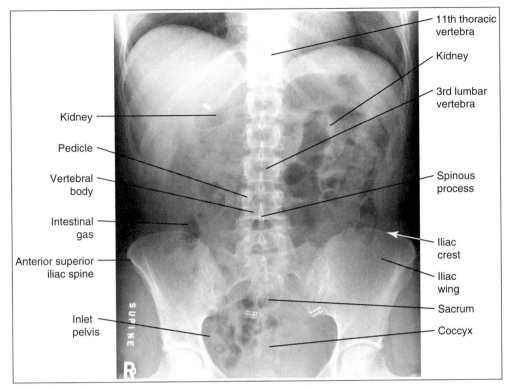

Figure 2-38. Supine abdominal image with accurate positioning.

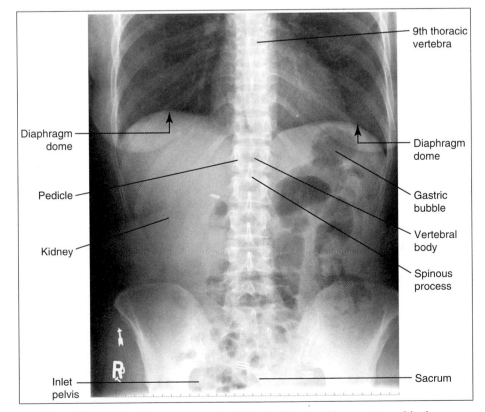

Figure 2-39. Upright anteroposterior abdominal image with accurate positioning.

Image Analysis

Density is uniform across abdomen.

- *Excessive abdominal soft tissue:* When an upright abdominal image is taken on a patient with *excessive abdominal soft tissue*, the soft tissue often drops down and forward. This movement results in a larger AP measurement at the lower abdominal level than at the upper abdominal level. For such patients, use two crosswise IRs to include all the abdominal structures, and take measurements of the lower *and* upper abdominal areas to ensure that accurate image density of each area will be obtained.

The abdominal image demonstrates an AP projection. The spinous processes are aligned with the midline of the vertebral bodies, and the distance from the pedicles to the spinous processes is the same on both sides. The sacrum is centered within the inlet of pelvis and is aligned with the symphysis pubis.

- To obtain an **AP supine abdominal image**, place the patient supine on the radiographic table. Position the shoulders and anterosuperior iliac spines at equal distances from the tabletop to prevent rotation, and draw the patient's arms away from the abdominal area to prevent them from being superimposed on the abdominal region (Figure 2-40).

- An **AP upright abdominal image** is obtained by placing the patient against an upright imaging tabletop. Position the shoulders and anterosuperior iliac spines at equal distances from the tabletop to prevent rotation, and draw the patient's arms away from the abdominal area to prevent them from being superimposed on the abdominal region (Figure 2-41).

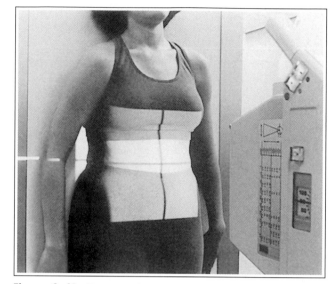

Figure 2-41. Proper patient positioning for upright anteroposterior abdominal image.

- *Demonstrating intraperitoneal air:* For intraperitoneal air to be best demonstrated, the patient should be positioned upright for 5 to 20 minutes before the image is taken. This allows enough time for the air to move away from the soft-tissue abdominal structures and rise to the level of the diaphragms (Figure 2-42). If a patient has come to the imaging department for a supine and upright abdominal series, begin with the upright image if the patient is ambulatory (able to walk) or transported by wheelchair. An ambulatory or wheelchair-using patient has been upright long enough for the air to rise, so it is not necessary to wait to take the image.

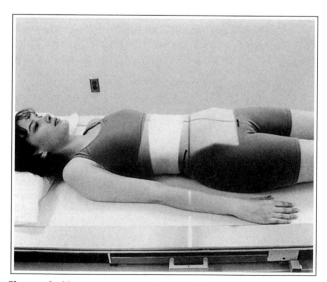

Figure 2-40. Proper patient positioning for supine abdominal image.

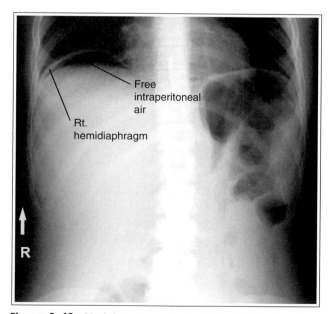

Figure 2-42. Upright anteroposterior abdominal image demonstrating free air under the right hemidiaphragm.

- *Detecting abdominal rotation:* Rotation of an abdominal image can decrease the visualization of fat lines that surround abdominal structures. For example, the psoas lateral muscles are outlined because of the fat that lies next to them. When the patient is rotated to one side, this fat shifts from lateral to anterior or posterior with respect to the muscle. The shift eliminates the subject contrast difference that exists when the muscle and fat are separated, hindering the usefulness of the psoas major muscles as diagnostic indicators. The upper and lower lumbar vertebrae can demonstrate rotation independently or simultaneously, depending on which section of the body is rotated. If the patient's thorax was rotated but the pelvis remained in an AP projection, the upper lumbar vertebrae and abdominal cavity demonstrate rotation. If the patient's pelvis was rotated but the thorax remained in an AP projection, the lower vertebrae and abdominal cavity demonstrate rotation. If the patient's thorax and pelvis were rotated simultaneously, the entire lumbar column and abdominal cavity demonstrate rotation. Rotation is effectively detected on an AP abdominal image by comparing the distance from the pedicles to the spinous processes on each side and by evaluating the centering of the sacrum within the inlet pelvis. If the distance from the pedicles to the spinous processes is greater on one side of the vertebrae than on the other, or if the sacrum is rotated toward one side of the inlet, pelvic rotation is present (see Image 34). The side with the smaller distance between the pedicles and spinous processes and toward which the sacrum is rotated is the side of the patient positioned farther from the tabletop and IR.

- *Distinguishing abdominal rotation from scoliosis:* In patients with scoliosis the lumbar bodies may appear rotated owing to the lateral twisting of the vertebrae. Scoliosis of the vertebral column can be very severe, demonstrating a large degree of lateral deviation, or it can be subtle, demonstrating only a small degree of deviation. Severe scoliosis is very obvious and is seldom mistaken for patient rotation, whereas subtle scoliotic changes can be easily mistaken for patient rotation (see Image 35). Although both demonstrate unequal distances between the pedicles and spinous processes, clues that can be used to distinguish subtle scoliosis from rotation are present. The long axis of a rotated vertebral column remains straight, whereas the scoliotic vertebral column demonstrates lateral deviation. When the lumbar vertebrae demonstrate rotation, it has been caused by the rotation of the upper or lower torso. The middle lumbar vertebrae (L3 and L4) cannot rotate unless the lower thoracic vertebrae or upper or lower lumbar vertebrae are also rotated. On the scoliotic image the middle lumbar vertebrae may demonstrate rotation without corresponding upper or lower vertebral rotation. This constitutes an acceptable image for a patient with this condition.

The long axis of the lumbar vertebral column is aligned with the long axis of the collimated field.

- Aligning the long axis of the lumbar vertebral column with the long axis of the collimated field ensures that the lateral abdominal cavity will not be clipped. To obtain proper upper abdominal alignment, align the xiphoid with the collimator's longitudinal light line. To obtain proper lower abdominal alignment, find the point midway between the patient's palpable anterior superior iliac spines (ASISs); then align this point with the collimator's longitudinal light line. Do not assume that the patient's navel is positioned directly above the vertebral column. Often it is shifted to one side.

The image was taken on expiration, and the diaphragm dome is located superior to the ninth posterior ribs.

- From full inspiration to expiration the diaphragm position moves from an inferior to a superior position. This movement also changes the pressure placed on the abdominal structures. On full expiration, the right side of the diaphragm dome is at the same transverse level as the eighth or ninth thoracic vertebra, whereas on inspiration, it may be found at the same transverse level as the ninth posterior rib. If the abdominal image is taken on inspiration, the inferior placement of the diaphragm places pressure on the abdominal organs, resulting in less space in the peritoneal cavity and greater abdominal density.

Supine position: The fourth lumbar vertebra is centered within the collimated field. The spinous process of the eleventh thoracic vertebra, the lateral body soft tissues, the iliac wings, and the symphysis pubis are included within the field.

- Including the spinous process of the eleventh thoracic vertebra ensures that the kidneys, tip of liver, and spleen, all of which lie inferior to it, will be present on the image. The symphysis pubis ensures that the inferior border of the peritoneal cavity is included on the image (see Image 36). To position the fourth lumbar vertebra in the center of the collimated field, use a 40- to 48-inch (102- to 120-cm) SID. Center a perpendicular central ray with the patient's midsagittal plane at the level of the iliac crest for the female patients and at a level 1 inch (2.5 cm) inferior to the iliac crest for male patients, to allow for the difference in size and longitudinal dimension between the female and male pelves.

- *Centering the central ray in males and females:* The centering determination measurements for male patients were taken from several male and female pelvic images, because (1) the patient is positioned in the same manner for a pelvic image as for an AP abdominal image, (2) the magnification factors (SID and OID) are identical to those used for an AP abdominal image, and (3) all pelvic anatomy was included and could be easily measured. The only difference in setup procedure between AP pelvic and AP abdominal images is the centering of the central ray. Although the superior centering used for the AP abdominal image projects the anteriorly located pelvic structures slightly more inferiorly than they appear on an AP pelvic image, the influence is the same on all abdominal IRs and affects the male and female pelves in the same manner. A measurement of each pelvic image was taken from the most superiorly located surface of the right iliac crest to the most inferior aspect of the right obturator foramen. Although slight variations of approximately $\frac{1}{4}$ inch (0.6 cm) did exist within each gender, the average female measurement was 8½ inches (21.25 cm) and the average male measurement was 9½ inches (24 cm). Because the IR length used for AP abdominal images is 17 inches (43 cm) and the pelvis is to fit on the lower half or 8½ inches (21.25 cm), one can understand why accurate central ray placement is important to include the needed structures.

- *IR size and direction:* A 14- × 17-inch (35- × 43-cm) lengthwise IR should be adequate to include all the required anatomical structures on *sthenic* and *asthenic* patients, as long as the transverse abdominal measurement is less than 14 inches (35 cm).

  If the spinous process of the eleventh thoracic vertebra is not included on this image, take a second image using an 11- × 14-inch (28- × 35-cm) crosswise IR. It is necessary for the second image to include approximately 2 to 3 inches (5 to 7.5 cm) of the same transverse section of the peritoneal cavity imaged on the first image, to ensure that no middle peritoneal information has been excluded. The top of the IR should extend to the patient's xiphoid (which is at the level of the tenth thoracic vertebra) to make sure that the spinous process of the eleventh thoracic vertebra is included. The longitudinal collimated field should remain fully open for both IRs. Transversely, collimate to within $\frac{1}{2}$ inch (1.25 cm) of the patient's lateral skinline.

  Use two 14- × 17-inch (35- × 43-cm) crosswise IRs on *hypersthenic* patients and on patients who have a transverse abdominal measurement of 14 inches (35 cm) or greater, to include all the necessary anatomical structures. Take the first image with the central ray centered to the midsagittal plane at a level halfway between the symphysis pubis and ASIS. Position the bottom of the second IR so that it includes 2 to 3 inches (5 to 7.5 cm) of the same transverse section of the peritoneal cavity imaged on the first image to ensure that no middle peritoneal information has been excluded. The top of the IR should extend to the patient's xiphoid (which is at the level of the tenth thoracic vertebra) to make sure that the spinous process of the eleventh thoracic vertebra is included.

- *Gonadal shielding:* Use gonadal shielding for supine images on all male patients and on female patients if two IRs are required and the upper abdomen is being imaged. Do not shield female patients if the lower abdomen is being imaged, because the shield may obscure needed information.

Upright position: The third lumbar vertebra is centered within the collimated field. Included within the field are the diaphragm, the ninth thoracic vertebra, the lateral body soft tissue, and the iliac wings.

- *Positioning and central ray:* The upright abdominal position is most often used to evaluate the peritoneal cavity for intraperitoneal air. For intraperitoneal air to be demonstrated, the diaphragm must be included in its entirety, because the air would be located directly inferior to the domes of the diaphragm (see Figure 2-42). When the image is taken on expiration, including the ninth thoracic vertebra will ensure demonstration of the diaphragm. To include the ninth thoracic vertebra at the top of the image and to center the third thoracic vertebra to the center of the collimated field, place the top of the IR (*not* the top of the collimator's light field) at a level of the axilla for the sthenic, slightly higher for the hypersthenic, and slightly lower for the asthenic patient. Use a 40- to 48-inch (102- to 120-cm) SID. Center a perpendicular central ray with the midsagittal plane and IR center. An upright abdominal image that does not include the entire diaphragm should be retaken (see Image 37).

- *IR size and direction:* A 14- × 17-inch (35- × 43-cm) lengthwise IR is adequate to include all the required anatomical structures on the *sthenic* and *asthenic* patient, as long as the patient's transverse abdominal measurement is less than 14 inches (35 cm). Open the longitudinal collimated field the full 17 inch (43 cm) field size and transversely collimate to within $\frac{1}{2}$ inch (1.25 cm) of the lateral skinline.

  Use two 14- × 17-inch (35- × 43-cm) crosswise IRs on *hypersthenic* patients and on sthenic and asthenic patients who have transverse abdominal measurement of 14 inches (35 cm) or greater, to include all the necessary anatomical structures. Take the first image with the top of the IR positioned as described above. Place the top of the second IR so it will include 2 to 3 inches (5 to 7.5 cm) of the same transverse section of the peritoneal cavity imaged on the first image, to ensure that no middle peritoneal information has been excluded. Center the central ray to the midsagittal plane for both images.

- *Gonadal shielding:* Use gonadal shielding for upright images on all male abdominal images and female patients if two IRs are required and the upper abdomen is being imaged. Do not shield female patients when the lower abdomen is imaged, because the shield may obscure needed information.

Anteroposterior Abdominal Image Analysis

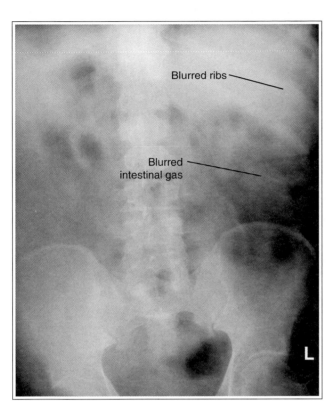

Image 31. Supine abdomen.

Analysis. The ribs and intestines are blurred, indicating that the patient moved and/or breathed during the exposure. The symphysis pubis is not included on the image. The central ray was positioned too superiorly. The lateral soft tissue is not entirely included on the image. Two crosswise images should have been taken.

Correction. Instruct the patient to halt respiration during the exposure. Using a short exposure time will also help if the patient has difficulty holding still. Repeat the examination using two crosswise IRs, making certain that the lower image includes the inferior peritoneal cavity.

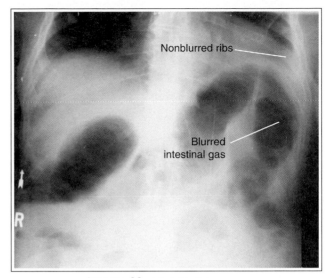

Image 32. Upright abdomen.

Analysis. This is the upper image of a crosswise abdominal image. The cortical outlines of the ribs and vertebral column are well defined without blur, whereas the intestinal structures demonstrate blur. This represents involuntary motion.

Correction. Repeat examination using the shortest possible exposure time.

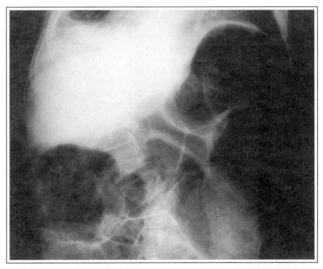

Image 33. Supine abdomen.

Analysis. This abdominal image is from a hypersthenic patient who had an excessive amount of bowel gas. In an attempt to demonstrate the areas superimposed with bowel gas, the exposure (mAs) was decreased. The decrease resulted in an underexposed area beneath the right diaphragm.

Correction. If this abdominal area is of importance, a second image should be taken with increased exposure. If the indication for the examination is to evaluate bowel gas, the image is acceptable.

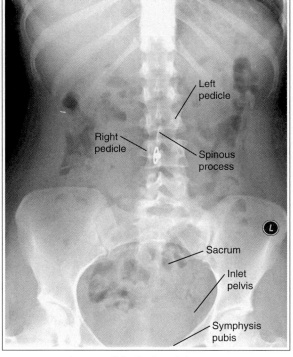

Image 34. Supine abdomen.

Analysis. The sacrum is not aligned with the symphysis pubis but is situated closer to the right hip, and the distance from the right pedicles to the spinous processes is less than the distance from the left pedicles to the spinous processes. The patient was rotated onto the left side (LPO).

Correction. Rotate the patient toward the right side until the shoulders and ASISs are positioned at equal distances from the IR.

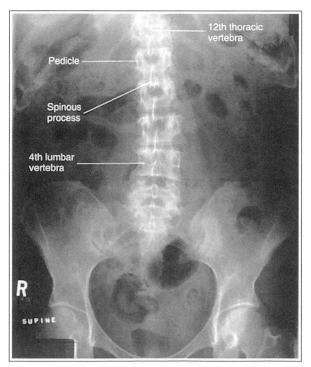

Image 35. Supine abdomen.

Analysis. The vertebral column deviates laterally at the level of the second through fourth lumbar vertebrae, the sacrum is centered within the inlet pelvis, and the distances from the pedicles to the spinous processes of the twelfth thoracic vertebra and fifth lumbar vertebra are equal. The vertebral column demonstrates subtle spinal scoliosis.

Correction. No correction movement is required for scoliosis. An AP abdominal image of a patient with scoliosis appears rotated.

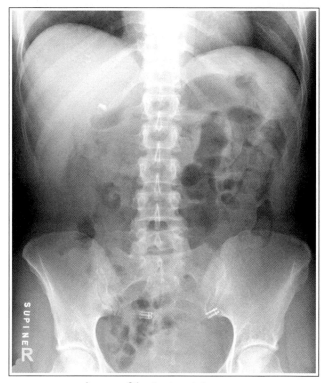

Image 36. Supine abdomen.

Analysis. The symphysis pubis is not included on the image. The central ray was centered too superiorly.

Correction. Because this is a male patient, center the central ray 1 inch (2.5 cm) inferior to the iliac crest.

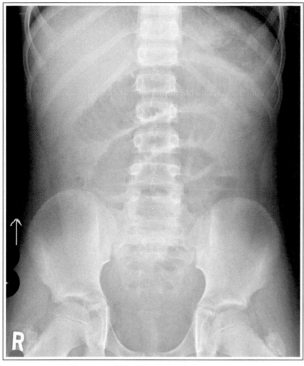

Image 37. Upright abdomen.

Analysis. This is an upright AP abdominal image. The domes of the diaphragm are not included on the image. The central ray was centered too inferiorly.

Correction. Center the central ray and IR approximately 2 inches (5 cm) superiorly.

ABDOMEN: LEFT LATERAL DECUBITUS POSITION (ANTEROPOSTERIOR PROJECTION)

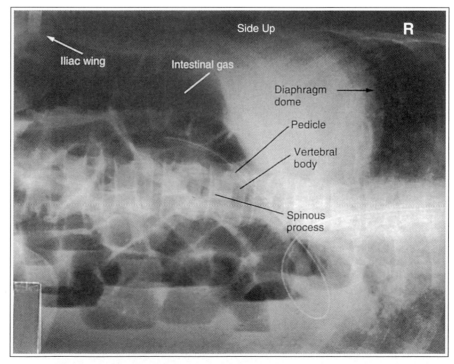

Figure 2-43. Decubitus abdominal image with accurate positioning.

Image Analysis

An arrow or "word" marker, indicating that the right side of patient was positioned up and away from the imaging table or cart, is present on image.

- Place an arrow or "word" marker indicating which side of the patient was positioned away from the tabletop or cart and in the collimated field.

Density is uniform across abdomen.

- *Using a wedge-compensating filter:* When a decubitus abdominal image from a patient with *excessive abdominal soft tissue* is taken, the soft tissue often drops toward the tabletop or cart. This movement results in a smaller AP measurement at the elevated right side than at the left side, which is positioned closer to the table-top or cart. To compensate for this thickness difference, a wedge-compensating filter may be used. The wedge filter absorbs some of the x-ray photons before they reach the patient, thereby decreasing the number of photons exposing the IR where the filter is located. The thick end of the wedge filter absorbs more photons than the thin end. When a wedge-compensating filter is used, attach it to the x-ray collimator head, with the thick end positioned toward the patient's right side and the thin end toward the left side. The collimator light projects a shadow of the compensating filter onto the patient. Position the shadow of the thin end at the level of the thickest part of the abdomen, allowing the thick end to extend toward the right side. Then use a technique that will accurately expose the thickest abdominal region. The wedge-compensating filter should absorb the needed photons to prevent overexposure of the thinner abdominal region. When the filter has been accurately positioned, radiographic density is uniform throughout the abdominal structures. Positioning the filter too close to or too far away from the thickest part of the abdomen results in an overexposed or underexposed area on the image, respectively.

The abdomen demonstrates an AP projection. The spinous processes are aligned with the midline of the vertebral bodies, the distance from the pedicles to the spinous processes is the same on both sides, and the iliac wings are symmetrical.

- A decubitus abdominal image is obtained by placing the patient in a left lateral recumbent position on the tabletop or cart, with the back resting against a grid cassette or the upright IR holder. Because intraperitoneal air migrates to the highest position, which is typically the elevated diaphragm or iliac wing, the left lateral position is chosen to position the gastric bubble away from the elevated diaphragm. To avoid rotation, align the shoulders, the posterior ribs, and the posterior pelvic wings perpendicular to the table-top or cart (Figure 2-44). Accomplish this alignment

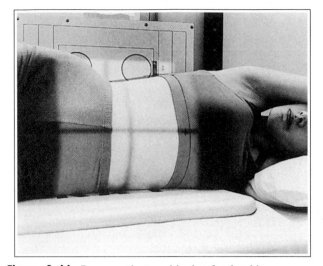

Figure 2-44. Proper patient positioning for decubitus abdominal image.

by resting your extended flat hand against each, respectively, and then adjusting the patient's rotation until your hand is positioned perpendicular to the tabletop or cart. It is most common for a patient to rotate the elevated thorax and pelvic wing anteriorly. A pillow or other support placed between the patient's knees may help to eliminate this forward rotation.

- *Demonstrating intraperitoneal air:* The lateral decubitus position is primarily used to confirm the presence of intraperitoneal air. For intraperitoneal air to be best demonstrated, the patient should be left in this position for 5 to 20 minutes before the image is taken, allowing enough time for the air to move away from the soft-tissue abdominal structures and rise to the level of the right diaphragm or iliac wing (Figure 2-45). To eliminate long waiting periods for patients who are scheduled to have a decubitus abdomen, have them transported to the imaging department in the left lateral decubitus position.

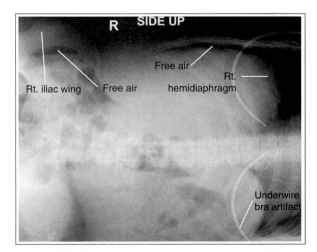

Figure 2-45. Decubitus abdominal image demonstrating free intraperitoneal air under right hemidiaphragm and at right iliac wing.

- ***Detecting abdominal rotation:*** The upper and lower lumbar vertebrae can demonstrate rotation independently or simultaneously, depending on which section of the body is rotated. If the patient's thorax is rotated but the pelvis remains in an AP projection, the upper lumbar vertebrae and abdominal cavity demonstrate rotation. If the patient's pelvis is rotated but the thorax remains in an AP projection, the lower vertebrae and abdominal cavity demonstrate rotation. If the patient's thorax and pelvis are rotated simultaneously, the entire lumbar column and abdominal cavity demonstrate rotation.

  Rotation is effectively detected on an AP abdominal image by comparing the distance from the pedicles to the spinous processes on each side and the symmetry of the iliac wings. If the distance from the pedicles to the spinous processes is greater on one side of the vertebrae than on the other side, the side with the smaller distance between the pedicles and spinous processes was the side of the patient positioned farther from the IR. If the iliac wings are not symmetrical, the wing demonstrating the least area is on the side of the patient positioned farther from the IR (see Image 38).

- ***Distinguishing rotation from scoliosis:*** In images from patients with spinal scoliosis the lumbar bodies may appear rotated owing to the lateral twisting of the vertebrae. An image on a patient with spinal scoliosis and a rotated decubitus abdomen demonstrates unequal distances between the pedicles and spinous processes. Clues are present that can be used to distinguish scoliosis from rotation. The long axis of a rotated vertebral column remains straight, whereas the scoliotic vertebral column demonstrates lateral deviation. When the lumbar vertebrae demonstrate rotation, it has been caused by the rotation of the upper or lower torso. The middle lumbar vertebrae (L3 and L4) cannot rotate unless the lower thoracic vertebrae or the upper or lower lumbar vertebrae are also rotated. On the scoliotic decubitus abdominal image the middle lumbar vertebrae may demonstrate rotation without corresponding upper or lower vertebral rotation.

The image was taken on expiration. The diaphragm domes are located superior to the ninth posterior rib.

- From full inspiration to expiration, the diaphragm moves from an inferior to a superior position. This movement also changes the pressure exerted on the abdominal structures. On full expiration the superior portion of the right upper diaphragm dome is at the same transverse level as the eighth or ninth thoracic vertebrae, whereas on inspiration, it may be found at the same transverse level as the ninth posterior rib. The left diaphragm is approximately ½ inch (1.25 cm) lower than the right diaphragm on both inspiration and expiration. When the decubitus abdominal image is taken on expiration, less pressure is exerted on the

peritoneal contents and greater space exists in the peritoneal cavity. If the decubitus position is taken on inspiration, the inferior placement of the diaphragm puts pressure on the abdominal organs, resulting in less space in the peritoneal cavity and greater abdominal density.

The third lumbar vertebra is centered within the collimated field. The right hemidiaphragm, ninth thoracic vertebra, right lateral soft tissues, and iliac wing are included within the field.

- The decubitus abdominal position is most often used to evaluate the peritoneal cavity for intraperitoneal air. To demonstrate intraperitoneal air, the right hemidiaphragm and iliac wing must be included. In the left lateral decubitus position, intraperitoneal air will rise to the highest level. In most patients the intraperitoneal air moves to the right upper quadrant just below the diaphragm, between the liver and abdominal wall. One exception to this placement of intraperitoneal air occurs in women with wide hips, whose highest level within the peritoneal cavity is just over the iliac bone (see Figure 2-45).

- ***IR size and direction:*** A 14- × 17-inch (35- × 43-cm) IR positioned lengthwise with respect to the patient should be adequate to include all the anatomical structures in asthenic and sthenic patients, as long as the transverse abdominal measurement is less than 14 inches (35 cm). To place the ninth thoracic vertebra at the top of the image and to center the third thoracic vertebra within the center of the collimated field, place the top of the IR at a level 2½ inches (6.25 cm) superior to the xiphoid (see Image 39). Use a 40- to 48-inch (102- to 120-cm) SID, and center a horizontal central ray with the midsagittal plane. Open the longitudinally and transversely collimated fields to the full 14- × 17-inch (35- × 43-cm) size. If the right lateral soft tissue does not appear to be included with this positioning, use two crosswise IRs instead of one lengthwise IR.

  Use two 14- × 17-inch (35- × 43-cm) IRs positioned crosswise with respect to the patient to include all the necessary anatomical structures in the hypersthenic patient and in sthenic and asthenic patients who have transverse abdominal measurements of 14 inches (35 cm) or greater. Take the first image with the top of the IR placed at a level 2½ inches (6.25 cm) superior to the xiphoid. Position the top of the second IR such that it includes approximately 2 to 3 inches (5 to 7.5 cm) of the same transverse section of the peritoneal cavity imaged on the first image, to ensure that no middle peritoneal information has been excluded. For both images, center a horizontal central ray with the midsagittal plane.

- ***Gonadal shielding:*** Use gonadal shielding on all male abdominal images and on female patients if two IRs are required and the upper abdomen is being imaged. Do not shield a female patient if the lower abdomen is imaged, because the shield may obscure needed information.

Lateral Decubitus Abdominal Image Analysis

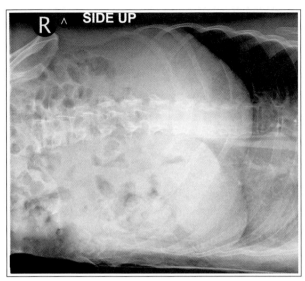

Image 38.

Analysis. The right iliac wing is narrower than the left iliac wing, and the distance from the right pedicles to the spinous processes is less than the distance from the left pedicles to the spinous processes. The patient's right side was positioned farther from the IR than the left side.

Correction. Rotate the patient's right side toward the IR until the shoulders and the ASISs are positioned at equal distances from the IR.

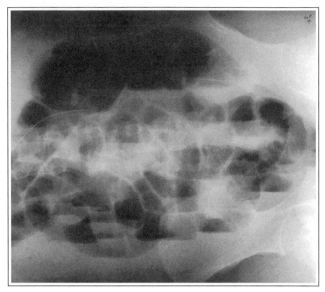

Image 39.

Analysis. The right hemidiaphragm is not included in the image. The IR and central ray were positioned too inferiorly.

Correction. Move the IR and central ray superiorly. Place the top of the IR at a level 2½ inches (6.25 cm) superior to the xiphoid, and center the central ray with the midsagittal plane and IR center.

PEDIATRIC CHEST

The following image analysis criteria are used for all pediatric chest images and should be considered when completing the analysis. Position- or projection-specific criteria relating to these topics are discussed with the other accompanying criteria for that position or projection.

Facility's identification requirements are visible on image as identified in Chapter 1.

- Neonates often require chest images to be taken daily for evaluation of lung development and ET placement. When so many images are involved, accurate date and time identification on images becomes essential.

A right or left marker, identifying the correct side of patient, is present on image and is not superimposed over anatomy of interest. Specific placement of marker is as described in Chapter 1.

Radiation protection practices, as defined in Chapter 1, have been followed.

No evidence of preventable artifacts, such as anatomical parts or removable monitoring leads, is present.

- Because lower kVp is used in pediatrics, clothing artifacts may be problematic in neonates and smaller children. The kVp used may not be high enough to burn out creases or folds, particularly in unlaundered material or flame-resistant clothing. It is best to image children without upper clothing or with a tee shirt when modesty is an issue. Skinfolds of neonates may also cause artifacts when they overlie the chest.

The lungs, diaphragm, heart, and bony structure outlines are sharply defined.

- Sharply defined recorded details are obtained when patient respiration and body movements are halted, when the least amount of OID is maintained, and when an optimal SID, as indicated in Table 2-3, is used. The long SID used in adult chest imaging is

TABLE 2-3 Pediatric Chest Technical Data				
Position or Projection	**kVp**	**Grid**		**SID**
Neonate: Supine or mobile AP projection	65-70			40-48 inches (100-120 cm)
Infant: Supine or mobile AP projection	70-75			40-48 inches (100-120 cm)
Child: PA projection	75-80	Grid (if AP measurement is over 5 inches [13 cm])		72 inches (183 cm)
Child: AP projection	70-75			40-48 inches (100-120 cm)
Neonate: Cross-table lateral position	65-70			40-48 inches (100-120 cm)
Infant: Cross-table lateral position	75-80			40-48 inches (100-120 cm)
Child: Lateral position	75-80	Grid (if side-to-side measurement is over 5 inches [13 cm])		72 inches (180 cm)
Neonate: Lateral decubitus position	65-70			40-48 inches (100-120 cm)
Infant: Lateral decubitus position	70-75			40-48 inches (100-120 cm)
Child: Lateral decubitus position	75-80	Grid (if AP measurement is over 5 inches [13 cm])		72 inches (183 cm)

AP, Anteroposterior; *kVp,* kilovolt peak; *PA,* posteroanterior; *SID,* source–image receptor distance.

not required in neonate and infant pediatrics examinations because heart magnification is minimal. Increased spatial resolution is also obtained when the smallest IR is selected for digital images.

Beam penetration is sufficient to faintly demonstrate the thoracic vertebrae and mediastinal structures. Contrast and density are adequate to demonstrate the internal lines and tubes when present and lung tissue (air-filled alveolar and linear connecting tissue) throughout the lung field.

- An optimal kVp technique, as shown in Table 2-3, sufficiently penetrates the chest structures and provides the contrast necessary to visualize the lung details. To obtain optimal density, set a manual mAs based on the patient's thorax thickness.
- The lungs of the neonate continue to grow for at least 8 years after birth. The growth results mainly from an increase in the number of respiratory bronchioles and alveoli. Only from one eighth to one sixth of the number of alveoli in adults are present in newborn infants, causing the lungs to be denser. Therefore on neonate and infant chest images the lungs demonstrate less image contrast within them and between them and the surrounding soft tissue than on adult chest images.
- *Internal lines and tubes:* Chest images are often taken to demonstrate the placement of internal lines and tubes. The accuracy of this placement is important for proper patient monitoring, treatment, and care. The radiographer plays an important role when imaging patients for the accuracy of tube and line placement. Small positioning variations during imaging, such as flexion or extension of the patient's neck, may result in questions arising about the accuracy of tube placement and in the need for the image to be retaken.

Neonates and infants require many of the same lines and tubes that adult patients need, such as the CV line (see Image 40) and chest tube (Figure 2-46).

Refer to the discussion in the adult AP chest section of this chapter on p. 69 for specifics on these lines and tubes. Following are listed some additional lines and tubes that should be considered when taking images of neonates and infants.

Endotracheal tube: The ET is discussed in the section on adult patients, also, but has been included again here for the discussion of specific placement as it pertains to neonatal and infant patients. The ET resides between the thoracic inlet and carina (level of T4 on neonate) and is used to inflate the lungs (see Image 41). With the distance from the thoracic inlet to the carina being minimal, the position of this tube is critical to within a few millimeters. When imaging for ET placement, the infant's face should be facing forward and the cervical vertebrae should be in a neutral position. With head rotation and cervical vertebrae flexion

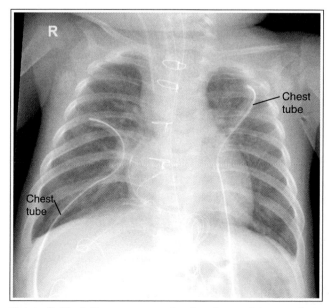

Figure 2-46. Infant anteroposterior chest image demonstrating a chest tube in each lung.

and extension the ET tip can move superiorly and inferiorly, respectively, making it more uncertain whether the tube is positioned in the correct location. Too superior positioning of the tube may place it in the esophagus, and too inferior placement may place the tube in the right main bronchus, causing hyperinflation of the right lung and collapse of the left lung. Images taken for ET placement should demonstrate penetration of the upper mediastinal region, and the longitudinal collimation should remain open enough (bottom of infant's lip) to include the upper airway.

Umbilical artery catheter (UAC): The UAC is found only in neonates, because the cord has dried up and fallen off in older infants. The UAC is used to measure oxygen saturation. Optimal location for the UAC is in the midthoracic aorta (T6 to T9) or below the level of the renal arteries, at approximately L1 to L2. On a lateral chest image the UAC is seen to lie posteriorly adjacent to the vertebral bodies because it courses in the aorta.

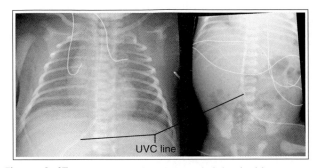

Figure 2-47. Anteroposterior chest and abdominal images demonstrating an umbilical vein catheter (*UVC*).

Umbilical vein catheter (UVC): The UVC is found only in neonates, because the cord has dried up and fallen off in older infants. The UVC is used to deliver fluids and medications. The UVC courses anteriorly and superiorly to the level of the heart. The ideal location of the UVC is at the junction of the right atrium and inferior vena cava (Figure 2-47).

NEONATE AND INFANT CHEST: ANTEROPOSTERIOR PROJECTION (SUPINE OR WITH MOBILE X-RAY UNIT)

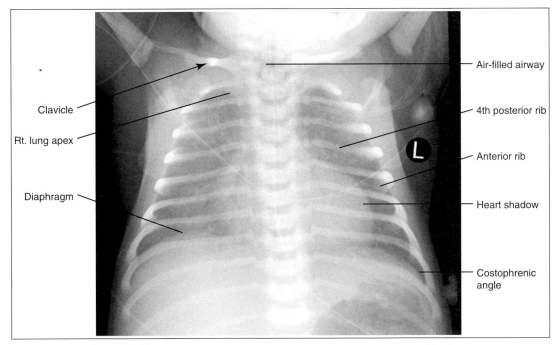

Figure 2-48. Neonate anteroposterior chest image with accurate positioning.

Image Analysis

The fourth thoracic vertebra is at the center of the collimated field. The upper airway, lungs, mediastinal structures, and costophrenic angles are included within the collimated field.

- Center the neonate or infant's chest to the center of an 8- × 10-inch (18- × 24-cm), lengthwise IR, and center

a perpendicular central ray to the midsagittal plane at the level of the mammary line (imaginary line connecting the nipples) for neonates and small infants. A larger IR and slightly inferior centering may be needed for larger infants. This IR and central ray placement centers the lung field on the image, permitting tight collimation on all sides of the lungs. Open the longitudinal collimation to include the upper airway (infant's bottom lip) and costophrenic angles (tenth posterior rib) and transversely collimate to within ½ inch (1.25 cm) of the lateral skinline.

- The lungs of the neonate continue to grow for at least 8 years after birth. The growth results mainly from an increase in the number of respiratory bronchioles and alveoli. As the lungs grow, the shape of the thoracic cavity changes from the neonate and infant's short, wide shape to the older child and adult's longer, narrower shape. The technologist must adjust the central ray centering point to accommodate the changing shape to avoid distortion and clipping lung structures when tightly collimating.

The chest demonstrates an AP projection. The distances from the vertebral column to the sternal ends of the clavicles are equal, and the lengths of the right and left corresponding posterior ribs are equal.

- Rotation on a supine or mobile chest image is caused by poor patient positioning or central ray alignment. To accurately position the infant without rotation, have an attendant use two hands for restraint. The thumb, forefinger, and middle finger of one hand are used to clasp the infant's wrists above his or her head, and the same digits of the other hand clasp the infant's ankles (Figure 2-49). The head and toes are positioned straight up. Head rotation is the most common cause of chest rotation in neonates and infants. The chest will rotate in the same direction in which the infant's head is rotated. Align the central ray perpendicular to the midsagittal plane and IR. To avoid rotation caused by poor central ray alignment, make certain the central ray is not angled toward the right or left lateral side of the infant instead of being perpendicular. If the central ray is angled toward the lateral side of the infant, the anatomical structures farthest from the IR (clavicles and anterior ribs) will be projected in the direction toward which the central ray is angled.
- *Detecting chest rotation:* Chest rotation is detected by evaluating the distance between the vertebral column

and the sternal ends of the clavicles and by comparing the length of the right and left inferior posterior ribs. The sternal clavicular end that is demonstrated farther from the vertebral column and the side of the chest that demonstrates the longer posterior ribs represents the side of the chest toward which the infant is rotated (see Image 41). If the cause of the rotation is poor central ray alignment, the sternal clavicular end that is demonstrated farther from the vertebral column and the side of the chest with the longer posterior ribs represents the side of the chest toward which the central ray angle was directed.

The anterior ribs are projecting downward and the posterior ribs demonstrate a gentle, cephalically bowed contour.

- The neonate or infant supine AP chest image tends to have a lordotic appearance because of the lack of kyphotic thoracic curvature that is seen in adults. Some facilities offset this appearance by angling the central ray 5 degrees caudally or tilting the foot end of the bed 5 degrees lower than the head end. Proper central ray centering will also help to reduce this lordotic appearance. Because the chest in neonates and infants is shorter than in adults, a common error is to center the central ray too inferiorly, resulting in an increase in the lordotic appearance.

  An AP neonate or infant chest image that demonstrates an excessively lordotic appearance will demonstrate cephalically projected anterior ribs and posterior ribs without the gentle, cephalically bowed contour (see Image 42). Such distortion foreshortens the lungs and mediastinal structures, causing the cardiac apex to appear uptilted and the main pulmonary artery to be concealed beneath the cardiac silhouette.

Neonate: Eight posterior ribs are demonstrated above the diaphragm, and the lungs demonstrate a fluffy appearance with linear-appearing connecting tissue, indicating full lung aeration for the neonatal chest image.

Infant: **At least nine posterior ribs are demonstrated above the diaphragm.**

- The appearance of the neonate's lungs may change with even one rib's difference in inflation. With dense substances such as blood, pus, protein, and cells filling the alveoli, it is the addition of the less dense air that will give the image the fluffy appearance, because the air is demonstrated on the image as a darker density among the lighter densities of blood, pus, protein, and cells. A lung that demonstrates a "white-out" appearance even though the diaphragm is below the eighth rib is filled with dense substances that do not allow air to fill the alveoli.

  For neonates and infants breathing without a respirator, observe the chest movement and expose the image after the infant takes a deep breath. Chest images

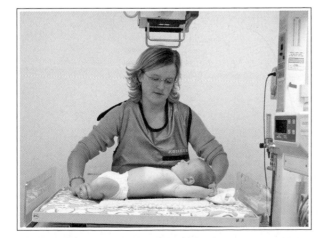

Figure 2-49. Proper patient positioning for anteroposterior neonate and infant chest image.

that are taken on expiration may demonstrate a decrease in image density, because a decrease in air volume increases the concentration of pulmonary tissues (see Image 40).

Respirators: For neonates and infants being ventilated with a conventional ventilator, observe the ventilator's pressure manometer (see Figure 2-25, *A*). The exposure should be taken when the manometer digital bar or analog needle moves to its highest position. If a high-frequency ventilator is being used, the exposure may be made at any time, because this ventilator maintains the lung expansion at a steady mean pressure without the bulk gas exchange of the conventional type (see Figure 2-25, *B*).

The chin does not obscure the airway or apical lung field.

- To prevent the chin from being superimposed on the airway and apical lung field, lift the neonate or infant's chin until the neck is in a neutral position. When the chin is superimposed on the airway and apical lung field, ET placement cannot be evaluated (see Image 43).

Neonate and Infant Anteroposterior Chest Analysis

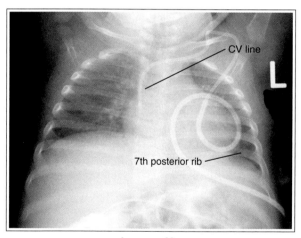

Image 40.

Analysis. The CV line is demonstrated in accurate position. Six posterior ribs are demonstrated above the diaphragm. Neonates should have at least eight and infants at least nine posterior ribs visible above the diaphragm. The lungs were not fully aerated.

Correction. If possible, take the exposure after the patient takes a deeper inspiration. If the patient is on a conventional ventilator, expose the image when the manometer is at its highest level, indicating a deep inspiration.

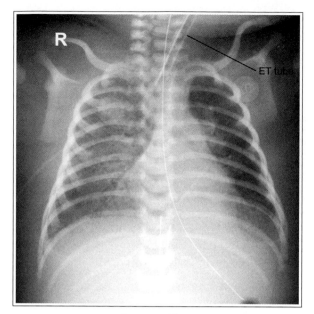

Image 41.

Analysis. The ET is demonstrated in an accurate position. The left sternal clavicular end is demonstrated farther from the vertebral column than the right sternal clavicular end, and the left lower posterior ribs are longer than the right. The patient's head is turned and the thorax rotated toward the left side.

Correction. Rotate the patient's face to a forward position, and rotate the thorax toward the right side until the midcoronal plane is parallel with the IR and perpendicular to the central ray.

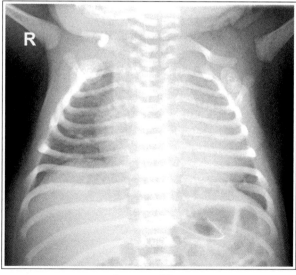

Image 42.

Analysis. The chest demonstrates an excessively lordotic appearance. The anterior ribs are projecting upwardly, and the posterior ribs do not demonstrate the slight upwardly bowed appearance, but are horizontal. The central ray was centered inferior to T4.

Correction. Move the central ray superiorly to better align it with the upper thorax. A 5-degree caudal angle may also be added to help better align the central ray and thorax.

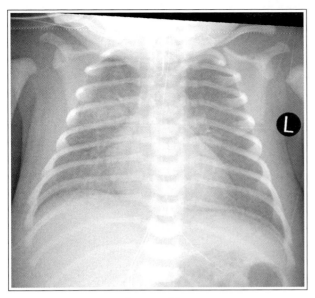

Image 43.

Analysis. The patient's chin is superimposed over the airway and apical lung field. The chin was not elevated to bring the neck into a neutral position.

Correction. Lift the chin until the patient's face is forward and the neck is in a neutral position.

CHILD CHEST: POSTEROANTERIOR AND ANTEROPOSTERIOR PROJECTIONS

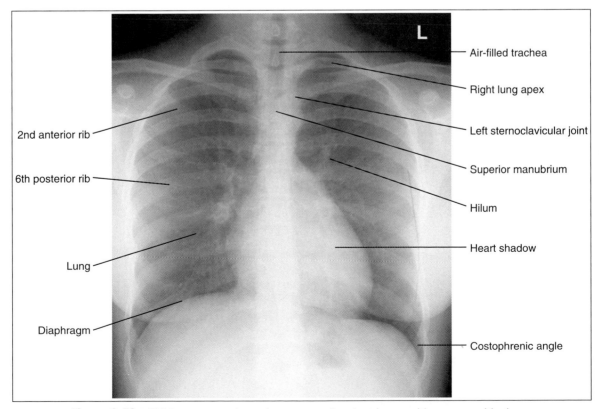

Figure 2-50. Child posteroanterior and anteroposterior chest image with proper positioning.

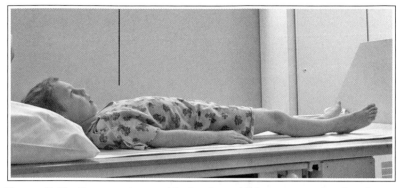

Figure 2-51. Proper patient positioning for a child posteroanterior chest image.

Image Analysis

The analysis of the child PA and AP chest images is the same as that for the infant or adult PA or AP chest, already discussed. The size of the child determines which criterion best meets the situation. For specifics on these topics, refer to the PA/AP chest discussion earlier in this chapter or the adult PA/AP sections in this chapter on pp. 54 and 68, respectively.

Child Chest PA and AP Image Analysis

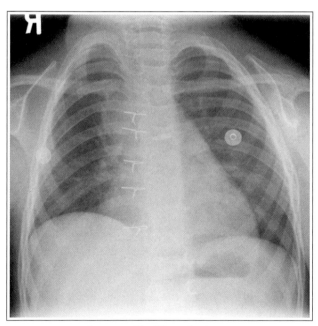

Image 44. PA projection.

Analysis. The right SC end is visible without superimposing the vertebral column superimposition, and the left sternal clavicular end superimposes the vertebral column. The patient was rotated into an RP position.

Correction. Rotate the left side of the patient's thorax toward the IR until the shoulders are at equal distances from the IR.

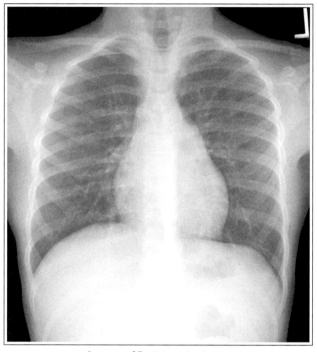

Image 45. PA projection.

Analysis. The manubrium is at the level of the second thoracic vertebra, and less than ½ inch (1.25 cm) of apical lung field is demonstrated superior to the clavicles. The patient's upper midcoronal plane was tilted posteriorly.

Correction. Anteriorly tilt the upper midcoronal plane until it is aligned parallel with the IR.

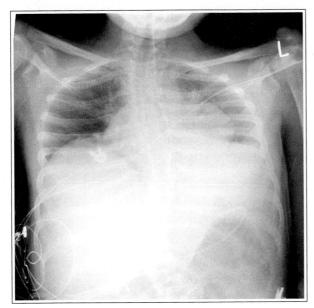

Image 46. AP projection.

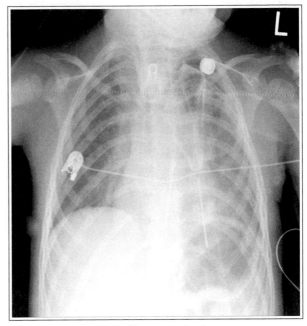

Image 47. AP projection.

Analysis. Only six posterior ribs are demonstrated above the diaphragm. The manubrium is superimposed over the second thoracic vertebra, the posterior ribs demonstrate a horizontal contour, and less than 1 inch (2.5 cm) of apical lung field is visible above the clavicles. The image was taken on expiration, and the central ray was angled too cephalically.

Correction. If the patient's condition allows, take the exposure after coaxing the patient into a deeper inspiration and adjust the central ray caudally until it is aligned perpendicular to the patient's midcoronal plane.

Analysis. The manubrium is superimposed over the fifth thoracic vertebra, the posterior ribs demonstrate a vertical contour, and more than 1 inch (2.5 cm) of apical lung field is visible above the clavicles. The central ray was angled too caudally.

Correction. Adjust the central ray cephalically until it is aligned perpendicular to the patient's midcoronal plane.

NEONATE AND INFANT CHEST: CROSS-TABLE LEFT LATERAL POSITION (SUPINE OR WITH MOBILE X-RAY UNIT)

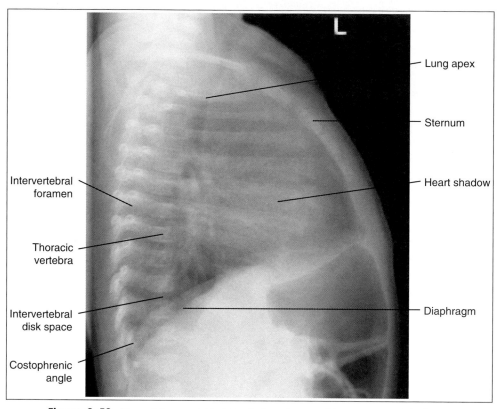

Figure 2-52. Neonatal cross-table lateral chest image with accurate positioning.

Image Analysis

The midcoronal plane, at the level of the fifth thoracic vertebra, is at the center of the collimated field. The entire lung field (including apices, costophrenic angles, and posterior ribs) and the airway are included within the field.

- Lateral chest images are useful in assessing the degree of inflation, permit confident recognition of cardiomegaly, and provide the clearest view of the thoracic vertebrae and sternum. The needed anatomical structures are placed on a lateral chest image when the neonate or infant is supine, and an 8- × 10-inch (18- × 24-cm), lengthwise IR is positioned against the neonate or infant's left lateral surface. The chest is placed in the middle of the IR by elevating the patient on a radiolucent sponge, and a horizontal central ray is positioned to the midcoronal plane at a level just inferior to the mammary line (Figure 2-53). A larger IR and slightly inferior centering may be needed for larger infants. This IR and central ray placement centers the lung field on the image, permitting tight collimation on all sides of the lungs. Open the longitudinal collimation to include the mid-cervical vertebrae and costophrenic

angles, and transversely collimate to within ½ inch (1.25 cm) of the lateral skinline.

Cross-table versus overhead lateral images: Neonates are very sensitive. Performing a cross-table lateral image on the neonate instead of the overhead lateral will reduce the amount of disturbance. Also, on overhead lateral images the lung adjacent to the IR tends to collapse, whereas the superior lung tends to overinflate.

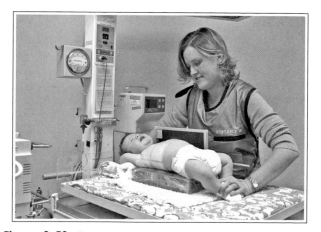

Figure 2-53. Proper patient positioning for a cross-table neonate and infant chest image.

The chest demonstrates no rotation when the posterior ribs are superimposed and the sternum is in profile.

- To avoid chest rotation, align an imaginary line connecting the shoulders, the posterior ribs, and the posterior pelvic wings perpendicular to the IR. Because the OID difference between the right and left lung fields is minimal on neonates and small infants, the posterior ribs on lateral chest images do not demonstrate the ½-inch (1.25-cm) separation that is seen on adult lateral chest images, but instead are directly superimposed.

- ***Detecting chest rotation:*** Chest rotation is effectively detected on a lateral chest image by evaluating the degree of superimposition of the posterior ribs. When the posterior ribs are demonstrated without superimposition, the chest was rotated for the image (see Image 48). One means of identifying the lung that is positioned posteriorly is to locate the most inferiorly demonstrated right and left corresponding ribs. The rib on the right side will be projected slightly more inferiorly than the rib on the left side because it is positioned farthest from the IR. The heart shadow may also be used as described in the discussion of the adult lateral chest image earlier in this chapter.

Humeral soft tissue is not superimposed over the anterior lung apices.

- Positioning the humeri upward, near the patient's head, prevents superimposition of the humeral soft tissue over the anterior lung apices (see Image 49).

The chin is not in the radiation field.

- Good radiation protection practices dictate that anatomical structures not evaluated on an image should not be included whenever possible. To prevent the chin from being included in the radiation field, lift it upward above the collimation field (see Image 50).

The hemidiaphragms form a gentle, cephalic curve.

- ***Respiration:*** For neonates and infants breathing without a respirator, observe the chest movement and take the exposure after the infant takes a deep breath. Chest images that are taken on expiration may demonstrate a decrease in image density, because a decrease in air volume increases the concentration of pulmonary tissues. With underaeration, the cephalic curve of the hemidiaphragms is exaggerated and their position is higher in the thorax (see Image 51).

- ***Respirators:*** For neonates and infants being ventilated with a conventional ventilator, expose the image when the manometer digital bar or analog needle moves to its highest position. If a high-frequency ventilator is being used, the exposure may be made at any time.

Neonate and Infant Lateral Chest Image Analysis

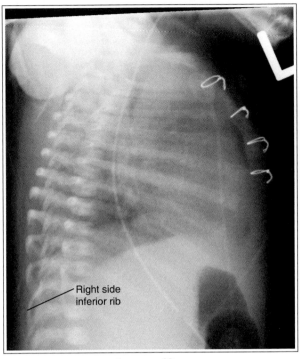

Right side inferior rib

Image 48.

Analysis. The posterior ribs are demonstrated without superimposition. The right lung is posterior to the left lung, as identified by the more inferior projection of the posterior rib on the right side compared with the left.

Correction. Rotate the right side of the thorax away from the bed or cart until the shoulders and posterior ribs are aligned perpendicular to the IR.

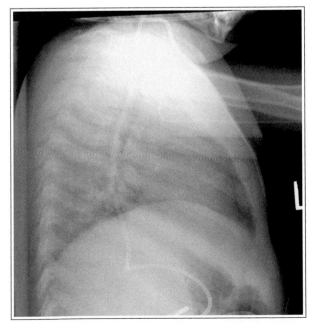

Image 49.

Analysis. The humeral soft tissue is superimposed over the anterior lung apices. The patient's arms were not elevated.

Correction. Raise the patient's arms until the humeri are next to the patient's head.

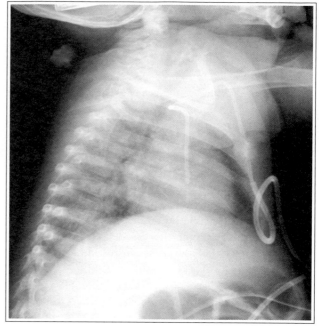

Image 51.

Analysis. The hemidiaphragms demonstrate an exaggerated cephalic curvature, and the humeral soft tissue is superimposed over the apical lung field. The lungs were not fully expanded, and the arms were not elevated to a position near the patient's head.

Correction. Expose the image after full inhalation, and raise the arms until they are adjacent to the patient's head.

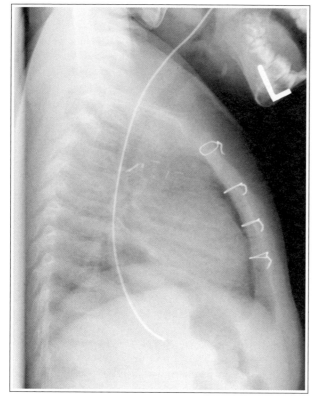

Image 50.

Analysis. The patient's chin is demonstrated within the collimated field. The chin was depressed.

Correction. Elevate the chin, outside the collimated field.

CHILD CHEST: LATERAL POSITION

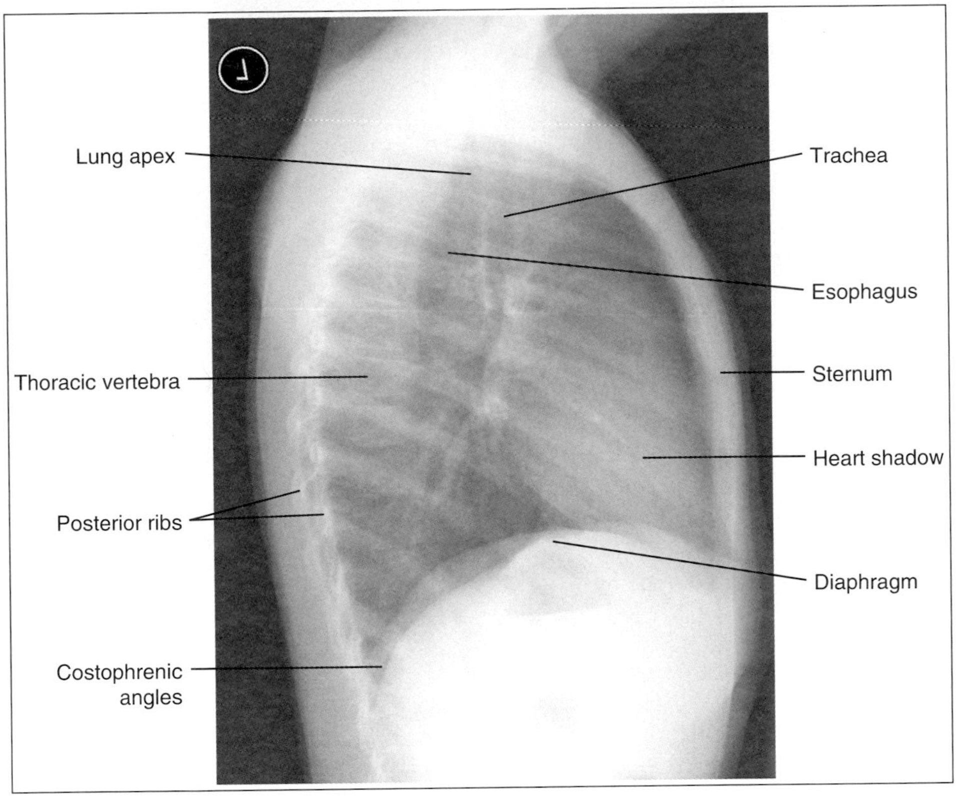

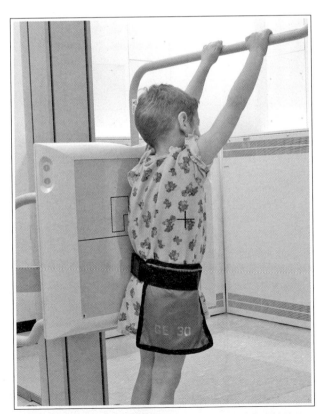

Figure 2-54. Child lateral chest image with accurate positioning.

Figure 2-55. Proper positioning for a child lateral chest image.

Image Analysis

The analysis of the child lateral chest image is the same as that of the infant or adult lateral chest image, already discussed. The size of the child determines which criterion best meets the situation. For specifics on this topic, refer to the discussion of infant lateral chest images earlier in this chapter or adult lateral chest images on p. 61.

Child Lateral Chest Image Analysis

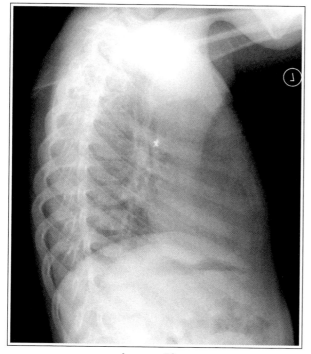

Image 52.

Analysis. More than ½ inch (1.25 cm) of separation is demonstrated between the posterior ribs. The gastric air bubble is adjacent to the anteriorly located lung, indicating that the left lung is anteriorly positioned. The chin is within the collimated field, and the humeral soft tissue is superimposed over the superior lung field. The chin and the humeri were not elevated.

Correction. Rotate the right side of the thorax anteriorly and the left side posteriorly until the shoulders and the posterior ribs are aligned perpendicular to the IR. Elevate the chin outside the collimated field, and raise the humeri next to the patient's head.

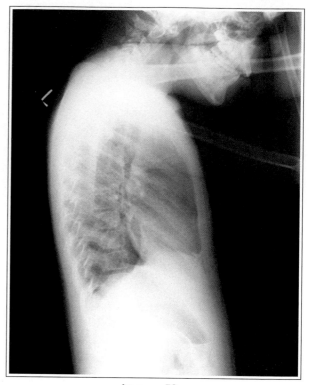

Image 53.

Analysis. Anatomical artifacts (patient's arms and mandible) are demonstrated on this image. Poor radiation protection practices are demonstrated.

Correction. Raise the patient's chin to bring it above the level of the chest and out of a properly collimated field. Increase the transverse collimation to within ½ inch (1.25 cm) of thorax skinline.

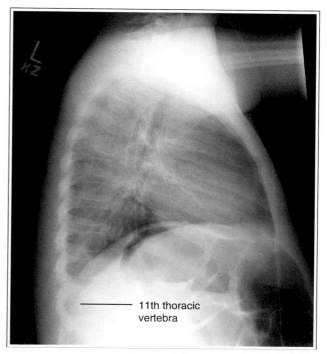

11th thoracic
vertebra

Image 54.

Analysis. The hemidiaphragms demonstrate an exaggerated cephalic curve, and they do not cover the entire eleventh thoracic vertebra. Full lung aeration is not demonstrated. The humeri are not elevated.

Correction. Coax the patient into taking a deeper inspiration. Elevate the humeri next to the patient's head.

NEONATE AND INFANT CHEST: LATERAL DECUBITUS POSITION (ANTEROPOSTERIOR PROJECTION)

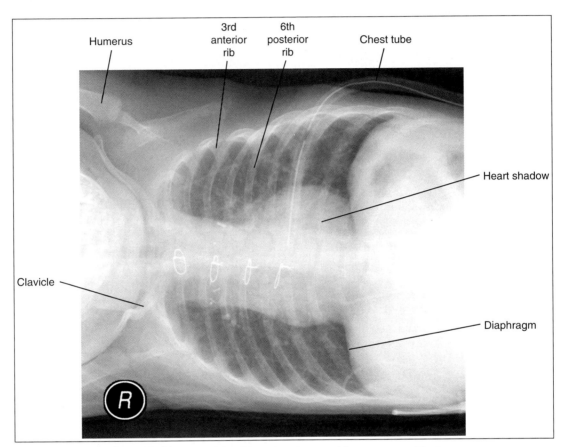

Figure 2-56. Lateral decubitus chest image with accurate positioning.

Image Analysis

Contrast and density are adequate to visualize fluid levels or the presence of air within the pleural cavity.

- *Positioning to demonstrate pleural air or fluid:* The lateral decubitus position is primarily used to confirm the presence of a pneumothorax or pleural effusion in the pleural cavity. To best demonstrate the presence of air, position the affected side of the thorax away from the bed or cart so that the air rises to the highest level in the pleural cavity. To best demonstrate fluid in the pleural cavity, position the affected side against the bed or cart. This positioning allows the fluid to move to the lowest level of the pleural cavity, away from the mediastinal structures (see Image 58).

The fourth thoracic vertebra is at the center of the collimated field. The upper airway, lungs, mediastinal structures, and costophrenic angles are included within the field.

- With the neonate or infant positioned on the lateral side that best demonstrates the condition of interest, place an 8- × 10-inch (18- × 24-cm), lengthwise IR against the patient's posterior surface and position the chest in the middle of the IR by elevating the patient on a radiolucent sponge. Center a horizontal central ray to the midsagittal plane at the level of the mammary line for neonates and small infants (Figure 2-57). A larger IR and slightly inferior centering may be needed for larger infants. This IR and central ray placement centers the lung field on the

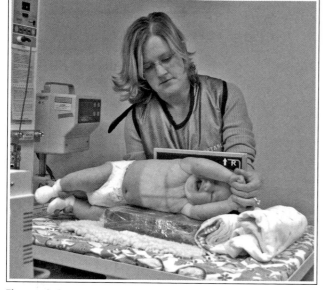

Figure 2-57. Proper patient positioning for lateral neonate and infant chest image.

image, permitting tight collimation on all sides of the lungs. Open the longitudinal collimation to include the upper airway (infant's bottom lip) and costophrenic angles (tenth posterior rib), and transversely collimate to within ½ inch (1.25 cm) of the lateral skinline.

The chest demonstrates an AP projection. The distances from the vertebral column to the sternal ends of the clavicles are equal, and the lengths of the corresponding right and left posterior ribs are equal.

- To avoid chest rotation, align the shoulders, the posterior ribs, and the posterior pelvic wings perpendicular to the bed or cart on which the neonate or infant is lying. This alignment positions the patient's shoulders and lungs at equal distances from the IR. Position the head straight ahead without rotation. The chest typically rotates in the same direction as the infant's head.
- *Detecting chest rotation:* Chest rotation is detected by evaluating the distance between the vertebral column and the sternal ends of the clavicles and by comparing the length of the right and left inferior posterior ribs. The sternal clavicular end that is superimposed over the least amount of the vertebral column, along with the side of the chest that demonstrates the longest inferior posterior ribs, represents the side of the chest toward which the infant is rotated (see Image 55).

The chin and arms are situated outside the lung field, and the lateral aspects of the clavicles are projected upward.

- To prevent the chin from being superimposed over the lung apices on the image, elevate the chin until the face is facing forward and the neck is in a neutral position (see Image 56). Placing the arms upward toward the patient's head positions them away from

the lung field and projects the lateral clavicles in an upward position (see Image 57).

The anterior ribs are projecting downward, and the posterior ribs demonstrate a gentle, bowed downward contour.

- The neonate or infant supine lateral decubitus chest image tends to have a lordotic appearance because of the lack of kyphotic thoracic curvature that is seen in adults. To reduce this lordotic appearance, align the central ray perpendicular to the midcoronal plane and center the central ray at the level of the mammary line. Because the chest in neonates and infants is shorter than in adults, a common error is to center the central ray too inferiorly, resulting in an increase in the lordotic appearance.
- An AP neonate or infant chest image that demonstrates an excessively lordotic appearance will demonstrate cephalically projected anterior ribs and posterior ribs without their gentle, cephalically bowed appearance (see Image 56).

Eight posterior ribs are demonstrated above the diaphragm and the lungs demonstrate a fluffy appearance with linear-appearing connecting tissue, indicating full lung aeration for the neonate or infant chest image.

- Observe the patient during quiet breathing, and expose the image when the lungs show expansion.
- *Respirators:* For neonates or infants being ventilated with a conventional ventilator, expose the image when the manometer digital bar or analog needle moves to its highest position. If a high-frequency ventilator is being used, the exposure may be made at any time.

The lung field positioned against the bed or cart is demonstrated without superimposition of the bed or cart pad. The midsagittal plane is demonstrated without lateral tilting.

- Elevating the neonate or infant on a radiolucent sponge prevents the chest from sinking into the cart pad. When the body is allowed to sink into the cart pad, artifact lines are seen superimposed over the lateral lung field of the side adjacent to the cart. Because fluid in the pleural cavity gravitates to the lowest level, it is in this area that the fluid will be demonstrated, and superimposition of the cart pad and the lower lung field may obscure fluid that has settled in the lowest level.

  Position the neonate or infant's entire body on the radiolucent sponge to align the midsagittal plane parallel with the bed or cart, preventing lateral tilting (see Image 58).

Neonate and Infant Lateral Decubitus Chest Image Analysis

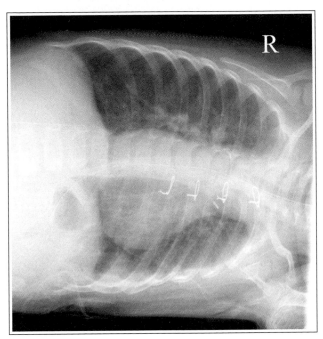

Image 55. AP projection.

Analysis. The left sternal clavicular end is demonstrated farther from the vertebral column than the right sternal clavicular end, and the left posterior ribs are longer than the right. The patient's head is turned, and the thorax is rotated toward the left side.

Correction. Rotate the patient's face to a forward position, and rotate the thorax toward the right side until the mid-coronal plane is parallel with the IR and perpendicular to the central ray.

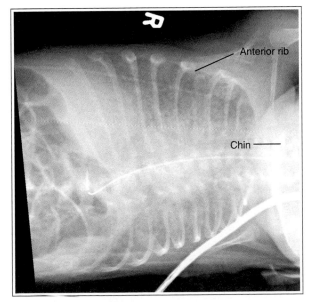

Image 56. AP projection.

Analysis. The chest demonstrates an excessively lordotic appearance. The anterior ribs are projecting cephalically, and the posterior ribs do not demonstrate the slight cephalically bowed contour but are horizontal. The central ray was centered inferiorly to T6. The right inferior ribs are longer than the left posterior ribs. The patient was rotated toward the right side. The chin is superimposed over the apices and upper airway.

Correction. Move the central ray superiorly to better align it with the upper thorax. A 5-degree caudal angle may also be added to help better align the central ray and thorax. Rotate the patient toward the right side until the shoulders and the posterior ribs are at equal distances to the IR. Elevate the chin until it is positioned outside the collimated field.

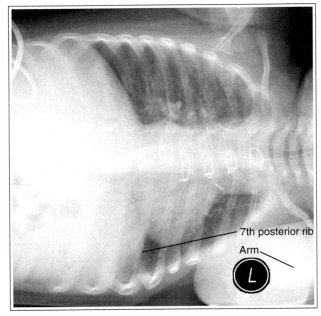

Image 57. AP projection.

Analysis. Seven posterior ribs are demonstrated above the diaphragm. Full lung aeration was not accomplished. The left arm is superimposed over a small portion of the left lateral lung field. The right clavicle is horizontal. The arms were not brought upward by the patient's head.

Correction. If possible, take the exposure after the patient takes a deep inspiration. If the patient is on a conventional ventilator, expose the image when the manometer is at it highest level, indicating a deep inspiration. Raise the patient's arms; bring them next to the patient's head.

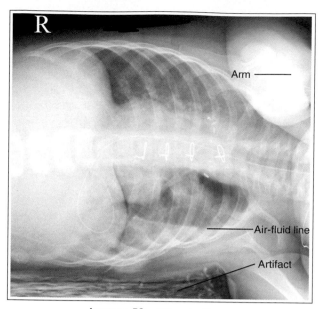

Image 58. AP projection.

Analysis. The device on which the patient is elevated is demonstrated adjacent to the left lateral lung field. Because the patient has not sunk into this device, it is not superimposed over the lateral lung field and is acceptable. The patient's upper midsagittal plane is laterally tilted toward the left side. The patient's upper thorax was allowed to hang over the elevating device. The patient's right arm is obscuring the lateral apical area. The right arm was not elevated to a position near the patient's head.

Correction. Place the entire thorax on the elevating device, positioning the midsagittal plane parallel with the bed or cart. Elevate the right arm so it is positioned next to the patient's head.

CHILD CHEST: LATERAL DECUBITUS POSITION (ANTEROPOSTERIOR OR POSTEROANTERIOR PROJECTION)

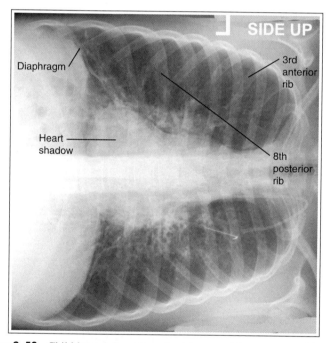

Figure 2-58. Child lateral decubitus chest image with accurate positioning.

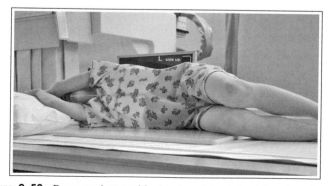

Figure 2-59. Proper patient positioning for a lateral decubitus chest image.

Image Analysis

The analysis of lateral decubitus chest images in children is the same as that of infant or adult lateral decubitus chest images, already discussed. The size of the child determines the criterion that best meets the situation. For specifics on this topic, refer to the discussion of lateral decubitus chest images earlier in this chapter or to the discussion of adult lateral decubitus chest images on p. 76.

Child Lateral Decubitus Chest Image Analysis

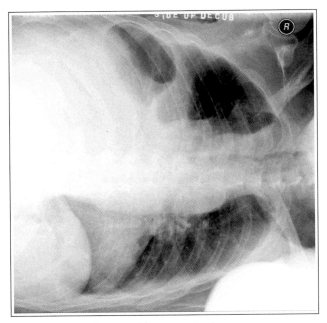

Image 59. AP projection.

Analysis. The left sternal clavicular end is superimposed over the vertebral column, the posterior ribs on the right side demonstrate the greater length, and the arms are superimposed over the right lateral lung apex. The patient was rotated toward the right side, and the left arm was at a 90-degree angle with thorax.

Correction. Rotate the patient's right side away from the IR, and elevate the left arm until it is positioned next to the patent's head.

PEDIATRIC ABDOMEN

A right or left marker identifying the correct side of the patient is present on the image. The markers are not superimposed on anatomy of interest.

Radiation protection practices, as defined in Chapter 1, have been followed.

No evidence of preventable artifacts is present (see Image 60).

The outlines of the diaphragm and the gases within the stomach and intestines are sharply defined.

- Sharply defined recorded details are obtained when patient motion is controlled, respiration is halted, a short exposure time is used, and a short OID is maintained. Increased spatial resolution is also obtained when the smallest IR is selected for digital imaging.

Contrast, density, and penetration are adequate to demonstrate the diaphragm, bowel gas pattern, and faint outline of bony structures.

- An optimal kVp technique, as shown in Table 2-4, sufficiently penetrates the bowel gas pattern and faintly outlines the bony structures. In infants and young children it is difficult to differentiate between the small and large bowels. The gas loops tend to look the same. Because little intrinsic fat is present, the abdominal organs (such as kidneys) are not well defined.

TABLE 2-4 Pediatric Abdominal Technical Data			
Position or Projection	kVp	Grid	SID
Neonate: AP Projection	65-75		40-48 inch (100-120 cm)
Infant: AP Projection	65-75		40-48 inch (100-120 cm)
Child: AP Projection	70-80	Grid (if AP measurement is over 5 inches [13 cm])	40-48 inch (100-120 cm)
Neonate: Lateral decubitus position	65-75		40-48 inch (100-120 cm)
Infant: Lateral decubitus position	65-75		40-48 inch (100-120 cm)
Child: Lateral decubitus position	70-80	Grid (if AP measurement is over 5 inches [13 cm])	40-48 inch (100-120 cm)

AP, Anteroposterior; *kVp*, kilovolt peak; *SID*, source–image receptor distance.

NEONATE AND INFANT ABDOMEN: ANTEROPOSTERIOR PROJECTION (SUPINE)

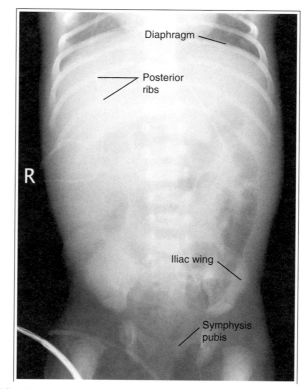

Figure 2-60. Neonatal anteroposterior abdominal image with accurate positioning.

Image Analysis

The abdomen demonstrates an AP projection. The inferior posterior ribs and the iliac wings are symmetrical.

- An AP abdominal image is obtained by placing the neonate or infant in a supine position with the IR centered beneath the abdomen. To avoid rotation, align the shoulders and the posterior pelvic wings at equal distances from the IR (Figure 2-61).
- *Detecting abdominal rotation:* The upper and lower lumbar vertebrae can demonstrate rotation independently or simultaneously, depending on

which section of the body is rotated. If the patient's thorax is rotated but the pelvis remains in an AP projection, the upper lumbar vertebrae and abdominal cavity demonstrate rotation. If the patient's pelvis is rotated but the thorax remains in an AP projection, the lower vertebrae and abdominal cavity demonstrate rotation. If the patient's thorax and pelvis are rotated simultaneously, the entire lumbar column and abdominal cavity demonstrate rotation.

Rotation is effectively detected on a decubitus abdominal image by comparing the symmetry of the inferior posterior ribs and the iliac wings (see Image 61). The ribs that demonstrate the longer

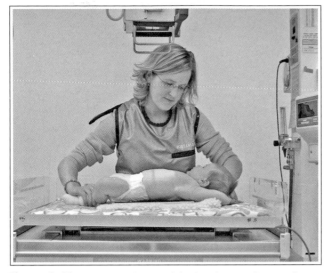

Figure 2-61. Proper patient positioning for anterioposterior neonate and infant abdominal image.

length and the iliac wing demonstrating the greater width are on the side toward which the patient is rotated.

The image was taken on expiration. The diaphragm domes are superior to the eighth posterior rib.

- From full inspiration to expiration, the diaphragm moves from an inferior to a superior position. This movement also changes the pressure placed on the abdominal structures. On full expiration the diaphragm dome is above the eighth posterior rib. When the decubitus abdominal image is taken on expiration, less pressure is exerted on the peritoneal contents and the space in the peritoneal cavity is greater. If the decubitus position is taken on inspiration, the inferior placement of the diaphragm puts pressure on the abdominal organs, resulting in less space in the peritoneal cavity and greater abdominal density (see Image 61).

- For neonates or infants being ventilated with a conventional ventilator, observe the ventilator's pressure manometer. The exposure should be taken when the manometer digital bar or analog needle moves to its highest position. If a high-frequency ventilator is being used, the exposure may be made at any time, because this ventilator maintains the lung expansion at a steady mean pressure without the bulk gas exchange of the conventional type.

The long axis of the lumbar vertebral column is aligned with the long axis of the collimated field.

- Aligning the long axis of the lumbar vertebral column with the long axis of the collimated field allows for tight transverse collimation (see Image 62).

The fourth lumbar vertebra is centered within the collimated field. The diaphragm, abdominal

structures, and symphysis pubis are included within the field.

- *IR size and centering:* With the neonate or infant positioned in supine AP projection, center an 8- × 10-inch (18- × 24-cm), lengthwise IR beneath the neonate or infant. Center a perpendicular central ray to the midsagittal plane at a transverse level approximately 2 inches (5 cm) superior to the iliac crest. A larger IR and slightly inferior centering may be needed for larger infants. This IR and central ray placement centers the abdomen on the image, permitting tight collimation on all sides of the lungs. Open the longitudinal collimation to include the diaphragm (1 inch [2.5 cm] inferior to mammary line) and symphysis pubis, and transversely collimate to within ½ inch (1.25 cm) of the lateral skinline.

- *Gonadal shielding:* Use gonadal shielding on all male abdominal images. Do not shield a female patient, because the shield may obscure needed information.

Neonate and Infant: Anteroposterior Abdominal Image Analysis

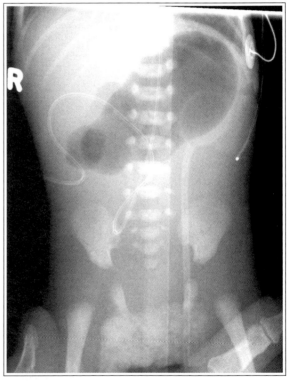

Image 60.

Analysis. The diaphragm is not included on the image, and anatomical artifacts (positioning attendant's fingers) are demonstrated on the image.

Correction. Move the central ray and IR 1 inch (2.5 cm) superiorly, and move the attendant's hands inferiorly outside of the collimated field.

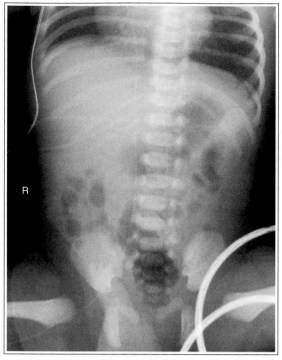

Image 61.

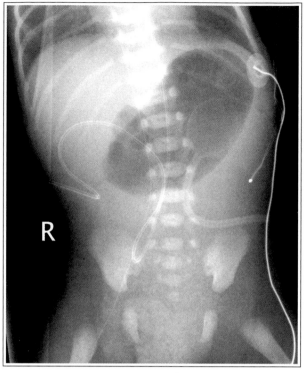

Image 62.

Analysis. The posterior ribs are longer on the right side than on the left, and the right iliac wing is wider than the left side posterior ribs. The diaphragm is at the level of the eighth posterior rib. The patient was rotated toward the right side, and the exposure was taken on inspiration.

Correction. Rotate the patient toward the left side until the shoulders and iliac wings are at equal distances to the IR, and expose the image after the patient exhales or the manometer is at its lowest level for conventional ventilators.

Analysis. The patient's upper vertebral column is tilted toward the right side. Tight collimation practices could not be followed.

Correction. Tilt the upper vertebral column toward the left side until the vertebral column is straight and aligned with the collimator's longitudinal light line. Increase transverse collimation to within $1/2$ inch (1.25 cm) from skinline.

CHILD ABDOMEN: ANTEROPOSTERIOR PROJECTION

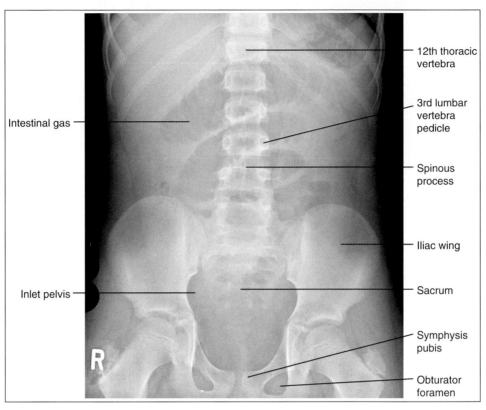

Intestinal gas

Inlet pelvis

12th thoracic vertebra

3rd lumbar vertebra pedicle

Spinous process

Iliac wing

Sacrum

Symphysis pubis

Obturator foramen

Figure 2-62. Child supine anteroposterior abdominal image with accurate positioning.

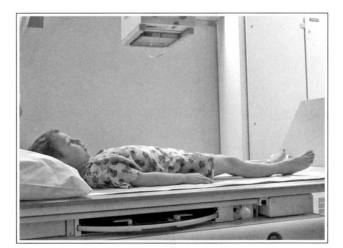

Figure 2-63. Proper positioning for a child supine anteroposterior abdominal image.

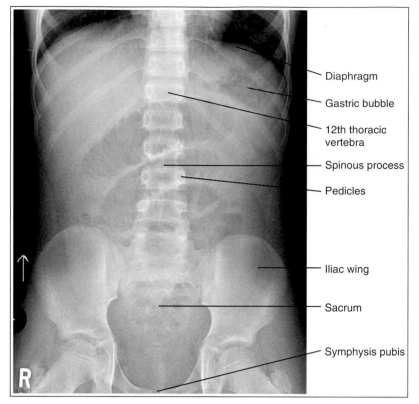

Figure 2-64. Child upright anteroposterior abdominal image with accurate positioning.

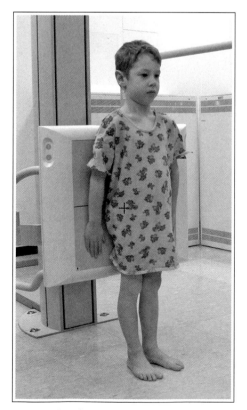

Figure 2-65. Proper positioning for a child upright anteroposterior abdominal image.

Image Analysis

The analysis of child AP abdominal images is the same as that of infant or adult AP abdominal images, already discussed. The size of the child determines which criterion best meets the situation. For specifics on this topic, refer to the discussion of infant AP abdominal images earlier in this chapter or the discussion of adult AP abdominal images on p. 88.

Child Anteroposterior Abdominal Image Analysis

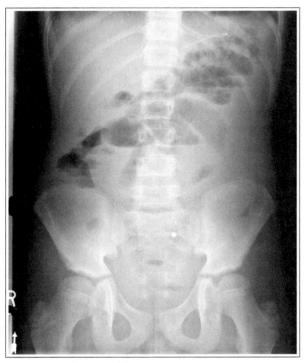

Image 63. Upright abdomen.

Analysis. The diaphragm is not included on this image. The central ray and IR are positioned too inferiorly.

Correction. The central ray and IR should be moved 2 inches (5 cm) superiorly.

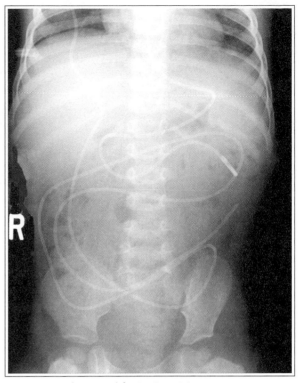

Image 64. Supine abdomen.

Analysis. The right posterior ribs are longer than the left, and the right iliac wing is wider than the left, indicating that the patient was rotated toward the right side.

Correction. Rotate the patient toward the left side until the shoulders and ASISs are at equal distances from the imaging table.

NEONATE AND INFANT ABDOMEN: LEFT LATERAL DECUBITUS POSITION (ANTEROPOSTERIOR PROJECTION)

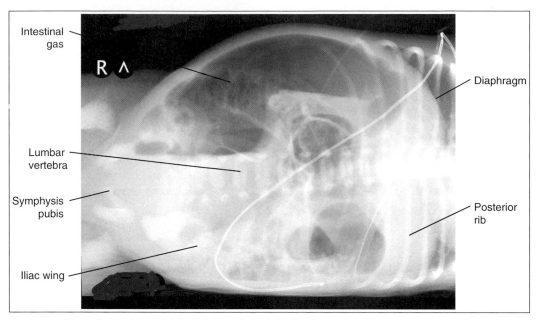

Figure 2-66. Neonatal lateral decubitus abdominal image with accurate positioning.

Image Analysis

An arrow or "word" marker, indicating that the right side of patient was positioned up and away from the bed or cart, is present on the image.

- Place an arrow or "word" marker indicating which side of the patient was positioned away from the tabletop or cart and in the collimated field.

The abdomen demonstrates an AP projection. The right and left corresponding posterior ribs and the iliac wings are symmetrical.

- A decubitus abdominal image is obtained by placing the neonate or infant in a left lateral recumbent position on the bed or cart with the posterior surface resting against a vertical IR. Because intraperitoneal air migrates to the highest position, which is typically the elevated diaphragm, the left lateral position is chosen to position the gastric bubble away from the elevated diaphragm. To avoid rotation, align the shoulders, the posterior ribs, and the posterior pelvic wings perpendicular to the bed or cart (Figure 2-67).
- *Demonstrating intraperitoneal air:* The lateral decubitus position is primarily used to confirm the presence of intraperitoneal air. To best demonstrate intraperitoneal air, the patient should be left in this position for a few minutes to allow enough time for the air to move away from the soft-tissue abdominal structures and rise to the level of the right diaphragm.

- *Detecting abdominal rotation:* The upper and lower lumbar vertebrae can demonstrate rotation independently or simultaneously, depending on which section of the body is rotated. If the patient's thorax is rotated but the pelvis remains in an AP projection, the upper lumbar vertebrae and abdominal cavity demonstrate rotation. If the patient's pelvis is rotated but the thorax remains in an AP projection, the lower vertebrae and abdominal cavity demonstrate rotation. If the patient's thorax and pelvis are rotated simultaneously, the entire lumbar column and abdominal cavity demonstrate rotation.

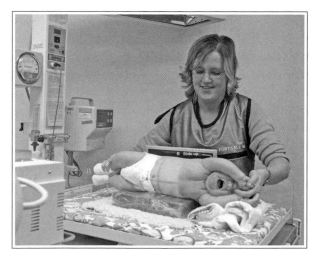

Figure 2-67. Proper patient positioning for lateral decubitus neonate and infant abdominal image.

Image labels for Figure 2-66: Intestinal gas, R ∧, Lumbar vertebra, Symphysis pubis, Iliac wing, Diaphragm, Posterior rib

Rotation is effectively detected on a decubitus abdominal image by comparing the symmetry of the posterior ribs and the iliac wings (see Image 65). The ribs that demonstrate the longer length and the iliac wing demonstrating the greater width are present on the side toward which the patient is rotated.

The image was taken on expiration. The diaphragm domes are superior to the eighth posterior rib.

- For neonates or infants being ventilated with a conventional ventilator, observe the ventilator's pressure manometer. The exposure should be taken when the manometer digital bar or analog needle moves to its highest position. If a high-frequency ventilator is being used, the exposure may be made at any time, because this ventilator maintains the lung expansion at a steady mean pressure without the bulk gas exchange of the conventional type.

  If the decubitus position is taken on inspiration, the inferior placement of the diaphragm puts pressure on the abdominal organs, resulting in less space in the peritoneal cavity and greater abdominal density.

The fourth lumbar vertebra is centered within the collimated field. The diaphragm and abdominal structures are included within the field.

- The decubitus abdominal position is most often used to evaluate the peritoneal cavity for intraperitoneal air. With the left lateral decubitus position, intraperitoneal air will rise to the highest level of the right hemidiaphragm, so it must be included (see Image 66).
- *IR size and centering:* With the neonate or infant positioned in a left lateral decubitus position, place an 8- × 10-inch (18- × 24-cm), lengthwise IR against the neonate or infant's posterior surface and position the abdomen in the middle of the IR. Center a horizontal central ray to the midsagittal plane at a transverse level 2 inches (5 cm) superior to the iliac crest. A larger IR and slightly inferior centering may be needed for larger infants. This IR and central ray placement centers the abdomen on the image, permitting tight collimation on all sides of the lungs. Open the longitudinal collimation to include the diaphragm (1 inch [2.5 cm]) inferior to the mammary line), and transversely collimate to within ½ inch (1.25 cm) of the lateral skinline.
- *Gonadal shielding:* Use gonadal shielding on all male abdominal images. Do not shield a female patient, because the shield may obscure needed information.

Neonate and Infant Lateral Decubitus Abdominal Image Analysis

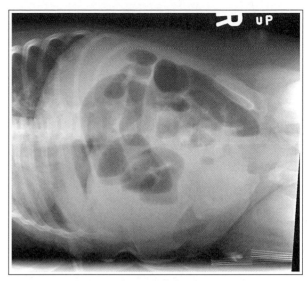

Image 65.

Analysis. The diaphragm is at the level of the eighth thoracic vertebra. The left posterior ribs are longer than the right, and the left iliac wing is wider than the right. The exposure was made after inspiration, and the patient was rotated toward the left side.

Correction. Take the exposure after patient exhales or manometer is at its lowest level, and rotate the patient toward the right side until the posterior ribs and the iliac wings are aligned perpendicular to the bed.

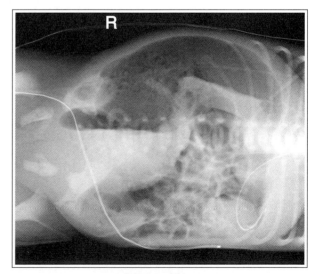

Image 66.

Analysis. The diaphragm is not included in its entirety. The central ray is positioned too inferiorly.

Correction. Move the central ray superiorly by ½ inch (1.25 cm).

CHILD ABDOMEN: LEFT LATERAL DECUBITUS POSITION (ANTEROPOSTERIOR PROJECTION)

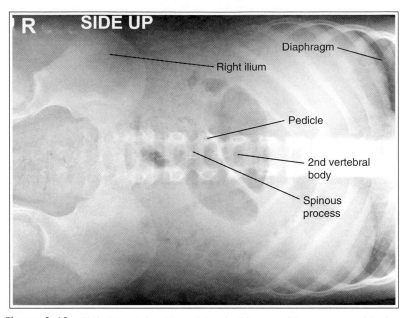

Figure 2-68. Child lateral decubitus abdominal image with accurate positioning.

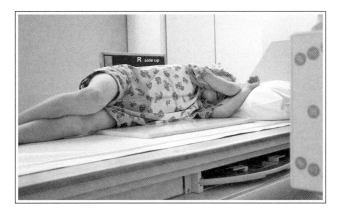

Figure 2-69. Proper positioning for a child lateral decubitus abdominal image.

Image Analysis

The analysis of the child lateral decubitus abdominal image is the same as that of the infant or adult lateral decubitus abdominal image, already discussed. The size of the child determines which criterion best meets the situation. For specifics on this topic, refer to the earlier discussion of infant lateral decubitus abdominal images or the discussion of adult AP abdominal images on p. 94.

Child Lateral Decubitus Abdominal Image Analysis

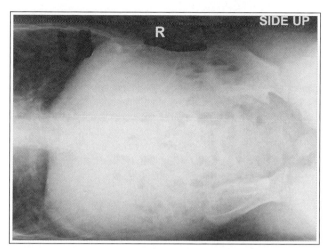

Image 67.

Analysis. The diaphragm is inferior to the tenth posterior rib, indicating that the examination was taken on inspiration.

Correction. Expose the image after patient has exhaled.

REFERENCE

1. Jeffrey B, Ralls P, Leung A, Brant-Zawadzke M: *Emergency imaging,* Philadelphia, 1999, Lippincott Williams & Wilkins.

CHAPTER 3

Image Analysis of the Upper Extremity

The following image analysis criteria are used for all upper extremity images and should be considered when completing the analysis.

Facility's identification requirements are visible on image as identified in Chapter 1.

A right or left marker, identifying the side being imaged, is present and is not superimposed on anatomy of interest. Specific placement of marker is as described in Chapter 1.

No evidence of preventable artifacts is present.

- If the patient's condition prevents removal, shift the artifact as far away from the affected area as possible and indicate the situation on the requisition (see Image 7).
- Consult with the ordering physician and the patient about whether bandages or splints can be removed.

The bony trabecular patterns and cortical outlines of the phalanx are sharply defined.

- Motion is the most common cause of poor definition on an image. Motion can be controlled by explaining the procedure so that the patient is aware of what is expected; by making the patient as comfortable as possible during the exam; and by using a short exposure time. When the patient is unable to control extremity movement, immobilization devices may be needed. Detail sharpness can also be increased by using a small focal spot and maintaining a short object–image receptor distance (OID). Increased spatial resolution is also obtained when the smallest image receptor (IR) is selected for digital images.

Contrast and density are adequate to demonstrate the surrounding soft-tissue and bony structures.

Penetration is sufficient to visualize the bony trabecular patterns and cortical outlines of the upper extremity.

- An optimal kilovolt-peak (kVp) technique (Table 3-1) sufficiently penetrates the bony and soft-tissue structures of the upper extremity and provides a contrast scale necessary to visualize the bony details. To obtain optimal density, set a manual milliampere per second (mAs) level based on the part thickness.

The long axis of the imaged structure is aligned with the long axis of the collimated field.

- Aligning the long axis of the imaged structure with the long axis of the collimator's longitudinal light line enables tight collimation without clipping needed anatomical structures.

TABLE 3-1	Upper Extremity Technical Data	
Part, Position, or Projection	**kVp**	**SID**
Finger	50-60	40-48 inches (100-120 cm)
Thumb	50-60	40-48 inches (100-120 cm)
PA projection, hand	50-60	40-48 inches (100-120 cm)
PA oblique position, hand	55-65	40-48 inches (100-120 cm)
Lateral position, hand	55-65	40-48 inches (100-120 cm)
Wrist	55-65	40-48 inches (100-120 cm)
Forearm	55-65	40-48 inches (100-120 cm)
Elbow	55-65	40-48 inches (100-120 cm)
Humerus	65-75	40-48 inches (100-120 cm)

kVp, Kilovolt peak; *PA*, posteroanterior; *SID*, source–image receptor distance.

FINGER: POSTEROANTERIOR PROJECTION

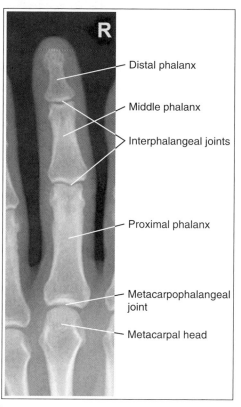

Distal phalanx

Middle phalanx

Interphalangeal joints

Proximal phalanx

Metacarpophalangeal joint

Metacarpal head

Figure 3-1. Posteroanterior finger image with accurate positioning.

Image Analysis

The finger demonstrates a posteroanterior (PA) projection. The soft-tissue width and the midpoint concavity are the same on both sides of the phalanges.

- Finger rotation is controlled by the amount of palm pronation. A PA projection is accomplished when the palm is positioned flat against the IR (Figure 3-2).

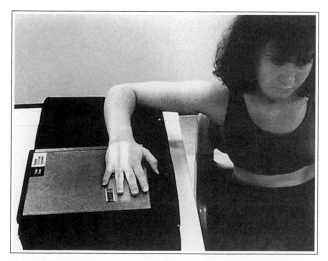

Figure 3-2. Proper patient positioning for posteroanterior finger image.

- *Detecting finger rotation:* Because the thumb prevents the hand from rotating laterally, medial rotation is the most common rotation error. Take a few minutes to study a finger skeleton, and note how the midpoints of the phalanges have equal side concavity when it is placed in a PA projection. Also note that the anterior surface is concave, whereas the posterior surface is slightly convex. As the skeleton is rotated internally or externally, the amount of concavity increases on the side toward which the anterior surface is rotated, whereas the side toward which the posterior surface rotates demonstrates less concavity. The same observations can be made about the soft tissue that surrounds the phalanges. More soft-tissue thickness is present on the anterior (palmar) hand surface than on the posterior surface, so the side demonstrating the greatest soft-tissue width on an image is the side toward which the anterior surface was rotated. Look for this midpoint concavity and soft-tissue width variation to indicate rotation on a finger image (see Image 1).

  Note on a hand skeleton that the second metacarpal is the longest of the finger digits and that the length decreases with each adjacent metacarpal. This knowledge can be used to determine whether the patient's finger was internally or externally rotated for a mispositioned PA finger image. If the finger was externally rotated, the aspect of the phalanges demonstrating the greater midpoint concavity faces the longer metacarpal (see Image 1). If the finger was internally rotated, the aspect of the phalanges demonstrating the greater midpoint concavity faces the shorter metacarpal.

No soft-tissue overlap from adjacent digits is present.

- Spreading the fingers slightly prevents soft-tissue overlapping from adjacent fingers. It is difficult to evaluate the soft tissue of an affected finger when superimposition of other soft tissue is present.

The interphalangeal (IP) and metacarpophalangeal (MP) joints are demonstrated as open spaces, and the phalanges are not foreshortened.

- The IP and MP joint spaces are open and the phalanges are not foreshortened if the finger is fully extended and the central ray is perpendicular and centered to the proximal IP (PIP) joint. This finger positioning and central ray placement align the joint spaces parallel with the central ray and perpendicular to the IR, as demonstrated in Figure 3-3, resulting in open joint spaces. It also prevents foreshortening of the phalanges, because their long axes are aligned parallel with the IR and perpendicular to the central ray. The alignment of the central ray and IR with the joint spaces and phalanges changes when the finger is flexed. In Figure 3-4, note how finger flexion causes the phalanges to foreshorten and be superimposed on the joint spaces (see Image 2).
- *Positioning the unextendable finger:* If the patient is unable to extend the finger, it may be necessary to use an anteroposterior (AP) projection to demonstrate open IP and MP joint spaces and to visualize the phalanges of greatest interest without foreshortening. In this case carefully evaluate the requisition to determine the phalanx and joint space of interest. Then supinate the patient's hand into an AP projection, elevating the proximal metacarpals until the phalanx of interest is parallel with the IR and the joint space of interest is perpendicular to the IR (Figure 3-5). Figures 3-6 and 3-7 demonstrate how patient positioning with respect to the central ray determines the anatomy that is visible. For Figure 3-6 the patient was imaged in a PA projection with fingers

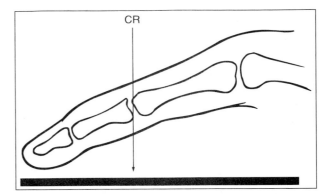

Figure 3-4. Poor alignment of joint space and central ray *(CR)*.

flexed. For Figure 3-7, the same patient was imaged in an AP projection with the proximal metacarpals elevated to place the affected proximal phalanges parallel with the IR. Note the difference in demonstration of the joint spaces and proximal phalanx fractures.

The PIP joint is at the center of the collimated field. The distal, middle, and proximal phalanges and half of the metacarpal are included within the field.

- Direct the central ray perpendicular to the PIP joint to place the joint in the center of the image. Open the longitudinal collimation to include the distal phalanx and the distal half of the metacarpal. Transverse collimation should be within $\frac{1}{2}$ inch (1.25 cm) of the finger skinline.
- One third of an 8- × 10-inch (18- × 24-cm) detailed screen-film or computed radiography IR placed crosswise should be adequate to include all the required anatomical structures. Digital imaging requires tight collimation, lead masking, and no overlap of individual exposures to produce optimal images.

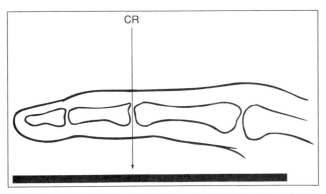

Figure 3-3. Accurate alignment of joint space and central ray *(CR)*.

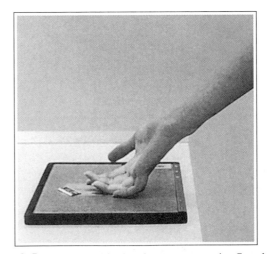

Figure 3-5. Patient positioning for anteroposterior flexed finger image.

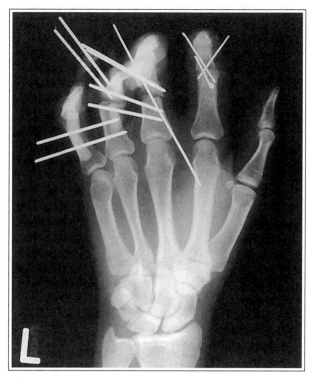

Figure 3-6. Posteroanterior projection with flexed fingers.

- Some facilities request that an unaffected adjacent digit be included on the image for comparison purposes. For a finger being imaged for the first time, some facilities want the entire metacarpal to be visualized on the image.

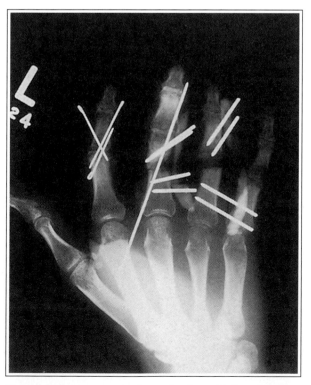

Figure 3-7. Anteroposterior projection with flexed fingers.

Posteroanterior Finger Image Analysis

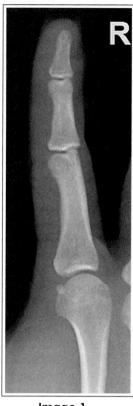

Image 1.

Analysis. The soft-tissue width and the concavity of the phalangeal midshafts on either side of the phalanx are not equal; the finger was rotated for the image. Because the side of the phalanges with the greater concavity and soft-tissue width is facing the longer metacarpal, the finger was rotated externally for the image.

Correction. Place the finger in a PA projection by rotating the finger slightly internally. The hand should be flat against the IR.

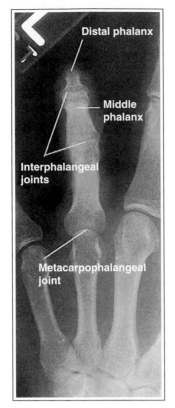

Image 2.

Analysis. The IP and MP joints are closed, and the distal and middle phalanges are foreshortened; the patient's finger was flexed.

Correction. Extend the patient's finger, and place the palm flat against the IR. If the patient is unable to extend the finger, image it in an AP projection, elevating the proximal metacarpals until the affected phalanx is parallel with the IR or the affected joint space is perpendicular to the IR (see Figure 3-5).

FINGER: POSTEROANTERIOR OBLIQUE PROJECTION

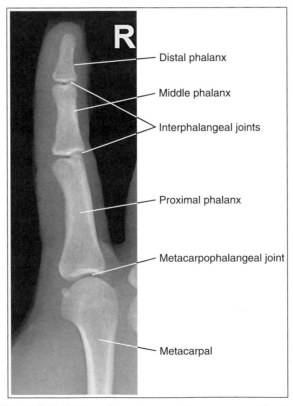

Figure 3-8. Oblique finger image with accurate positioning.

Image Analysis

The digit has been placed in a 45-degree oblique position. Twice as much soft-tissue width is demonstrated on one side of the digit as on the other side, and more concavity is demonstrated on one aspect of the phalangeal midshafts than on the other.

- An oblique finger position is accomplished by rotating the affected finger 45 degrees from the PA projection (Figure 3-9). It is most common and comfortable for a patient to rotate the finger and hand into an external oblique position for an oblique finger image, although an internal oblique position may be used when the second digit is imaged, to prevent a long OID.
- Examine a finger skeleton in a PA projection and in oblique and lateral positions. Note how the phalangeal midshaft concavity varies as the digit is rotated from a PA projection and that the anterior surface is concave whereas the posterior surface is slightly convex. As the skeleton is rotated internally or externally, the amount of concavity increases on the side toward which the anterior surface is rotated, whereas the side toward which the posterior surface is rotated will demonstrate less concavity. Similar observations can be made about the soft tissue that surrounds the phalanges. More soft-tissue thickness is present on the anterior (palmar) hand surface than the posterior surface, so the side demonstrating the greatest soft-tissue width on an image will be the side toward which the anterior surface is rotated.
- *Assessing accuracy of oblique positioning:* Study the amount of phalangeal midshaft concavity and soft-tissue width demonstrated on oblique finger images to verify the accuracy of rotation and to determine the proper repositioning movement needed when an oblique digit image shows too much or too little obliquity. A 45-degree oblique digit image demonstrates more phalangeal midshaft concavity and soft-tissue width on the side positioned away from the IR. Use the soft-tissue width to assess the degree of digital obliquity. If twice as much soft-tissue width is present on one side of the digit as on

the other, a 45-degree oblique position has been obtained. If the phalangeal midshaft concavity and soft-tissue width on both sides of the digit are more nearly equal, the finger was not rotated enough for the image (see Image 3). If the soft-tissue width on one side of the digit is more than twice as much as that on the other, and when one aspect of the phalangeal midshaft is concave but the other aspect is convex, the angle of obliquity was more than 45 degrees (see Image 4).

No soft-tissue overlap from adjacent digits is present.

- Slightly spread the patient's fingers to prevent overlapping of the adjacent finger's soft tissue onto that of affected finger. Superimposition of these soft tissues makes it difficult to evaluate the soft tissue of the affected finger (see Image 5).

The IP and MP joints are visualized as open spaces, and the phalanges are not foreshortened.

- The IP and MP joint spaces are open and the phalanges are not foreshortened if the finger is fully extended and positioned parallel with the IR and perpendicular to the central ray. When the hand and fingers are positioned obliquely, some of the fingers are no longer placed against the IR but are positioned at varying OIDs. In this position the distal phalanges naturally tilt toward the IR.

  To keep the affected finger parallel with the IR and to maintain open joint spaces, it may be necessary to place an immobilization device beneath the distal phalanx. This is especially true when the second and third digits are imaged, for they are at the greatest OID. It is also necessary to center a perpendicular central ray to the PIP joint to maintain open joint spaces. Failure to position the affected finger parallel with the IR and perpendicular to the central ray foreshortens the phalanges and closes the joint spaces (see Image 6).

The PIP joint is at the center of the collimated field. The distal, middle, and proximal phalanges and half of the metacarpal of the affected digit are included within the field.

- Direct a perpendicular central ray to the PIP joint to place it in the center of the image. Open the longitudinal collimation to include the distal phalanx and the distal half of the metacarpal. Transversely collimate to within ½ inch (1.25 cm) of the finger skinline.
- One third of an 8- × 10-inch (18- × 24-cm) detailed screen-film or computed radiography IR placed crosswise should be adequate to include all the required anatomical structures. Digital imaging requires tight collimation, lead masking, and no overlap of individual exposures to produce optimal images.
- Some facilities require an unaffected adjacent digit to be included on the image for comparison purposes. Also, for a finger being imaged for the first time, some facilities want the entire metacarpal to be visualized on the image.

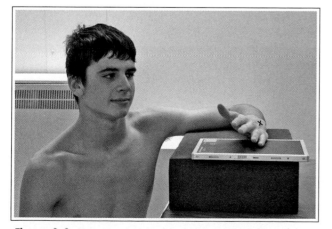

Figure 3-9. Proper patient positioning for oblique finger image.

Oblique Finger Image Analysis

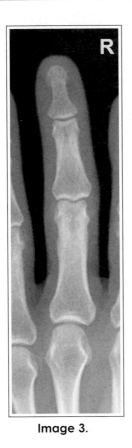

Image 3.

Analysis. On both sides of the phalanx the soft-tissue width and midshaft concavity are nearly equal; the patient's finger was positioned at less than 45 degrees of obliquity for the image.

Correction. Increase the finger obliquity to 45 degrees. Keep the finger parallel with the IR.

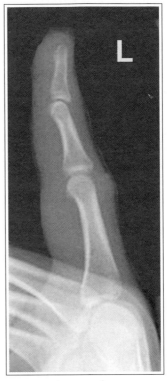

Image 4.

Analysis. More than twice as much soft-tissue width is present on one side of the phalanges as on the other. One aspect of the midshafts of the phalanges is concave, and the other aspect is slightly convex. Obliquity was more than 45 degrees for this image.

Correction. Decrease the finger obliquity to 45 degrees.

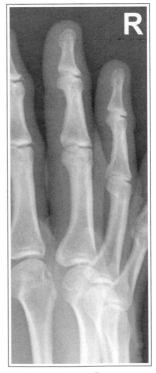

Image 5.

Analysis. Soft tissue from an adjacent digit is superimposed over the affected digit's soft tissue; fingers were not spread apart.

Correction. Spread the fingers until the adjacent fingers are positioned away from the affected finger.

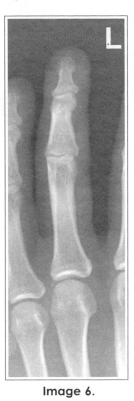

Image 6.

Analysis. The IP joint spaces are closed, and the distal and middle phalanges are foreshortened; the finger was not positioned parallel with the IR.

Correction. Position the finger parallel with the IR. It may be necessary to position an immobilization device beneath the distal phalanx to maintain accurate finger positioning. If the distal phalanx is of interest and the patient is unable to extend the finger, image it in a posterior oblique position, elevating the proximal metacarpals until the affected phalanx is aligned parallel with the IR and rotated 45 degrees.

FINGER: LATERAL POSITION

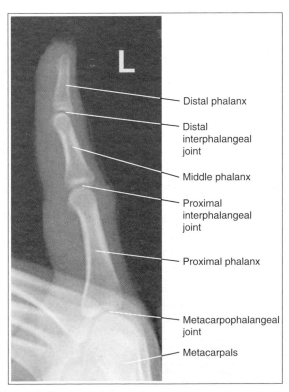

Figure 3-10. Lateral finger image with accurate positioning.

Image Analysis

The digit of interest is in a lateral position. The anterior aspect of the middle and proximal phalanges demonstrates midshaft concavity, and the posterior aspects of the phalanges show slight convexity.

- A lateral finger position is accomplished by rotating the affected finger 90 degrees from the PA projection (Figure 3-11). Whether the hand is rotated internally or externally to obtain this goal depends on which direction will bring the finger closer to the IR. Typically, when the second and third fingers are imaged the hand is rotated internally and when the fourth and fifth fingers are imaged the hand is rotated externally.
- *Distinguishing lateral position from rotated position:* To understand the difference between a truly lateral digit position and a position that is rotated, study a finger skeleton in lateral and anterior oblique positions. Note how the midshaft concavity of the middle and proximal phalanges varies as the digit is rotated. In a lateral position the anterior aspect of these phalanges is concave, but the posterior aspect demonstrates slight convexity. In an oblique position, both sides of the middle and proximal phalangeal midshafts demonstrate concavity, but the side toward which the anterior surface is rotated demonstrates a greater degree of concavity than the side toward which the posterior surface is rotated. The soft-tissue width at either side of the phalanx also changes in the lateral and oblique positions. More soft tissue is present on the side of the phalanges toward which the anterior surface is rotated (see Image 8).

No soft-tissue overlap from adjacent digits is present.

- Flex the unaffected fingers into a tight fist, allowing the finger of interest to remain extended. To visualize the proximal phalanx, it may be necessary to extend the affected finger with an immobilization device or to tape the unaffected fingers away from the affected finger.

If the unaffected fingers are not drawn away from the proximal phalanx of the affected finger, they will be superimposed on the area, preventing adequate visualization (see Image 7). An immobilization device should not be used if a fracture of this area is suspected and the device causes stress to the area.

The IP joints are visible as open spaces, and the phalanges are not foreshortened.

- The IP joints are open, and the phalanges are demonstrated without foreshortening as long as the finger was positioned parallel with the IR and the central ray was perpendicular to and centered with the PIP joint.
- When the third and fourth digits are imaged, they are positioned at a greater OID than the second and fifth digits. To keep the third and fourth digits parallel with the IR, it may be necessary to place an immobilization device beneath their distal phalanges. When a finger is not positioned parallel with the IR and perpendicular to the central ray, the IP joint spaces are closed and the phalanges are foreshortened.

The PIP joint is at the center of the collimated field. The distal, middle, and proximal phalanges and the metacarpal head of the affected digit are included within the field.

- Center a perpendicular central ray to the PIP joint to place it in the center of the image. Open the longitudinal collimation to include the distal phalanx and the metacarpal head. Transversely collimate to within ½ inch (1.25 cm) of the finger skinline.
- One third of an 8- × 10-inch (18- × 24-cm) detailed screen-film or computed radiography IR placed crosswise should be adequate to include all the required anatomical structures. Digital imaging requires tight collimation, lead masking, and no overlap of individual exposures to produce optimal images.

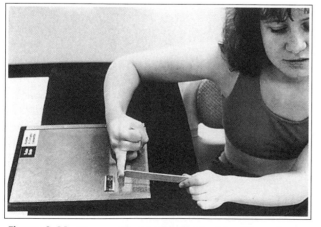

Figure 3-11. Proper patient positioning for lateral finger image.

Lateral Finger Image Analysis

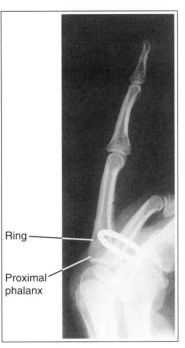

Image 7.

Image 8.

Analysis. The unaffected fingers were not flexed enough to prevent soft-tissue or bony superimposition of the affected digit's proximal phalanx. An unaffected finger has a ring artifact that is superimposed over the digit of interest.

Correction. Tightly flex the unaffected fingers away from the affected finger. Hyperextending the affected finger with an immobilization prop may also help to increase demonstration of the proximal phalanx if a fracture of this area is not suspected. Remove the ring if possible.

Analysis. Concavity is demonstrated on both sides of the middle and proximal phalangeal midshafts, indicating that the finger was not adequately rotated for this image.

Correction. Increase the degree of finger rotation until the finger is in a lateral position.

THUMB: ANTEROPOSTERIOR PROJECTION

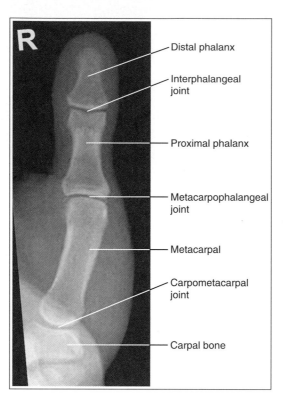

Figure 3-12. Anteroposterior thumb image with accurate positioning.

Image Analysis

The first digit demonstrates an AP projection. The concavity on both sides of the phalangeal and metacarpal midshafts is equal, as is soft-tissue width on both sides of the phalanges.

- An AP projection is accomplished by internally rotating the patient's hand until the thumb is positioned in an AP projection (Figure 3-13). The thumbnail can be used as a reference to determine when the thumb is truly positioned anteroposteriorly. The nail should be positioned directly against the IR and should not be visible on either side of the thumb. A nonrotated AP thumb image demonstrates equal concavity on both sides of the phalangeal and metacarpal midshafts as well as equal soft-tissue widths on both sides of the phalanges.

- *Detecting thumb rotation:* When the thumb is rotated away from an AP projection, the amount of midshaft concavity increases on the side of the thumb toward which the anterior surface rotates and decreases on the side toward which the posterior surface rotates. The same observation can be made about the soft tissue surrounding the phalanges when the thumb is rotated. More soft-tissue width is evident on the side toward which the anterior surface is rotated, and less soft-tissue width is seen on the side toward which the posterior surface is rotated (see Image 9).

The long axis of the thumb is aligned with the long axis of the collimated field.

- Aligning the long axis of the thumb with the long axis of the collimator's longitudinal light line enables you to collimate tightly without clipping the distal phalanx or proximal metacarpal (see Image 10).

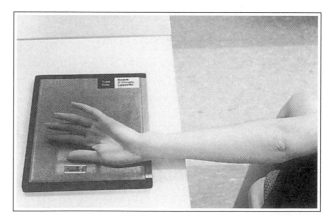

Figure 3-13. Proper patient positioning for anteroposterior thumb image.

The IP, MP, and carpometacarpal (CM) joints are visible as open joint spaces, and the phalanges are not foreshortened.

- The IP, MP, and CM joint spaces are open, and the phalanges are demonstrated without foreshortening as long as the thumb is positioned flat against and placed parallel with the IR and the central ray was perpendicular to and centered with the MP joint space. This positioning aligns the joint spaces parallel with the central ray and perpendicular to the IR and positions the long axes of the distal phalanges perpendicular to the central ray and parallel with the IR. These relationships change when the thumb is flexed or extended for the image. Thumb flexion and extension foreshortens the phalanges and superimposes them over the joint spaces (see Image 11).

Superimposition of the medial palm soft tissue over the proximal first metacarpal and the CM joint is minimal.

- When the thumb is in an AP projection, the medial palm soft tissue is superimposed over the proximal first metacarpal and the CM joint. Only a small amount of this soft-tissue overlap occurs when the medial palm surface is drawn away from the thumb. It may be necessary to use the patient's other hand as an immobilization device to maintain good positioning of the medial palmar surface. If the medial surface of the palm is not drawn away from the thumb, the soft tissue and possibly the fourth and fifth metacarpals obscure the proximal first metacarpal and CM joint (see Image 12).
- *Evaluating a PA thumb image:* The principles of AP thumb image analysis can be used to evaluate a PA projection thumb image (Figure 3-14), with the following modifications. First, the medial palm soft tissue does not overlap the proximal first metacarpal and CM joint. Second, on a PA projection, the CM joint is closed.

The MP joint is at the center of the collimated field. The distal and proximal phalanges, the metacarpal, and the CM joint are included within the field.

- Center a perpendicular central ray to the MP joint, which is located where the palm's interconnecting skin attaches to the thumb, to place it in the center of the image. Open the longitudinal collimation to include the distal phalanx and CM joint. Transversely collimate to within 1/2 inch (1.25 cm) of the thumb skinline.
- One third of an 8- × 10-inch (18- × 24-cm) detailed screen-film or computed radiography IR placed crosswise should be adequate to include all the required anatomical structures. Digital imaging requires tight collimation, lead masking, and no overlap of individual exposures to produce optimal images.

Anteroposterior Thumb Image Analysis

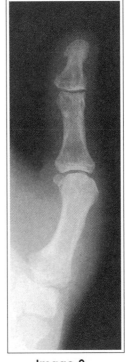

Image 9.

Analysis. The soft-tissue width and the concavity of the phalangeal and metacarpal midshafts are not the same on both sides. The side next to the fingers demonstrates more concavity. The hand was internally rotated too far, demonstrating the thumb in an oblique position.

Correction. Decrease the internal hand rotation until the thumb is in an AP projection. The thumbnail should be resting against the IR and should not be visible on either side of the thumb.

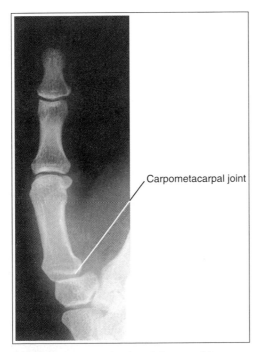

Carpometacarpal joint

Figure 3-14. Posteroanterior thumb image with accurate positioning.

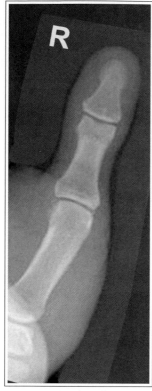

Image 10.

Analysis. The long axis of the thumb is not aligned with the long axis of the collimated field. Note that the proximal metacarpal and the CM joint are clipped.

Correction. Align the long axis of the thumb with the long axis of the collimated field.

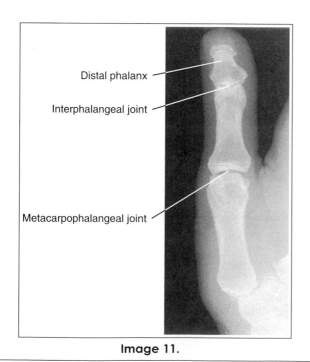

Image 11.

Analysis. The distal phalanx is foreshortened, and the IP joint space is closed. The distal thumb was flexed or extended.

Correction. Position the thumb flat against and parallel with the IR.

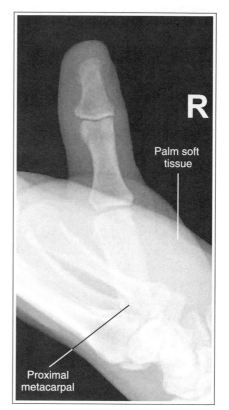

Image 12.

Analysis. The fifth metacarpal and the medial palm soft tissue are superimposed over the proximal first metacarpal and CM joint. The medial metacarpal and palmar surface have not been drawn away from the thumb.

Correction. Using the patient's other hand or another immobilization device, draw the medial side of the hand and palmar surface away from the thumb. Make sure that the thumb does not rotate away from an AP projection with this movement and that the patient's opposite hand is not included in the collimated field.

THUMB: LATERAL POSITION

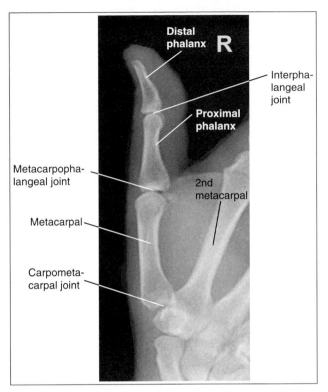

Figure 3-15. Lateral thumb image with accurate positioning.

Image Analysis

The thumb demonstrates a lateral position. The anterior aspect of the proximal phalanx and metacarpal demonstrates midshaft concavity, and the posterior aspect of the proximal phalanx and metacarpal demonstrates slight convexity.

- To accomplish lateral thumb positioning, place the patient's hand flat against the IR; then flex the hand and fingers only until the thumb naturally rolls into a lateral position (Figure 3-16). Overflexion causes superimposition of the second and third proximal metacarpals onto the proximal first metacarpal, obscuring it (see Image 13). When the hand and fingers are accurately flexed and the thumb is in a lateral position, the midshaft of the proximal phalanx and metacarpal demonstrates concavity on their anterior aspects and convexity on their posterior aspects. If the patient's hand is not rotated enough to place the thumb in a lateral position, the posterior aspects of these midshafts show some degree of concavity (see Image 14).

The IP, MP, and CM joints are visible as open spaces, and the phalanges are not foreshortened.

- The IP, MP, and CM joints are open and the phalanges are visible without foreshortening if the entire thumb

rests against and is positioned parallel with the IR and a perpendicular central ray is centered to the MP joint.

The proximal first metacarpal is only slightly superimposed by the proximal second metacarpal.

- Whenever possible, the anatomical part of interest should be demonstrated without superimposition. For a lateral thumb image, the proximal metacarpal can be demonstrated with

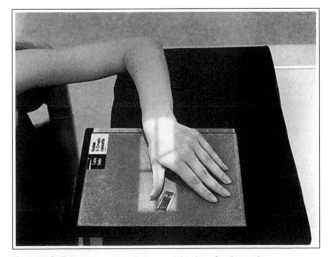

Figure 3-16. Proper patient positioning for lateral thumb image.

only a very small amount of superimposition if the thumb is abducted away from the palm. Failure to abduct the thumb results in a significant amount of first and second proximal metacarpal overlap and obstruction of the CM joint (see Image 15).

The first MP joint is at the center of the collimated field. The distal and proximal phalanges, the metacarpal, and the CM joint are included within the field.

- Center a perpendicular central ray to the MP joint, which is located where the palm's interconnecting skin attaches to the thumb, to place it in the center of the image. Open the longitudinal collimation to include the distal phalanx and CM joint. Transversely collimate to within $\frac{1}{2}$ inch (1.25 cm) of the thumb skinline.
- One third of an 8- × 10-inch (18- × 24-cm) detailed screen-film or computed radiography IR placed crosswise should be adequate to include all the required anatomical structures. Digital imaging requires tight collimation, lead masking, and no overlap of individual exposures to produce optimal images.

Lateral Thumb Image Analysis

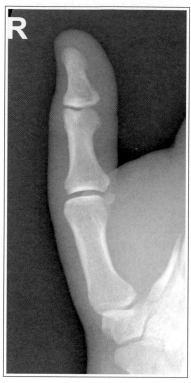

Image 14.

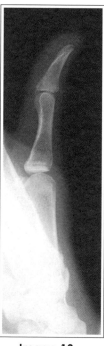

Image 13.

Analysis. The second and third proximal metacarpals are superimposed over the first proximal metacarpal. The hand was overflexed.

Correction. Abduct the thumb away from the hand, and decrease the amount of hand flexion while maintaining a lateral thumb position.

Analysis. The thumb is not in a lateral position. The posterior aspect of the proximal phalanx and metacarpal midshafts demonstrate concavity, indicating that the hand was not adequately flexed.

Correction. Increase the degree of hand flexion until the thumb rolls into a lateral position.

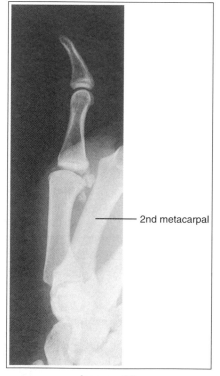

2nd metacarpal

Image 15.

Analysis. The proximal metacarpal is superimposed by the proximal second metacarpal. The thumb was not abducted.

Correction. Abduct the thumb.

THUMB: POSTEROANTERIOR OBLIQUE PROJECTION

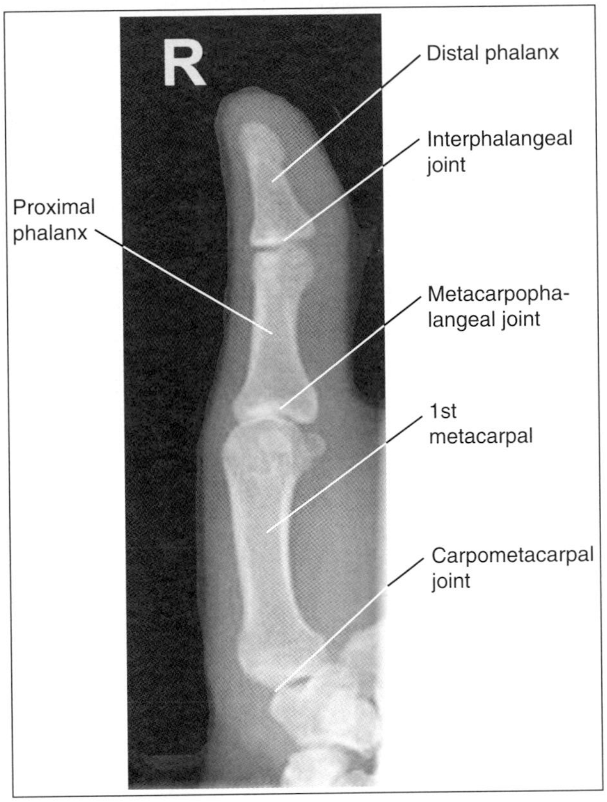

R

Distal phalanx

Interphalangeal joint

Proximal phalanx

Metacarpophalangeal joint

1st metacarpal

Carpometacarpal joint

Figure 3-17. Oblique thumb image with accurate positioning.

Image Analysis

The thumb is in a 45-degree oblique position. Twice as much soft tissue and more phalangeal and metacarpal midshaft concavity are present on the side of the thumb next to the fingers than on the other side.

- When the hand is extended and the palmar surface is placed flat against the IR, the thumb is rotated into a 45-degree lateral oblique position (Figure 3-18). In this position, more midshaft concavity is present on one side of the phalanges and metacarpal than on the other side. If the hand is not placed flat against the IR, the thumb rolls toward a lateral position. The more flexed the fingers are, the closer the thumb is to a lateral position. Such positioning can be identified on an image by noting the concavity of the anterior aspect and the convexity of the posterior aspect of the proximal phalanx and metacarpal (see Image 16).

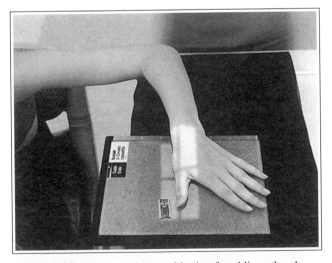

Figure 3-18. Proper patient positioning for oblique thumb image.

The long axis of the thumb is aligned with the long axis of the collimated field.

- Aligning the long axis of the thumb with the long axis of the collimation light field enables you to collimate tightly without clipping the distal phalanx or proximal metacarpal (see Image 17).

The IP, MP, and CM joints are visible as open joint spaces, and the phalanges are not foreshortened.

- The IP, MP, and CM joint spaces are open and the metacarpal and phalanges are visible without foreshortening when the first proximal metacarpal palmar surface remains flat against the IR. If the hand is medially rotated, the palmar surface is lifted off the IR, causing the thumb to tilt downward. The downward tilt closes the IP and MP joint spaces and foreshortens the phalanges (see Image 18).

The first MP joint is at the center of the collimated field. The distal and proximal phalanges, metacarpal, and CM joint are included within the field.

- Center a perpendicular central ray to the MP joint, which is located where the palmar interconnecting skin attaches to the thumb, to place it in the center of the image. Open the longitudinal collimation to include the distal phalanx and CM joint. Transversely collimate to within ½ inch (1.25 cm) of the thumb skinline.
- One third of an 8- × 10-inch (18- × 24-cm) detailed screen-film or computed radiography IR placed crosswise should be adequate to include all the required anatomical structures.

Oblique Thumb Image Analysis

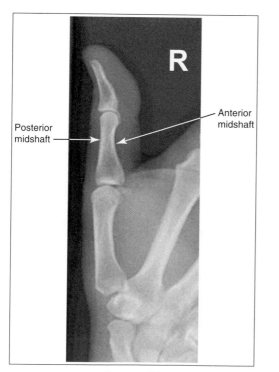

Image 16.

Analysis. The midshafts of the proximal phalanx and metacarpal demonstrate slight convexity on their posterior surfaces and concavity on their anterior surfaces. The thumb was positioned at more than 45 degrees of obliquity. The patient's palm was not placed flat against the IR.

Correction. Extend the patient's hand and place the palm flat against the IR.

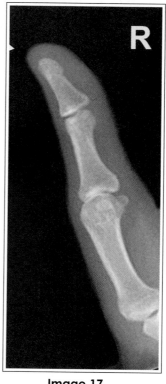

Image 17.

Analysis. The long axis of the thumb is not aligned with the long axis of the collimated field. Note that the proximal metacarpal and the CM joint are partially clipped.

Correction. Align the long axis of the thumb with the long axis of the collimation field.

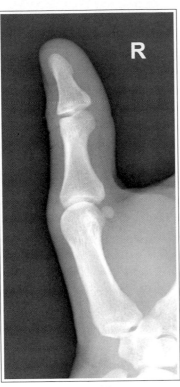

Image 18.

Analysis. The IP and MP joints are closed, and the phalanges are foreshortened. The lateral aspect of the palmar surface was not positioned against the IR, and the thumb was tilting down toward the IR.

Correction. Place the palmar surface and thumb against the IR.

HAND: POSTEROANTERIOR PROJECTION

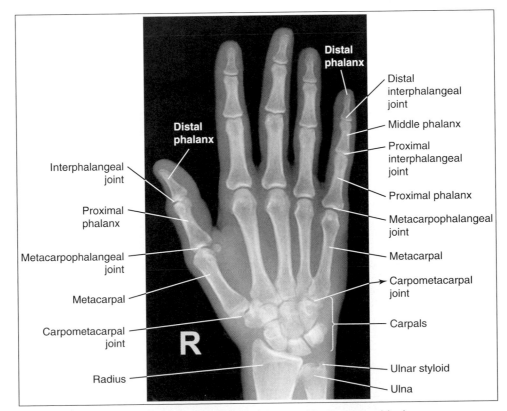

Figure 3-19. Posteroanterior hand image with accurate positioning.

Image Analysis

The digits and metacarpals demonstrate a PA projection. The soft-tissue outlines of the second through fifth phalanges are uniform, the distance between the metacarpal heads is equal, and the same midshaft concavity is demonstrated on both sides of the phalanges and metacarpals of the second through fifth digits.

- A PA projection of the hand is obtained when the patient fully extends the hand and rests the palmar surface (pronation) flat against the IR (Figure 3-20).
- *PA versus external oblique hand position:* If the hand is not fully extended but is slightly flexed, it often relaxes into an external oblique position when it is resting against the IR. A medial oblique hand image is signified by slight superimposition of the third through fifth metacarpal heads and unequal soft-tissue thickness and midshaft concavity on the sides of the phalanges. The metacarpals also show unequal midshaft concavity and spacing (see Image 19). Abducting the patient's arm and placing the forearm and humerus on the same horizontal plane, with the elbow flexed 90 degrees, assists in preventing a medial oblique position. When the patient has been positioned in this manner, the ulnar styloid appears in profile on the image. Internal rotation of the hand is seldom a problem, because the thumb prevents this movement.

No soft-tissue overlap of adjacent digits is present.

- Fingers should be spread slightly to prevent soft-tissue overlapping.

The IP, MP, and CM joints are visible as open spaces, and the phalanges and metacarpals are not foreshortened. The thumb is demonstrated in a 45-degree oblique position.

- When the hand and fingers are fully extended and a perpendicular central ray is centered to the third MP joint space, the phalanges and metacarpals are aligned parallel with and the joints spaces perpendicular to the IR and the phalanges and metacarpals are aligned perpendicular to the joint spaces and parallel with the central ray. These alignments result in the IP, MP, and CM joints demonstrated as open spaces and the phalanges and metacarpals seen without foreshortening on the PA hand image.

- Flexion of the hand causes poor alignment of the phalanges, metacarpals and IP and CM joint spaces with the IR and central ray, resulting in closed joint spaces and foreshortening of the phalanges and metacarpals (see Image 20). The position of the first digit also changes when the image is taken with the hand flexed, because flexion rotates the first digit into a lateral position.

The third MP joint is at the center of the collimated field. The distal, middle, and proximal phalanges, the metacarpals, the carpals, and approximately 1 inch (2.5 cm) of the distal radius and ulna are included within the field.

- Center a perpendicular central ray to the third MP joint to place it in the center of the collimated light field. This MP joint is situated just slightly distal to the head of the third metacarpal. Once the central ray is centered, open the longitudinal collimation to include the distal phalanx and 1 inch (2.5 cm) of the distal forearm. Transversely collimate to within $\frac{1}{2}$ inch (1.25 cm) of the first and fifth finger's skinline.

- Either one half of a 10- × 12-inch (24- × 30-cm) detailed screen-film IR placed crosswise or a single 8- × 10-inch (18- × 24-cm) digital IR placed lengthwise should be adequate to include all the required anatomical structures.

- *Pediatric bone age assessment:* A bone-age image is obtained to assess the skeletal versus the chronological age of a child. Because bones develop in an orderly pattern, skeletal age may be assessed from infancy through adolescence. Illness, metabolic or endocrine dysfunction, and taking certain types of medications and therapies are all reasons why a pediatric patient's skeletal and chronological age may not correspond. A left PA hand and wrist image is typically the image of choice because bony developmental changes are readily visible and easily evaluated. For skeletal age to be evaluated, the phalanges, metacarpals, carpals, and distal radius and ulna must be included in their entirety (see Figure 1-21, page 13).

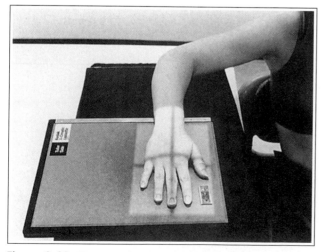

Figure 3-20. Proper patient positioning for posteroanterior hand image.

Posteroanterior Hand Image Analysis

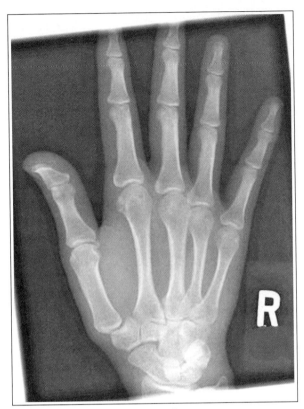

Image 19.

Analysis. The hand was externally rotated (in a medial oblique position), as indicated by the superimposition of the third and fourth metacarpal heads, the unequal midshaft concavity on either side of the phalanges and metacarpals, and the uneven spacing of the metacarpal heads. The tip of the second and third fingers has been collimated off, and less than 1 inch (2.5 cm) of the distal radius and ulna is included.

Correction. Internally rotate the hand until the palm and fingers are placed flat against the IR, and open the longitudinally collimated field to include the second and third fingertips and 1 inch (2.5 cm) of the distal radius and ulna.

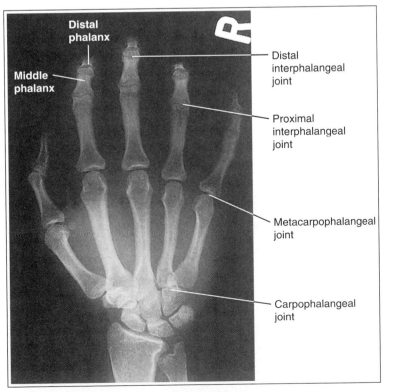

Image 20.

Analysis. The IP and CM joints are closed, and the phalanges and metacarpals are foreshortened. The first digit demonstrates a lateral position. The hand and fingers were flexed for this image.

Correction. Fully extend the patient's hand and fingers, then place them flat against the IR.

HAND: POSTEROANTERIOR OBLIQUE PROJECTION (EXTERNAL ROTATION)

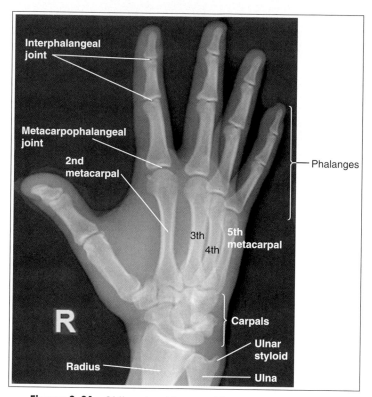

Figure 3-21. Oblique hand image with accurate positioning.

Image Analysis

**The hand has been externally rotated 45 degrees.
Each of the second through fifth metacarpal midshafts
demonstrate more concavity on one side than on the
other and have varying amounts of space between them.
The first and second metacarpal heads are not superimposed, and the third through fifth metacarpal heads
are slightly superimposed, and a slight space is present
between the fourth and fifth metacarpal midshafts.**

- To accomplish a medial oblique hand position, begin
  with the hand in a PA projection. Then, externally rotate
  the hand until it forms a 45-degree angle with the IR
  (Figure 3-22).
- To confirm the 45-degree angle, it is best to image the
  hand and not the wrist. The wrist will demonstrate more
  than 45 degrees of obliquity when the hand is in a
  45-degree oblique position, so using the wrist can result
  in a miscalculation of the amount of obliquity. This is
  especially true if the humerus and forearm have not been
  placed on the same horizontal plane. When the patient
  has been positioned with the arm on the same horizontal
  plane, the ulnar styloid is demonstrated in profile medially on the image. A radiolucent immobilization device
  can be used to help maintain this position.
- *Verifying oblique hand position:* A 45-degree oblique
  hand image can be recognized by the amount of

metacarpal midshaft and metacarpal head superimposition. If the hand has not been rotated enough, the
metacarpal relationship is similar to that demonstrated on
a PA projection image of the hand: The midshafts of the
metacarpals are nearly evenly spaced, and the metacarpal
heads are not superimposed (see Image 21). On a
45-degree oblique hand image a space should be maintained between the fourth and fifth metacarpal midshafts.
If the hand is rotated more than 45 degrees, this space is

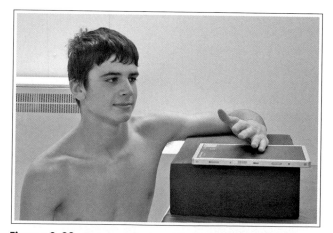

Figure 3-22. Proper patient positioning for oblique hand
image with extended fingers.

obscured and the fourth and fifth metacarpals demonstrate some degree of superimposition (see Image 22).

No soft-tissue overlap of adjacent digits is present.

- Fingers should be spread slightly to prevent soft-tissue overlapping (see Image 23).

The IP and MP joints are visible as open spaces, and the phalanges are demonstrated without foreshortening. The thumb's position may vary from a lateral to an oblique position.

- The IP and MP joint spaces are open and the phalanges are not foreshortened when the hand and fingers are fully extended and aligned parallel with the IR. An immobilization device should be used to help the patient maintain this positioning.
- *Disadvantages of using fingers as props:* A common positioning error in oblique hand imaging is to use the patient's fingers instead of an immobilization device to maintain the oblique position. For this positioning, the fingers are flexed until the fingertips touch the IR to prop the hand for the oblique position (Figure 3-23). Such positioning closes the IP joint spaces and foreshortens the phalanges (see Images 22 and 24).

The third MP joint is at the center of the collimated field. The distal, middle, and proximal phalanges, the metacarpals, the carpals, and approximately 1 inch (2.5 cm) of the distal radius and ulna are included within the field.

- Center a perpendicular central ray to the third MP joint to place it in the center of the collimated light field. The MP joint is situated just slightly distal to the head of the third metacarpal. Once the central ray is centered, open the longitudinal collimation to include the distal phalanges and the distal forearm. Transversely collimate to within ½ inch (1.25 cm) of the first and fifth finger's skinline.

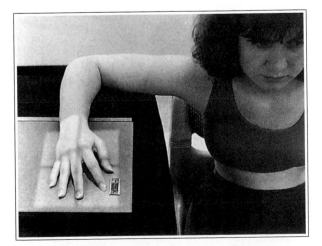

Figure 3-23. Proper patient positioning for oblique hand image with flexed fingers.

- Either one half of a 10- × 12-inch (24- × 30-cm) detailed screen-film IR placed crosswise or a single 8- × 10-inch (18- × 24-cm) digital IR placed lengthwise should be adequate to include all the required anatomical structures.

Oblique Hand Image Analysis

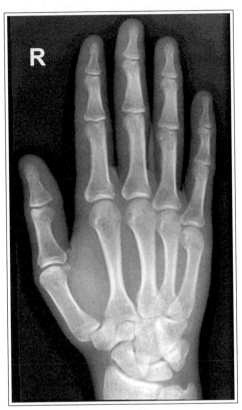

Image 21.

Analysis. The metacarpal heads demonstrate only slight superimposition, the metacarpal midshaft concavities are fairly uniform, and the spaces between the metacarpal midshafts are nearly equal. The hand was not rotated enough.

Correction. Externally rotate the hand until the metacarpals and the IR form a 45-degree angle.

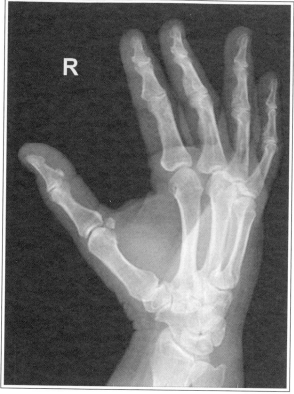

Image 22.

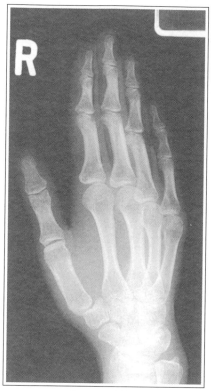

Image 23.

Analysis. The midshafts of the third through fifth metacarpals are superimposed. The patient's hand was placed at more than 45 degrees of obliquity. The phalanges are foreshortened, and the IP joints spaces are closed. The fingers were not positioned parallel with the IR, but instead were used to prop the hand (see Figure 3-23).

Correction. Internally rotate the hand until the metacarpals and the IR form a 45-degree angle and extend the fingers, placing them parallel with the IR.

Analysis. Soft-tissue and bony structure overlap of the digits is present. The fingers were not spread apart.

Correction. Spread all fingers enough to prevent soft-tissue overlap.

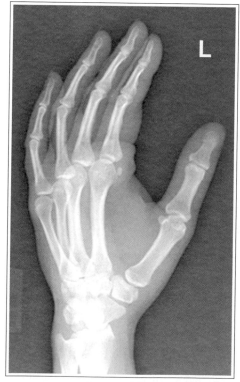

Image 24.

Analysis. The distal and middle phalanges are foreshortened, and the IP joint spaces are closed. The fingers were not positioned parallel with the IR, but were instead used to prop the hand (see Figure 3-23).

Correction. Extend the fingers and place them parallel with the IR. It may be necessary to situate an immobilization device beneath the fingers to maintain this positioning.

HAND: "FAN" LATERAL POSITION (LATEROMEDIAL PROJECTION)

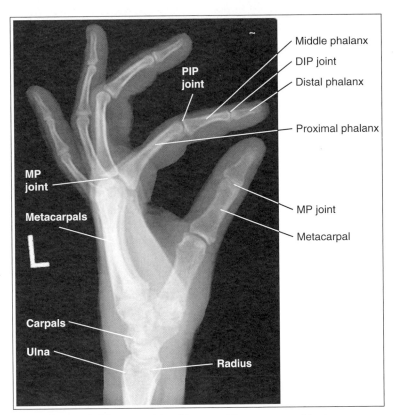

Figure 3-24. Lateral hand image with accurate positioning.

Image Analysis

Density is adequate to demonstrate the surrounding metacarpal soft tissue and bony structures of the hand.

- For the "fan" lateral hand image, it is difficult to simultaneously demonstrate the phalanges and the metacarpals with optimal density because of the difference in thickness between the two body parts when the fingers are separated. Evaluate the requisition to determine what anatomy of the hand is of interest so the mAs can be adjusted to obtain optimal density in that area.

The second through fifth digits are separated, demonstrating little superimposition of the proximal bony or soft-tissue structures. The thumb is demonstrated without superimposition of the other digits. Its position may vary from a PA projection to a slightly oblique position.

- For a lateral hand position, place the medial hand surface resting against the IR; then fan or spread the fingers as far apart as possible without superimposing the thumb. The fingers are fanned most effectively by drawing the second and third fingers anteriorly and the fourth and fifth fingers posteriorly. The amount of finger separation obtained will depend on the patient's mobility (Figure 3-25). Immobilization devices are available to help maintain proper positioning. When the fingers are fanned, they can be individually studied. If the fingers are not adequately separated, they superimpose one another on the image (see Image 25).

The second through fifth metacarpals are superimposed.

- Superimpose the second through fifth metacarpals by palpating the patient's knuckles and placing them directly on top of one another.
- *Verifying a lateral hand position:* On a lateral hand image a true lateral wrist position, represented by superimposition of the ulna and radius, is not always accomplished when the metacarpal midshafts are superimposed. Instead, the ulna is demonstrated slightly posterior to the radius.

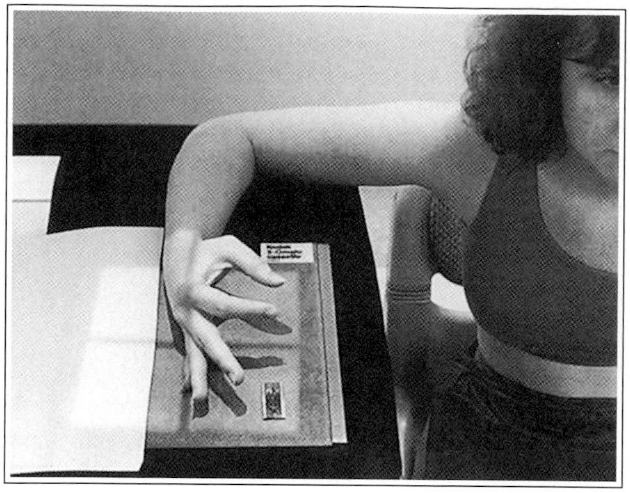

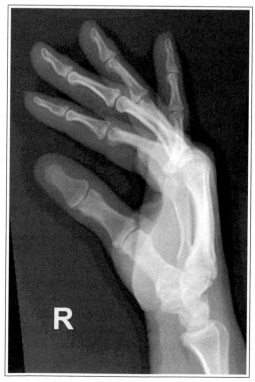

Figure 3-25. Proper patient positioning for lateral hand image.

Because of this variation, a true lateral position of the hand should be determined by judging the degree of superimposition of the second through fifth metacarpal midshafts and not the degree of ulnar and radial super-imposition. If the metacarpal midshafts are not superimposed and the fifth metacarpal is demonstrated anterior to the second through fourth metacarpals, the hand was slightly externally rotated or supinated (see Image 25). The fifth metacarpal can be identified by its length; it is the shortest of the second through fifth metacarpals. If the metacarpal midshafts are not superim-posed and the second metacarpal is demonstrated anterior to the third through fifth metacarpals, the hand was slightly internally rotated or pronated (see Image 26). The second metacarpal can also be identified by its length: it is the longest.

The IP joints are open, and the phalanges are not foreshortened.

- The IP joint spaces are open and the phalanges are visible without foreshortening when the thumb is depressed and positioned parallel with the IR.

The MP joints are at the center of the collimated field. The distal, middle, and proximal phalanges, the metacarpals, the carpals, and approximately 1 inch (2.5 cm) of the distal radius and ulna are included within the field.

- Center a perpendicular central ray to the second MP joint to place it in the center of the collimated light field. Once the central ray is centered, open the longi-tudinal collimation to include the distal phalanges and the distal forearm. Transversely collimate to within ½ inch (1.25 cm) of the first and fifth finger's skinline.
- Either one half of a 10- × 12-inch (24- × 30-cm) detailed screen-film IR placed crosswise or a single 8- × 10-inch (18- × 24-cm) screen-film or computed radiography IR placed lengthwise should be adequate to include all the required anatomical structures.

OPTIONAL DIGIT POSITIONING: lateral hand in extension

The second through fifth digits are fully extended and superimposed. (See Image 27.) Density of the second through fifth digits and metacarpals is uniform, but the first metacarpal density is overexposed. The positioning analysis for the metacarpals is the same as for the "fan" lateral image.

- Extending the hand and fingers until they are aligned on the same plane places the hand in extension. It has been suggested that foreign bodies of the palm can be better localized when the lateral hand image is taken in extension.

OPTIONAL DIGIT POSITIONING: lateral hand in flexion

The second through fifth digits are flexed and superimposed (see Image 28).

Density of the second through fifth digits and metacarpals is uniform, but the first metacarpal density is overexposed. The positioning for the metacarpals is the same as for the "fan" lateral image.

- Flex the second through fifth fingers until they meet the first finger but do not superimpose it. It has been sug-gested that this position of the lateral hand is used to distinguish the degree of anterior or posterior displace-ment of a fractured metacarpal.

Lateral Hand Image Analysis

Image 25.

Analysis. The second through fifth metacarpal midshafts are not superimposed, and the shortest (fifth) metacarpal is anterior to the third through fourth metacarpals. The hand was externally rotated or supinated. This image may also result if the central ray was positioned anterior to the MP joints to increase transverse collimation.

Correction. Internally rotate or pronate the patient's hand until the metacarpals are superimposed. Center the central ray to the MP joints.

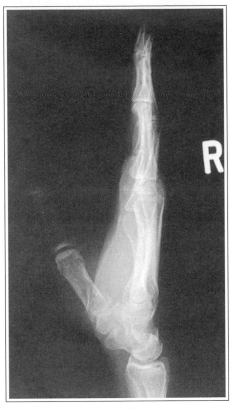

Image 27.

Analysis. The digits are superimposed. This image was taken with the hand and fingers in full extension.

Correction. If an extension lateral hand image is desired, no correction is required. If a "fan" lateral hand image is desired, fan or spread the fingers as far apart as possible by drawing the second and third fingers anteriorly and the fourth and fifth fingers posteriorly.

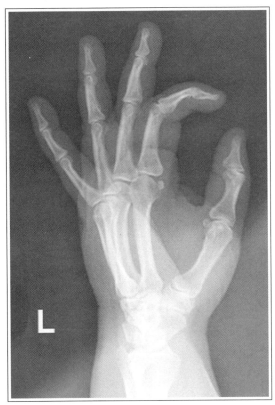

Image 26.

Analysis. The second through fifth metacarpal midshafts are not superimposed, and the longest (second) metacarpal is anterior to the third through fifth metacarpals. The hand was internally rotated or pronated.

Correction. Externally rotate or supinate the patient's hand until the metacarpals are superimposed.

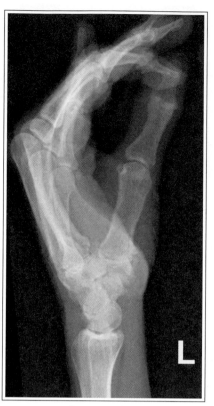

Image 28.

Analysis. The digits are superimposed. This image was taken with the hand and fingers flexed.

Correction. If a flexed lateral hand image was desired, no correction is required. If a "fan" lateral hand was desired, fan or spread the fingers as far apart as possible by drawing the second and third fingers anteriorly and the fourth and fifth fingers posteriorly.

WRIST: POSTEROANTERIOR PROJECTION

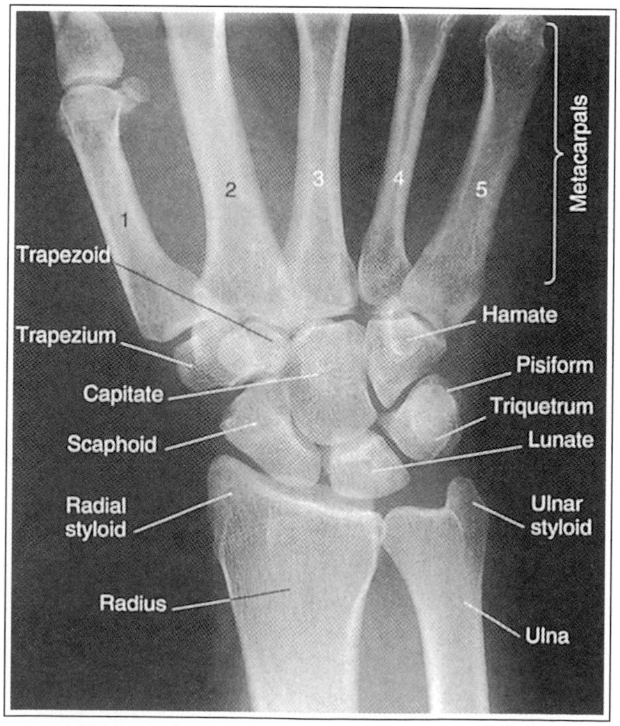

Figure 3-26. Posteroanterior wrist image with accurate positioning.

Image Analysis

Contrast and density are adequate to demonstrate the scaphoid fat stripe.

- *Significance of the scaphoid fat stripe:* The scaphoid fat stripe is one of the soft-tissue structures that should be visible on all PA wrist images (Figure 3-27). It is convex and is located just lateral to the scaphoid in an uninjured wrist. A change in the convexity of this stripe may indicate to the reviewer the presence of joint effusion or of a radial side fracture of the scaphoid, radial styloid process, or proximal first metacarpal.

The wrist is positioned in a PA projection. The radial and ulnar styloids are at the extreme lateral and medial edges, respectively, of each bone. The radioulnar articulation is open, and superimposition of the metacarpal bases is limited.

- Rotation of the wrist and forearm is controlled by the position of the hand, elbow, and humerus. A PA projection is accomplished by abducting the humerus until it is positioned parallel with the IR and the elbow is in a lateral position. The hand is then pronated, placing the wrist in a PA projection (Figure 3-28).
- *Detecting wrist rotation and radial styloid position:* When the hand and wrist are rotated externally into a medial oblique position, the carpal bones and the metacarpal bases located on the medial aspect of the wrist are superimposed, whereas those located laterally are not. The lateral interconnecting carpal and metacarpal joint spaces are also demonstrated (see Image 29). Internal rotation (or lateral oblique position) of the hand and wrist causes the laterally located carpal bones and the metacarpal bases to be superimposed and increases visibility of the pisiform and hamate hook (see Image 30).

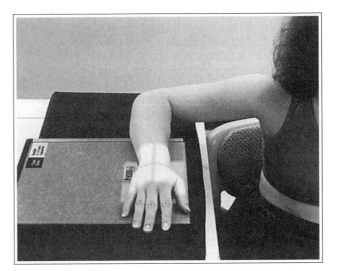

Figure 3-28. Proper patient positioning for posteroanterior wrist image.

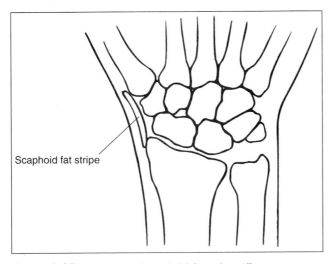

Figure 3-27. Location of scaphoid fat stripe. *(From Martensen K II: Radiographic positioning and analysis of the wrist, In-Service Reviews in Radiologic Technology, 16[5], 1992.)*

External and internal hand and wrist rotation also cause the radial styloid to rotate out of profile and closes the radioulnar articulation.

- *Humerus and elbow positioning and ulnar styloid visualization:* Humerus and elbow positioning determines the placement of the ulnar styloid. Abducting the humerus to position the elbow in a lateral position with the humeral epicondyles aligned perpendicular to the IR brings the ulnar styloid in profile and aligns the radius and ulna parallel with each other. The ulna and radius cross each other if the humerus is not abducted but is allowed to remain in a vertical position with the humeral epicondyles closer to parallel with the IR. This inaccurate positioning can be identified on a PA wrist image by viewing the ulnar styloid, which is no longer demonstrated in profile (see Image 36).

The distal radius is demonstrated without foreshortening. The anterior and posterior articulating margins of the radius are nearly superimposed.

- The distal radial carpal articular surface is concave and slants approximately 11 degrees from posterior to anterior. Because the forearm is positioned parallel with the IR for a PA wrist image, the slant of the distal radius causes the posterior radial margin to project slightly ($\frac{1}{4}$ inch or 0.6 cm) distal to the anterior radial margin, obscuring the radiocarpal joints.
- *Distal radius superimposition:* If an image is obtained that demonstrates an excessive amount of the radial articulating surface, or if open radioscaphoid and radiolunate joint spaces are desired, view the distal radioulnar articulation to determine the correcting movement. The posterior edge of this surface is blunt, whereas the anterior edge is rounded. Study the distal end of a radial skeletal bone to better familiarize yourself with this difference. If an image is obtained that demonstrates

the posterior radial margin distal to the anterior margin, the proximal forearm was elevated higher than the distal forearm (see Images 29 and 31). It should also be noted that when the wrist is medially rotated the posterior radial surface is superimposed over the ulna. If the anterior radial margin is demonstrated distal to the posterior margin, the proximal forearm was positioned lower than the distal forearm. To superimpose the distal radial margins and to demonstrate radioscaphoid and radiolunate joints as open spaces (see Image 30), the proximal aspect of the forearm should be positioned slightly (5 to 6 degrees from horizontal) lower than the distal forearm.

- *Positioning patient with thick proximal forearm:* On a patient with a large muscular or thick proximal forearm, it may be necessary to allow the proximal forearm to extend off the IR or table in order to position the forearm parallel with the IR. If the patient is not positioned in this manner, the radius will be foreshortened, demonstrating an excessive amount of radial articular surface, and superimposition of the scaphoid and lunate onto the radius will be greater (see Image 31).

The second through fifth CM joint spaces are open. The scaphoid is only slightly foreshortened, and the lunate is trapezoidal.

- When the wrist is placed in a neutral, nonflexed position, these three image appearances are achieved. To place the wrist in a neutral position, flex the patient's fingers, flexing the hand until the metacarpals are angled to approximately 10 to 15 degrees with the IR.

- *Effect of flexion and extension on carpal bones:* View your own wrist in a PA projection with the hand extended flat against a hard surface. Note how the wrist is slightly flexed. Next, begin slowly flexing your hand and notice how the wrist moves from a flexed to an extended position with increased hand flexion. To understand how carpal bone position varies with wrist flexion and extension, study the drawings of the scaphoid, capitate, and lunate bones in Figure 3-29. Note how the positions of these carpals change with each movement. Also study the position of the CM joint space in reference to a perpendicular central ray. Images 32 and 33 demonstrate a PA wrist in flexion (the hand was extended) and extension (the hand was overflexed), respectively. Compare these images with the properly positioned wrist in the image in Figure 3-26. Wrist flexion resulted in obscured third through fifth CM joint spaces, a severely foreshortened scaphoid that has taken a signet ring configuration (a large circle with a smaller circle within it), and a triangular lunate (see Image 32). Wrist extension has resulted in foreshortened metacarpals, closed second through third CM joint spaces, decreased scaphoid foreshortening, and a triangular lunate (see Image 33). Because the metacarpals are different lengths and may be positioned at different angles with the IR when the hand is flexed, to open all of the CM joints it is necessary to position each metacarpal at a 10- to 15-degree angle to the IR.

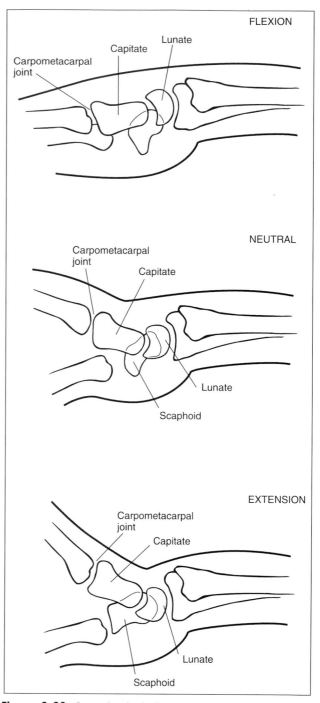

Figure 3-29. Lateral wrist in flexion *(top)*, neutral position *(middle)*, and extension *(bottom)*. *(From Martensen K II: Radiographic positioning and analysis of the wrist, In-Service Reviews in Radiologic Technology, 16[5], 1992.)*

The long axes of the third metacarpal and the midforearm are aligned with the long axis of the collimated light field. The scaphoid and half of the lunate are positioned distal to the radius.

- If the long axes of the third metacarpal and the mid forearm are aligned with the long axis of the collimated

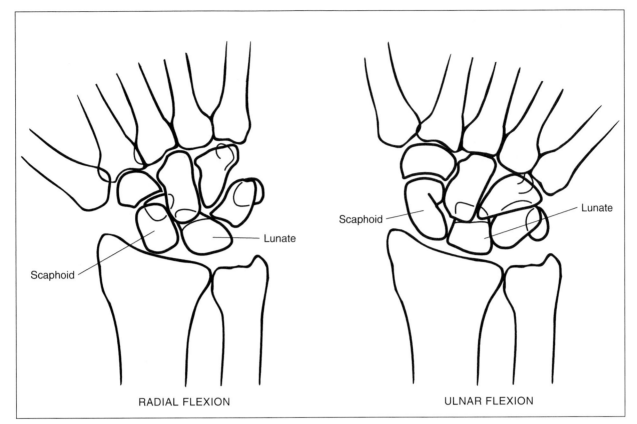

Figure 3-30. Posteroanterior wrist in radial flexion *(left)* and ulnar flexion *(right)*. *(From Martensen K II: Radiographic positioning and analysis of the wrist, In-Service Reviews in Radiologic Technology, 16[5], 1992.)*

light field, the patient's wrist has been placed in a neutral position. If a neutral position is not maintained for a PA projection wrist image, the shapes of the scaphoid and the position of the lunate are altered (Figure 3-30 and Images 34 and 35). Radial flexion of the wrist causes the distal scaphoid to shift anteriorly (toward the palmar surface) and to demonstrate increased foreshortening as it forms a signet ring configuration. The lunate will shift medially, toward the ulna. In ulnar flexion the distal scaphoid tilts posteriorly (dorsally) and demonstrates decreased foreshortening, and the lunate shifts laterally, toward the radius. Radial flexion and ulnar flexion images of the wrist may be specifically requested to demonstrate wrist joint mobility.

The carpal bones are at the center of the collimated field. The carpal bones, one fourth of the distal ulna and radius, and half of theproximal metacarpals are included within the field.

- The wrist joint is located at a level just distal to the palpable ulnar styloid. To obtain an image of the carpal bones with the least amount of distortion, place a perpendicular central ray at this level and centered to the midwrist area. Open the longitudinal collimation to include half of the metacarpals. Transversely collimate to within ½ inch (1.25 cm) of the wrist skinline.

- Either one half of an 8- × 10-inch (18- × 24-cm) detailed screen-film or computed radiography IR or one third of a 10- × 12-inch (24- × 30-cm) detailed screen-film IR placed crosswise should be adequate to include all the required anatomical structures.

- ***Wrist examination taken to include more than one fourth of the forearm:*** When a wrist examination is requested to include more than one fourth of the distal forearm, the central ray should remain on the wrist joint, and the collimation field should be opened to demonstrate the desired amount of forearm. This method will result in an extended, unnecessary radiation field distal to the metacarpals. A lead strip placed over this extended radiation field protects the patient's phalanges and prevents backscatter from reaching the IR. The advantage of this method over centering the central ray proximal to the wrist joint is an undistorted demonstration of the carpal bones.

EFFECT OF UPPER EXTREMITY MOVEMENTS ON BONY COMPONENTS OF THE WRIST

The wrist is a very complex joint with numerous bony components and movement possibilities. In an attempt to simplify the effect that different upper extremity movements have on the bony components, the following summary is offered. The positions of the elbow and hand affect forearm and wrist rotation and can be identified by the positions of the ulnar and radial styloid, respectively. When the elbow is in a lateral position (humeral epicondyles aligned perpendicular to IR), the ulnar styloid is in profile. When the hand is in a PA projection, the radial styloid is in profile.

It is the hand position that varies the shape of the scaphoid. If the wrist is flexed as a result of hand extension or is radially flexed, the scaphoid is foreshortened. If the wrist is extended as a result of hand flexion or is ulnar-flexed, the scaphoid is demonstrated with decreased foreshortening. The shape and location of the lunate also vary with the position of the wrist and hand. It becomes triangular with hand extension and flexion and changes position in reference to the distal radius with radial and ulnar flexion. In radial flexion the lunate is positioned distal to the radioulnar articulation, whereas in ulnar flexion it is positioned distal to the radius.

Because the shapes of the scaphoid and lunate can be changed with more than one positioning movement, it is necessary to evaluate mispositioned images carefully to determine which movement is causing the misposition. It is also possible for two corrections to be needed simultaneously to obtain accurate positioning. The accuracy of hand flexion and extension are easily identified by evaluating the CM joints. Wrist ulnar or radial deviation are identified by evaluating the alignment of the third metacarpal with the radius.

Posteroanterior Wrist Image Analysis

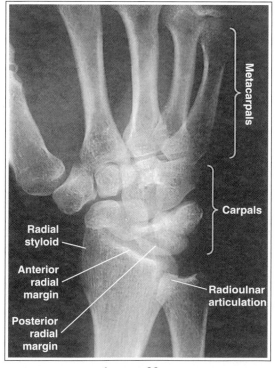

Image 29.

Analysis. The medially located carpal bones and metacarpals are superimposed, whereas the laterally located carpal and metacarpal joint spaces are open. The radioulnar articulation is closed, and the radial styloid is not in profile. The wrist was externally rotated (in a medial oblique position). The posterior margin of the distal radius is too far distal to the anterior margin. The proximal forearm was slightly elevated. The ulnar styloid is in profile, indicating that the elbow and humerus were accurately positioned.

Correction. Internally rotate the hand until the wrist is in a true PA projection, and depress the proximal forearm. For a patient with a thick proximal forearm, allow the proximal forearm to hang off the IR and/or the table.

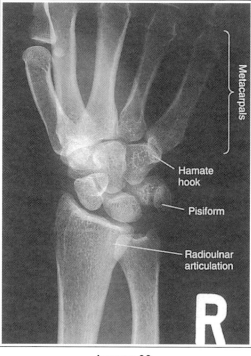

Image 30.

Analysis. The laterally located carpals and metacarpals are superimposed, and the pisiform and hamate hook are visualized. The radioulnar articulation is closed. The wrist was internally rotated (in a lateral oblique position). The ulnar styloid is in profile, indicating accurate elbow and humerus positioning, and the distal radial articular surfaces are directly superimposed over each other, demonstrating open radiolunate and radioscaphoid joint spaces. The proximal forearm was positioned slightly lower than the distal forearm.

Correction. Rotate the hand externally until the wrist is in a PA projection.

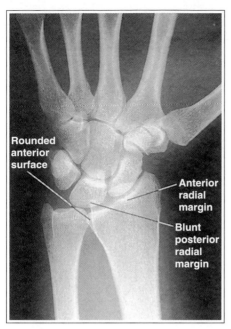

Image 31.

Analysis. The posterior margin of the distal radius is too far distal to the anterior margin. The posterior margin can be identified by the blunt, posterior ulnar articulating edge. The forearm was foreshortened, with the proximal forearm positioned higher than the distal forearm.

Correction. Lower the proximal forearm until it is parallel with the IR. If you desire a superimposed distal radial articular surface, which will demonstrate open radiolunate and radioscaphoid joint spaces, position the proximal forearm slightly (5 to 6 degrees from horizontal) lower than the distal forearm. For a patient with a thick proximal forearm, allow the proximal forearm to extend beyond the IR and/or table.

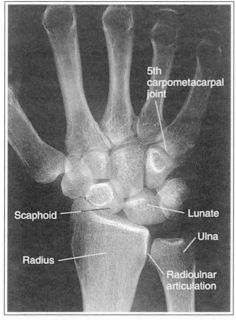

Image 32.

Analysis. The scaphoid demonstrates excessive foreshortening and has a signet ring configuration, the CM joints are obscured, and the lunate is triangular but is properly positioned distal to the radius. Two hand mispositions will cause this scaphoid shape: radial deviation and hand extension. Because the third metacarpal is aligned with the midforearm and the lunate is properly positioned distal to the radius, radial deviation can be eliminated as the positional problem. Hand extension (wrist flexion) is the cause of this mispositioning.

Correction. Curl the patient's fingers, flexing the hand until the second through fifth metacarpals are angled at approximately 10 to 15 degrees with the IR.

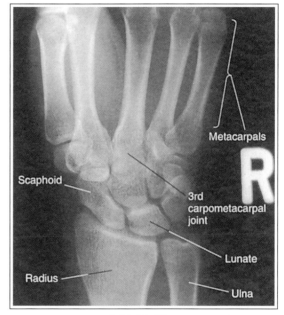

Image 33.

Analysis. The scaphoid is demonstrated with decreased foreshortening, and the second through third metacarpals are superimposed over the CM joints. The lunate is properly positioned distal to the radioulnar articulation. Two hand mispositions will cause this scaphoid shape: ulnar deviation and hand overflexion (metacarpals angled at more than 10 to 15 degrees with the IR). Because the third metacarpal is aligned with the midforearm and the lunate is properly positioned distal to the radioulnar articulation, ulnar deviation can be eliminated as the positional problem. Hand overflexion (wrist extension) is the cause of this misposition. The fifth CM joint is open because the fifth metacarpal is shorter and was placed at less of an angle to the IR than the other metacarpals when the hand was flexed.

Correction. Extend fingers and hand until the second through fifth metacarpals are angled at 10 to 15 degrees with the IR.

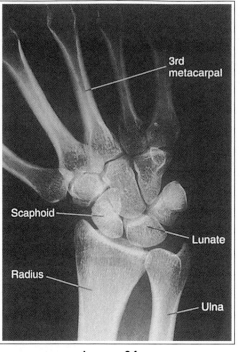

Image 34.

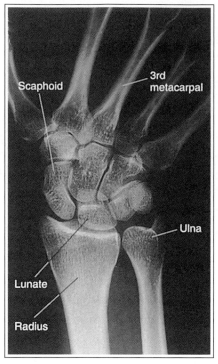

Image 35.

Analysis. The scaphoid demonstrates increased foreshortening, the lunate is positioned mostly distal to the ulna, and the third metacarpal is not aligned with the long axis of the midforearm. Because the scaphoid foreshortens with both hand extension and radial deviation, you can determine the correct repositioning movement for this image by evaluating the alignment of the third metacarpal with the midforearm and the openness of the CM joint spaces. The third metacarpal is not aligned with the midforearm and the scaphoid demonstrates increased foreshortening, so you can conclude that the patient was in radial deviation. Because the CM joint spaces are open, the hand was properly flexed.

Correction. Ulnar-deviate the wrist until the third metacarpal and the midforearm are aligned, placing the hand and wrist in a neutral position. If a radial deviation wrist image is desired to evaluate patient mobility, no correction movement is required.

Analysis. The scaphoid is demonstrated with decreased foreshortening, the lunate is entirely positioned distal to the radius, and the third metacarpal is not aligned with the midforearm. All of these positioning points indicate that the wrist was in ulnar deviation for the image. Because the CM joint spaces are open, you can conclude that the hand was accurately flexed.

Correction. Radially deviate the wrist until the third metacarpal is aligned with the midforearm, placing the hand and wrist in a neutral position. If an ulnar deviation wrist image is desired to evaluate patient mobility, no correcting movement is required.

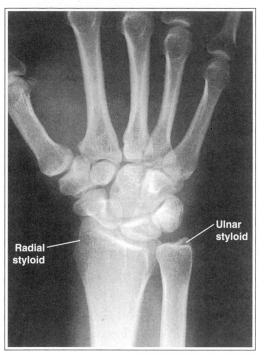

Image 36.

Analysis. This image has many positioning problems. First, the radioulnar articulation is closed and the lateral intercarpal joints are open while the medial intercarpal joints are closed, indicating that the hand and wrist were externally rotated. Second, the ulnar styloid is not in profile, indicating that the elbow and humerus were mispositioned. Next, the distal radius is foreshortened. Note how the articulating surface is demonstrated with the posterior margin far too distal to the anterior margin. The proximal forearm was positioned higher than the distal forearm. Finally, the scaphoid demonstrates excessive foreshortening, and the fourth and fifth CM joints are obscured. The image was taken with the wrist in slight external rotation, with the fourth and fifth metacarpals positioned at less than a 10- to 15-degree angle to the IR, although the second and third distal metacarpals were elevated accurately.

Correction. Flex the elbow and abduct the humerus 90 degrees, placing the entire arm on the same horizontal plane. Internally rotate the hand and wrist until they are positioned in a true AP projection. Curl the fingers, flexing the hand until all the metacarpals are angled at 10 to 15 degrees to the IR.

WRIST: POSTEROANTERIOR OBLIQUE PROJECTION (EXTERNAL ROTATION)

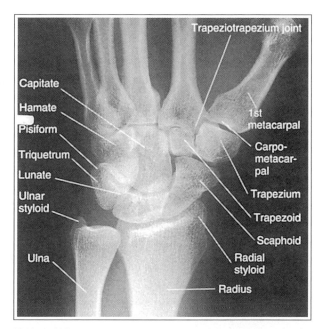

Figure 3-31. Oblique wrist image with accurate positioning.

Image Analysis

Contrast and density are adequate to demonstrate the scaphoid fat stripe.

- The scaphoid fat stripe is one of the soft-tissue structures that should be visible on all oblique wrist images.

It is convex and is located just lateral to the scaphoid on an uninjured wrist (Figure 3-32). A change in the shape of this fat stripe or in its proximity to the scaphoid may indicate joint effusion or a radial side fracture.

The wrist has been placed in a 45-degree lateral (external) oblique position. The trapezoid and trapezium are

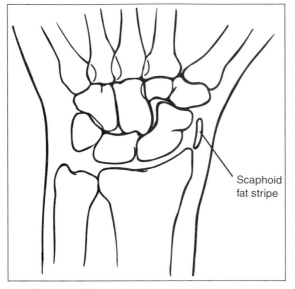

Figure 3-32. Location of scaphoid fat stripe.

demonstrated without superimposition, and the trapeziotrapezoidal joint space is open. The scaphoid tuberosity and waist are demonstrated in profile. Only a small degree of trapezoid and capitate superimposition is present.

- To accomplish an oblique wrist image, begin with the wrist in a PA projection with the humerus and the forearm on the same horizontal plane. Externally rotate the hand and wrist until the wrist forms a 45-degree angle with the IR (Figure 3-33). When judging the degree of wrist obliquity, it is best to view the wrist and not the hand. The obliquity of the hand and wrist are not always equal when they are rotated, especially if the humerus and forearm are not positioned on the same horizontal plane for the image.
- *Determining the accuracy of wrist obliquity:* On a PA projection image (see Image 37), the trapezoid and

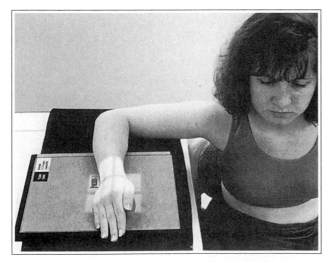

Figure 3-33. Proper patient positioning for oblique wrist image.

trapezium are superimposed. Placing the wrist in a medial oblique position draws the trapezium from beneath the trapezoid, providing clear visualization of both carpal bones and the joint space (trapeziotrapezoidal) between them. The medial oblique position also rotates the scaphoid tuberosity and waist into profile. The relationships between the trapezoid and trapezium and the trapezoid and capitate are used to discern an accurate oblique wrist position. If the wrist is underrotated, the trapezoid and trapezium are superimposed, the trapeziotrapezoidal joint space is obscured, and the trapezoid demonstrates minimal capitate superimposition (see Image 38). If wrist obliquity is more than 45 degrees, the trapezium demonstrates minimal trapezoidal superimposition, the capitate is superimposed by the trapezoid, and the trapeziotrapezoidal joint space is obscured (see Image 39).

The second CM and the scaphotrapezium joint spaces are demonstrated.

- For the PA projection of the wrist, the CM joints are opened by flexing the hand until the metacarpals are at a 10- to 15-degree angle to the IR. When the hand and wrist are placed in obliquity, the same metacarpal tilt must be maintained to open the second CM and scaphotrapezium joint spaces. If the distal metacarpals are allowed to tilt toward the IR, these two joints are obscured (see Image 38).

The long axes of the third metacarpal and midforearm are aligned with the long axis of the collimated field. The scaphoid tuberosity and waist are demonstrated in profile and are not positioned directly next to the radius.

- If the long axes of the third metacarpal and the midforearm are aligned with the long axis of the collimation field, the patient's wrist is placed in a neutral position. Radial deviation increases the foreshortening of the scaphoid, preventing visualization of the scaphoid tuberosity and waist, and positions the scaphoid directly next to the radius (see Image 40). Ulnar deviation decreases scaphoid foreshortening (see Image 41).

The distal radius is demonstrated without foreshortening. The anterior and posterior margins of the radius are nearly superimposed.

- The distal radial carpal articular surface is concave and slants approximately 11 degrees from posterior to anterior when the radius and ulna are positioned parallel with the IR. Because the forearm is positioned parallel with the IR for an oblique wrist image, the slant of the distal radius causes the posterior margin to be projected slightly ($\frac{1}{4}$ inch or 0.6 cm) distal to the anterior radial margin, obscuring the radiocarpal joints.

  If an image is obtained that demonstrates an excessive amount of the radial articulating surface, or if open radioscaphoid and radiolunate joint spaces are desired, you should view the distal radioulnar articulation to determine the correcting movement. The radial surface superimposed over the ulna is associated with the posterior radial margin.

- **Distal radius margin superimposition:** If an image is obtained that demonstrates the posterior radial margin too far distal to the anterior margin, the proximal forearm was elevated higher than the distal forearm (see Image 41). If the anterior radial margin is demonstrated distal to the posterior margin, the proximal forearm was positioned lower than the distal forearm. To demonstrate open radioscaphoid and radiolunate joint spaces (see Image 42), position the proximal forearm slightly (5 to 6 degrees) lower than the distal forearm.

- *Positioning patient with thick proximal forearm:* For the patient with a large muscular or thick proximal forearm, allow the proximal forearm to extend beyond the IR or table to position it parallel with the IR. If the patient is not positioned in this manner, the radius is foreshortened, demonstrating an excessive amount of radial articular surface, and superimposition of the scaphoid and lunate onto the radius is increased.

The ulnar styloid is in profile at the far medial edge.

- The position of the humerus and elbow determines the placement of the ulnar styloid. The ulnar styloid is demonstrated in profile when the patient's humerus is abducted to align the humeral epicondyles perpendicular to the IR and place the elbow in a lateral position. If the humerus is not abducted to this degree, the ulnar styloid is no longer demonstrated in profile.

The carpal bones are at the center of the collimated field. The carpal bones, one fourth of the distal ulna and radius, and half of the proximal metacarpals are included within the field.

- The wrist joint is located at a level just distal to the first proximal metacarpal. To obtain an oblique image of the carpal bones with the least amount of distortion, place a perpendicular central ray at this level and centered with the midwrist area. Open longitudinal collimation to include half of the metacarpals. Transversely collimate to within ½ inch (1.25 cm) of the wrist skinline.
- Either half of an 8- × 10-inch (18- × 24-cm) detailed screen-film or computed radiography IR or one third of a 10- × 12-inch (24- × 30-cm) detailed screen-film IR placed crosswise should be adequate to include all the required anatomical structures. Digital images require tight collimation without overlapping of individual exposures.

Oblique Wrist Image Analysis

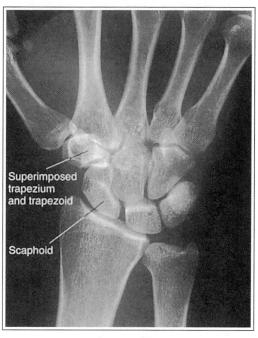

Image 37.

Analysis. The trapezoid and trapezium are superimposed, and the scaphoid tuberosity is not demonstrated in profile. This is a PA projection.

Correction. Externally rotate the wrist until it forms a 45-degree angle with the IR.

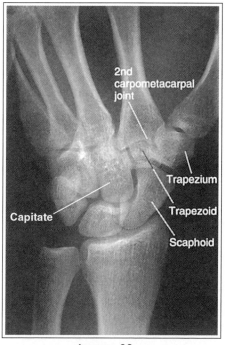

Image 38.

Analysis. The trapezoid and trapezium are partially superimposed, obscuring the trapeziotrapezoidal joint space.

Trapezoid capitate superimposition is minimal. The wrist was rotated less than 45 degrees. The second CM and scaphotrapezoidal joint spaces are closed. The distal second metacarpal was positioned too far away from the IR.

Correction. Externally rotate the wrist until it forms a 45-degree angle with the IR. Depress the distal second metacarpal until it is positioned at a 10- to 15-degree angle to the IR.

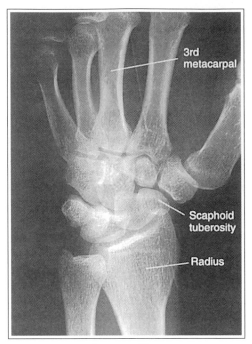

Image 40.

Analysis. The third metacarpal and midforearm are not aligned, the scaphoid is foreshortened, and the scaphoid tuberosity is situated next to the radius. The wrist was radially flexed.

Correction. Ulnar-deviate the wrist until the long axes of the third metacarpal and the midforearm are aligned.

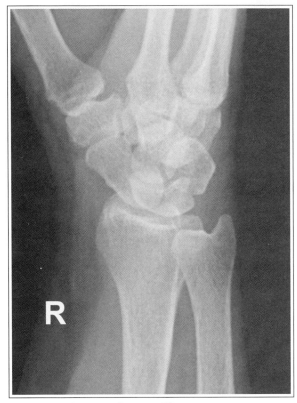

Image 39.

Analysis. Trapezoid and trapezium are partially superimposed, obscuring the trapeziotrapezoidal joint space. The trapezoid demonstrates excessive capitate superimposition. The wrist obliquity was more than 45 degrees.

Correction. Internally rotate the wrist until it forms a 45-degree angle with the IR.

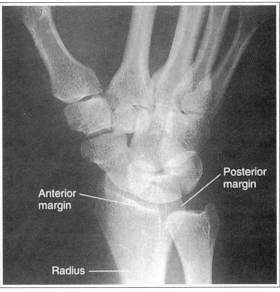

Image 41.

Analysis. The posterior margin of the distal radius is quite distal to the anterior margin, the third metacarpal and midforearm are not aligned, and the scaphoid demonstrates little foreshortening. The proximal forearm was elevated, and the wrist was ulnar-flexed.

Correction. Lower the proximal forearm until the forearm is parallel with the IR. For a patient with a muscular or thick proximal forearm, it may be necessary to allow the proximal forearm to hang off the IR or table in order to obtain a parallel forearm. Radial-deviate the wrist until the third metacarpal and midforearm are aligned.

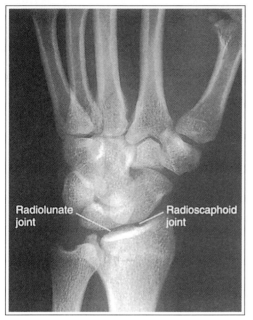

Image 42.

Analysis. The anterior and posterior margins of the distal radius are superimposed, demonstrating open radiolunate and radioscaphoid joint spaces. The proximal forearm was positioned slightly (5 to 6 degrees from horizontal) lower than the distal forearm.

Correction. This is an acceptable image. No correction movement is needed.

WRIST: LATERAL POSITION (LATEROMEDIAL PROJECTION)

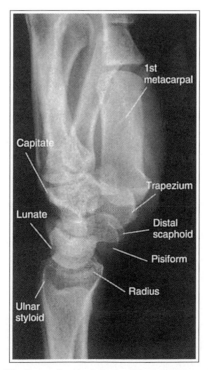

Figure 3-34. Lateral wrist image with accurate positioning.

Image Analysis

Contrast and density are adequate to demonstrate the pronator fat stripe and surrounding posterior wrist soft tissue.

- The pronator fat stripe is one of the soft-tissue structures that should be demonstrated on all lateral wrist images (Figure 3-35). It is located parallel to the anterior (volar) surface of the distal radius, is normally convex, and lies within ¼ inch (0.6 cm) of the radial cortex. Bowing or obliteration of this fat stripe may be the only indication of a subtle radial fracture.
- The soft tissue that surrounds the posterior (dorsal) aspect of the wrist should also be visible. This posterior soft tissue is convex on the uninjured wrist. To the reviewer a straightening or concave appearance of this surface may indicate swelling and injury.

The wrist is in a lateral position. The distal end of the scaphoid and the pisiform, as well as the radius and ulna, are superimposed.

- A lateral position of the wrist is accomplished by flexing the elbow 90 degrees and abducting the humerus until it is parallel with the IR, placing the entire arm on the same horizontal plane. Rotate the wrist into a lateral position with its ulnar (medial) aspect against the IR (Figure 3-36).
- To ensure true lateral positioning, place the palmar aspect of your thumb and forefinger against the anterior and posterior aspects, respectively, of the patient's wrist joint, as demonstrated in Figure 3-37. Adjust wrist rotation until your thumb and finger are aligned perpendicular to the IR.
- *Detecting wrist rotation:* The relationship between the pisiform and the distal aspect of the scaphoid can best be used to discern whether a lateral wrist position has been obtained. On a lateral image, these two carpals should be superimposed and should be demonstrated anterior to the capitate and lunate. When the wrist is

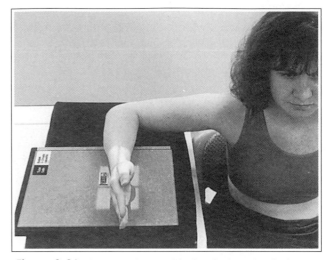

Figure 3-36. Proper patient positioning for lateral wrist image.

rotated, the AP relationship between the distal scaphoid and pisiform changes, and the pronator fat stripe is obscured. If the wrist is rotated externally (hand supinated), the distal scaphoid is visible posterior to the pisiform (see Image 43). If the wrist is rotated internally (hand pronated), the distal scaphoid is visible anterior to the pisiform (see Image 44). A second method of determining how to reposition a rotated lateral wrist image uses the radius and ulna. Because the exact amount of superimposition of the radius and ulna depends on the position of the humerus, you should always view the pisiform and distal scaphoid relationship when determining whether the wrist is truly lateral. If the distal scaphoid and pisiform are not superimposed and the ulna is positioned anterior to the radius, the patient's wrist was externally rotated (hand supinated) (see Image 43). If the distal scaphoid and pisiform are not superimposed and the ulna is positioned posterior to the radius, the patient's wrist was internally rotated (hand pronated) (see Image 44).

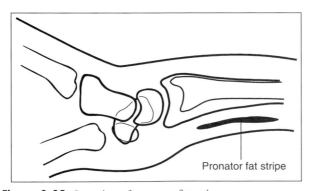

Figure 3-35. Location of pronator fat stripe.
(From Martensen K II: Radiographic positioning and analysis of the wrist, In-Service Reviews in Radiologic Technology, 16[5], 1992.)

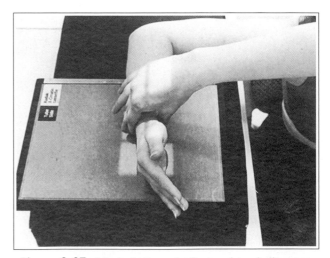

Figure 3-37. Manipulating wrist for true lateral alignment.

- *Mediolateral wrist image:* Routinely, the lateral wrist position is taken with the ulnar side of the wrist against the IR. If, instead, the radial side of the wrist was placed against the IR (mediolateral projection), the ulna and pisiform are visualized anterior to the radius and scaphoid, respectively, and the ulnar styloid is demonstrated in profile anteriorly (see Image 45).

The carpal bones do not indicate radial or ulnar deviation. The distal scaphoid is superimposed over the pisiform.

- To obtain a neutral lateral wrist image, align the long axes of the third metacarpal and the midforearm parallel with the IR. When the proximal forearm is higher or lower than the distal forearm, the wrist is radial-flexed or ulnar-flexed, respectively. In radial and ulnar deviation the distal scaphoid moves but the pisiform's position remains relatively unchanged. Radial deviation of the wrist forces the distal scaphoid anteriorly (Figure 3-38), resulting in demonstration of the pisiform distal to the scaphoid (see Image 46). Ulnar deviation shifts the distal scaphoid posteriorly (see Figure 3-38), resulting in demonstration of the pisiform proximal to the scaphoid (see Image 47). The degree of pisiform and distal scaphoid separation is usually very small, because you would be unlikely to position a patient in maximum wrist deviation without being aware of the positioning error. To obtain optimal lateral wrist images, however, we must learn to eliminate even small degrees of deviation.

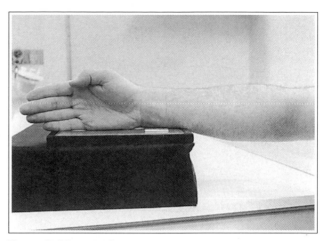

Figure 3-39. Positioning of patient with thick proximal forearm.

- *Positioning patient with thick proximal forearm:* For a patient with a large muscular or thick proximal forearm, it may be necessary to allow the proximal forearm to hang off the IR or table to maintain a neutral wrist position (Figure 3-39). If the patient is not positioned in this manner, radial deviation of the wrist will result. If the proximal forearm does not remain level but is allowed to depress lower than the distal forearm in this situation, ulnar deviation will result.

The long axis of the first metacarpal is aligned parallel with the forearm.

- If the long axis of the first metacarpal is positioned adjacent to the second metacarpal and aligned parallel with the forearm, the patient's wrist is placed in a neutral position.
- When the wrist is flexed or extended, the positions of the scaphoid and lunate are altered. In wrist flexion the lunate and the distal scaphoid tilt anteriorly (see Image 48). In wrist extension the lunate and distal scaphoid tilt posteriorly (see Image 49). Flexion and extension images of the wrist may be specifically requested to demonstrate wrist joint mobility.

The ulnar styloid is demonstrated in profile posteriorly.

- When the humerus and elbow are positioned, the placement of the ulna styloid changes. The ulnar styloid is demonstrated in profile when the patient's elbow is in a lateral position, with the humerus abducted and the humeral epicondyles aligned perpendicular to the IR. If the humerus is not abducted to this degree the ulnar styloid will not be demonstrated in profile (see Images 43 and 50).
- *Lateral wrist position with no forearm rotation:* In contrast to positioning the forearm and humerus on the same horizontal plane for a lateral wrist image, Epner and colleagues[1] suggest that a lateral wrist image be taken with zero forearm rotation. For this to be accomplished, the humerus is not abducted and the elbow is placed in an AP projection (Figure 3-40). Such positioning rotates

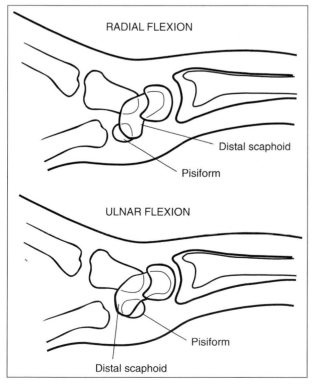

Figure 3-38. Lateral wrist in radial deviation *(top)* and ulnar deviation *(bottom).*

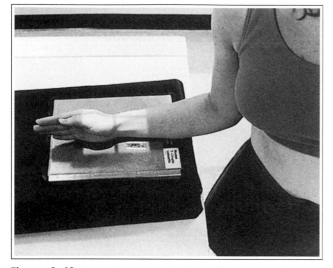

Figure 3-40. Lateral wrist positioning without humeral abduction.

the ulnar styloid out of profile, demonstrating it distal to the midline of the ulnar head (see Images 43 and 50). Because forearm rotation has been eliminated, the ulnar head also shifts closer to the lunate. Epner states that this positioning allows for more accurate measuring of the ulnar length. Department policy determines which humerus positioning is performed in your facility.

The trapezium is demonstrated without superimposition of the first proximal metacarpal.

• To obtain optimal demonstration of the trapezium, lower the distal first metacarpal until it is at the same level as the second metacarpal. This positioning places the trapezium and metacarpal parallel with the IR, demonstrating them without superimposition. If the distal first metacarpal is not lowered, it is foreshortened, and its proximal aspect is superimposed over the trapezium (see Image 51).

The carpal bones are at the center of the collimated field. The carpal bones, one fourth of the distal ulna and radius, and half of the proximal metacarpals are included within the field.

• In a lateral position the wrist joint is located just proximal to the first metacarpal base. To obtain an image of the carpal bones with the least amount of distortion, place a perpendicular central ray at this level and centered to the midwrist area. Open the longitudinal collimation to include half of the metacarpals. Transversely collimate to within ½ inch (1.25 cm) of the wrist skinline.
• Either half of an 8- × 10-inch (18- × 24-cm) detailed screen-film or computed radiography IR or one third of a 10- × 12-inch (24- × 30-cm) detailed screen-film IR placed crosswise should be adequate to include all the required anatomical structures. Digital imaging requires tight collimation without overlapping of individual exposures.

• **Wrist examination that includes more than one fourth of the forearm:** When a wrist examination is requested to include more than one fourth of the distal forearm, the central ray should remain on the wrist joint, and the collimation field should be opened to demonstrate the desired amount of forearm. This method results in an extended, unnecessary radiation field distal to the metacarpals. A lead strip placed over this extended radiation field protects the patient's phalanges and prevents any possible backscatter from reaching the IR. The advantage of this method over centering the central ray proximal to the wrist joint is an undistorted demonstration of the carpal bones. A lateral wrist image taken with the central ray positioned proximal to the wrist joint demonstrates the distal scaphoid projecting distal to the pisiform (see Image 47).

Lateral Wrist Image Analysis

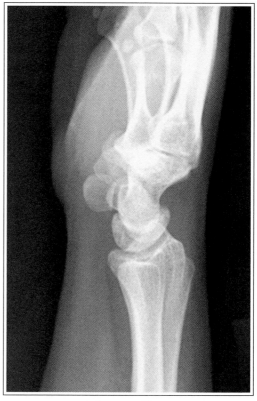

Image 43.

Analysis. The wrist is not in a lateral position. The pisiform is shown anterior to the scaphoid, and the ulna anterior to the radius. The wrist was externally rotated (hand supinated). The proximal first metacarpal is partially superimposed over the trapezium. The first metacarpal was not positioned parallel with the forearm. The ulnar styloid is not positioned in profile but is demonstrated projecting distal to the midline of the ulnar head. This ulnar positioning indicates that the humerus was positioned without abduction as demonstrated in Figure 3-40.

Correction. Internally rotate the wrist (pronate the hand) until the wrist is in a lateral position, and depress the distal metacarpal until the metacarpal is aligned parallel with the forearm. Adjust the patient's humerus to meet your department protocol. If the ulnar styloid is to be demonstrated in profile, abduct the humerus and flex the elbow 90 degrees, placing the forearm and humerus on the same horizontal plane. If department protocol requires that a lateral wrist image be taken without humeral abduction, no correction movement is needed. Consistency in arm position is important to evaluating ulnar length.

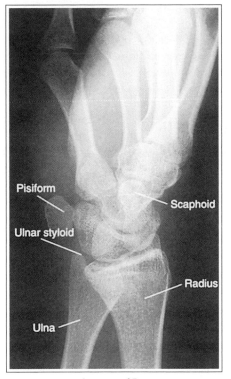

Image 45.

Analysis. The ulna and pisiform are demonstrated anterior to the radius and scaphoid, respectively, and the ulnar styloid is demonstrated in profile anteriorly. The radial side of the wrist was placed against the IR (mediolateral projection).

Correction. Externally rotate the hand and wrist until the ulnar side of the wrist is placed against the IR if a lateromedial projection is desired.

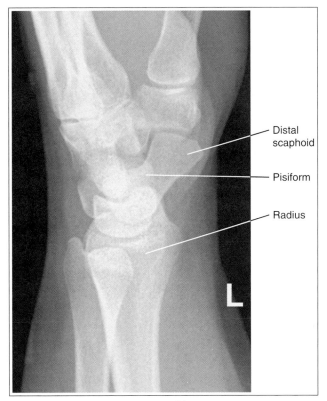

Image 44.

Analysis. The wrist is not in a lateral position. The distal scaphoid is anterior to the pisiform, and the radius is anterior to the ulna. The wrist was internally rotated (hand pronated).

Correction. Externally rotate the wrist (supinate the hand) until the wrist is in a true lateral position.

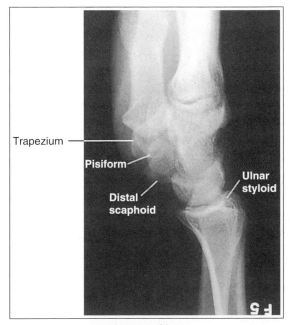

Image 46.

Analysis. The pisiform is demonstrated distal to the scaphoid. Two possible positioning errors cause such an image. Either the central ray was not centered with the wrist joint but was positioned distally, or the wrist was in radial deviation. Note that the ulnar styloid is not in profile but is projecting distal to the midline of the ulnar head. This ulnar positioning indicates that the patient was positioned without humerus abduction as demonstrated in Figure 3-40. The proximal first metacarpal is partially superimposed over the trapezium. The metacarpal was not aligned parallel with the IR.

Correction. Center the central ray with the wrist joint, which is located just proximal to the trapezium. Position the wrist in neutral deviation by aligning the long axes of the third metacarpal and the midforearm parallel with the IR. Depress the distal metacarpal until the first metacarpal is aligned parallel with the IR.

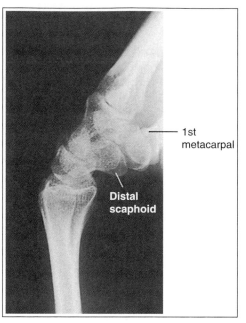

Image 48.

Analysis. The first metacarpal is not aligned parallel with the midforearm. The wrist was flexed anteriorly.

Correction. If a neutral position is desired, align the long axis of the first metacarpal parallel with the midforearm. If a wrist flexion image was taken to evaluate wrist mobility, no correction movement is required.

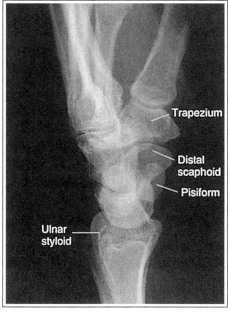

Image 47.

Analysis. The distal scaphoid is demonstrated distal to the pisiform. Two possible positioning errors cause such a problem. Either the wrist was in ulnar deviation or the central ray was not centered with the wrist joint but was positioned to the midforearm.

Correction. Place the wrist in a neutral position by aligning the long axes of the third metacarpal and the midforearm parallel with the IR. Center the central ray with the wrist joint, which is located just proximal to the trapezium.

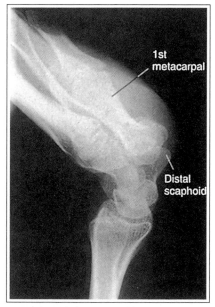

Image 49.

Analysis. The first metacarpal is not aligned parallel with the midforearm. The wrist is extended posteriorly.

Correction. If a neutral position is desired, align the first metacarpal parallel with the midfoream. If a wrist extension image was taken to evaluate wrist mobility, no correction movement is required.

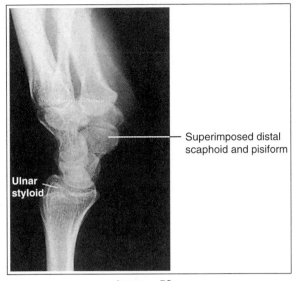

Image 50.

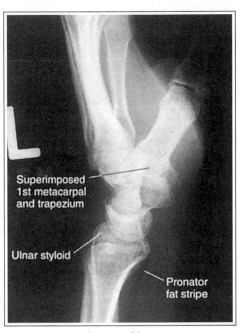

Image 51.

Analysis. The pisiform and the distal scaphoid are positioned accurately for a lateral wrist image. The ulnar styloid is not positioned in profile but is demonstrated projecting distal to the midline of the ulnar head. This ulnar positioning indicates that the humerus was positioned without abduction as demonstrated in Figure 3-40.

Correction. Adjust the patient's humerus to meet your department protocol. If the ulnar styloid is to be demonstrated in profile, abduct the humerus and flex the elbow 90 degrees, placing the forearm and humerus on the same horizontal plane. If department protocol requires that a lateral wrist image be taken without humeral abduction, no correction movement is needed. Consistency in arm position is important to evaluating ulnar length.

Analysis. The first proximal metacarpal is superimposed over the trapezium. The thumb was not positioned parallel with the midforearm but was pointing upward. The ulnar styloid is not in profile.

Correction. Depress the patient's distal thumb until the metacarpal is aligned parallel with the midforearm. Adjust the patient's humerus to meet your department protocol. If the ulnar styloid is to be demonstrated in profile, abduct the humerus and flex the elbow 90 degrees, placing the forearm and humerus on the same horizontal plane. If department protocol requires that a lateral wrist image be taken without humeral abduction, no correction movement is needed.

WRIST: ULNAR-DEVIATION, POSTEROANTERIOR AXIAL PROJECTION (SCAPHOID)

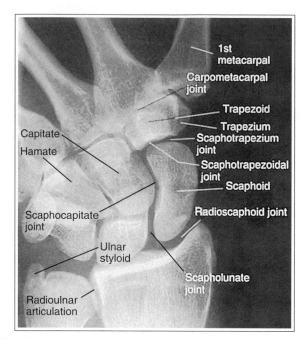

Figure 3-41. Ulnar-deviated posteroanterior wrist image with accurate positioning.

Image Analysis

Contrast and density are adequate to demonstrate the scaphoid fat stripe.

- The scaphoid fat stripe is one of the soft-tissue structures that should be visible on all scaphoid images (Figure 3-42). It is convex and is located just lateral to the scaphoid in an uninjured wrist. A change in the convexity of this stripe may signify to the reviewer joint effusion or a scaphoid fracture.

The scaphotrapezium and scaphotrapezoidal joint spaces are open.

- To obtain accurate scaphoid positioning, abduct the humerus until it is positioned parallel with the IR and place the elbow in a flexed, lateral position. Then pronate the extended hand, place the wrist in ulnar deviation, and ensure the wrist is rotated medially approximately 25 degrees (Figure 3-43).
- The scaphotrapezium and scaphotrapezoidal joints are aligned at a 15-degree angle to the IR when the patient's hand is in full extension. These joints will be open when a 15-degree proximally angled central ray is used. If the hand is not extended so that the palm is placed flat against the IR, but rather is flexed, the second metacarpal is superimposed over the trapezoid and trapezium and closes the scaphotrapezium and scaphotrapezoidal joint spaces (see Image 52).

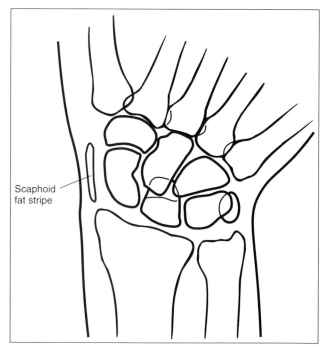

Figure 3-42. Location of scaphoid fat stripe. *(From Martensen K II: Radiographic positioning and analysis of the wrist, In-Service Reviews in Radiologic Technology, 16[5], 1992.)*

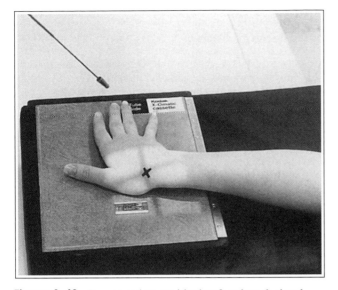

Figure 3-43. Proper patient positioning for ulnar-deviated, posteroanterior wrist image. *X* indicates location of scaphoid.

The wrist is in maximum ulnar deviation, as demonstrated by the alignment of the long axis of the first metacarpal and the radius, and the position of the lunate distal to the radius. The scaphoid is demonstrated without foreshortening or excessive elongation. When a scaphoid fracture is indicated, the fracture line is demonstrated.

- To demonstrate the scaphoid without foreshortening, position the patient's wrist in maximum ulnar deviation; then direct a 15-degree proximal (toward the elbow) central ray angulation to the long axis of the scaphoid. Maximum ulnar deviation has been accomplished when the first metacarpal is aligned with the radius. In a neutral PA projection of the nonflexed wrist, the distal scaphoid tilts anteriorly approximately 20 degrees. This tilt results in foreshortening of the scaphoid image (Figures 3-26 and 3-44). To offset some of this foreshortening and demonstrate all aspects of the scaphoid, place the wrist in ulnar deviation. In ulnar deviation the distal scaphoid moves posteriorly, decreasing the degree of foreshortening (Figure 3-44).

  Adequate ulnar deviation and central ray angulation place the central ray perpendicular to the long axis of the scaphoid (Figure 3-45). Because 70% of the fractures occur at the waist, most scaphoid fractures should be visualized with this positioning and angulation (see Image 53).
- ***Compensating for inadequate ulnar deviation:*** The position of the distal scaphoid changes with ulnar wrist deviation. Many patients with suspected scaphoid fractures are unable to achieve maximum ulnar wrist deviation. Without adequate ulnar deviation, the distal scaphoid is positioned more anteriorly. To compensate for this increased anterior tilt, the central ray angulation should be increased to approximately 20 degrees to

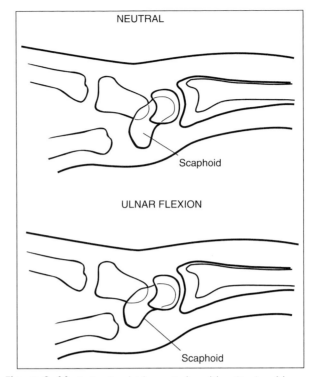

Figure 3-44. Lateral wrist in neutral position *(top)* and in ulnar flexion *(bottom).*

place the central ray and scaphoid long axis perpendicular to each other.
- ***Scaphoid elongation:*** The goal of the scaphoid image is to demonstrate the scaphoid without foreshortening or elongation. A slight amount of elongation of the scaphoid occurs on scaphoid images because the IR is not positioned parallel with the long axis of the scaphoid and the central ray is not aligned perpendicular with the IR (see Figure 3-45). Excessive elongation of the scaphoid results when the central ray is angled more than needed to align it perpendicular to the long axis of the scaphoid.

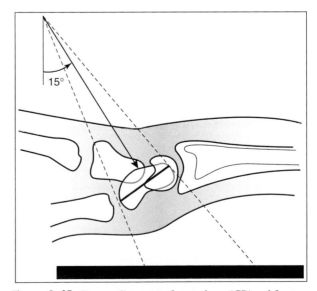

Figure 3-45. Proper alignment of central ray *(CR)* and fracture.

- *Mechanics of scaphoid fracture:* The scaphoid is the most commonly fractured carpal bone. One reason for this is its location among the other carpal bones. Two rows of carpal bones exist, a distal row and a proximal row, with joint spaces between them that allow the wrist to flex. The long scaphoid bone, however, is aligned partially with both of these rows with no joint space. When an individual falls on an outstretched hand the wrist is hyperextended, causing the proximal and distal carpal rows to flex at the joints, and a great deal of stress is placed on the narrow waist of the scaphoid. This stress may result in a fracture.

- Three areas of the scaphoid may be fractured: the waist, which sustains approximately 70% of the fractures; the distal end, which sustains 20% of the fractures; and the proximal end, which sustains 10% (Figure 3-46). Because scaphoid fractures can be at different locations on the scaphoid, precise positioning and central ray angulation are essential to obtain the optimum demonstration of this bone.

- *Demonstrating fractures of distal and proximal scaphoid:* When a fracture is suspected because of persistent pain and obliteration of the fat stripe but has not been demonstrated on routine images, it may be necessary to use different angles to position the central ray parallel with these fractures sites (Figure 3-47). A decrease of 5 to 10 degrees in central ray angulation better demonstrates the proximal scaphoid. Compare Figures 3-48 and 3-49. These images demonstrate a proximal fracture. Figure 3-48 was taken with the typical 15-degree proximal angle, and Figure 3-49 was taken with a 5-degree proximal angle.

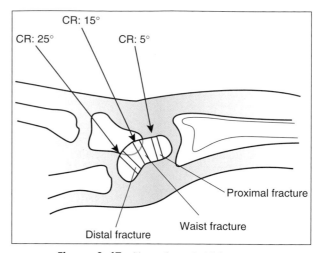

Figure 3-47. Sites of scaphoid fracture.

Note the increase in fracture line visualization in Figure 3-49. Decrease the central ray angle by 5 to 10 degrees, with a maximum of 25 degrees, to best demonstrate a distal scaphoid fracture (Figure 3-50). Angulations greater than 25 degrees project the proximal first metacarpal onto the distal scaphoid, obscuring the area of interest (see Image 54).

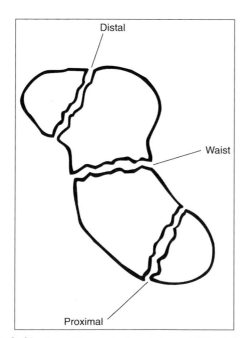

Figure 3-46. Poor alignment of central ray *(CR)* and fracture.

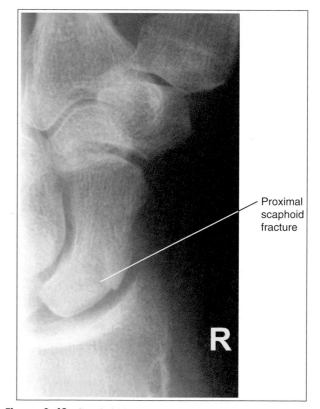

Figure 3-48. Scaphoid image taken with a 15-degree proximal CR angle and demonstrating a proximal scaphoid fracture.

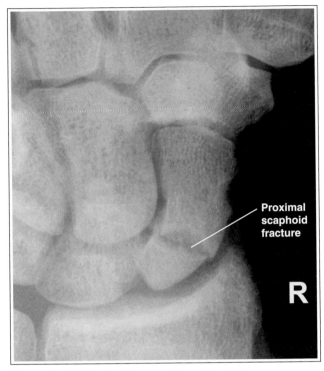

Figure 3-49. Scaphoid image taken with a 5-degree proximal CR angle and demonstrating a proximal scaphoid fracture.

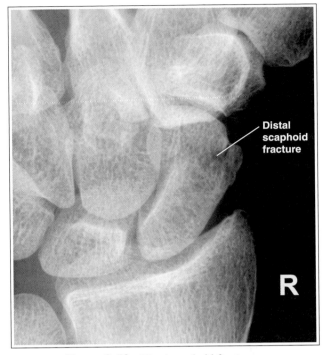

Figure 3-50. Distal scaphoid fracture.

The scaphocapitate and scapholunate joints are open. The ulnar styloid is in profile medially.

- The scaphocapitate and scapholunate joints are open when the wrist is medially rotated approximately 25 degrees. This obliquity is accomplished somewhat naturally as the patient's wrist is ulnar-flexed, with the humerus abducted and positioned parallel with the IR, and the elbow placed in a flexed, lateral position.

  If the scaphocapitate joint space is closed and the capitate and hamate are demonstrated without superimposition, the degree of obliquity was insufficient (see Image 55). If the scapholunate joint space is closed and the capitate and hamate demonstrate some degree of superimposition the wrist was rotated more that needed (see Image 56). Excessive medial wrist obliquity often occurs when the humerus and forearm are not positioned on the same horizontal plane and the elbow is placed in a lateral position. On an image, one can judge accurate humerus, forearm, and elbow positioning by evaluating the ulnar styloid. Accurate positioning places the ulnar styloid in profile medially. If the arm is not positioned accurately, the ulnar styloid is demonstrated distal to the midline of the ulnar head (see Image 57).

The radioscaphoid joint space is open.

- The distal radial carpal articular surface is concave and slants approximately 11 degrees from posterior to anterior when the forearm is positioned parallel with the IR.

On a PA projection without a central ray angulation, the posterior radial margin is demonstrated slightly distal to the anterior margin if the forearm is placed parallel with the IR. When a 15-degree proximal central ray angulation is employed for the scaphoid position, the posterior margin is projected slightly proximal to the anterior margin (Figure 3-51). To demonstrate an open radioscaphoid joint, the anterior and posterior margins of the distal radius should be superimposed. This superimposition is accomplished by elevating the proximal forearm very slightly (2 degrees) above the distal forearm.

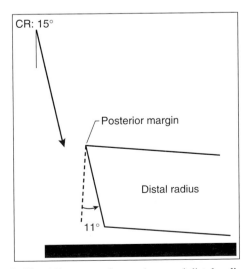

Figure 3-51. Alignment of central ray and distal radius to obtain open radioscaphoid joint.

The scaphoid is at the center of the collimated field. The carpal bones, the radioulnar articulation, and the proximal first through fourth metacarpals are included within the field.

- To place the scaphoid at the center of the collimated field, center the central ray with the scaphoid. In ulnar deviation, the scaphoid can be palpated halfway between the first metacarpal base and the radial styloid. After the central ray is centered, open the longitudinal collimation to include the first through fourth metacarpal bases and the distal radius. Transversely collimate to within ½ inch (1.25 cm) of the wrist skinline.

    Avoid collimating too tightly. It is difficult to determine how to reposition the patient when an image reveals poor positioning if key anatomical structures are not included.

- Half of an 8- × 10-inch (18- × 24-cm) detailed screen-film or computed radiography IR placed crosswise should be adequate to include all the required anatomical structures.

Posteroanterior Axial (Scaphoid) Image Analysis

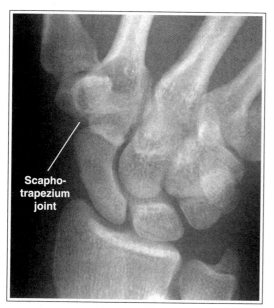

Image 52.

Analysis. The scaphotrapezium, scaphotrapezoidal, and CM joint spaces are closed. The hand and fingers were not positioned flat against the IR.

Correction. Extend the patient's fingers, placing the hand flat against the IR.

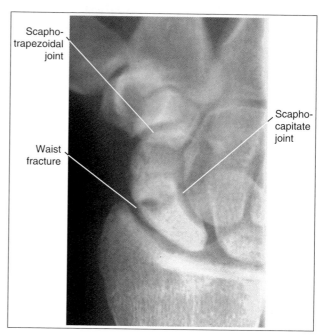

Image 53.

Analysis. This image demonstrates a scaphoid waist fracture. The scaphotrapezium, scaphotrapezoidal, and CM joint spaces are closed. The hand and fingers were not positioned flat against the IR. The scaphocapitate and radioscaphoid joints are closed, indicating that the degree of obliquity was inadequate and the proximal forearm was slightly depressed, respectively.

Correction. Extend the patient's fingers, placing the hand flat against the IR, and slightly increase the amount of external wrist obliquity and elevate the proximal forearm.

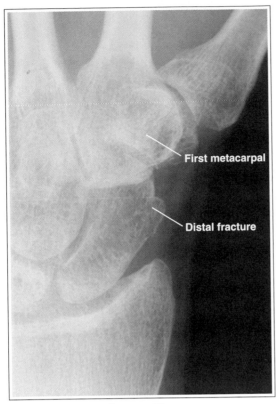

Image 54.

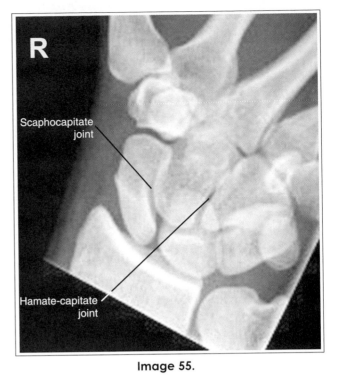

Image 55.

Analysis. A 30-degree proximal central ray angle was used, with the hand and fingers positioned flat against the IR. A distal scaphoid fracture is present. The proximal first metacarpal is superimposed over the distal scaphoid, and the radioscaphoid joint is closed. The central ray angulation was too great, and the proximal forearm was slightly depressed.

Correction. To best demonstrate a distal scaphoid fracture, decrease the amount of central ray angulation. A maximum 25-degree angle should be used to demonstrate a distal scaphoid fracture. Compare this image with the image in Figure 3-50, which was taken on the same patient with a 25-degree angle. Slightly elevate the proximal forearm to open the radioscaphoid joint.

Analysis. The scaphocapitate joint is closed and the hamate-capitate joint is open. The wrist was not externally rotated enough.

Correction. Increase the degree of external wrist rotation.

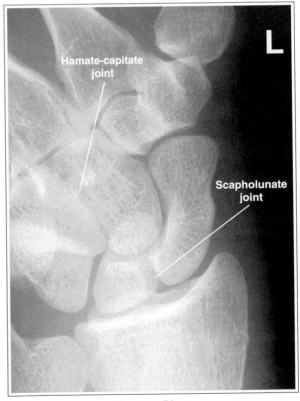

Image 56.

Analysis. The scapholunate and hamate-capitate joints are closed. The wrist was externally rotated more than needed.

Correction. Decrease the amount of external wrist rotation.

Hamate-capitate joint

Ulnar styloid

Scapholunate joint

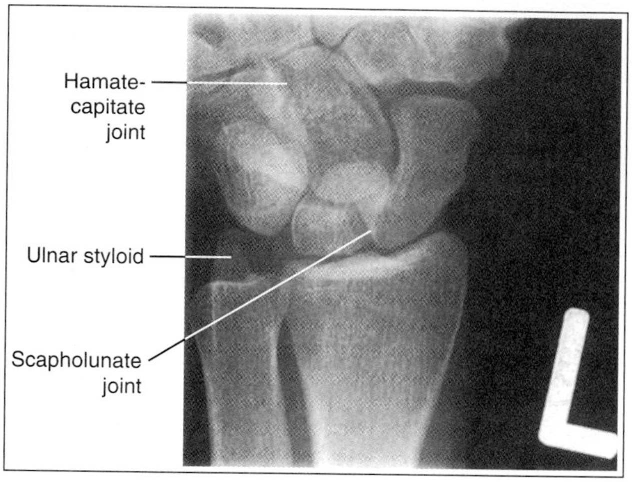

Image 57.

Analysis. The scapholunate and hamate-capitate joints are closed. The wrist was externally rotated more than needed. The styloid process is demonstrated distal to the ulnar head midline. The humerus was not abducted with the elbow in a flexed, lateral position. The scaphoid is not in the center of the field, and the proximal metacarpals are not included on the image.

Correction. Decrease the amount of external wrist rotation and abduct the humerus, placing the elbow in a flexed, lateral position. Move the central ray ½ inch (1.25 cm) distally.

WRIST: CARPAL CANAL (TUNNEL) (TANGENTIAL, INFEROSUPERIOR PROJECTION)

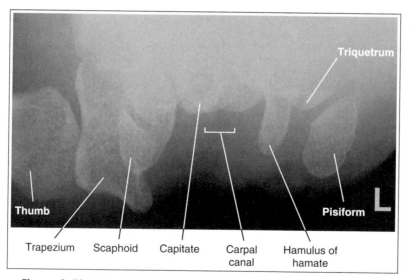

Triquetrum

Thumb

Pisiform

Trapezium   Scaphoid   Capitate   Carpal canal   Hamulus of hamate

Figure 3-52. Carpal canal image of the wrist with accurate positioning.

Image Analysis

The pisiform is demonstrated without superimposition of the hamulus of the hamate, and the carpal canal is clearly demonstrated.

- The carpal canal position of the wrist is accomplished by placing the distal forearm and wrist on the IR in a

PA projection, then hyperextending (dorsiflex) the wrist until the long axis of the metacarpals are close to vertical, while the wrist remains in contact with the IR. To obtain adequate wrist hyperextension have the patient grasp the fingers with the opposite hand and gently pull them posteriorly (Figure 3-53).

- The carpal canal position is used to evaluate the carpal canal for the narrowing that gives rise to carpal canal

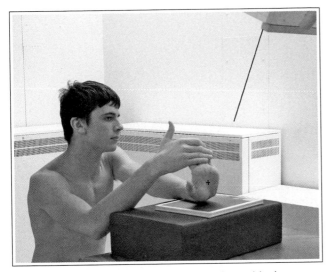

Figure 3-53. Proper carpal canal wrist positioning.

syndrome and demonstrate fractures of the pisiform and hamulus of the hamate. The carpal canal is a passageway formed anteriorly by the flexor retinaculum, posteriorly by the capitate, laterally by the scaphoid and trapezium, and medially by the pisiform and hamate (Figure 3-54). Fractures of the pisiform and hamulus process are best demonstrated when they are seen without superimposition. This is accomplished by rotating the patient's hand 10 degrees internally (toward radial side) until the fifth metacarpal is aligned perpendicular to the IR. If the hand is not internally rotated the pisiform will be superimposed over the hamulus process on the image (see Image 58).

The carpal canal is visualized in its entirety, and the carpal bones are demonstrated with only slight elongation.

- To show the carpal canal and demonstrate the carpals with only slight elongation, the patient's hand is positioned vertically and the central ray is angled 25 to 30 degrees

proximally. (Use a 25-degree angle if the patient is able to place the hand vertically, and use a 30-degree angle if the patient is unable to bring the hand to a completely vertical position, but can bring it within 15 degrees of vertical.) If the angle between the central ray and metacarpals is too great, the carpal canal will not be fully demonstrated and the carpal bones will be foreshortened (see Image 59). If the angle between the central ray and metacarpals is too small, the bases of the hamulus process, pisiform, and scaphoid are obscured by the metacarpal bases (see Image 60).

- **Insufficient wrist extension:** When imaging a patient who is unable to extend the wrist enough to place the metacarpals to within 15 degrees of vertical, the central ray angle needs to be increased. To determine the degree of angulation, first align the central ray so it is parallel with the patient's palmar surface, then increase the angle an additional 15 degrees proximally (Figure 3-55). The resulting image will demonstrate adequate visualization of the carpal bones and carpal canal, though they will demonstrate excessive elongation because of the angle formed between the central ray and IR (see Image 61).

The carpal canal is at the center of the collimated field. The trapezium, distal scaphoid, pisiform and hamulus of the hamate are included within the field.

- The carpal canal is positioned in the center of the collimated field by centering the central ray to center of the palm of the hand. After the central ray is centered, open the longitudinal and transverse collimations to within $\frac{1}{2}$ inch (1.25 cm) of the wrist skinline.

- One half of an 8- × 10-inch (18- × 24-cm) detailed screen-film or computed IR placed crosswise should be adequate to include all the required anatomical structures.

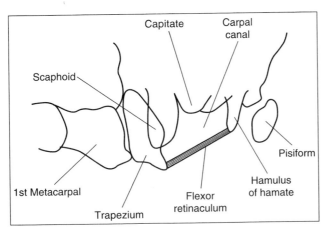

Figure 3-54. Carpal canal anatomy.

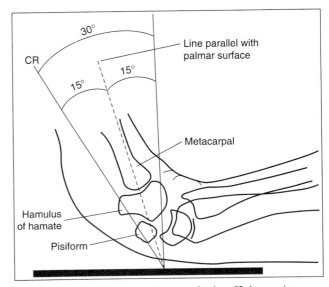

Figure 3-55. Central ray alignment for insufficient wrist extension.

Carpal Canal Image Analysis

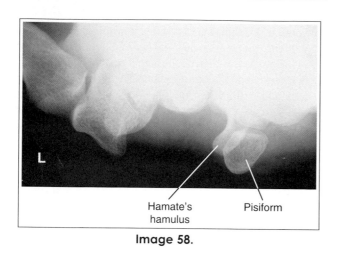

Image 58.

Hamate's hamulus   Pisiform

Analysis. The pisiform is superimposed over the hamulus of the hamate. The patient's wrist and distal forearm were either in a PA projection or in slight external (toward the ulnar side) rotation.

Correction. Rotate the hand internally (toward the radius) until the fifth metacarpal is vertical.

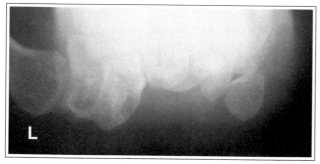

Image 59.

Analysis. The carpal canal is not demonstrated in its entirety, and the carpal bones are foreshortened. The angle between the central ray and metacarpals was too great.

Correction. Decrease the central ray angle until it is within 15 degrees of the metacarpals (see Figure 3-55).

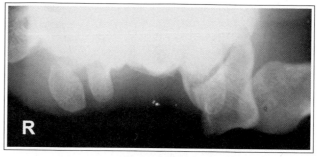

Image 60.

Analysis. The metacarpal bases obscure the bases of the hamate's hamulus process, pisiform, and scaphoid. The angle between the central ray and metacarpals was too small.

Correction. Increase the central ray angle until it is within 15 degrees of the metacarpals (see Figure 3-55), or increase the amount of wrist hyperextension by pulling the fingers posteriorly until the metacarpals are vertical.

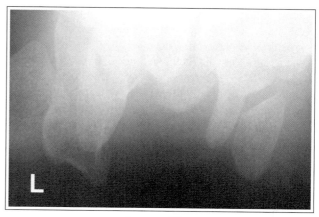

Image 61.

Analysis. The carpal bones and carpal canal demonstrate excessive elongation because of the angle formed between the central ray and IR.

Correction. Increase the amount of wrist hyperextension by pulling the fingers posteriorly until the metacarpals are vertical, if the patient is able to, and then adjust the central ray until it is within 15 degrees of the metacarpals (see Figure 3-55).

FOREARM: ANTEROPOSTERIOR PROJECTION

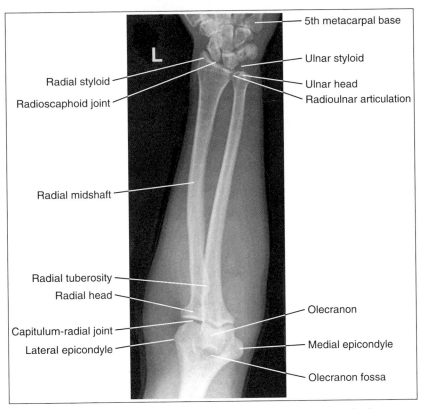

Figure 3-56. Anteroposterior forearm image with accurate positioning.

Image Analysis

Image density is uniform across entire forearm.

- *Anode-heel effect:* To use the anode-heel effect to obtain uniform density across the forearm, position the thinner wrist (distal forearm) at the anode end of the tube and the thicker elbow (proximal forearm) at the cathode end. Set an exposure (mAs) that will adequately demonstrate the midpoint of the forearm.

The long axis of the forearm is aligned with the long axis of the collimated field.

- Aligning the long axis of the forearm with the long axis of the collimated field enables you to collimate tightly without clipping the distal or proximal forearm.

The forearm midpoint is at the center of the collimated field. The wrist and elbow joints and forearm soft tissue are included within the field.

- A perpendicular central ray is centered to the midpoint of the forearm to place it in the center of the image.
- When the wrist and elbow joints are included on the image, the degree of radiation beam divergence used to image a long body part needs to be considered (Figure 3-57).

- *IR length for the forearm:* Choose an IR that is long enough to allow at least 1 inch (2.5 cm) of IR to extend beyond each joint space; half of a 14- × 17-inch (35- × 43-cm) IR placed lengthwise should be adequate. To ensure that the IR extends beyond the elbow joint, palpate the medial epicondyle, which is located approximately ¾ inch (2 cm) proximal to the elbow joint. To ensure that the IR extends beyond the wrist joint, palpate the base of the first metacarpal; the wrist joint is located just proximal to this base. Digital imaging requires tight collimation without overlapping of individual exposures.
- *Central ray centering and collimation:* Once the forearm is accurately positioned in relation to the IR, center the central ray with the midpoint of the forearm and open the longitudinal collimation field until it extends just beyond the elbow and the wrist. If the collimation does not extend beyond the joints, adjust the centering point of the central ray until both the elbow and the wrist joint are included within the collimated field without demonstrating an excessive field beyond them. Transverse collimation should be within ½ inch (1.25 cm) of the forearm skinline.

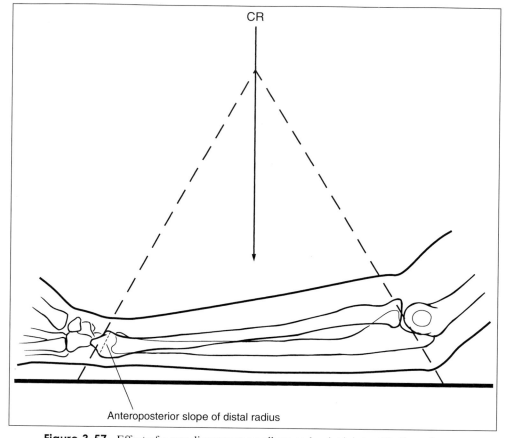

CR

Anteroposterior slope of distal radius

Figure 3-57. Effect of x-ray divergence on elbow and wrist joints. *CR,* Central ray.

DISTAL FOREARM POSITIONING
The distal and proximal forearm is positioned in an AP projection. The radial styloid is demonstrated in profile laterally, and superimposition of the metacarpal bases and of the radius and ulna is minimal.

- To obtain an AP projection of the distal forearm, supinate the hand and place the second through fifth metacarpal heads against the IR (Figure 3-58).
- *Detecting distal forearm rotation:* Rotation of the distal forearm results from inaccurate positioning of the hand and wrist. If the wrist and hand are not positioned in an AP projection but are rotated, the radial styloid is no longer in profile and the distal radius and ulna and the metacarpal bases are superimposed. To identify which way the wrist is rotated, evaluate the metacarpal and carpal bones. When the wrist and hand are medially (internally) rotated, the laterally located first and second metacarpal bases and carpal bones are superimposed, and the medially located metacarpals, pisiform, and hamate hook are better demonstrated (see Images 62 and 64). If the wrist and hand are laterally (externally) rotated, the medially located fourth and fifth metacarpal bases and carpal bones will be superimposed, whereas the laterally located metacarpals and carpal bones will demonstrate less superimposition.

- *Distal forearm positioning for fracture:* Patients with known or suspected fractures may be unable to position both the wrist and elbow joints into an AP projection simultaneously. In such cases, position the joint closer to the fracture in a true position. When the fracture is situated closer to the wrist joint, the wrist joint and distal forearm should meet the requirements for an AP

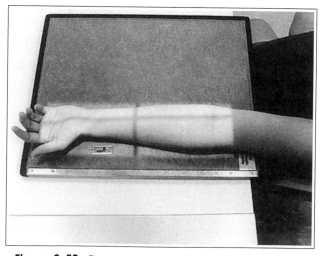

Figure 3-58. Proper anteroposterior forearm positioning.

projection, but the elbow and proximal forearm may demonstrate an oblique or lateral position. It may be necessary to position the distal forearm in a PA projection when an AP projection is difficult for the patient. The wrist joint and distal forearm should still be positioned as previously described (see Image 63).

The ulnar styloid is projected distally to the midline of the ulnar head.

- The position of the ulnar styloid is determined by the position of the humerus and elbow. When the humerus and elbow positions are adjusted but the wrist position is maintained, it is the ulna that rotates and changes position. Positioning the humeral epicondyles parallel with the IR for the AP projection of the forearm places the ulnar styloid posterior to the head of the ulna. If the elbow is rotated internally (medially) and the wrist remains in an AP projection, the ulnar styloid is demonstrated laterally, next to the radius. If the elbow is rotated externally (laterally) and the wrist remains in an AP projection, the ulnar styloid is demonstrated in profile medially.

The anterior and posterior carpal articulating surfaces of the distal radius are superimposed, and the radioscaphoid and radiolunate joint spaces are open.

- The distal radial carpal articular surface is concave and slants at approximately 11 degrees from posterior to anterior. When the forearm is placed parallel with the IR in an AP projection and the central ray is centered to the midforearm, diverged x-rays record the image (see Figure 3-57) much as if the central ray were angled toward the wrist joint. If this angle of divergence is parallel with the AP slant of the distal radius, the resulting image shows superimposed distal radial margins and open radioscaphoid and radiolunate joint spaces.

PROXIMAL FOREARM POSITIONING

The proximal forearm is positioned in an AP projection. The radial head is superimposed over the lateral aspect of the proximal ulna by approximately $1/4$ inch (0.6 cm). If included on the IR, the medial and lateral humeral epicondyles are demonstrated in profile at the extreme medial and lateral edges of the distal humerus.

- An AP proximal forearm projection is obtained by palpating the humeral epicondyles and aligning them parallel with the IR, placing the proximal radius anterior to the ulna (see Figure 3-58).
- *Detecting proximal forearm rotation:* Proximal forearm rotation results when the humeral epicondyles are poorly positioned. Rotation can be identified on the image when the radial head demonstrates more or less than $1/4$ inch (0.6 cm) superimposition on the ulna and when the humeral epicondyles are not visualized in profile. When more than $1/4$ inch (0.6 cm) of the radial head is

superimposed over the ulna, the elbow has been medially (internally) rotated (see Image 71). When less than $1/4$ inch (0.6 cm) of radial head is superimposed over the ulna, the elbow has been laterally (externally) rotated (see Image 64).

- *Proximal forearm positioning for fracture:* Patients with known or suspected fractures may be unable to position both the wrist and elbow joint into an AP projection simultaneously. In such cases, position the joint closer to the fracture in the truer position. When the fracture is situated closer to the elbow joint, the elbow joint and proximal forearm should meet the requirements for an AP projection, whereas the wrist and distal forearm may demonstrate obliquity.

The capitulum-radius joint is either partially or completely closed, and the radial head articulating surface is demonstrated. The olecranon process is situated within the olecranon fossa, and the coronoid process is visible on end.

- The elbow image on an AP forearm image is slightly different from an AP elbow image, owing to the difference in centering of the central ray. The central ray is placed directly over the elbow joint for an AP elbow image, but it is centered distal to the elbow joint, at the midforearm, for an AP forearm image. With distal centering, diverged rays record the elbow joint image instead of straight central rays, much the same as if the central ray were angled toward the elbow joint (see Figure 3-57). Imaging the elbow with diverged rays projects the radial head into the capitulum-radius joint and causes the anterior margin of the radial head to project beyond the posterior margin, demonstrating its articulating surface.
- *Effect of elbow flexion:* The positions of the olecranon process and fossa and the coronoid process are determined by the amount of elbow flexion. Accurate forearm positioning requires us to position the elbow in full extension, which places the olecranon process within the olecranon fossa and demonstrates the coronoid process on end. When a forearm image is taken with the elbow flexed and the proximal humerus elevated (Figure 3-59), the olecranon process moves away from the olecranon fossa and the coronoid process shifts proximally. How far the olecranon process is from the fossa depends on the degree of elbow flexion. The greater the elbow flexion, the farther the olecranon process is positioned away from the fossa and the more foreshortened is the distal humerus.

The radial tuberosity is demonstrated in profile medially, and the radius and ulna appear parallel.

- When the distal humerus is positioned with the epicondyles parallel with the IR, the relationship of the radius and ulna is controlled by wrist positioning. To place the radius and ulna parallel and the radial

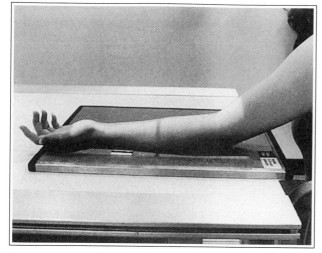

Figure 3-59. Patient positioned for anteroposterior forearm image with flexed humerus.

tuberosity in profile medially, position the wrist and hand in an AP projection. When the hand and wrist are pronated, the radius crosses over the ulna, and the radial tuberosity is rotated posteriorly, out of profile (see Image 65).

Anteroposterior Forearm Image Analysis

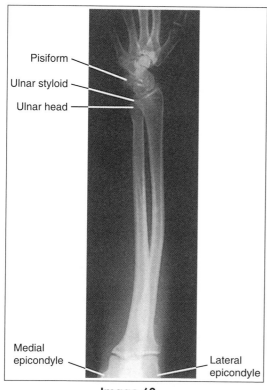

Image 62.

Analysis. The humeral epicondyles are demonstrated in profile, and the ulnar styloid is demonstrated distal to the

midline of the ulnar head. The elbow has been accurately positioned. The first and second metacarpal bases and the laterally located carpal bones are superimposed, and the medially located carpal bones and pisiform are well demonstrated. The radial styloid is not visible in profile. The wrist was internally rotated.

Correction. While maintaining the AP projection of the elbow, rotate the wrist and hand externally until the hand is supinated and the wrist is in an AP projection.

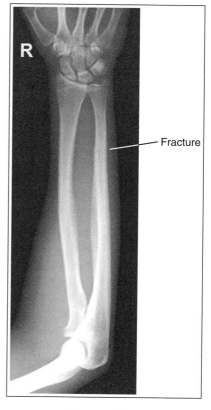

Image 63.

Analysis. A fracture is located at the distal forearm. The wrist demonstrates a PA projection, whereas the elbow is in a lateral position.

Correction. Because the joint closer to the fracture is in the true projection, no repositioning movement is needed.

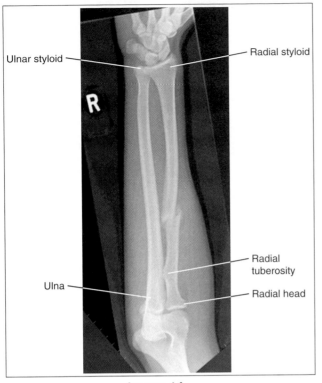

Image 64.

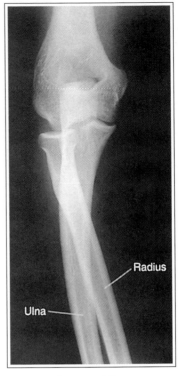

Image 65.

Analysis. The radial styloid is not demonstrated in profile, the laterally located first and second metacarpal bases and carpal bones are superimposed, and the medially located carpals are better demonstrated. The wrist was medially (internally) rotated. Less than $1/4$ inch (0.6 cm) of the radial head is superimposed over the ulna. The elbow was laterally (externally) rotated.

Correction. Rotate the wrist and hand laterally (externally) until they are in an AP projection, and rotate the elbow medially (internally) until the humeral epicondyles are parallel with the IR.

Analysis. The radius and ulna are not parallel. The radius is crossed over the ulna, and the radial tuberosity is not demonstrated in profile. For this image, the elbow is in an AP projection but the wrist and hand are positioned in a PA projection. The distal forearm and wrist joint were not included on the image.

Correction. While maintaining an AP projection of the elbow, externally rotate the wrist and hand until they are in an AP projection. Center the central ray more distally, and open the longitudinal collimation to include the wrist joint.

FOREARM: LATERAL POSITION (LATEROMEDIAL PROJECTION)

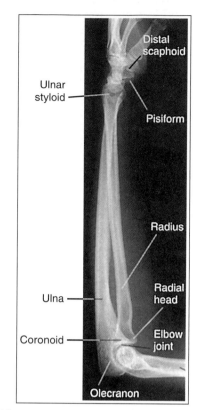

Figure 3-60. Lateral forearm image with accurate positioning.

Image Analysis

Density is uniform across the entire forearm, and contrast and density are adequate to demonstrate the elbow fat structures.

- *Anode-heel effect:* To use the anode-heel effect to obtain uniform density across the forearm, position the thinner wrist (distal forearm) at the anode end of the tube and the thicker elbow (proximal forearm) at the cathode end. Set an exposure (mAs) that will adequately demonstrate the midpoint of the forearm.

- *Soft-tissue structures on lateral forearm image:* Soft-tissue structures of interest are the anterior and posterior fat pads and the supinator fat stripe at the elbow and the pronator fat stripe at the wrist (Figure 3-61). The elbow's anterior fat pad is situated anterior to the distal humerus, and the elbow's supinator fat stripe is visible parallel to the anterior aspect of the proximal radius. A change in the shape or placement of these fat structures indicates joint effusion and elbow injury. The elbow's posterior fat pad is normally obscured on a negative lateral forearm image owing to its location within the olecranon fossa. On elbow injury, joint effusion

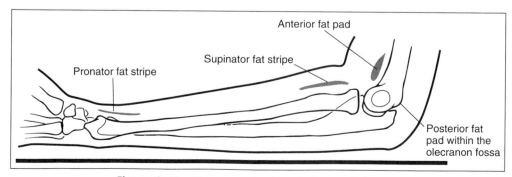

Figure 3-61. Placement of wrist and elbow soft tissue.

pushes this pad out of the fossa, allowing it to be visualized proximal and posterior to the olecranon process. The wrist's pronator fat stripe is demonstrated parallel to the anterior surface of the distal radius. Bowing or obliteration of this fat stripe may be the only indication of subtle radial fractures.

The forearm midpoint is at the center of the collimated field. The radius and ulna, wrist and elbow joints, and forearm soft tissue are included within the field.

- A perpendicular central ray is centered to the midpoint of the forearm to place the forearm in the center of the image.

   When the wrist and elbow joints are included on the image, the degree of radiation beam divergence used to image a long body part needs to be considered (Figure 3-62).
- *IR length for the forearm:* Choose an IR that is long enough to allow at least 1 inch (2.5 cm) of IR to extend beyond each joint space; half of a 14- × 17-inch (35- × 43-cm) screen-film or computed radiography IR placed lengthwise should be adequate. To ensure that the IR extends beyond the elbow, palpate the medial epicondyle, which is located ¾ inch (2 cm) proximal to the elbow joint. To ensure that the IR extends beyond the wrist joint, palpate the base of the first metacarpal; the wrist joint is located just proximal to this base. Digital imaging requires tight collimation without overlapping of individual exposures.
   - *Central ray centering and collimation:* Once the forearm is accurately positioned in relation to the IR,

center the central ray to the midpoint of the forearm, and open the longitudinal collimation field until it extends just beyond the elbow and wrist joints. If collimation does not extend beyond the joints, adjust the centering point of the central ray until both the elbow and the wrist joint are included within the collimated field without demonstrating an excessive field beyond them. Transverse collimation should be within ½ inch (1.25 cm) of the forearm skinline.

DISTAL FOREARM POSITIONING
The distal forearm is in a lateral position.
The AP aspect of the distal scaphoid and pisiform are aligned with each other, and the distal scaphoid is demonstrated slightly distal to the pisiform. The distal radius and ulna are superimposed.

- A lateral position of the wrist and distal forearm is obtained by rotating the wrist into a lateral position with its ulnar aspect against the IR (Figure 3-63). To ensure true lateral positioning, place the palmar aspect of your thumb and forefinger against the anterior and posterior aspects of the patient's wrist joint. Then adjust the rotation until your thumb and finger are aligned perpendicular to the IR.
- *Distal forearm positioning for fracture:* Patients with known or suspected fractures may be unable to position both the wrist and elbow joint into a lateral position simultaneously. In such cases position the joint closer to the fracture in a true position. When the fracture is situated closer to the wrist joint, the wrist and distal forearm should meet the lateral positioning requirements, indicating a true lateral position, but the elbow and proximal forearm may demonstrate obliquity (see Image 66).
- *Verifying a lateral forearm position:* The pisiform and distal scaphoid relationship can be used to discern whether a true lateral wrist and distal forearm are demonstrated. On a lateral forearm image with accurate

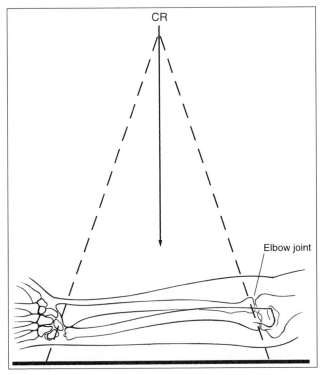

Figure 3-62. Alignment of x-ray divergence on distal forearm. *CR,* Central ray.

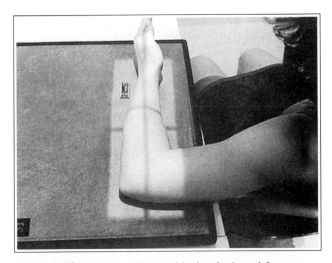

Figure 3-63. Proper patient positioning for lateral forearm image.

positioning, these two bones should be visible anterior to the capitate and lunate, with their anterior aspects aligned and the distal scaphoid projecting distal to the pisiform. It is the diverged x-ray beams used to image the pisiform and scaphoid that causes the distal scaphoid to be projected distal to the pisiform. When the wrist and distal forearm are rotated, the anterior alignment of the scaphoid and pisiform, as well as of the radius and ulna, changes. If the wrist and distal forearm have been externally rotated (supinated), the pisiform is visible anterior to the distal scaphoid, and the ulna appears anterior to the radius. The radial tuberosity will also be visible anteriorly if the elbow is placed in a true lateral position (see Image 67). If the wrist and distal forearm have been internally rotated (pronated), the distal scaphoid is visible anterior to the pisiform and the radius appears anterior to the ulna (see Image 68).

The ulnar styloid is demonstrated in profile posteriorly.

- When the humerus and elbow are mispositioned, the placement of the ulna changes. The ulnar styloid is put in profile by placing the elbow in a lateral position and abducting the humerus until it is parallel with the IR, aligning the entire arm on the same horizontal plane. If the humerus is not abducted, nor the elbow positioned laterally, the ulnar styloid is positioned medially, out of profile.

PROXIMAL FOREARM AND DISTAL HUMERUS POSITIONING
Elbow is flexed 90 degrees.

- When the elbow is flexed 90 degrees, displacement of the anterior or posterior fat pads can be used as a sign to determine diagnosis. Poor elbow positioning, however, also displaces these fat pads and consequently simulates joint pathology. When the elbow is extended, nonpathological displacement of the anterior and posterior fat pads may result from intraarticular pressure and the olecranon's position within the olecranon fossa.

The distal humerus is in a lateral position. The distal humerus demonstrates three concentric (having the same center) arcs, formed by the trochlear sulcus, capitulum, and medial aspect of the trochlea. The elbow joint space is open, and the radial head is superimposed over the coronoid process.

- A lateral proximal forearm image is obtained by placing the elbow in a lateral position and abducting the humerus until it is parallel with the IR, thereby putting the entire arm on the same horizontal plane. The wrist and hand are then placed in a lateral position, and the medial (ulnar) aspect of the forearm rests against the IR (see Figure 3-63). Even though the capitulum is placed anterior to the medial trochlea and the humeral epicondyles are not superimposed for this position, an open joint space may still be obtained. Because the central ray is centered to

the midforearm, the diverged x-rays used to image the distal humerus align parallel with the slant of the capitulum and medial trochlea (see Figure 3-62). The result of this parallelism is an open elbow joint space.

- **Effect of muscular or thick forearm:** Because the patient's forearm rests on its medial (ulnar) surface, the size of the proximal and distal forearm affects the appearance of the elbow joint space. For a patient with a muscular or thick proximal forearm, which is therefore elevated higher than the distal forearm, the capitulum is positioned too far anteriorly and the medial trochlea too posteriorly to align with the x-ray beam divergence. The resulting image demonstrates a closed elbow joint space, and the radial head is positioned distal to the coronoid process (see Image 69).

- **Forearm and humeral positioning for fracture:** Patients with known or suspected fractures may be unable to position both the wrist and elbow joint into a lateral position simultaneously. In such cases position the joint closer to the fracture in the true position. When the fracture is situated closer to the elbow joint, the elbow joint and proximal forearm should meet the requirements for a lateral position, whereas the wrist and distal forearm may demonstrate obliquity.

- **Effect of poor humeral positioning:** Misalignment of the capitulum and medial trochlea as well as of the radial head and coronoid process is also the result of poor humeral positioning. When the distal surface of the capitulum appears quite distal to the distal surface of the medial trochlea and the radial head is positioned posterior to the coronoid process, the proximal humerus was elevated (Figure 3-64 and Image 70). When the distal surface of the capitulum appears proximal to the distal surface of the medial trochlea and the radial head is positioned too anteriorly on the coronoid process, the proximal humerus was positioned lower than the distal humerus.

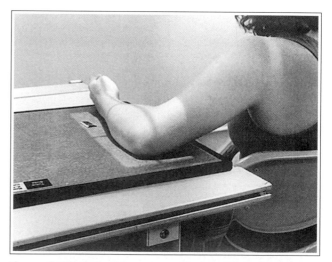

Figure 3-64. Lateral forearm positioning with elevated proximal humerus.

Lateral Forearm Image Analysis

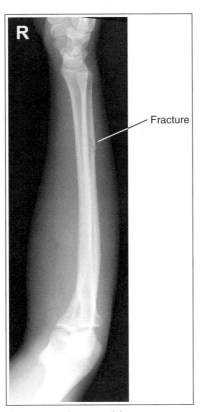

Image 66.

Analysis. A fracture is located at the distal forearm. The wrist demonstrates a lateral position, but the elbow is rotated.

Correction. Because the joint closer to the fracture is in the true projection, no repositioning movement is needed.

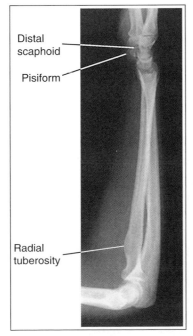

Image 67.

Analysis. On this image the elbow has been accurately positioned. The pisiform is demonstrated anterior to the scaphoid and the radial tuberosity is shown anteriorly in profile, indicating that the wrist and distal forearm were slightly externally rotated (supinated).

Correction. While maintaining accurate elbow positioning, internally rotate (pronate) the wrist and distal forearm into a lateral position. This movement will rotate the scaphoid toward the pisiform, aligning their anterior aspects.

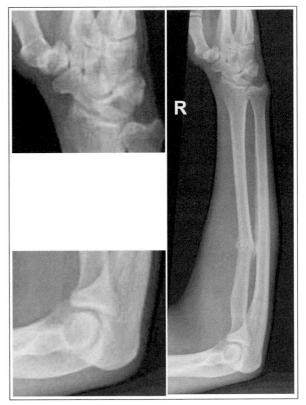

Image 68.

Analysis. The distal scaphoid is anterior to the pisiform and the radius is anterior to the ulna, indicating that the wrist and hand were internally rotated (pronated).

Correction. If the patient is able, externally rotate (supinate) the hand and wrist until they are in a true lateral position. This may not be possible because of the radial fracture.

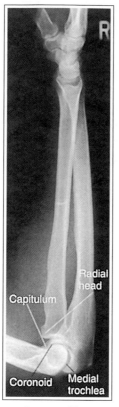

Image 69.

Analysis. The capitulum is positioned too far anterior to the medial trochlea, and the radial head is positioned distal to the coronoid process. The proximal forearm was elevated higher than the distal forearm, possibly because the patient has a muscular or thick proximal forearm.

Correction. Raise the distal forearm until the forearm is positioned parallel with the IR, or, if the patient's proximal forearm is muscular or thick, no positioning adjustment is needed.

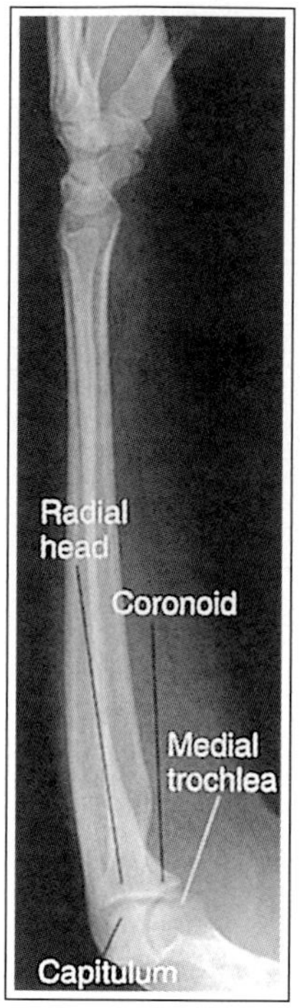

Image 70.

Analysis. The wrist is accurately positioned. The distal end of the capitulum is shown distal to the medial trochlea, and the radial head is posterior to the coronoid process. The proximal humerus was elevated as demonstrated in Figure 3-64.

Correction. While maintaining accurate wrist positioning, depress the proximal humerus until the humerus is parallel with the IR.

ELBOW: ANTEROPOSTERIOR PROJECTION

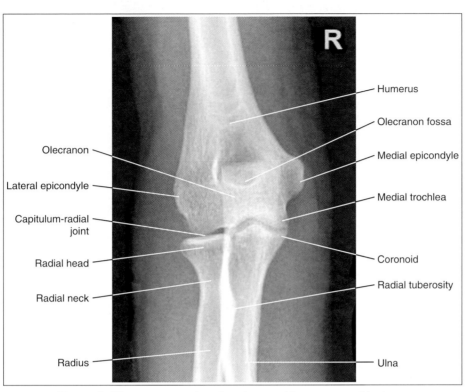

Figure 3-65. Anteroposterior elbow image with accurate positioning.

Image Analysis

The elbow is positioned in an AP projection. The medial and lateral humeral epicondyles are demonstrated in profile at the extreme medial and lateral edges of the distal humerus, and the radial head is superimposed over the lateral aspect of the proximal ulna by approximately ¼ inch (0.6 cm). The coronoid process is demonstrated on end.

- An AP projection of the elbow is obtained by supinating the patient's hand and externally rotating the forearm and humerus until an imaginary line drawn between the humeral epicondyles is parallel with the IR (Figure 3-66). This positioning places the proximal radius anterior to the ulna.

- *Detecting elbow rotation:* Rotation of the elbow is a result of poor humeral epicondyle positioning and can be identified on an image when (1) the epicondyles are not visualized in profile, (2) the radial head is demonstrated with more or less than ¼ inch (0.6 cm) superimposition of the ulna, and (3) the coronoid process is seen in profile. The smaller, lateral humeral epicondyle is more sensitive to rotation, moving out of profile with only a slight degree of elbow rotation. If the epicondyles are not demonstrated in profile, evaluate the degree of radial head superimposition of the ulna to determine how to reposition for an AP projection. If more than ¼ inch

(0.6 cm) of radial head is superimposed over the ulna, the elbow has been medially (internally) rotated (see Image 71). If less than ¼ inch (0.6 cm) of the radial head is superimposed over the ulna, the elbow has been laterally (externally) rotated (see Image 72).

The radial tuberosity is demonstrated in profile medially, and the radius and ulna are parallel.

- The alignment of the radius and ulna is determined by the position of the humerus and the wrist. When the humerus is positioned with the humeral epicondyles

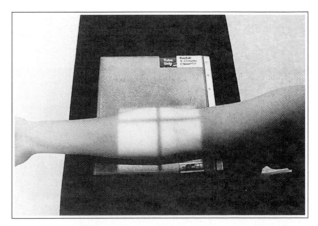

Figure 3-66. Proper patient positioning for anteroposterior elbow image.

parallel with the IR, the radial and ulnar relationship can be adjusted with wrist rotation. For an AP projection of the elbow, the hand and wrist should also be positioned in an AP projection by supinating the hand. This positioning places the radial tuberosity medially in profile and eliminates crossing of the radius and ulna. As the hand and wrist are pronated, the radius crosses over the ulna, and the radial tuberosity is rotated posteriorly, out of profile (see Image 73).

The capitulum-radius joint is open, the radial head articulating surface is not demonstrated, the olecranon process is situated within the olecranon fossa, and the coronoid process is demonstrated on end.

- You must use accurate central ray placement and position the forearm parallel with the IR to obtain an open capitulum-radius joint space. When the central ray is centered proximal to the elbow joint space, the capitulum is projected into the joint; when the central ray is centered distal to the elbow joint, the radial head is projected into the joint space (see Image 74). Poor central ray placement also distorts the radial head, causing its articulating surface to be demonstrated. The degree of joint closure depends on how far the central ray is positioned from the elbow joint. The farther away from the joint the central ray is centered, the more the capitulum-radial joint space is obscured and the more the radial head articulating surface is demonstrated.

- **Effect of elbow flexion:** Flexion of the elbow joint also distorts the AP elbow image. With elbow flexion, the capitulum-radial joint closes, the olecranon process moves away from the olecranon fossa, and the coronoid process shifts proximally. How a flexed elbow is positioned with respect to the IR determines which elbow structures are distorted on the image. If a flexed elbow is resting on the posterior point of the olecranon, with the proximal humerus and the distal forearm elevated as demonstrated in Figure 3-67, both the humerus and the forearm are foreshortened and the capitulum-radial

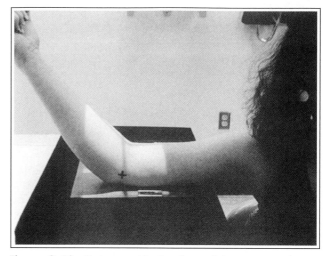

Figure 3-68. Patient positioning for partial anteroposterior elbow projection: humerus parallel with image receptor.

joint is obscured (see Image 75). Foreshortening of the proximal humerus is signified on the image by an oval olecranon fossa that is clearly demonstrated, without the olecranon within it. Foreshortening of the distal forearm is demonstrated if the radial head articulating surface is imaged partially on end. The severity of the distortion increases with increased elbow flexion.

- **Compensating for a nonextendable elbow (partial AP projections):** An elbow that cannot be fully extended should be imaged using separate exposures to image the distal humerus and the proximal forearm—a method referred to as *partial AP projections*.

  Figure 3-68 demonstrates how the patient should be positioned for an undistorted AP distal humerus image to be obtained. Note that the humerus is placed parallel with the IR. The resulting image demonstrates an undistorted image of the distal humerus, whereas the proximal forearm is severely distorted and the capitulum-radial joint space is obscured (see Image 76). Figure 3-69

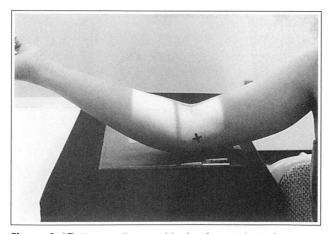

Figure 3-67. Proper elbow positioning for a patient who cannot fully extend the elbow but can extend to at least 30 degrees.

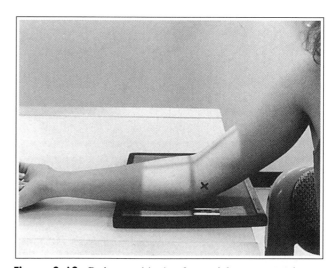

Figure 3-69. Patient positioning for partial anteroposterior elbow projection: forearm parallel with image receptor.

demonstrates how the patient should be positioned for an undistorted AP proximal forearm image to be obtained. Note that the forearm is placed parallel with the IR. The resulting image demonstrates an undistorted image of the proximal forearm and an open capitulum-radial joint, but the distal humerus is severely distorted (see Image 77). The capitulum-radial joint space is visible on the image only if the forearm is positioned parallel with the IR.

The elbow joint is at the center of the collimated field. The elbow joint, one fourth of the proximal forearm and distal humerus, and the lateral soft tissue are included within the field.

- The elbow joint is located ¾ inch (2 cm) distal to the easily palpable medial epicondyle. To obtain an image of the elbow joint with the least amount of distortion, place a perpendicular central ray at this level and centered to the mid-elbow. Open longitudinal collimation to include one fourth of the proximal forearm and distal humerus. Transverse collimation should be within ½ inch (1.25 cm) of the elbow skinline.
- Half of a 10- × 12-inch (24- × 30-cm) detailed screen-film IR placed crosswise or an 8- × 10-inch (18- × 24-cm) computed radiography IR placed lengthwise should be adequate to include all the required anatomical structures.

Anteroposterior Elbow Image Analysis

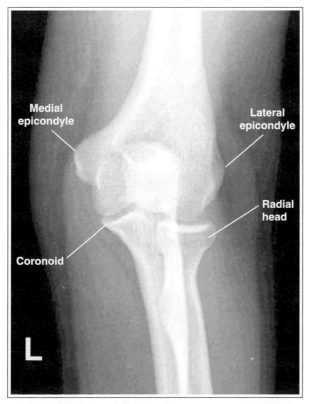

Image 71.

Analysis. The humeral epicondyles are not in profile. The radial head is superimposing more than ¼ inch (0.6 cm) of the ulna, and the coronoid process is visible medially. The elbow was medially (internally) rotated. The capitulum-radial joint space is closed. The distal forearm was slightly elevated.

Correction. Rotate the elbow laterally (externally) until the humeral epicondyles are parallel with the IR, and position the forearm parallel with the IR.

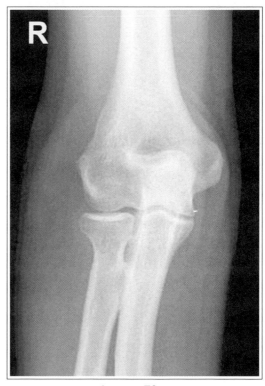

Image 72.

Analysis. The humeral epicondyles are not in profile, and less than ¼ inch (0.6 cm) of the radial head is superimposing the ulna. The image was taken with the elbow in lateral (external) rotation.

Correction. Rotate the elbow medially (internally) until the humeral epicondyles are parallel with the IR.

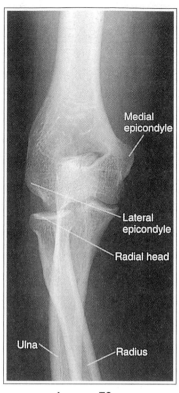

Image 73.

Analysis. The radius is crossed over the ulna, and the radial tuberosity is not demonstrated in profile. The hand and wrist were pronated for this image.

Correction. Supinate the hand and wrist into an AP projection.

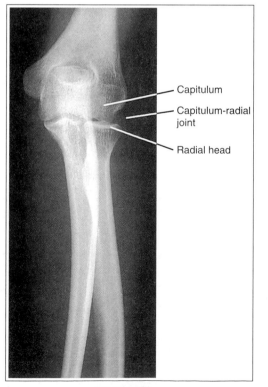

Image 74.

Analysis. The capitulum-radial joint space is closed, and the radial head articulating surface is demonstrated. The central ray was centered distal to the joint space.

Correction. Center the central ray to the mid-elbow at a level ¾ inch (2 cm) distal to the medial epicondyle.

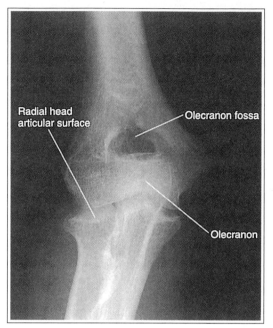

Image 75.

Analysis. The capitulum-radial joint space is closed, and the proximal forearm and distal humerus are foreshortened. The elbow was flexed (40 degrees), and the arm was resting on the posterior point of the elbow with the distal forearm and proximal humerus elevated.

Correction. If possible, fully extend the elbow. If the patient is unable to extend the elbow, take two partial AP exposures, one with the forearm and one with the humerus positioned parallel with the IR, as demonstrated in Figures 3-68 and 3-69.

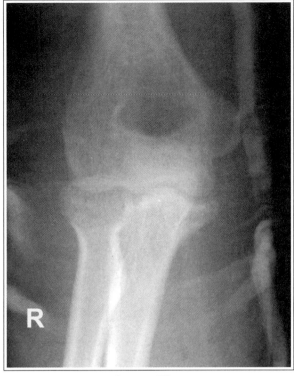

Image 76.

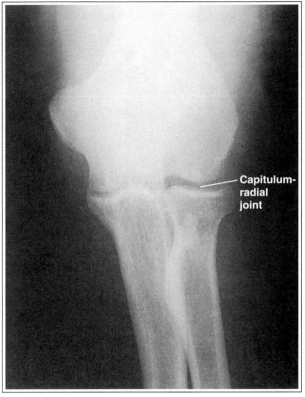

Image 77.

Analysis. The distal humerus is demonstrated without fore-shortening, but the proximal forearm is severely distorted. The humerus was positioned parallel with the IR, but the distal forearm was elevated as demonstrated in Figure 3-68.

Correction. If possible, fully extend the elbow. If the patient is unable to extend the elbow, this is an acceptable image of the distal humerus. A second AP projection of the elbow should be taken with the forearm positioned parallel with the IR, as demonstrated in Figure 3-69.

Analysis. The distal forearm is demonstrated without fore-shortening, and the capitulum-radial joint space is open, but the distal humerus is severely distorted. The forearm was positioned parallel with the IR, whereas the proximal forearm was elevated as demonstrated in Figure 3-69.

Correction. If possible, fully extend the elbow. If the patient is unable to extend the elbow, this is an acceptable image of the proximal forearm. A second AP projection of the elbow should be taken with the humerus positioned parallel with the IR, as demonstrated in Figure 3-68.

ELBOW: ANTEROPOSTERIOR OBLIQUE PROJECTIONS (INTERNAL AND EXTERNAL ROTATION)

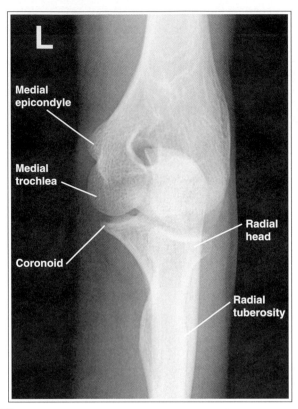

Figure 3-70. Internally rotated oblique elbow image with accurate positioning.

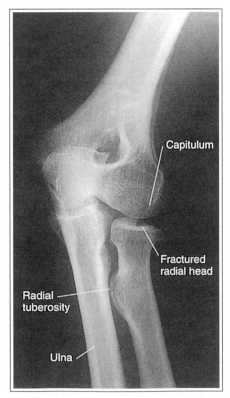

Figure 3-71. Externally rotated oblique elbow image with accurate positioning.

Image Analysis

External Oblique Position: **The capitulum-radial joint is open, and the radial head articulating surface is not demonstrated.**

Internal Oblique Position: **The trochlea-coronoid process joint is open, and the coronoid process articulating surface is not demonstrated.**

- To obtain an open capitulum-radial and trochlear-coronoid process joint spaces, you must use accurate central ray placement and position the elbow with the forearm parallel with the IR. When the central ray is centered proximal to the elbow joint spaces, the structures of the distal humerus are projected into the joint; when the central ray is centered distal to the elbow joint, the structures of the proximal forearm are projected into the joint space. Poor central ray positioning also distorts the radial head and coronoid process, causing their articulating surface to be visualized. The degree of joint closure and radial head and coronoid process distortion depends on how far the central ray is positioned from the elbow joint. The farther away from the joint the central ray is centered, the more the joint spaces will be obscured, and the more the articulating surfaces of the radial head and coronoid process will be demonstrated.
- *Effect of elbow flexion:* Flexion of the elbow joint also distorts the oblique elbow image. With elbow flexion, the olecranon process moves away from the olecranon fossa and the coronoid process shifts proximally. How the flexed elbow is positioned with respect to the IR determines which elbow structures are distorted on the image. If a flexed elbow is resting on the posterior point of the olecranon, with the proximal humerus and the distal forearm elevated, both the humerus and the forearm are foreshortened and the capitulum-radial and trochlear-coronoid process joints are obscured. Foreshortening of the proximal humerus is demonstrated on an image by an oval olecranon fossa that is clearly demonstrated but without the olecranon process within it. Foreshortening of the distal forearm is demonstrated on the image if the radial head and trochlear articulating surfaces are visualized.

  The severity of the distortion depends on the degree of elbow flexion. If the humerus is positioned parallel with the IR and the distal forearm is elevated, the image shows an undistorted distal humerus, but the proximal forearm is severely distorted and the capitulum-radial joint is obscured (see Image 78). If the forearm is positioned parallel with the IR and the proximal humerus is elevated, the image shows an undistorted proximal forearm and an open capitulum-radial and trochlear-coronoid process joints, but the distal humerus is severely distorted.
- *Oblique positioning of the nonextendable elbow:* For oblique elbow images, if the patient's condition prevents full elbow extension, the anatomical structure (forearm or humerus) of interest should be positioned parallel with the IR. If the radial head or coronoid process is

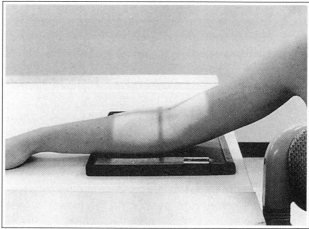

Figure 3-72. Proper patient positioning for oblique elbow image with a flexed elbow.

of interest, position the forearm parallel with the IR (Figure 3-72). If the capitulum or medial trochlea is of interest, position the humerus parallel with the IR. The degree and direction of elbow obliquity are the same as those used for an extended elbow.

INTERNAL OBLIQUE POSITION
The elbow has been positioned with 45 degrees of internal obliquity. The coronoid process, the trochlear notch, and the medial aspect of the trochlea are demonstrated in profile. The trochlear-coronoid process articulation is open, and the radial head and neck are superimposed over the ulna.

- An accurately positioned internal oblique elbow image is obtained by placing the arm in an AP elbow projection, then internally rotating the hand and humerus until the humeral epicondyles are at a 45-degree angle to the IR (Figure 3-73). When the elbow obliquity is correct, the

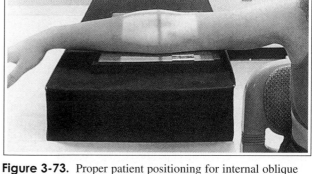

Figure 3-73. Proper patient positioning for internal oblique elbow image.

coronoid process is demonstrated in profile and the radial head and tuberosity are superimposed over the ulna. If the humeral epicondyles are at less than 45 degrees of obliquity, the radial head is demonstrated lateral to the coronoid process and does not entirely superimpose the ulna (see Image 79). If the humeral epicondyles are at more than 45 degrees of obliquity, the radial head is partially visualized anterior to the coronoid process (see Image 80).

EXTERNAL OBLIQUE POSITION

The elbow has been positioned at 45 degrees of external obliquity. The capitulum and radial tuberosity are demonstrated in profile; the radial head, neck, and tuberosity are visualized without superimposing the ulna; and the radioulnar articulation is demonstrated.

- Accurate positioning for an external oblique elbow image is achieved by positioning the arm in an AP projection, then externally rotating the humerus and forearm until the humeral epicondyles form a 45-degree angle with the IR (Figure 3-74). This positioning rotates the radius away from the ulna, demonstrating it without superimposition. If the humeral epicondyles are at less than 45 degrees of obliquity, the radial head and tuberosity still partially superimpose the ulna (see Image 81). If the humeral epicondyles are at more than 45 degrees of obliquity, the coronoid process is partially superimposed over the radial head, and the radial neck and tuberosity are free of superimposition; the radial tuberosity is no longer in profile (see Image 82).

The elbow joint is at the center of the collimated field. The elbow joint, one fourth of the proximal forearm and distal humerus, and surrounding soft tissue are included within the field.

- The elbow joint is located ¾ inch (2 cm) distal to the easily palpable medial humeral epicondyle. To obtain an undistorted image of the elbow joint, place a perpendicular central ray at this level and centered to the mid-elbow. Open longitudinal collimation to include one fourth of the proximal forearm and distal humerus. Transverse collimation should be within ½ inch (1.25 cm) of the elbow skinline.

- Half of a 10- × 12-inch (24- × 30-cm) detailed screen-film IR placed crosswise or an 8- × 10-inch (18- × 24-cm) computed radiography IR placed lengthwise should be adequate to include all the required anatomical structures.

Oblique Elbow Image Analysis

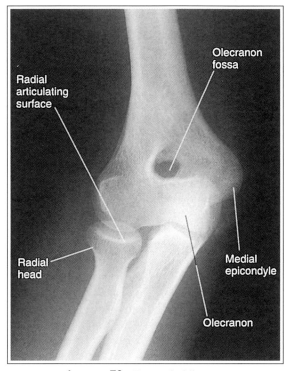

Image 78. External oblique.

Analysis. The elbow has been positioned at a 45-degree external oblique position. The olecranon process is drawn slightly away from the olecranon fossa, the capitulum-radial joint space is closed, and the radial articulating surface is demonstrated. The forearm was not positioned parallel with the IR.

Correction. If possible, fully extend the elbow. If the patient is unable to fully extend the elbow and the radial head is of interest, position the forearm parallel with the IR, and allow the proximal humerus to be elevated, as demonstrated in Figure 3-72.

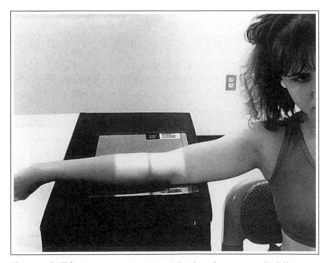

Figure 3-74. Proper patient positioning for external oblique elbow image.

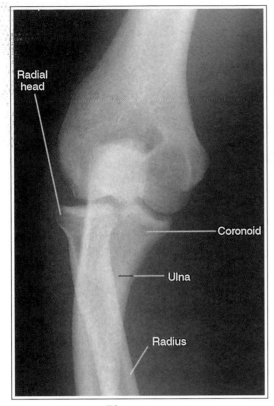

Image 79. Internal oblique.

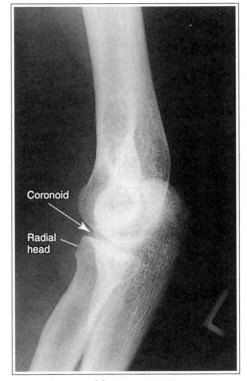

Image 80. Internal oblique.

Analysis. The radial head is demonstrated lateral to the coronoid process without complete superimposition of the ulna, and the most proximal aspect of the olecranon is not demonstrated in profile. The degree of elbow obliquity is less than 45 degrees.

Correction. Increase the degree of internal obliquity until the humeral epicondyles are angled at 45 degrees with the IR.

Analysis. The radial head is partially demonstrated anterior to the coronoid process, without complete superimposition of the ulna. The degree of elbow obliquity is more than 45 degrees.

Correction. Decrease the degree of internal obliquity until the humeral epicondyles are angled at 45 degrees with the IR.

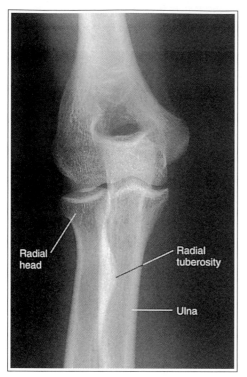

Image 81. External oblique.

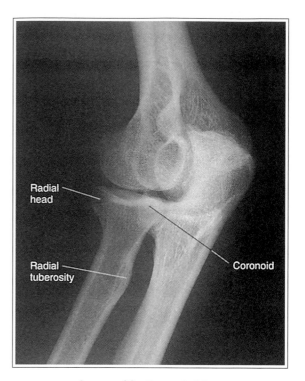

Image 82. External oblique.

Analysis. The radial head and tuberosity are partially superimposed over the ulna, and the radioulnar articulation is obscured. The degree of elbow obliquity is less than 45 degrees. The forearm was not positioned parallel with the IR.

Correction. Increase the degree of external obliquity until the humeral epicondyles are angled at 45 degrees with the IR, and position the forearm parallel with the IR.

Analysis. The coronoid process is partially superimposed over the radial head, but the radial neck and tuberosity are free of superimposition. The radial tuberosity is not demonstrated in profile. The elbow was rotated more than 45 degrees.

Correction. Decrease the degree of lateral obliquity until the humeral epicondyles are angled at 45 degrees with the IR.

ELBOW: LATERAL POSITION (LATEROMEDIAL PROJECTION)

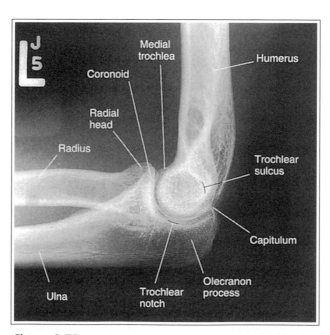

Figure 3-75. Lateral elbow image with accurate positioning.

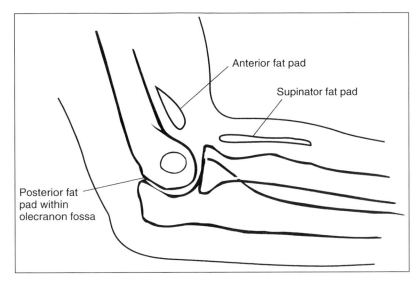

Figure 3-76. Locations of fat pads on lateral elbow projection. *(From Martensen K III:* The elbow, *In-Service Reviews in Radiologic Technology, 14[11], 1992.)*

Image Analysis

Contrast and density are adequate to demonstrate the anterior, posterior, and supinator fat pads, surrounding soft tissue, and bony structures.

- *Fat pads on lateral elbow image:* To evaluate a lateral elbow image, the reviewer not only analyzes the bony structure, but also studies the placement of the soft-tissue fat pads. Three fat pads of interest are present on a lateral elbow image: the anterior and posterior fat pads and the supinator fat stripe. The anterior fat pad should routinely be seen on all lateral elbow images when adequate exposure factors are used. This pad is formed by the superimposed coronoid process and radial pads and is situated immediately anterior to the distal humerus (Figure 3-76). A change in the shape or placement of the anterior fat pad may indicate joint effusion and elbow injury. The posterior fat pad is normally obscured on a negative lateral elbow image owing to its location within the olecranon fossa (Figure 3-76). When an injury occurs, joint effusion pushes this pad out of the fossa, allowing it to be visualized proximal and posterior to the olecranon fossa. The supinator fat stripe is visible parallel to the anterior aspect of the proximal radius (see Figure 3-76). Displacement of this fat stripe is useful in diagnosing fractures of the radial head and neck.

The elbow is flexed 90 degrees.

- When the elbow is flexed 90 degrees, the forearm can be elevated to properly align the anatomical structures of the distal humerus, and displacement of the anterior and posterior fat pads can be used as signs to determine diagnosis. If the elbow is not adequately flexed, these fat pads can be displaced by poor positioning instead of joint pathology, interfering with their diagnostic usefulness. When the arm is extended, nonpathological displacement

of the anterior fat pad results from intraarticular pressure placed on the joint. Nonpathological displacement of the posterior fat pad is a result of positioning of the olecranon within the olecranon fossa, which causes proximal and posterior displacement of the pad (see Image 83).

The elbow is in a lateral position. The distal humerus demonstrates three concentric arcs, which are formed by the trochlear sulcus, capitulum, and medial trochlea. The elbow joint space is open, and the radial head is superimposed over the coronoid process.

- A lateral elbow image is obtained when the humeral epicondyles are positioned directly on top of each other, placing an imaginary line drawn between them perpendicular to the IR. To obtain this humeral epicondyle positioning, place the humerus parallel with the IR and elevate the distal forearm until the palpable medial and lateral epicondyles are superimposed (Figure 3-77). This positioning aligns the trochlear

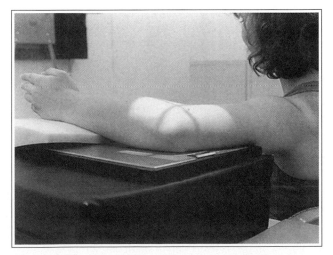

Figure 3-77. Proper patient positioning for lateral elbow image.

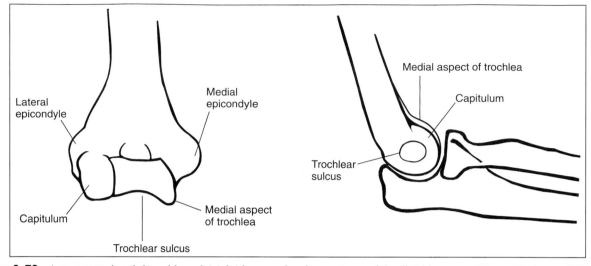

Figure 3-78. Anteroposterior *(left)* and lateral *(right)* images showing anatomy of the distal humerus. *(From Martensen K III: The elbow,* In-Service Reviews in Radiologic Technology, *14[11], 1992.)*

sulcus, capitulum, and medial trochlea into three concentric (having the same center) arcs (Figure 3-78). The trochlear sulcus is the small center arc. It moves very little when a positional change is made and works like a pivoting point between the capitulum and the medial aspect of the trochlea. The largest of the arcs is the medial aspect of the trochlea. It is demonstrated very close to and slightly superimposed on the curve of the trochlear notch. The intermediate-sized arc is the capitulum. When these three arcs are in accurate alignment, the elbow joint is visualized as an open space and the anterior and proximal surfaces of the radial head and coronoid process are aligned.

- *Importance of accurate positioning:* The distal humerus, radial head, and coronoid process are misaligned when the proximal humerus and distal forearm are inaccurately positioned. Proximal humerus positioning determines the alignment of the distal surfaces of the capitulum and medial trochlea, whereas distal forearm positioning determines the AP alignment of the capitulum and medial trochlea. Proximal humerus and distal forearm positioning also determines the alignment of the radial head and coronoid process. Depression or elevation of the proximal humerus moves the radial head anteriorly or posteriorly on the coronoid process, respectively. Depression or elevation of the distal forearm shifts the radial head distally or proximally, respectively, to the coronoid process.

To help understand how the distal humerus and radial head move together, remember that ligaments connect the capitulum and the radial head, so any movement in one causes an equal amount of movement in the other. Precise positioning is a must to obtain a true lateral elbow image. It takes only a small amount of inaccurate

positioning to misalign the distal humerus and close the elbow joint space.

- *Mispositioning of the proximal humerus:* If the proximal humerus is elevated (Figure 3-79), the radial head is positioned too far posteriorly on the coronoid process, and the distal capitulum surface is demonstrated too far distal to the distal surface of the medial trochlea (see Image 84). If the proximal humerus is positioned lower than the distal humerus (Figure 3-80), the radial head is positioned too far anteriorly on the coronoid process, and the distal capitulum surface is demonstrated too far proximal to the distal medial trochlear surface (see Image 85).

- *Mispositioning of the distal forearm:* When the distal forearm is positioned too low (Figure 3-81), the image shows the radial head distal to the coronoid process and the capitulum too far anterior to the medial trochlea

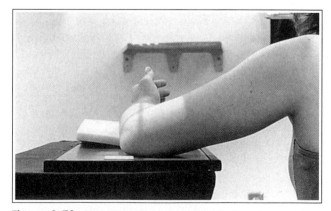

Figure 3-79. Patient positioned for lateral elbow image with elevated proximal humerus.

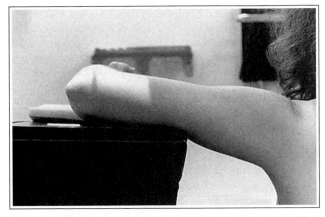

Figure 3-80. Patient positioned for lateral elbow image with depressed proximal humerus.

(see Image 86). When the distal forearm is positioned too high (Figure 3-82), the image shows the radial head proximal to the coronoid process and the capitulum too far posterior to the medial trochlea (see Image 87). Carefully evaluate images that show poor positioning. Often, both forearm and humeral corrections are needed to obtain accurate positioning.

The radial tuberosity is superimposed by the radius and is not demonstrated in profile.

- Visibility of the radial tuberosity is determined by the position of the wrist and hand. When the wrist and hand are placed in a lateral position, the radial tuberosity is situated on the medial aspect of the radius. Because a lateral elbow image is taken in a lateromedial projection, the radius is superimposed over the radial tuberosity. If the wrist and hand are not placed in a lateral position, placement of the radial tuberosity changes. When the wrist and hand are supinated (externally rotated), the

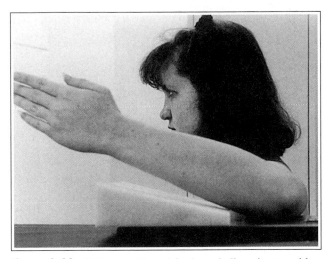

Figure 3-82. Patient positioned for lateral elbow image with elevated distal forearm.

radial tuberosity is demonstrated in profile anteriorly (see Image 88). Pronation (internal rotation) of the wrist and hand shows the radial tuberosity in profile posteriorly (see Image 89).

- Lateral elbow images using the different hand and wrist positions just described are often taken to study the circumference of the radial head and neck for fractures; they are referred to as *radial head images.*

The elbow joint is at the center of the collimated field. The elbow joint, one fourth of the proximal forearm and distal humerus, and the surrounding soft tissue are included within the field.

- The elbow joint is located ¾ inch (2 cm) distal to the lateral epicondyle. To obtain an undistorted image of the elbow joint, place a perpendicular central ray at this level and centered to the midelbow. Open longitudinal collimation to include one fourth of the proximal forearm and distal humerus. Transverse collimation should be within ½ inch (1.25 cm) of the elbow skinline.
- Half of a 10- × 12-inch (24- × 30-cm) detailed screen-film IR placed crosswise or an 8- × 10-inch (18- × 24-cm) computed radiography IR placed lengthwise should be adequate to include all the required anatomical structures.

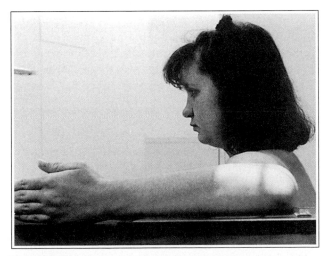

Figure 3-81. Patient positioned for lateral elbow image with depressed distal forearm.

Lateral Elbow Image Analysis

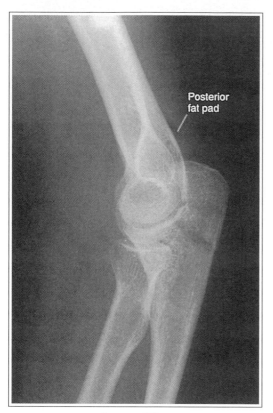

Image 83.

Analysis. The elbow is extended. The olecranon is positioned within the olecranon fossa, and the posterior fat pad is demonstrated proximal to the olecranon process. The radial tuberosity is demonstrated in profile posteriorly, indicating that the hand and wrist were pronated.

Correction. If possible, flex the elbow 90 degrees. Position the hand and wrist in a lateral position.

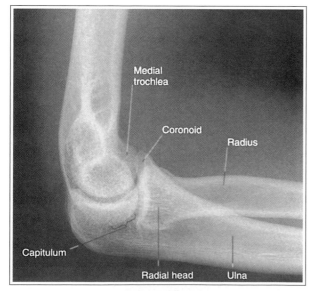

Image 84.

Analysis. The radial head is positioned too far posteriorly on the coronoid process, and the distal surface of the capitulum is demonstrated too far distal to the distal surface of the medial trochlea. The patient was positioned with the proximal humerus elevated, as demonstrated in Figure 3-79.

Correction. Lower the proximal humerus until the humeral epicondyles are superimposed and the humerus is positioned parallel with the IR. This change will move the capitulum proximally and the medial trochlea distally. Because the capitulum and the trochlea move simultaneously, the amount of adjustment needed is only half of the distance demonstrated between where the two distal surfaces should be on a lateral elbow image with accurate positioning and where they are on this image. On this image this distance is approximately ½ inch (1 cm), so the repositioning adjustment needed is only ¼ inch (0.6 cm).

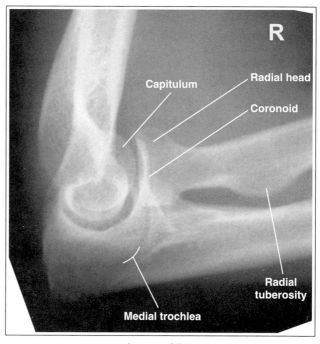

Image 85.

Analysis. The radial head is positioned anterior on the coronoid process, and the distal surface of the capitulum is too far proximal to the distal surface of the medial trochlea. The patient was positioned with the proximal humerus depressed, as demonstrated in Figure 3-80. The radial tuberosity is demonstrated posteriorly, indicating that the hand and wrist were pronated.

Correction. Elevate the proximal humerus until the humeral epicondyles are superimposed and the humerus is positioned parallel with the IR. Because the radial head and coronoid process, the capitulum, and the trochlea move simultaneously, the amount of adjustment required is only half the distance demonstrated between the two anterior and distal surfaces, respectively. Externally rotate the hand and wrist into a lateral position.

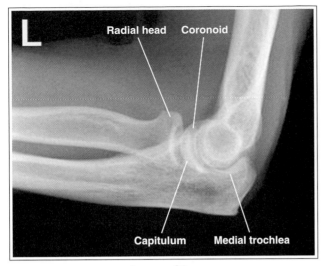

Image 86.

Analysis. The radial head is distal to the coronoid process, and the capitulum appears too far anterior to the medial trochlea. The patient was placed with the distal forearm positioned too close to the IR, as demonstrated in Figure 3-81.

Correction. Elevate the distal forearm until the humeral epicondyles are superimposed. This change will move the capitulum posteriorly and the medial trochlea anteriorly. Because the radial head and coronoid process, the capitulum, and the trochlea move simultaneously, the amount of adjustment required is only half the distance demonstrated between the two distal and anterior surfaces, respectively.

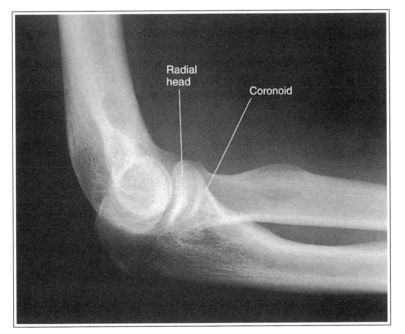

Image 87.

Analysis. The radial head is proximal to the coronoid process, and the capitulum appears too far posterior to the medial trochlea. The patient was positioned with the distal forearm placed too far away from the IR, as demonstrated in Figure 3-82. The radial tuberosity is visible anteriorly. The distal forearm was externally rotated.

Correction. Lower the distal forearm until the humeral epicondyles are superimposed, and internally rotate the distal forearm until the wrist is in a lateral position.

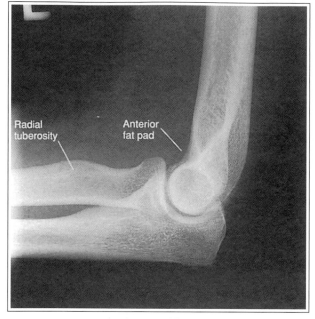

Image 88.

Analysis. The elbow joint space is open, and the distal humerus demonstrates accurate alignment. The radial tuberosity is demonstrated in profile anteriorly, indicating that the wrist and hand were supinated (externally rotated).

Correction. If the circumference of the radial head and neck is being evaluated and the medial aspect of the radial head in profile is desired, the radial tuberosity should be demonstrated in profile anteriorly and no repositioning movement is needed. If a true lateral elbow image is desired, the distal forearm should be internally rotated until the wrist is in a lateral position.

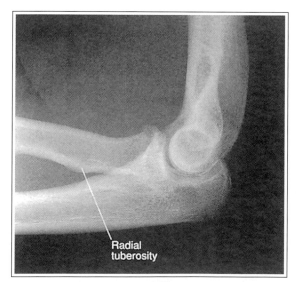

Image 89.

Analysis. The elbow joint space is open, and the distal humerus demonstrates accurate alignment. The radial tuberosity is demonstrated in profile posteriorly, indicating that the hand and wrist were pronated (internally rotated).

Correction. If the circumference of the radial head and neck is being evaluated and the medial aspect of the radial head in profile is desired, the radial tuberosity should be seen in profile anteriorly and no repositioning movement is needed. If a true lateral elbow image is desired, the distal forearm should be externally rotated until the wrist is in a lateral position.

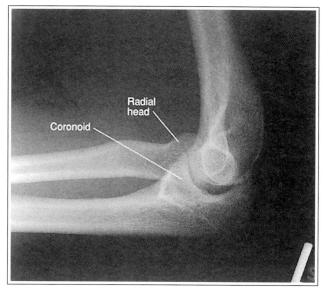

Image 90.

Analysis. Two positional problems on this image are preventing the distal humerus from demonstrating accurate alignment. The radial head is positioned anterior and proximal to the coronoid process, and the capitulum is positioned too far proximal and posterior to the medial trochlea. The proximal humerus was positioned too low, and the distal forearm was positioned too high, a combination of the errors demonstrated in Figures 3-80 and 3-82.

Correction. Raise the proximal humerus and lower the distal forearm until the humeral epicondyles are superimposed.

ELBOW: RADIAL HEAD AND CAPITULUM

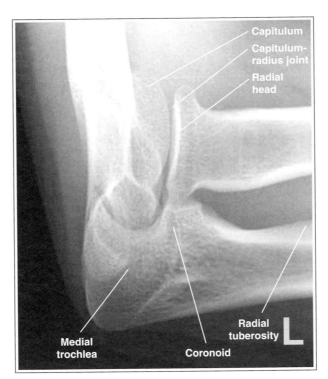

Figure 3-83. Radial head and capitulum image with accurate positioning.

The radial head and capitulum image is a special projection taken when a fracture of the radial head or capitulum is suspected.

Image Analysis

The elbow is flexed 90 degrees.

- If the elbow is flexed 90 degrees, the forearm can be elevated to properly align the anatomical structures of the distal humerus.

The capitulum and medial trochlea are demonstrated without superimposition, and the radial head is superimposed on only the anterior tip of the coronoid process.

- This position is obtained by placing the patient in a lateral position with the humeral epicondyles aligned perpendicular to the IR and placing a 45-degree proximal (toward the shoulder) angle on the central ray (Figure 3-84). It is this humerus and central ray positioning that accurately separates the capitulum and trochlea of the distal humerus and positions the radial head anterior to the coronoid process. The combination of positioning and angulation projects the anatomical structures (radial head and capitulum) situated farther from the IR proximal to those structures (coronoid process and medial trochlea) situated closer to the IR.
- *Effects of errors in positioning or angulation:* If the central ray is angled accurately but the proximal

humerus is depressed lower than the distal humerus, the medial trochlea and capitulum cortices are not clearly defined, the coronoid process is free of radial head superimposition, and the radial neck and tuberosity are superimposed by the ulnar supinator crest (a sharp, prominent ridge running along the lateral margin of the ulna that divides the ulna's anterior and posterior surfaces) (see Image 91). The same image can result if the patient is accurately positioned but the central ray is angled more than 45 degrees.

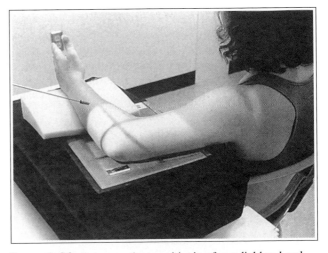

Figure 3-84. Proper patient positioning for radial head and capitulum image.

If the central ray is accurately angled but the proximal humerus is elevated, the medial trochlea demonstrates some capitular superimposition and the radial head is superimposed over a greater portion of the coronoid process (see Image 92). The same image can result if the patient is accurately positioned but the central ray is angled less than 45 degrees.

The capitulum-radial joint is open, and the proximal radial head and coronoid process are aligned.

- An accurately aligned radial head and coronoid process and an open capitulum-radial head joint is obtained when the elbow is in a lateral position. A lateral elbow position is accomplished when the humeral epicondyles are positioned directly on top of each other, placing them perpendicular to the IR (see Figure 3-84).
- *Effect of distal forearm mispositioning:* The alignment of the proximal surfaces of the radial head and coronoid process is affected when the distal forearm is positioned. Precise positioning is a must to obtain accurate alignment. It takes only a small degree of inaccurate positioning to close the capitulum-radius joint. If the distal forearm is positioned too low, the image shows a closed capitulum-radius joint space and shows the capitulum too far anterior to the medial trochlea and the radial head distal to the coronoid process (see Image 93). If the distal forearm is positioned too high, the image shows the capitulum too far posterior to the medial trochlea and the radial head proximal to the coronoid process.

The radial head surface of interest is demonstrated in profile.

- The position of the wrist determines which surface of the radial head is placed in profile.
- *Effect of wrist position:* When the patient's elbow is placed in a lateral position, wrist rotation causes the radius to rotate around the ulna. This rotation places different radial head surfaces in profile. To determine which surfaces are in profile, one should become familiar with the relationship between the wrist position and visualization of the radial tuberosity. The radial tuberosity is adjacent to the medial aspect of the radius. If the tuberosity is demonstrated, the medial aspect of the radial head is also shown on that same surface and the lateral aspect of the radial head is visible on the opposite surface. If the patient's wrist is positioned in a PA projection, the radial tuberosity and medial radial head are demonstrated posteriorly and the lateral radial head appears in profile anteriorly (see Image 93). If the wrist is in a lateral position, the radial tuberosity is not demonstrated in profile but is superimposed by the radius. In this position the anterior radial head is demonstrated in profile anteriorly, and the posterior surface is shown in profile posteriorly (see Image 91).

The radial head is at the center of the collimated field. The proximal forearm, distal humerus, and surrounding soft tissue are included within the field.

- To place the radial head in the center of the collimated field, center the central ray ¾ inch (2 cm) distal (toward the wrist) to the lateral epicondyle. Open the longitudinally and transversely collimated fields to within ½ inch (1.25 cm) of the posterior elbow skinline.
- An 8- × 10-inch (18- × 24-cm) detailed screen-film or computed radiography IR placed lengthwise should be adequate to include all the required anatomical structures.

Radial Head and Capitulum Image Analysis

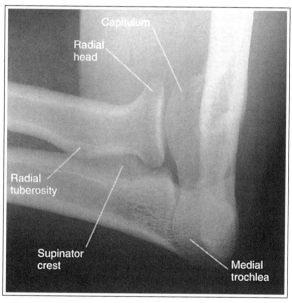

Image 91.

Analysis. The distal medial trochlea and capitulum cortices are not clearly defined, the coronoid process is free of radial head superimposition, and the radial neck and tuberosity are superimposed by the ulnar supinator crest. The proximal humerus was depressed lower than the distal humerus.

Correction. Elevate the proximal humerus until the humeral epicondyles are perpendicular to the image.

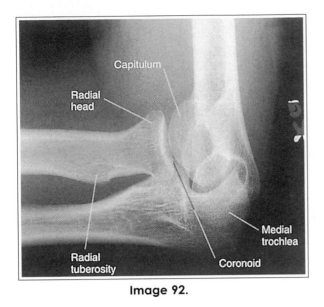

Image 92.

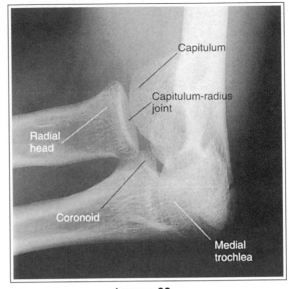

Image 93.

Analysis. The capitulum-radius joint space is closed, the radial head is demonstrated distal to the coronoid process, and the capitulum is demonstrated too far anterior to the medial trochlea, indicating that the distal forearm was depressed. The radial head is superimposed over more than just the tip of the coronoid process, and the medial trochlea and capitulum would demonstrate slight super-imposition if the distal forearm had been accurately positioned; the proximal humerus was elevated. The radial tuberosity is demonstrated in profile posteriorly and the lateral surface of the radial head is demonstrated in profile anteriorly, whereas the medial surface is in profile poste-riorly; the wrist was placed in a PA projection.

Correction. Elevate the distal forearm and depress the proximal humerus until the humeral epicondyles are aligned perpendicular to the IR. If you want the anterior and posterior surfaces of the radial head to be demon-strated in profile, place the wrist in a lateral position.

Analysis. The capitulum-radius joint space is closed, and the radial head is demonstrated distal to the coronoid process. The radial tuberosity is not demonstrated in profile, the anterior surface of the radial head is in profile anteriorly, and the posterior surface is in profile posteriorly; the wrist was placed in a lateral position.

Correction. Elevate the distal forearm until the humeral epicondyles are aligned perpendicular to the IR. The amount of movement needed is half the difference between how close the anterior surfaces of the capitulum and medial trochlea should be on a radial head and capitulum image with accurate positioning and how close they are located on this image. If the lateral and medial surfaces of the radial head should be demonstrated in profile, the patient's wrist needs to be placed in a PA projection.

HUMERUS: ANTEROPOSTERIOR PROJECTION

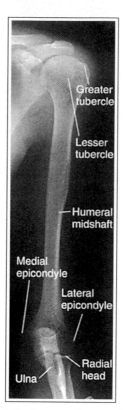

Figure 3-85. Anteroposterior humerus image with accurate positioning.

Image Analysis

Scatter radiation is controlled. Image density is uniform across the humerus.

- If the patient's upper arm AP thickness measures less than 5 inches (13 cm), a grid is not required. For such a patient, a high-contrast, low (below 70) kVp technique sufficiently penetrates the bony and soft-tissue structures of the humerus without causing excessive scatter radiation to reach the IR and hinder image contrast. If the upper arm measures more than 5 inches (13 cm), a grid should be used, because this thickness would produce enough scatter radiation to negatively affect the image contrast. When a grid is used, increase the kVp to above 70 to penetrate the thicker humerus and to provide an adequate scale of contrast. If the technique is manually set, increase the exposure (mAs) by the standard density conversion factor for the grid ratio (number used to express a grid's scatter-eliminating ability) being used, to compensate for the scatter and the primary radiation that the grid will absorb.

- *Anode-heel effect:* To take advantage of the anode-heel effect, position the thinner elbow (distal humerus) at the anode end of the tube and the thicker (proximal humerus) at the cathode end. Set an exposure (mAs) that will adequately demonstrate the midpoint of the humerus.

The humerus is in an AP projection. The medial and lateral humeral epicondyles are demonstrated in profile, and the radial head and tuberosity are superimposed over the lateral aspect of the proximal ulna by approximately ¼ inch (0.6 cm). The greater tubercle is demonstrated in profile laterally, the humeral head is demonstrated medially in profile, and the vertical cortical margin of the lesser tubercle is visible approximately halfway between the greater tubercle and the humeral head.

- An AP projection is obtained by placing the patient in either a supine or an upright AP projection with the affected arm extended. Supinate the hand and externally rotate the elbow until an imaginary line drawn between the palpable humeral epicondyles is aligned parallel with the IR (Figure 3-86). This positioning places the proximal radius anterior to the ulna, causing the radial head and tuberosity to be superimposed over the lateral ulna by approximately ¼ inch (0.6 cm), and places the greater tuberosity in profile.

- *Detecting humeral rotation:* Rotation of the humerus is a result of poor humeral epicondyle positioning. When the humeral epicondyles and the greater tuberosity are not demonstrated in profile, measure the amount of radial head and tuberosity superimposition of the ulna to determine how the patient should be repositioned. If less

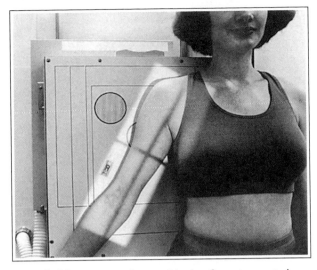

Figure 3-86. Proper patient positioning for anteroposterior humerus image: collimator head rotated.

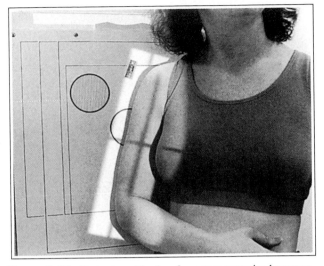

Figure 3-87. Patient positioning for anteroposterior humerus image when fracture is located close to shoulder.

than ¼ inch (0.6 cm) of the radial head and tuberosity are superimposed over the ulna, the elbow and humerus have been excessively laterally (externally) rotated (see Image 94). If more than ¼ inch (0.6 cm) of the radial head and tuberosity are superimposed over the ulna, the elbow and humerus have been medially (internally) rotated (see Image 95).

- *Forearm positioning for humeral fracture:* When a fracture of the humerus is suspected or a follow-up image is being taken to assess healing of a humeral fracture, the patient's forearm should not be externally rotated to obtain the AP projection because external rotation of the forearm increases the risk of radial nerve damage. For such an examination the joint closer to the fracture should be aligned in the true AP projection. If the fracture site is situated closer to the shoulder joint and the arm cannot be externally rotated, the greater tuberosity is placed in profile by rotating the patient's body toward the affected humerus 35 to 40 degrees (Figure 3-87). Depending on the amount of humeral rotation at the fracture site, the distal humerus may or may not be an AP projection (see Image 96). If the fracture is situated closer to the elbow joint, extend the arm and rotate the patient's body toward the affected humerus until the humeral epicondyles are aligned parallel with the IR. Depending on the amount of humeral rotation at the fracture site, the greater tuberosity may or may not be in profile.

The long axis of the humerus is aligned with the long axis of the collimated field.

- If the humerus can remain aligned with the long axis of the IR while including the elbow and shoulder joints, align the long axis of the collimated light field with the long axis of the humerus to allow for tight transverse collimation.
- For many adult humeral images, it may be necessary to position the humerus diagonally on the IR to include

the elbow and shoulder joint. For this positioning the collimator head or tube column should be turned or rotated to align the long axis of the collimated light field with the long axis of the humerus. (If a grid is used, the collimator head may be rotated, but do not rotate the tube column, or grid cutoff—unwanted absorption of primary radiation—will result.)

- If the collimator head or tube column cannot be adjusted for a diagonal positioning, leave the transversely collimated field open enough to include the shoulder joint and elbow. With this setup the collimated field includes a large portion of the patient's thorax. Therefore the thorax is exposed to unnecessary radiation but can be protected by use of a contact shield across it. Remember to leave at least 3 inches (7.5 cm) of space between the humeral head and the shield to allow for magnification, so the shoulder joint is not obscured by the shield (Figure 3-88).

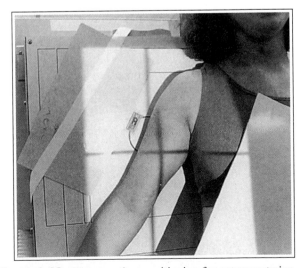

Figure 3-88. Proper patient positioning for anteroposterior humerus image using shields when collimator head cannot be rotated.

The humeral midpoint is at the center of the collimated field. The shoulder and elbow joints and the lateral humeral soft tissue are included within the field.

- To place the humeral midpoint in the center of the image, palpate the coracoid process and the medial epicondyle and position the central ray halfway between these two palpable landmarks. When the elbow and shoulder joints are included on the image, the degree of radiation beam divergence that is used for a long body part needs to be considered.

- *IR length and positioning:* Choose an IR that is long enough to allow at least 1 inch (2.5 cm) of IR to extend beyond each joint space; a 14- × 17-inch (35- × 43-cm) screen-film or computed radiography IR placed lengthwise should be adequate. For a patient with a long humerus, it may be necessary to position the humerus diagonally on the IR to obtain the needed IR length. Palpate the two joints to ensure that the IR extends beyond them. The elbow is located approximately ¾ inch (2 cm) proximal to the medial epicondyle. The shoulder joint is located at the same level as the palpable coracoid.

- *Central ray centering and collimation:* Once the humerus is accurately positioned with the IR, center a perpendicular central ray to the humeral midpoint, and the longitudinal collimated field is opened until it extends 1 inch (2.5 cm) beyond the elbow and shoulder joint. If the collimation does not extend beyond both joints, adjust the centering point of the central ray until both the elbow and the shoulder joint are included within the collimated field without demonstrating an excessive light field beyond them. Transverse collimation should be to within ½ inch (1.25 cm) of the skinline laterally and the coracoid medially.

Anteroposterior Humeral Image Analysis

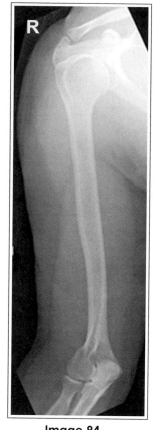

Image 94.

Analysis. The humeral epicondyles are not demonstrated in profile, the radial head and tuberosity do not superimpose the ulna, and the cortical margin of the lesser tuberosity is not shown halfway between the greater tuberosity and the humeral head. The arm was externally rotated more than the required amount.

Correction. Internally rotate the arm until the humeral epicondyles are positioned parallel with the IR.

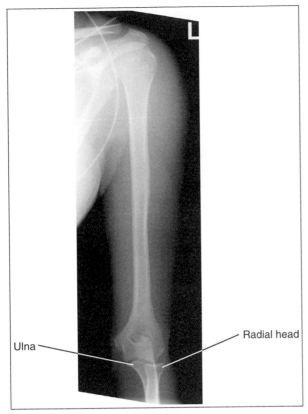

Image 95.

Analysis. Neither the humeral epicondyles nor the greater tuberosity is demonstrated in profile, and the radial head and tuberosity are superimposed over more than ¼ inch (0.6 cm) of the ulna. The arm was internally rotated.

Correction. Externally rotate the arm until the humeral epicondyles are positioned parallel with the IR.

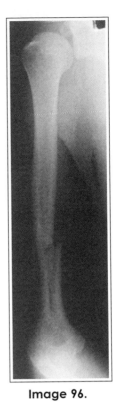

Image 96.

Analysis. A fracture is present at the distal humerus. The glenohumeral joint space is demonstrated, indicating that this image was taken with the patient rotated toward the humerus.

Correction. Because the joint closer to the fracture is in a true projection, no repositioning movement is needed.

HUMERUS: LATERAL POSITION

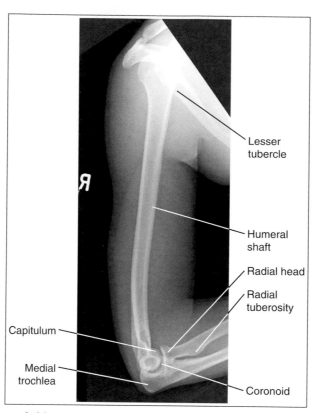

Figure 3-89. Mediolateral humerus image with accurate positioning.

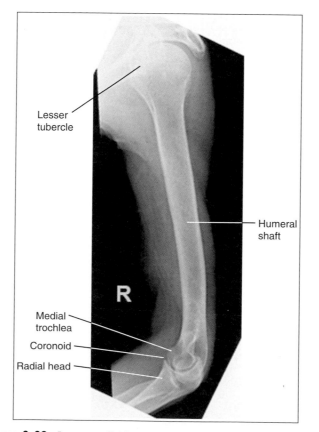

Figure 3-90. Lateromedial humerus image with accurate positioning.

Image Analysis

Scatter radiation is controlled. Image density is uniform across the humerus.

- If the patient's upper arm AP thickness measures less than 5 inches (13 cm), a grid is not required, but a grid is required if the patient's upper arm measures more than 5 inches (13 cm). When a grid is used, increase the penetration to above 70 kVp to penetrate the thicker humerus and to provide an adequate scale of contrast. If the technique is manually set, increase the exposure (mAs) by the standard density conversion factor for the grid ratio used to compensate for the absorption of the scatter and primary radiation that occurs.
- *Anode-heel effect:* To take advantage of the anode-heel effect, position the thinner elbow (distal humerus) at the anode end of the tube and the thicker (proximal humerus) at the cathode end. Set an exposure (mAs) that will adequately demonstrate the midpoint of the humerus.

The humerus is in a lateral position. The lesser tubercle is demonstrated in profile medially, and the humeral head and greater tubercle are superimposed. For a *mediolateral projection*, most of the radial head is demonstrated anterior to the coronoid process, the radial tuberosity is demonstrated in profile, and the capitulum is visualized proximal to the medial trochlea (Figure 3-89). For a *lateromedial projection*, the radial head and coronoid process are superimposed, the radial tuberosity is not demonstrated in profile, and the capitulum is visible distal to the medial trochlea (Figure 3-90).

- Two methods can be used to position the patient for a lateral humerus image: mediolateral and lateromedial. The first method positions the patient's body in an upright PA projection, with the elbow flexed 90 degrees and the forearm and humerus internally rotated until an imaginary line connecting the humeral epicondyles is perpendicular to the IR; this is a *mediolateral projection* (Figure 3-91). Have the patient rotate the humerus internally while the body maintains a PA projection. Do not allow the patient to rotate the body toward the affected humerus instead. Such body obliquity would cause a decrease in density of the proximal humerus compared with the distal humerus (see Image 97), because the shoulder tissue would be superimposed over the proximal humerus. If body rotation cannot be avoided, an increase in exposure (mAs) is required to adequately demonstrate the upper humerus.
- The second method positions the patient's body in an AP projection. The hand is positioned against the patient's side, the elbow is slightly flexed, and the forearm and humerus are internally rotated until an imaginary line connecting the humeral epicondyles is perpendicular to the IR; this is a *lateromedial projection* (Figure 3-92).

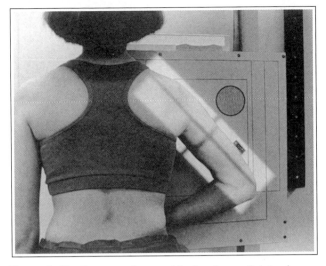

Figure 3-91. Proper patient positioning for mediolateral humerus image.

If the patient's forearm is positioned across the body in an attempt to flex the elbow 90 degrees and the distal humerus is not brought away from the IR enough to position the humeral epicondyles perpendicular to the IR (Figure 3-93), the image demonstrates the capitulum posterior to the medial trochlea, a distorted proximal forearm, and the lesser tubercle in partial profile (see Image 98).

The difference in the anatomical relationship of the distal humerus between the mediolateral and lateromedial projections is a result of x-ray beam divergence. For a lateral humerus image, the central ray is centered to the midhumeral shaft, which is located approximately 5 inches (13 cm) from the elbow joint. Because the elbow joint is placed so far away from the central ray, diverged x-ray beams are used to image the elbow joint. This causes the anatomical structures positioned farthest

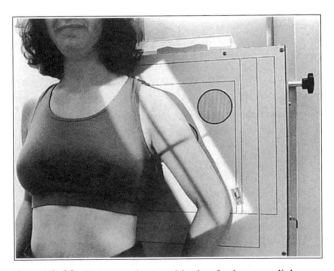

Figure 3-92. Proper patient positioning for lateromedial humerus image.

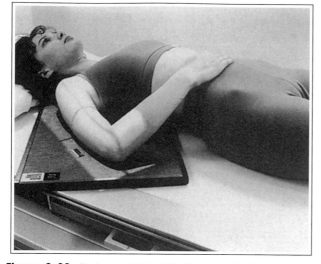

Figure 3-93. Patient positioned for lateromedial humerus image with poor distal humerus alignment.

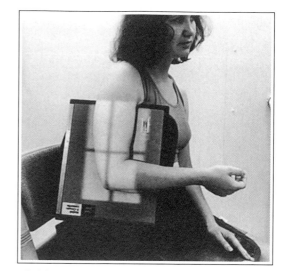

Figure 3-94. Proper patient positioning for distal humerus fracture.

from the IR to be diverged more distally than the anatomical structures positioned closest to the IR. In the mediolateral projection the medial trochlea is placed farther from the IR than the capitulum. Consequently, x-ray beam divergence will project the medial trochlea distal to the capitulum. In the lateromedial projection the capitulum is situated farther from the IR; therefore the x-ray beam divergence will project it distal to the medial trochlea.

- **Positioning for a humeral fracture:** When a fracture of the humerus is suspected or a follow-up image is being taken to assess healing of a fracture, the patient's forearm or humerus should not be rotated to obtain a lateral position. Rotation of the forearm and humerus would increase the risk of radial nerve damage and displacement of the fracture fragments. Because the forearm should not be rotated for a trauma examination, a lateral image of the proximal and distal humerus must be obtained by positioning the patient differently.

- *Distal humeral fracture:* Obtain a lateral distal humerus image by gently sliding an IR between the patient and the distal humerus. Adjust the IR until the epicondyles are positioned perpendicular to the IR. Place a flat contact protecting shield between the patient and the IR to absorb any radiation that would penetrate the IR and expose the patient. Finally, center the central ray perpendicular to the IR and distal humerus (Figure 3-94). This positioning should demonstrate a true lateral position of the distal humerus with superimposition of the epicondyles and of the radial head and coronoid process (see Image 99).

- *Proximal humeral fracture:* A lateral image can be achieved by positioning the patient in one of two ways.

  The first method is best done with the patient in an upright position. This position is known as the *scapular Y* position. Begin by placing the patient in a PA upright projection with the humerus positioned as is, and then

rotate the patient toward the affected humerus (approximately 45 degrees) until the scapular body is in a lateral position (Figure 3-95 and Image 100). Precise positioning and evaluating points for this image can be studied by referring to the discussion of the anterior oblique position on p. 230.

The second method of obtaining a lateral image of the proximal humerus can be accomplished with either an upright or a recumbent position. It is known as the *transthoracic lateral position* (Figure 3-96). The patient's body is placed in a lateral position with the affected humerus resting against the grid IR, and the unaffected arm is raised above the patient's head. To prevent superimposition of the shoulders on the image, either (1) elevate the unaffected shoulder by tilting the upper midsagittal plane toward the IR and using a horizontal

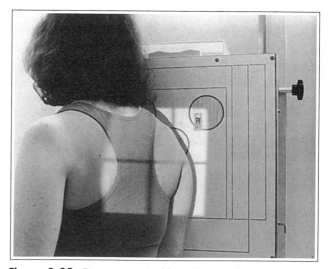

Figure 3-95. Proper scapular Y positioning of patient for proximal humerus fracture.

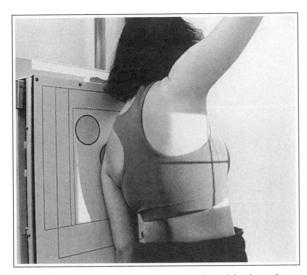

Figure 3-96. Proper transthoracic lateral positioning of patient for proximal humerus fracture.

central ray or (2) position the shoulders on the same transverse plane and angle the central ray 10 to 15 degrees cephalically.

For both positions, direct the central ray to the midthorax at the level of the affected shoulder. Use *breathing technique* to blur the vascular lung markings and axillary ribs: A long exposure time (3 seconds) is used while the patient breathes shallowly (costal breathing) during the exposure. A transthoracic image with accurate positioning should sharply demonstrate the affected proximal humerus halfway between the sternum and the thoracic vertebrae, without superimposition of the unaffected shoulder (see Image 101).

The long axis of the humerus is aligned with the long axis of the collimated field.

- If the patient's humerus can remain aligned with the long axis of the IR while the elbow and shoulder joints are included on the IR, align the long axis of the collimated light field with the long axis of the humerus to allow for tight transverse collimation. For many adult humeral images, it may be necessary to position the humerus diagonally on the IR to include the elbow and shoulder joint. For this positioning the collimator head or tube column should be turned or rotated to align the long axis of the collimated light field with the long axis of the humerus. (If a grid is used, do not rotate the tube column, or grid cutoff—unwanted absorption of primary radiation—will result.)
- If the collimator head or tube column cannot be adjusted for diagonal positioning, leave the transversely collimated field open enough to include the elbow and shoulder joint. With this setup the collimated field includes a large portion of the patient's thorax. Therefore the thorax is exposed to unnecessary radiation but can be protected by laying a flat contact shield across it. Remember to leave at least 3 inches (7.5 cm)

of space between the humeral head and the shield to allow for magnification, so the shoulder joint is not obscured by the shield.

The humeral midpoint is at the center of the collimated field. The shoulder and elbow joints, the proximal humerus and forearm, and the lateral humeral soft tissue are included within the field.

- To place the humeral midpoint in the center of the image, palpate (1) the acromion angle (Figure 3-97) for a mediolateral projection or (2) the coracoid process for a lateromedial projection and the medial epicondyle. Position the central ray with the humeral midpoint at a level halfway between the two palpable landmarks. To include the elbow and shoulder joints on the image, the degree of radiation beam divergence that is used when imaging a long body part needs to be considered.
- *IR length and positioning:* Choose an IR that is long enough to allow at least 1 inch (2.5 cm) of IR to extend beyond each joint space; a 14- × 17-inch (35- × 43-cm) screen-film or computed radiography IR placed lengthwise should be adequate. On a patient with a long humerus, it may be necessary to position the humerus diagonally on the IR to obtain the needed IR length. Palpate the joints to ensure that the IR extends beyond them. The elbow is located approximately ¾ inch (2 cm) distal to the medial epicondyles. The shoulder joint is located at the same level as the palpable coracoid and acromion angle.
- *Central ray centering and collimation:* Once the humerus is accurately positioned with the IR and the central ray is centered to the humeral midpoint, open the longitudinal collimated field until it extends 1 inch (2.5 cm) beyond the elbow and shoulder joint. If the collimation

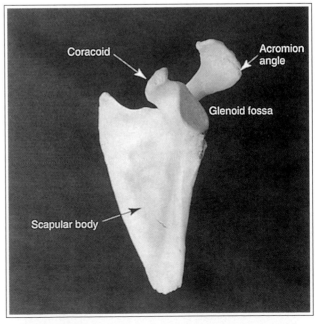

Figure 3-97. Location of acromion angle and coracoid.

does not extend beyond both joints, adjust the centering point of the central ray until both the elbow and the shoulder joint are included within the collimated field without demonstrating an excessive light field beyond them. Transverse collimation should be within ½ inch (1.25 cm) of the skinline laterally and to (1) the lateral scapular border for the mediolateral projection or (2) the coracoid for the lateromedial projection.

Lateral Humeral Image Analysis

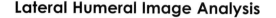

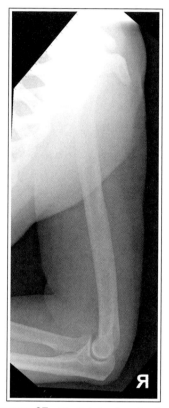

Image 97. Mediolateral projection.

Analysis. The density is lighter at the proximal humerus than at the distal humerus. The torso was not in a PA projection but was rotated toward the humerus, increasing the tissue thickness at the proximal humerus.

Correction. Rotate the torso away from the proximal humerus into a PA projection.

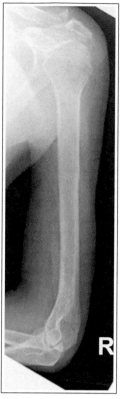

Image 98. Lateromedial projection.

Analysis. The humerus is not in a lateral position. The epicondyles are not superimposed, the capitulum is posterior to the medial trochlea, and the proximal forearm is distorted. The forearm was positioned across the patient's body and the distal humerus was not drawn away from the table to place the epicondyles perpendicular to the IR, as demonstrated in Figure 3-93.

Correction. Position the patient as demonstrated in Figure 3-92, with the distal humerus positioned adjacent to the IR, aligning the humeral epicondyles perpendicular to the IR.

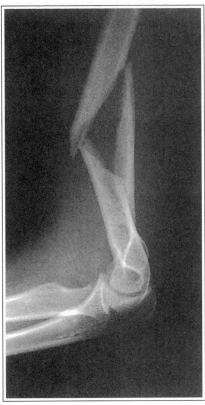

Image 99.

Analysis. This is a fractured lateral distal humeral image. The patient was accurately positioned.

Correction. No correction movement is required.

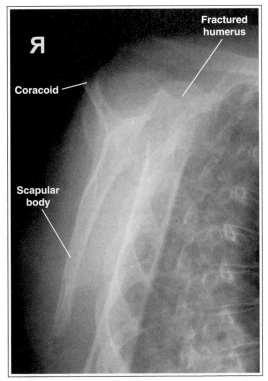

Image 100.

Analysis. This is a scapular Y image of a fractured proximal humerus. The image demonstrates accurate positioning. The scapular body is in a true lateral position. The scapular body, acromion, and coracoid form a Y, with the scapular body as the leg and the acromion and coracoid as the arms.

Correction. No correction movement is required.

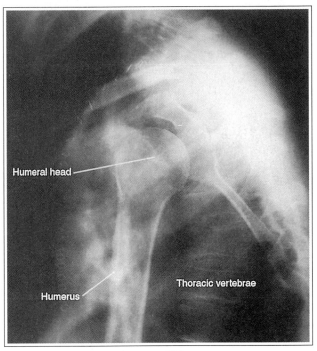

Image 101.

Analysis. This figure is a transthoracic image of the proximal humerus. The image demonstrates accurate positioning. The unaffected shoulder is superior to the affected shoulder, and the humerus is clearly demonstrated halfway between the thoracic vertebrae and the sternum.

Correction. No correction movement is required.

REFERENCE

1. Epner RA, Bowers WH, Guilford WB: Ulnar variance—the effect of wrist positioning and roentgen filming techniques, *J Hand Surg* 7:298-305, 1982.

Image Analysis of the Shoulder

The following image analysis criteria are used for all shoulder images and should be considered when the analysis is completed. Position- or projection-specific criteria relating to these topics are discussed with the other accompanying criteria for that position or projection.

Facility's patient identification requirements are visible on image.

A right or left marker, identifying correct side of patient, is present on the image and is not superimposed over anatomy of interest. Specific placement of marker is as described in Chapter 1.

No evidence of preventable artifacts, such as gown snaps, undergarments, slings, and splints, is present.

- Consult with the ordering physician and the patient about whether slings or splints can be removed.

The bony trabecular patterns and cortical outlines of the proximal humerus and shoulder girdle are sharply defined.

- Sharply defined image details are obtained when patient motion and respiration are halted, when a small focal spot is used, and when a short object–image receptor distance (OID) is maintained. Increased spatial resolution is also obtained when the smallest image receptor (IR) is selected for digital images.

Contrast and density are adequate to demonstrate the surrounding soft tissue and bony structures. Density is uniform throughout shoulder. Penetration is sufficient to visualize the bony trabecular patterns and cortical outlines of the required shoulder structures.

- An optimal kilovolt-peak (kVp) technique, as shown in Table 4-1, sufficiently penetrates the shoulder structures

TABLE 4-1 **Shoulder Technical Data**				
Position or Projection	**kVp**	**Grid**	**AEC Chamber(s)**	**SID**
AP projection, shoulder	65-75	Grid	Center	40-48 inches (100-120 cm)
Inferosuperior (axial) projection, shoulder	65-75			40-48 inches (100-120 cm)
Posterior oblique position (Grashey), shoulder	65-75	Grid	Center	40-48 inches (100-120 cm)
Anterior oblique position (scapular Y), shoulder	65-75	Grid		40-48 inches (100-120 cm)
AP axial projection (Stryker), shoulder	65-75	Grid		40-48 inches (100-120 cm)
Tangential projection (outlet), shoulder	65-75	Grid		40-48 inches (100-120 cm)
AP and axial projections, clavicle	65-75	Grid		40-48 inches (100-120 cm)
AP projection, AC joint	60-70 65-70	Nongrid Grid		72 inches (183 cm)
AP projection, scapula	65-75	Grid	Center	40-48 inches (100-120 cm)
Lateral position, scapula	70-75	Grid		40-48 inches (100-120 cm)

AEC, Automatic exposure control; *AP*, anteroposterior; *kVp*, kilovolt peak; *SID*, source–image receptor distance.

and provides the contrast scale necessary to visualize the shoulder details. If the anteroposterior (AP) or inferosuperior shoulder thickness measurement is over 5 inches (13 cm), a grid should be employed to absorb the scatter radiation produced by the shoulder, increasing detail visibility. To obtain optimal density, set a manual milliampere-seconds (mAs) level based on the patient's shoulder thickness or choose the appropriate automatic exposure control (AEC) chamber when recommended (Table 4-1).

- For AP projections of the shoulder, clavicle, and acromioclavicular (AC) joints, uniform density throughout the shoulder is obtained through the use of a compensating filter. When an exposure (mAs) is set or the AEC is accurately positioned over the glenohumeral joint to provide adequate shoulder density, often the laterally located acromion process and clavicular end are overexposed because of the difference in AP body thickness between these two regions. A compensating filter placed over or under the lateral clavicle region can be used to obtain uniform density across the entire shoulder (Figure 4-1). The filter should be positioned as described in Chapter 1 on p. 39.

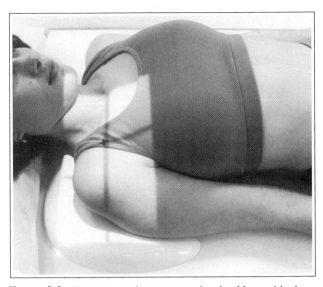

Figure 4-1. Proper neutral anteroposterior shoulder positioning with compensating filter.

SHOULDER: ANTEROPOSTERIOR PROJECTION

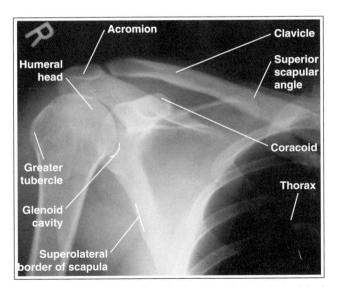

Figure 4-2. Anteroposterior shoulder image with accurate positioning.

Image Analysis

The shoulder girdle is in an AP projection. The scapular body demonstrates transverse foreshortening, showing the glenoid cavity; the superolateral border of the scapula is visible without thorax superimposition; and the clavicle is demonstrated horizontally, with the medial end of the clavicle positioned next to the lateral vertebral column. When the humeral head is not dislocated, the posterior portion of the glenoid cavity and the medial margin of the humeral head are superimposed.

- An AP shoulder projection is achieved by placing the patient in either a supine or an upright AP projection, with the shoulders positioned at equal distances from the imaging table or upright grid holder (Figures 4-1 and 4-3). When the patient is positioned in an AP projection, the clavicle should be demonstrated horizontally, with the medial end positioned next to the lateral vertebral column

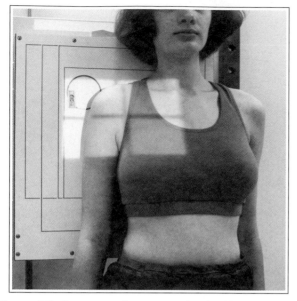

Figure 4-3. Proper neutral anteroposterior shoulder positioning.

without excessive curvature or longitudinal foreshortening, and the scapular body is at 35 to 45 degrees of obliquity, with the lateral scapula situated more anteriorly than the medial scapula, and the glenoid cavity is visible.

- The amount of scapular obliquity and glenoid fossa demonstration depends on the degree of shoulder retraction. Retraction or backward movement of the shoulder is a result of the gravitational pull placed on the shoulder when the patient is in a supine position and patient spinal straightening and backward shoulder movement when the patient is in an upright position. It causes the scapular body to be positioned more nearly parallel with the image.
- *Upright positioning for kyphosis:* The kyphotic patient will have less discomfort if in an upright position while the image is taken. If it is not possible to place the kyphotic patient in an upright position, use angled sponges under the shoulders and thorax to place the shoulders at equal distances from the imaging table. An imaging table sponge also helps ease patient discomfort.
- *Detecting rotation:* Rotation on an AP shoulder image is detected by evaluating the details of the scapular body, glenoid cavity, and clavicle. When the patient is rotated toward the affected shoulder (places affected shoulder closer to IR than unaffected shoulder), the scapular body is positioned closer to or parallel with the IR and appears wider on the image. The thorax is superimposed over the superolateral scapular region, the glenoid cavity and scapular neck are positioned more in profile, and the clavicle is longitudinally foreshortened, with the medial clavicular end shifted away from the vertebral column (see Image 1). When the patient is rotated away from the affected shoulder, the scapular body demonstrates increased transverse foreshortening, the thorax is superimposed over a smaller amount of the scapula, the glenoid cavity is better demonstrated, and the medial clavicular end is superimposed over the vertebral column (see Image 2).

- *Effect of shoulder dislocation:* The AP shoulder projection is taken to detect shoulder fractures, as well as humeral head dislocations. When the shoulder is not dislocated, the humeral head is centered to and slightly superimposed over the glenoid cavity. Shoulder dislocation can result in positioning of the humeral head either anterior or posterior and inferior to the glenoid cavity. Anterior dislocation, which is more common (95%), results in the humeral head being demonstrated anteriorly, beneath the coracoid process (see Image 3). Posterior dislocations, which are uncommon (2% to 4%), result in the humeral head being demonstrated posteriorly, beneath the acromion process or spine of the scapula.

The scapular body is demonstrated without longitudinal foreshortening. The superior scapular angle is superimposed by the midclavicle.

- The tilt of the midcoronal plane determines the degree of longitudinal scapular foreshortening. When the midcoronal plane is vertical and positioned parallel with the IR, the scapula is demonstrated without foreshortening.
- *Detecting scapular foreshortening:* If the upper midcoronal plane is tilted anteriorly (forward) the superior scapular angle will be demonstrated superior to the midclavicle (see Image 4). If the upper midcoronal plane is tilted posteriorly (backward) the superior scapular angle will be shown inferior to the midclavicle (see Image 5). The severity of foreshortening will increase with an increase in the degree of midcoronal plane tilt.
- *Compensating for kyphosis:* For the kyphotic patient, little can be done to improve patient positioning, but a cephalic central ray angulation can be used to offset the forward angle of the scapula. The central ray should be angled perpendicular to the scapular body.

The humerus is aligned parallel with the body, and the glenoid cavity faces laterally.

- Proper AP shoulder positioning is accomplished with zero humeral abduction. When the humerus is abducted, it is demonstrated away from the body, the glenoid cavity shifts superiorly, and the scapular body glides around the thorax, moving anteriorly (see Image 6). This scapular movement increases as humeral abduction increases beyond 60 degrees.

The glenohumeral joint space and the coracoid process are at the center of the collimated field. The glenohumeral joint, the lateral two thirds of the clavicle, the proximal third of the humerus, and the superior scapula are included within the field.

- When the central ray is centered 1 inch (2.5 cm) inferior to the palpable coracoid process, the glenohumeral joint is centered within the collimated field. The coracoid process can be palpated 1 inch (2.5 cm) inferior to the midpoint of the lateral half of the clavicle and medial to the humeral head (Figure 4-4). Even on very muscular patients, the concave pocket formed inferior to the

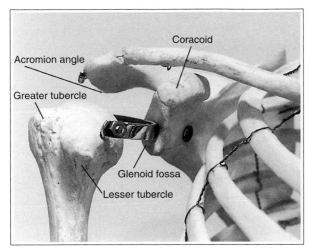

Figure 4-4. Location of coracoid process.

lateral half of the clavicle and medial to the humeral head can be used to center the central ray.

- Center the IR to the central ray and open the longitudinal collimation enough to include the top of the shoulder. Transversely collimate to within ½ inch (1.25 cm) of lateral humeral skinline.
- An 8- × 10-inch (18- × 24-cm) or 10- × 12-inch (24- × 30-cm) IR placed crosswise should be adequate to include all the required anatomical structures. The IR may be placed lengthwise to demonstrate more of the humerus.

HUMERAL HEAD POSITIONING

The position of the humeral epicondyles with respect to the IR determines which anatomical aspect of the humeral head is demonstrated in profile.

- ***Positioning for suspected fracture or dislocation:*** On a patient with suspected shoulder dislocations or humeral fractures the humerus should not be rotated. Take the exposure with the humerus positioned as it is.

In *neutral rotation,* the greater tubercle is partially demonstrated in profile laterally and the humeral head is partially demonstrated in profile medially (see Figure 4-1).

- Accurate neutral humeral head rotation is accomplished by placing the patient's palm against the thigh, which will align the humeral epicondyles at a 45-degree angle with the IR (see Figure 4-3).

In *external rotation,* the greater tubercle is demonstrated in profile laterally, the humeral head is demonstrated in profile medially, and the vertical cortical outline of the lesser tubercle is visible approximately halfway between the greater tubercle and the medial aspect of the humeral head (see Image 7).

- Accurate external humeral head rotation is obtained by externally rotating the patient's arm until the humeral epicondyles are aligned parallel with the IR (Figure 4-5).

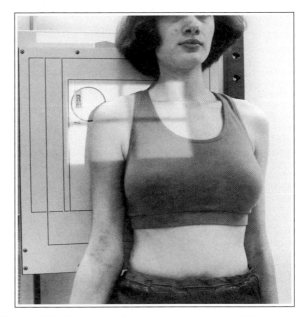

Figure 4-5. Proper external anteroposterior shoulder positioning.

- An arrow or word marker should be used to indicate external humeral rotation. If the arrow is used, it should point laterally.

Locating the Greater and Lesser Tubercles and Humeral Head

- A method of determining where the greater tubercle and humeral head will be positioned on an image is to use the palpable humeral epicondyles. The lateral epicondyle is aligned with the greater tubercle, and the medial epicondyle is aligned with the humeral head. This means that when the humeral epicondyles are in profile, the greater tubercle and humeral head also will be. The lesser tubercle is anteriorly located at a right angle to the greater tubercle.

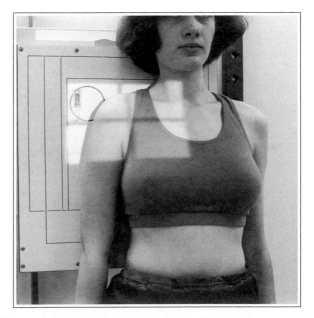

Figure 4-6. Proper internal anteroposterior shoulder positioning.

In *internal rotation,* the lesser tubercle is demonstrated in profile medially and the humeral head is superimposed by the greater tubercle (see Image 8).

- Accurate internal humeral head rotation is obtained by internally rotating the patient's arm until the humeral epicondyles are aligned perpendicular with the IR (Figure 4-6).
- Internal humeral rotation may also cause the scapula to move anteriorly, transversely foreshortening the scapular body, and may cause the humeral head to demonstrate increased glenoid fossa superimposition.
- An arrow or word marker should be used to indicate internal humeral rotation. If the arrow is used, it should point medially.

Anteroposterior Shoulder Image Analysis

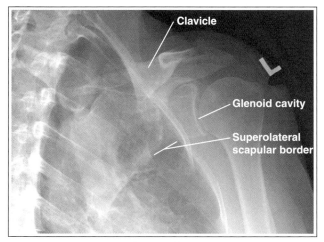

Image 1.

Analysis. The glenoid cavity is nearly in profile, with only a small amount of the articulating surface demonstrated, the superolateral border of the scapula is superimposed by the thorax, and the clavicle is longitudinally foreshortened. The patient was rotated toward the affected shoulder.

Correction. Rotate the patient away from the affected shoulder into an AP projection, with the shoulders positioned at equal distances from the imaging table.

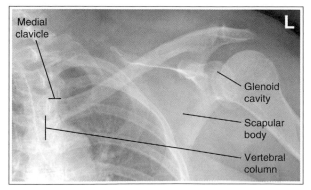

Image 2.

Analysis. The scapular body is drawn from beneath the thorax and is foreshortened, the glenoid cavity is demonstrated on end, and the medial clavicular end is superimposed over the vertebral column. The patient was rotated toward the unaffected shoulder.

Correction. Rotate the patient toward the affected shoulder into an AP projection, with the shoulders positioned at equal distances from the imaging table.

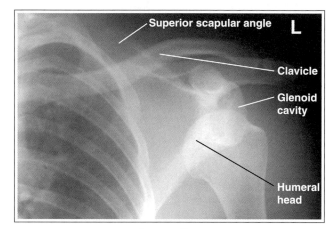

Image 3.

Analysis. The humeral head is demonstrated below the coracoid process, and the superior scapular angle is shown superior to the clavicle. The patient's shoulder is dislocated, and the upper midcoronal plane was tilted anteriorly.

Correction. Do not adjust humeral positioning. Tilt the upper midcoronal plane toward the IR.

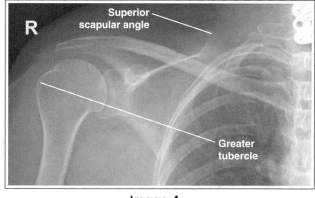

Image 4.

Analysis. The superior scapular angle is demonstrated superior to the clavicle. The patient's upper midcoronal plane was tilted anteriorly. The greater tubercle is in profile laterally.

Correction. Tilt the upper midcoronal plane posteriorly. For a kyphotic patient whose vertebral column cannot be straightened, bring the central ray perpendicular to the scapular body by angling it cephalically. No corrective movement is necessary if the greater tubercle is wanted in profile.

If a neutral position is desired, position the humeral epicondyles at a 45-degree angle with the IR (see Figure 4-3). To demonstrate the lesser tubercle in profile, internally rotate the arm until the humeral epicondyles are perpendicular to the IR (see Figure 4-6).

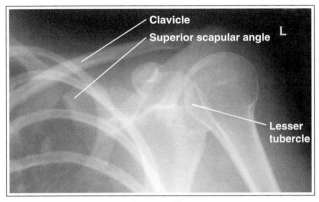

Image 5.

Analysis. The superior scapular angle is demonstrated inferior to the clavicle. The patient's upper midcoronal plane was tilted posteriorly. The lesser tubercle is demonstrated in profile medially, and the greater tubercle and humeral head are superimposed. The patient's humerus was internally rotated until the humeral epicondyles were perpendicular to the IR.

Correction. Tilt the upper midcoronal plane anteriorly. No corrective movement is necessary if the lesser tubercle is wanted in profile. If a neutral position is desired, position the humeral epicondyles at a 45-degree angle to the IR (see Figure 4-3). To demonstrate the greater tubercle in profile, externally rotate the arm until the humeral epicondyles are parallel with the IR (see Figure 4-5).

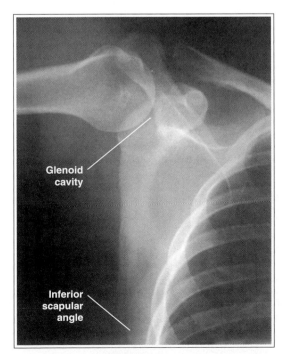

Image 6.

Analysis. The humerus is demonstrated at a 90-degree angle with the body, the glenoid cavity faces superiorly, and the lateral scapular body is drawn away from the thorax. The humerus was abducted.

Correction. Position the humerus next to the patient's body.

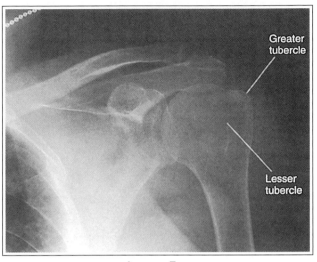

Image 7.

Analysis. The greater tubercle is demonstrated in profile laterally, the humeral head is demonstrated medially, and the cortical margin of the lesser tubercle is visible approximately halfway between the greater tubercle and the humeral head. The patient's humerus was externally rotated until the humeral epicondyles were parallel with the IR.

Correction. No corrective movement is necessary if the greater tubercle is wanted in profile. If a neutral position is desired, position the humeral epicondyles at a 45-degree angle with the IR (see Figure 4-3). To demonstrate the lesser tubercle in profile, internally rotate the arm until the humeral epicondyles are perpendicular to the IR (see Figure 4-6).

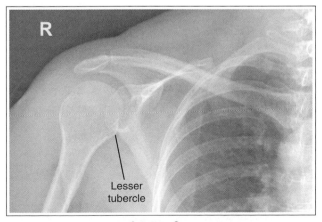

Image 8.

Analysis. The lesser tubercle is demonstrated in profile medially, and the greater tubercle and humeral head are superimposed. The patient's humerus was internally rotated until the humeral epicondyles were perpendicular to the IR.

Correction. No corrective movement is necessary if the lesser tubercle is wanted in profile. If a neutral position is desired, position the humeral epicondyles at a 45-degree angle with the IR (see Figure 4-3). To demonstrate the greater tubercle in profile, externally rotate the arm until the humeral epicondyles are parallel with the IR (see Figure 4-5).

SHOULDER: INFEROSUPERIOR (AXIAL) PROJECTION

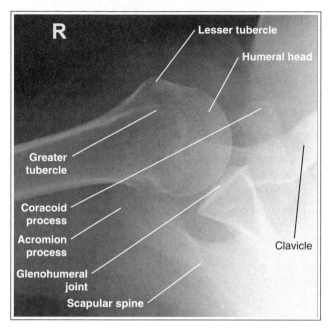

Figure 4-7. Axillary shoulder image with accurate positioning obtained with humeral epicondyles positioned parallel with floor.

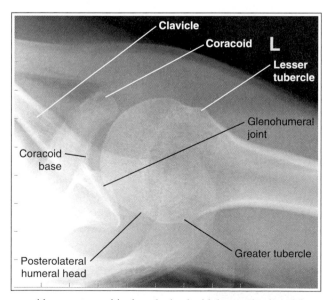

Figure 4-8. Axillary shoulder image with accurate positioning obtained with humeral epicondyles positioned at 45 degrees with floor.

Image Analysis

The inferior and superior margins of the glenoid cavity are nearly superimposed, with only a small amount of humeral head superimposition. The lateral edge of the coracoid process base is aligned with the inferior glenoid cavity margin.

- The axial position of the shoulder is obtained by placing the patient supine on the imaging table in an AP projection with the affected shoulder next to the lateral edge of the imaging table. The patient's arm is then abducted 90 degrees from the body, and a horizontal beam is directed to the axilla, parallel with the glenohumeral joint space (Figure 4-9).
- *Effect of humeral abduction on central ray alignment:* Because no palpable structures are present to help align the central ray with the glenohumeral joint, we must rely on our knowledge of scapular movement on humeral abduction to align it. Abduction of the arm is accomplished by combined movements of the glenohumeral joint and the scapula as it glides around the thoracic cavity. The ratio of movement in these two articulations is two parts glenohumeral to one part scapulothoracic, with the initial movement being primarily glenohumeral. If the patient's arm is not abducted, the glenoid cavity is angled **approximately** 20 degrees with the lateral body surface.
- In a patient who is not experiencing severe pain with the 90-degree humeral abduction, the scapular movement angles the glenoid cavity to approximately 30 to 35 degrees with the lateral body surface (Figure 4-10). Consequently, to align the central ray parallel with the glenohumeral joint on such a patient, the angle between the lateral body surface and central ray should be 30 to 35 degrees. This angle is best accomplished by first determining the 23- and 45-degree angles as discussed in Chapter 1, then aligning the central ray between these two angles. Thirty-four degrees is halfway between the 23- and 45-degree angles (see Figure 4-9).
- Because the glenoid cavity faces superiorly when the arm is abducted, if a patient is unable to fully abduct the

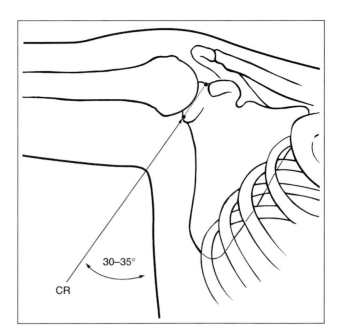

Figure 4-10. Placement of glenoid cavity with arm abducted 90 degrees. *CR*, Central ray.

arm, the angle between the lateral body surface and central ray needs to be decreased to align it parallel with the glenohumeral joint (Figure 4-11). Because the first 60 degrees of humeral abduction involves primarily movement of the glenohumeral joint without accompanying scapular movement, the angle between the central ray and lateral body surface should be **approximately** 20 degrees when the humerus is abducted up to 60 degrees.

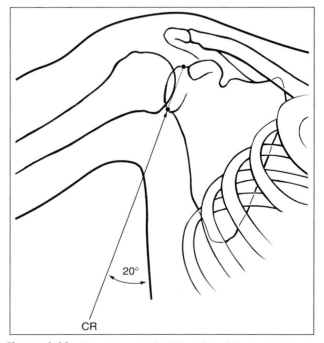

Figure 4-11. Placement of glenoid cavity with arm abducted less than 90 degrees. *CR*, Central ray.

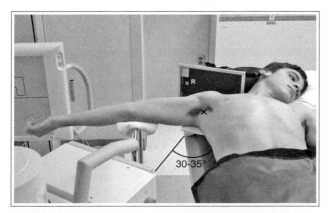

Figure 4-9. Proper inferosuperior axillary shoulder positioning.

- ***Detecting inaccurate central ray alignment:*** Inaccurate alignment of the central ray with the glenohumeral joint space can be signified on an image by the increased demonstration of the articulating surface of the glenoid cavity and misalignment of the inferior glenoid cavity margin with the lateral edge of the coracoid process base. Whether the angle between the central ray and the lateral body surface should be increased or decreased can be determined by viewing the relationship of the coracoid process base to the inferior glenoid cavity margin. Because the inferior glenoid cavity margin is situated farther from the IR, it will be projected to one side of the coracoid process base instead of being aligned with it if the central ray is aligned inaccurately. If the central ray to lateral body surface angle is too small, the inferior glenoid cavity margin will be projected lateral to the lateral edge of the coracoid process base. (Closely compare the coracoid process base and glenoid cavity relationships in Figure 4-7 and Image 9.) If the angle is too large, the inferior margin will be projected medial to the lateral edge of the coracoid process base (see Image 10).

The proximal humerus is demonstrated without distortion, and the long axis of the humeral shaft is demonstrated with limited foreshortening.

- Poor alignment of the IR with the central ray and with the humerus results in image distortion. Distortion caused by poor IR and central ray alignment can be eliminated by aligning the central ray with the patient's glenohumeral joint and then positioning the IR vertically at the top of the affected shoulder so it is perpendicular to the central ray. Distortion of the humeral shaft and head can be reduced when the patient's humerus is placed in 90-degree abduction. If the patient is unable to abduct the arm to 90 degrees, the humeral shaft and head demonstrate foreshortening (see Image 11). The severity of the distortion depends on how close to 90 degrees the patient was able to abduct the humerus. The more the humerus is abducted, the less distortion is demonstrated.

The proximal humerus is positioned as indicated by your facility.

When humeral epicondyles are positioned *parallel* with the floor, the lesser tubercle is demonstrated in profile anteriorly (see Figure 4-7).

- The lesser tubercle is placed in profile when the arm is extended, then externally rotated until an imaginary line connecting the epicondyles is positioned parallel with the floor.

When humeral epicondyles are positioned at a 45-degree angle with the floor, the lesser tubercle is demonstrated in partial profile anteriorly and the posterolateral aspect of the humeral head is in profile posteriorly (see Figure 4-8).

- The lesser tubercle is placed in partial profile, and the posterolateral aspect of the humeral head is positioned in profile when the arm is extended and then externally rotated until an imaginary line connecting the humeral epicondyles is placed at a 45-degree angle with the floor (see Figure 4-9). The lateral epicondyle is positioned closer to the floor. This humerus positioning is especially helpful in identifying a compression fracture of the posterolateral aspect of the humeral head. This compression fracture, a result of an anterior shoulder dislocation, is known as the *Hill-Sachs defect.*

- If the humeral epicondyles are positioned at an angle greater than 45-degrees with the floor, or if the patient's elbow is flexed so the hand of the affected arm can be used to hold the IR in place, the lesser tubercle and posterolateral humeral head will not be demonstrated. The greater tubercle will be demonstrated in profile posteriorly and the humeral head anteriorly when the humerus is externally rotated enough to place the humeral epicondyles perpendicular to the floor (see Image 12).

The entire coracoid process is demonstrated in profile.

- The coracoid process is demonstrated in profile when the scapular body is placed parallel with the imaging table, as the patient is positioned supine. With excessive external arm rotation the inferior scapula tilts anteriorly as the vertebral column arches to accomplish this arm rotation. This tilting results in the base of the coracoid process moving beneath the glenoid cavity, decreasing its visibility (see Image 13).

The humeral head is centered within the collimated field. The glenoid cavity, coracoid process, scapular spine, acromion process, and a third of the proximal humerus are included within the field.

- ***Including the posterior surface:*** To ensure that the scapular spine is included within the image, elevate the patient's shoulder 2 to 3 inches (5 to 7.6 cm) from the imaging table with a sponge or folded washcloth. If the shoulder is not elevated, the posterior portion of the humerus and shoulder may not be included on the image (see Image 14).

- ***Including the coracoid:*** To include the coracoid process on the image, instruct the patient to turn the face away from the affected shoulder then laterally flex the neck, tilting the head toward the unaffected shoulder. Place an IR at the top of the patient's shoulder perpendicular to the imaging table and resting snugly against the patient's neck. If the IR is not positioned snugly against the patient's neck, the coracoid process and possibly the glenoid cavity and proximal humerus may not be included on the image (see Image 15).

- ***Centering the humeral head:*** To align the central ray with the glenohumeral joint, center the central ray horizontally to the midaxillary region at the same level as the coracoid process. (Palpate to locate the coracoid process before humeral abduction.) The humeral head is centered in the collimated field for the axial shoulder even though the central ray is centered to the glenohumeral joint, because the IR cannot be positioned medially enough to center the joint in the center.

- Open the longitudinal collimation slightly beyond the coracoid process, and transversely collimate to within ½ inch (1.25 cm) of the proximal humeral skinline.
- An 8- × 10-inch (18- × 24-cm) IR placed crosswise should be adequate to include all the required anatomical structures.

Axillary Shoulder Image Analysis

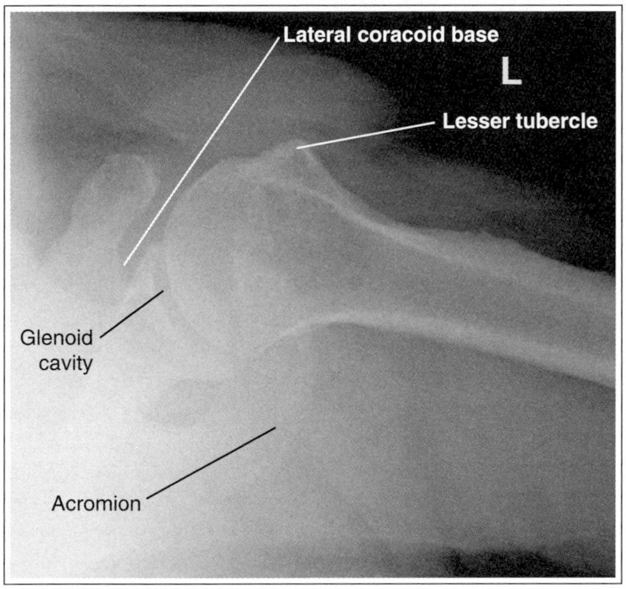

Image 9.

Analysis. The glenohumeral joint is closed, and the inferior glenoid cavity margin is demonstrated lateral to the coracoid process base. The angle formed between the lateral body surface and the central ray was less than required to align the central ray parallel with the glenohumeral joint.

Correction. Increase the angle between the lateral body surface and the central ray to 30 to 35 degrees.

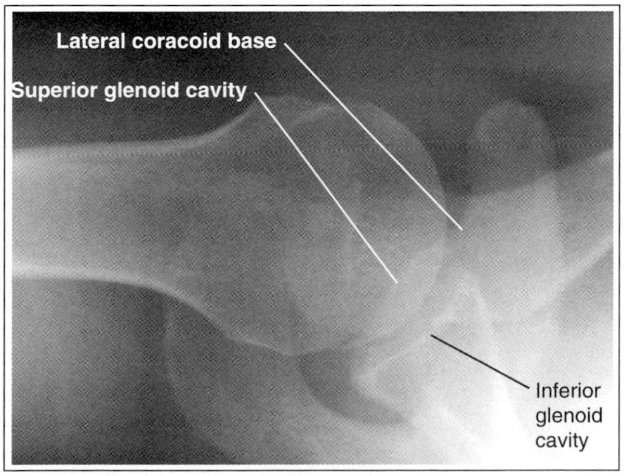

Image 10.

Analysis. The glenohumeral joint is closed, and the inferior glenoid cavity margin is demonstrated medial to the lateral edge of the coracoid process base and superior glenoid cavity margin, indicating that the angle between the lateral body surface and the central ray was too large. The humeral head is distorted. The humerus was not abducted to a 90-degree angle with the body.

Correction. Decrease the angle between the lateral body surface and central ray. If the patient is able to abduct the arm to 90 degrees, the lateral body surface and central ray angle should be 30 to 35 degrees. If the patient is unable to abduct the arm, a smaller angle is required (see Figure 4-11).

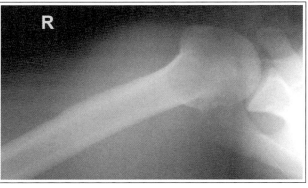

Image 11.

Analysis. The glenoid cavity and coracoid process are accurately demonstrated, but the humerus is foreshortened and the humeral head is distorted. The arm was not abducted 90 degrees from the body.

Correction. If possible, have the patient abduct the humerus 90 degrees from the body. If the patient cannot abduct the humerus, no corrective movement is necessary.

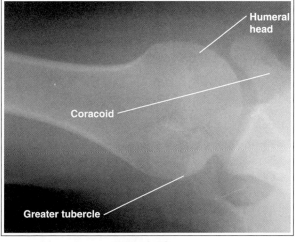

Image 12.

Analysis. The greater tubercle is in profile posteriorly. The entire coracoid process is demonstrated in profile. The humerus was externally rotated enough to position the humeral epicondyles perpendicular to the floor.

Correction. Internally rotate the humerus until the epicondyles are at a 45-degree angle with the floor if the posterolateral humeral head is desired in profile or until they are parallel with the floor if the lesser tubercle is desired in profile.

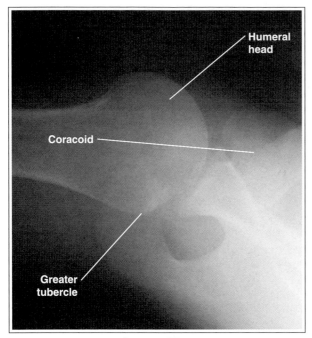

Image 13.

Analysis. The greater tubercle is in profile posteriorly, and the coracoid process base is partially obscured by the glenoid cavity. The humerus was externally rotated enough to position the humeral epicondyles perpendicular to the floor, and the inferior scapula was tilted anteriorly.

Correction. Internally rotate humerus until the epicondyles are at a 45-degree angle with floor if the posterolateral humeral head is desired in profile and until they are parallel with the floor if the lesser tubercle is desired in profile. This arm movement will also result in the scapula being positioned parallel with the imaging table, increasing coracoid process visibility.

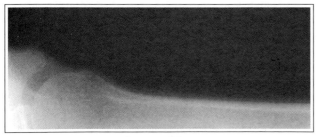

Image 14.

Analysis. The acromion process, scapular spine, and posterior aspect of the proximal humerus are not included on the image. The patient's shoulder was not adequately elevated off the imaging table.

Correction. Elevate the shoulder 2 to 3 inches (5 to 7.6 cm) off the imaging table with a sponge or folded washcloth.

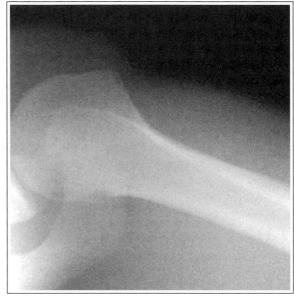

Image 15.

Analysis. The coracoid process and a portion of the glenoid cavity are not included on the image. The patient's head was not turned or the neck laterally flexed toward the unaffected shoulder enough to adequately position the IR medially.

Correction. Turn the patient's face, and laterally flex the neck and tilt the head toward the unaffected shoulder. Then snugly position the edge of the IR against the patient's neck.

SHOULDER: POSTERIOR OBLIQUE POSITION (GRASHEY METHOD)

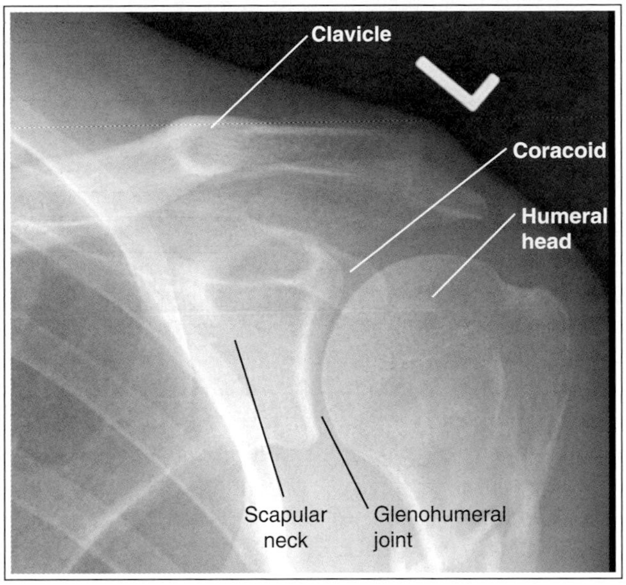

Figure 4-12. Posterior oblique (Grashey) shoulder image with accurate positioning.

Image Analysis

The glenoid cavity is demonstrated in profile with the glenohumeral joint space open, the lateral coracoid process demonstrates approximately $1/4$ inch (0.6 cm) of superimposition of the humeral head, the glenoid cavity is shown without thorax superimposition, and the clavicle is longitudinally foreshortened.

- To obtain an image that demonstrates the glenoid cavity in profile and an open glenohumeral joint space, the patient's scapular body must be positioned parallel with the IR. This is accomplished by placing the patient in an upright AP projection, then rotating the patient's body approximately 35 to 45 degrees toward the affected shoulder (Figure 4-13). A 35- to 45-degree posterior oblique position routinely opens the glenohumeral joint space as long as the patient is upright and the affected shoulder is in a neutral position without protraction.
- **Effect of shoulder protraction on the required degree of patient obliquity:** Protraction or forward movement of the shoulder occurs as a result of pressure that is placed on the affected shoulder when the patient leans against the upright IR holder. The sternoclavicular and AC joints function cooperatively to allow the shoulder to be drawn anteriorly. When the shoulder is drawn anteriorly, the scapula glides around the thorax, moving the lateral portion of the scapula anteriorly. This increase in anterior shoulder positioning places the scapular body at a larger angle with the IR, therefore requiring an increase in patient obliquity to bring the scapular body

parallel with the IR for the Grashey method. An image taken with the patient leaning against the IR holder will demonstrate an open glenohumeral joint, but a portion of the thorax will be superimposed over the glenoid cavity (see Image 16).

- An increase in patient obliquity is also necessary when the examination is performed on a kyphotic or recumbent patient. Because of the vertebral column curvature, the kyphotic patient's shoulders are situated anteriorly, aligning them similarly to protracted shoulders. In this

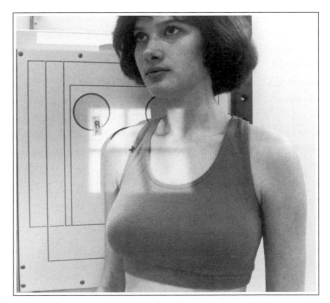

Figure 4-13. Proper positioning for posterior oblique (Grashey) shoulder image.

situation an image can be obtained that demonstrates the glenoid cavity in profile and an open glenohumeral joint space, although the thorax often is superimposed over them. In the recumbent position the pressure of the body on the shoulder forces the shoulder of interest anteriorly and superiorly when the patient is rotated. Images taken with the patient in this position demonstrate the glenoid cavity situated slightly superiorly and the clavicle aligned more vertically (see Image 17).

- *Recommended method of determining degree of body obliquity:* The most accurate method of determining the amount of patient obliquity necessary for all Grashey shoulder images is to palpate the patient's coracoid process and acromion angle, then rotate the patient toward the affected shoulder until the coracoid process is superimposed over the acromion angle, aligning an imaginary line connecting them perpendicular to the IR (Figure 4-14).

- *Detecting incorrect obliquity:* Incorrect body obliquity will be identified on an image as a closed glenohumeral joint space. Whether the body has been rotated too much or too little to accomplish this closed joint can be determined by evaluating the relationship of the coracoid process with the humeral head, the degree of thorax superimposition on the glenoid cavity and scapular neck, and the longitudinal clavicle foreshortening. If obliquity was excessive, the glenohumeral joint space is closed, more than $\frac{1}{4}$ inch (0.6 cm) of the lateral tip of the coracoid process is superimposed over the humeral head, the thorax demonstrates increased glenoid cavity and scapular neck superimposition, and the clavicle demonstrates excessive longitudinal foreshortening (see Image 18). If obliquity was insufficient, the glenohumeral joint

space is closed, the lateral tip of the coracoid process demonstrates less than $\frac{1}{4}$ inch (0.6 cm) of humeral head superimposition, the thorax is not superimposed over the scapular neck, and the clavicle demonstrates little foreshortening (see Image 19).

- *Evaluating the recumbent patient's image:* When evaluating a Grashey image on a recumbent patient, you cannot use clavicular foreshortening as a guide to determine repositioning because it is vertically positioned, although you can evaluate its proximity to the scapular neck. If obliquity was excessive, the glenohumeral joint is closed, the lateral tip of the coracoid process is superimposed over more than $\frac{1}{4}$ inch (0.6 cm) of the humeral head, and the clavicle is superimposed over the scapular neck (see Image 20). If the obliquity was insufficient, then the glenohumeral joint is closed, the lateral tip of the coracoid process is superimposed over less than $\frac{1}{4}$ inch (0.6 cm) of the humeral head, and the clavicle is not superimposed over the scapular neck (see Image 21).

- *Repositioning for Grashey image:* When repositioning for an excessive or insufficient obliquity on a Grashey image, remember that the glenohumeral joint space is narrow and that the necessary repositioning movement is only half of the distance demonstrated between the anterior and posterior margins of the glenoid cavity. In most cases you need to move the patient only a few degrees to obtain an open joint space, so it is important to carefully evaluate and make mental notes on how the patient was positioned for the initial exam. If a repeat is necessary, start with the patient position used for the initial exam, then adjust the position from this starting point.

The glenohumeral joint is at the center of the collimated field. The glenoid cavity, humeral head, coracoid and acromion processes, and distal clavicle are included within the field.

- Center a perpendicular central ray at a level 1 inch (2.5 cm) inferior and medial to the palpable coracoid process to place the glenohumeral joint at the center of the collimated field. The coracoid process can be palpated $\frac{3}{4}$ inch (2 cm) inferior to the midpoint of the lateral half of the clavicle and medial to the humeral head. Even on very muscular patients the concave pocket formed inferior to the lateral half of the clavicle and medial to the humeral head can be used to center the central ray.

- Center the IR to the central ray and open the longitudinal collimated field enough to include the shoulder top and transversely collimate to the lateral humeral skinline.

- An 8- × 10-inch (18- × 24-cm) IR placed crosswise should be adequate to include all the required anatomical structures.

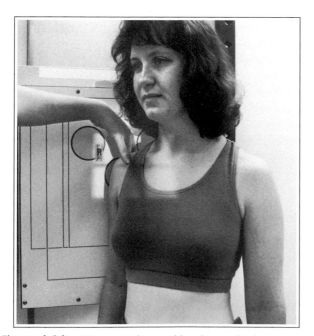

Figure 4-14. Alignment of coracoid and acromion processes for posterior oblique (Grashey) shoulder image.

Posterior Oblique (Grashey) Shoulder Image Analysis

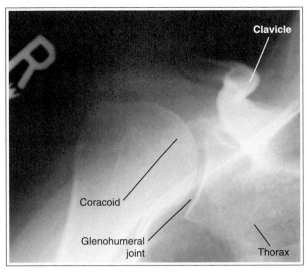

Image 16.

Analysis. The glenohumeral joint space is open, and the lateral tip of the coracoid process is superimposed over the humeral head by approximately ¼ inch (0.6 cm). The clavicle demonstrates excessive longitudinal foreshortening, and the thorax is superimposed over the inferior glenohumeral joint space. The image was taken with the shoulder protracted and the patient rotated more than 45 degrees to obtain an open glenohumeral joint space. Shoulder protraction results when the patient leans against the upright IR holder or is in a supine position. Because the clavicle is not vertical, it can be determined that this examination was conducted with the patient leaning against the upright holder.

Correction. Position the patient's upper midcoronal plane in a vertical position, and place the affected shoulder in a neutral position. Do not allow the patient to lean against the upright IR holder. Less patient obliquity will be required with this new positioning.

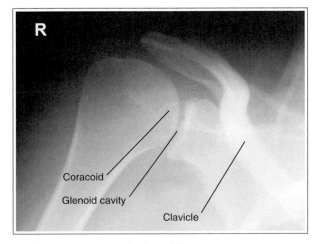

Image 17.

Analysis. The glenohumeral joint space is open, the glenoid cavity is situated slightly superiorly, and the clavicle is aligned somewhat vertically. This examination was taken with the patient in a recumbent position.

Correction. No positioning change is required. The goal of the examination is to obtain an image with an open and unobstructed glenohumeral joint space.

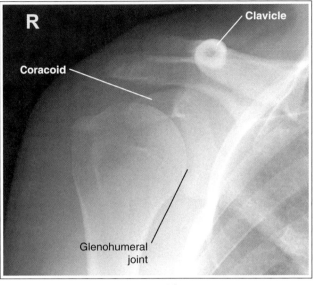

Image 18.

Analysis. The glenohumeral joint space is closed, more than ¼ inch (0.6 cm) of the lateral tip of the coracoid process is superimposed over the humeral head, and the clavicle demonstrates excessive longitudinal foreshortening. Patient obliquity was excessive.

Correction. Decrease the degree of patient obliquity. The amount of decrease required is only half of the distance between the anterior and posterior margins of the glenoid cavity.

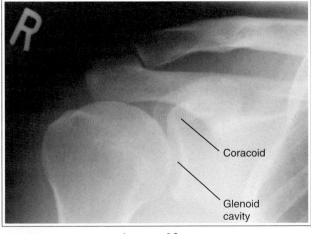

Image 19.

Analysis. The glenohumeral joint space is closed, the lateral tip of the coracoid process does not superimpose the humeral head, and the clavicle demonstrates little fore-shortening. Patient obliquity was insufficient.

Correction. Increase the degree of patient obliquity, thereby moving the coracoid process toward the humeral head and shifting the anterior and posterior margins of the glenoid cavity toward each other.

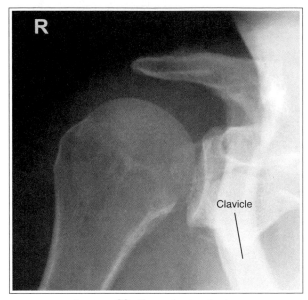

Image 20. Recumbent patient.

Analysis. The glenohumeral joint space is closed, more than ¼ inch (0.6 cm) of the coracoid process tip is superimposed

over the humeral head, and the clavicle is superimposed over the scapular neck. Patient obliquity was excessive.

Correction. Decrease the degree of patient obliquity.

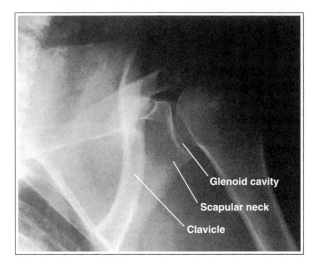

Image 21. Recumbent patient.

Analysis. The glenohumeral joint space is closed, less than ¼ inch (0.6 cm) of the coracoid process tip is superimposed over the humeral head, and the clavicle is not superimposed over the scapular neck. Patient obliquity was insufficient.

Correction. Increase the degree of patient obliquity.

SHOULDER: ANTERIOR OBLIQUE POSITION (SCAPULAR Y)

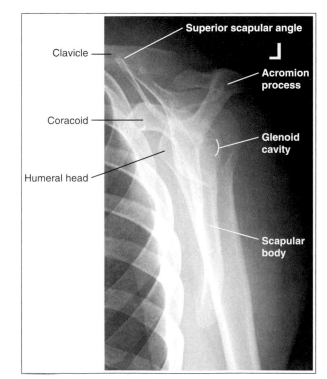

Figure 4-15. Anterior oblique (scapular Y) shoulder image with accurate positioning.

Image Analysis

The scapula demonstrates the least amount of magnification.

- The standing anterior oblique patient position places the scapula closer to the IR, resulting in the least amount of scapular magnification and the greatest scapular detail.

The scapular body is in a lateral position. The lateral and vertebral scapular borders are superimposed, and the scapular body is not superimposed over the thoracic cavity. The scapular body and the acromion and coracoid processes form a Y, with the scapular body as the leg and the acromion and coracoid processes as the arms. The glenoid cavity is demonstrated on end at the converging point of the arms and leg of the Y.

- To place the scapular body in a lateral position, begin by placing the patient in an upright posteroanterior (PA) projection, with the affected arm hanging freely. This nonelevated arm position aligns the vertebral border of the scapula parallel with the IR when the scapula is in a lateral position, allowing the coracoid and acromion processes to be demonstrated in profile. From this PA projection, rotate the patient's body 45 to 60 degrees toward the affected scapula until the lateral and vertebral scapular borders are superimposed (Figure 4-16).
- ***Amount of body obliquity required:*** The degree of body obliquity required to superimpose the scapular borders for the scapular Y position has been questioned. Some textbooks state that the midcoronal plane should form a 60-degree angle with the IR. This degree of obliquity originated from the observations made by Rubin and colleagues of the Y shoulder formation while they were

evaluating 60-degree oblique chest images.[1] A later study of the scapular Y position presented by De Smet in 1979 found that a 45-degree anterior obliquity was the optimal obliquity for this image.

The controversy between these two observations may lie in the position of the humerus. For a 60-degree anterior oblique chest image, the patient's humerus is abducted and the hand is placed on the patient's crest. When the patient is rotated, the shoulder is retracted (drawn backward). This humerus and shoulder positioning causes the scapula to glide around the thoracic cavity, moving toward the spinal column. When the scapula is in this posterior position, the patient's body needs to be rotated more to bring the scapular body lateral. The 1979 report by De Smet states that the humerus is to hang freely.[2] Because the humerus and shoulder are not forced backward when the arm hangs freely, the scapula is positioned slightly more anteriorly, therefore needing less obliquity to bring it into a lateral position.

- ***Using scapular palpation to determine accurate degree of body obliquity:*** Accurate patient obliquity can be obtained by palpating the scapular anatomy. First, palpate the coracoid process and the acromion angle, and locate the midpoint of an imaginary line drawn between them. Next, locate the vertebral border of the scapula. Rotate the patient toward the affected shoulder until the vertebral scapular border is aligned with a point midway between the acromion and coracoid processes. This positioning sets up the Y formation, with the scapular body positioned between the acromion and coracoid processes. Once the correct obliquity is determined, have the patient step toward the IR until the patient's shoulder just touches the upright grid and IR holder. The exact degree of obliquity varies from patient to patient, depending on shoulder roundness, arm position, and pressure placed on the shoulder when the patient touches the IR holder.
- ***Posterior oblique positioning:*** For a patient who is supine, the scapular Y image can be obtained by means of a posterior oblique position. Palpate the acromion and coracoid processes and vertebral scapular borders in the same way as described for the standing anterior oblique position, and rotate the patient toward the unaffected shoulder until the vertebral scapular border lies midway between the acromion and coracoid processes. The anatomical relationship of the bony structures of the scapula should be aligned identically on anterior and posterior oblique Y images. The posterior oblique image, however, demonstrates increased magnification of the scapula and humerus (see Image 22).
- ***Detecting mispositioning:*** If the patient obliquity is not accurate for the scapular Y position, the Y formation of the scapula is not formed, the medial and lateral borders of the scapular body are not superimposed but are visualized next to each other, and the glenoid cavity is not demonstrated on end.
- To determine whether patient obliquity needs to be increased or decreased to superimpose the medial and

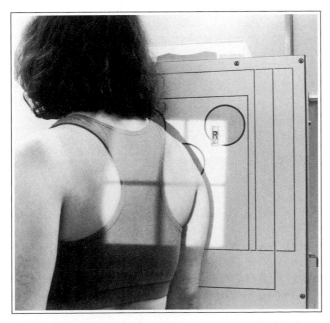

Figure 4-16. Proper anterior oblique (scapular Y) positioning.

lateral borders of scapular body and position the glenoid cavity on end, identify the borders of the scapula. The lateral border is thick, with two cortical outlines that are separated by approximately ¼ inch (0.6 cm), whereas the cortical outline of the vertebral border demonstrates a single thin line. If the lateral border is demonstrated next to the ribs, and the vertebral border is visualized laterally, patient obliquity was excessive (see Image 23). If the vertebral border is demonstrated next to the ribs and the lateral border is visible laterally, patient obliquity was insufficient to superimpose the borders (see Image 24).

If the shoulder is *not* dislocated, the humeral head and glenoid cavity and the humeral shaft and scapular body are superimposed. If the shoulder is dislocated, the humeral head and shaft are shown either anterior or posterior to the glenoid cavity and scapular body, respectively. If the proximal humerus is fractured, the humeral head and glenoid cavity are superimposed, but the midshaft will be demonstrated anteriorly or posteriorly to the scapular body. Each of these situations should demonstrate the scapular Y formation described previously.

- Two indications for the scapular Y position are to determine whether a shoulder dislocation or proximal humeral fracture exists. The position of the humeral head and shaft in relation to the glenoid cavity and scapular body should not be a positioning concern to the imaging technologist. As long as the scapula is positioned in a Y formation, proper positioning has been obtained. When the shoulder is being imaged to rule out a dislocation or proximal humeral fracture, the patient's humerus should not be moved.

- *Detecting shoulder dislocation:* The cortical outline of the glenoid cavity is visible as a circular density at the junction of the coracoid and acromion processes and the scapular body. Normally the humeral head is superimposed over this junction. When the humeral head is not positioned over the glenoid cavity, a shoulder dislocation exists and will result in positioning of the humeral head either anterior or posterior and inferior to the glenoid cavity. An anterior dislocation, which is more common (95%), results in the humeral head's being demonstrated anteriorly, beneath the coracoid process (see Image 25). A posterior dislocation, which is uncommon (2% to 4%), results in the humeral head's being demonstrated posteriorly, beneath the acromion process (Figure 4-17).

- *Detecting proximal humeral fracture:* The scapular Y position will demonstrate the alignment of the humeral head and shaft in a lateral position without requiring the patient to move the arm. An image taken of a patient with a proximal humeral fracture will demonstrate superimposition of the humeral head and glenoid cavity, but the humeral shaft will be positioned anteriorly or posteriorly to the scapular body (see Image 26). It is important that correct alignment of the scapula is accomplished when a fracture is suspected, because poor alignment may result

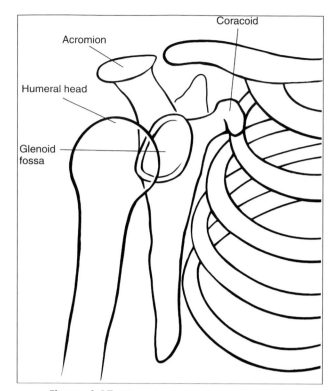

Figure 4-17. Posterior dislocation of shoulder.

in misdiagnosis. Images 26 and 27 are from the same patient. Compare the accuracy of the scapular Y formation and the alignment of the humeral head and shaft on these images.

The scapula is demonstrated without longitudinal foreshortening, and the superior scapular angle is superimposed over the clavicle.

- Longitudinal foreshortening of the scapula is prevented when the midcoronal plane remains vertical. Foreshortening is a result of leaning the patient's upper midcoronal plane and shoulder toward the IR. This forward position causes the glenoid cavity and the acromion and coracoid processes to move inferiorly and the superior scapular angle and spine to move superiorly. A longitudinally foreshortened scapula image demonstrates the superior scapular angle above the clavicle (see Image 28).

- *Positioning for kyphosis:* On a patient with spinal kyphosis the scapula is longitudinally foreshortened because of the forward curvature of the vertebral column. To offset this curvature and obtain a scapula without foreshortening, the central ray may be angled perpendicular to the vertebral scapular border. This angulation can be obtained by palpating the vertebral scapular border and aligning the central ray perpendicular to it. For anterior oblique images, the angulation would be caudal, and for posterior oblique images, the angulation would be cephalad.

The midscapular body is at the center of the collimated field. The entire scapula, which includes the inferior angle, the coracoid and acromion processes, and the proximal humerus, are included within the field.

- To place the midscapular body in the center of the collimated field, center a perpendicular central ray to the vertebral border of the scapula halfway between the inferior scapular angle and the acromial angle. Each of these anatomical structures is palpable and should be used to ensure accurate positioning.
- Center the IR to the central ray, and open the longitudinal collimation enough to include the acromion process and inferior scapular angles. Transversely collimate to within the lateral humeral skinline.
- A 10- × 12-inch (24- × 30-cm) IR placed lengthwise should be adequate to include all the required anatomical structures.

Anterior Oblique (Scapular Y) Shoulder Image Analysis

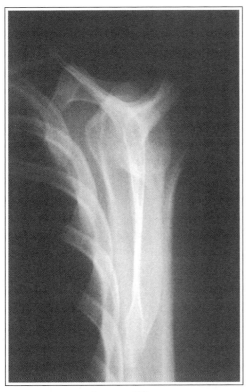

Image 22.

Analysis. The vertebral and lateral borders of the scapular body are superimposed, the coracoid and acromion processes form the upper arms of a Y, and the cortical outline of the glenoid cavity is visualized at the Y's arm and leg junction. The patient was accurately positioned. Note the increased amount of magnification of the scapula and humerus compared with the image shown in Figure 4-15. This image was taken with the patient in a posterior oblique position.

Correction. No corrective movement is necessary. If the patient can stand, the anterior oblique position would demonstrate less magnification.

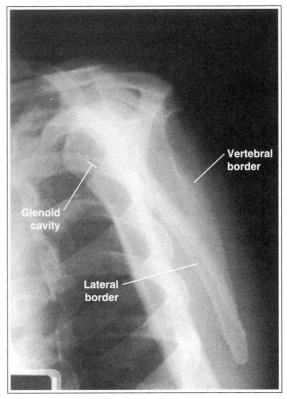

Image 23.

Analysis. The lateral and vertebral borders of the scapula are demonstrated without superimposition, and the glenoid cavity is not demonstrated on end but is shown medially. The lateral scapular border is demonstrated next to the ribs, and the vertebral border is visible laterally. The patient was rotated more than necessary to superimpose the borders of scapular body.

Correction. Decrease the patient obliquity. The amount of decrease is half the distance demonstrated between the vertebral and lateral scapular borders. The measurement should be taken at the midscapular body region.

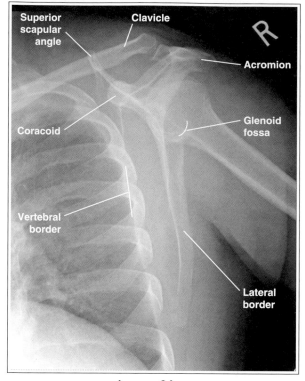

Image 24.

Analysis. The lateral and vertebral borders of the scapula are demonstrated without superimposition, and the glenoid cavity is not demonstrated on end but appears laterally. The vertebral scapular border is demonstrated next to the ribs, whereas the lateral border is visible laterally. The patient was not rotated enough to superimpose the borders of the scapular body.

Correction. Increase the patient obliquity.

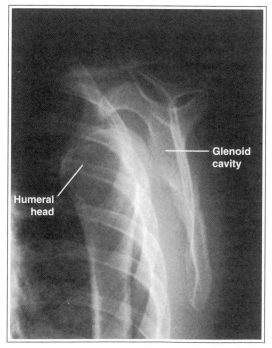

Image 25.

Analysis. The scapular body and acromion and coracoid processes are accurately positioned into a Y formation, and the cortical outline of the glenoid cavity is demonstrated at the junction of the arms and leg of the Y. The humeral head and shaft are demonstrated anterior to the glenoid cavity and scapular body, respectively. The shoulder is anteriorly dislocated.

Correction. No corrective movement is required.

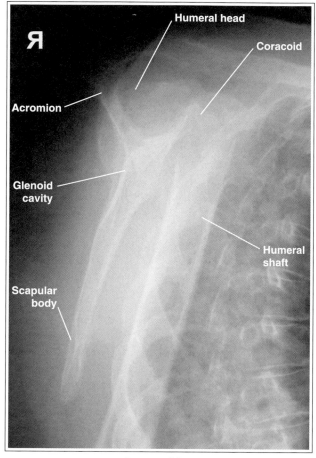

Image 26.

Analysis. The scapular body and acromion and coracoid processes are accurately positioned into a Y formation, and the cortical outline of the glenoid cavity is demonstrated at the junction of the arms and leg of the Y. The humeral head and glenoid cavity are superimposed, and the humeral shaft is anterior to the scapular body. The proximal humerus is fractured.

Correction. No corrective movement is required.

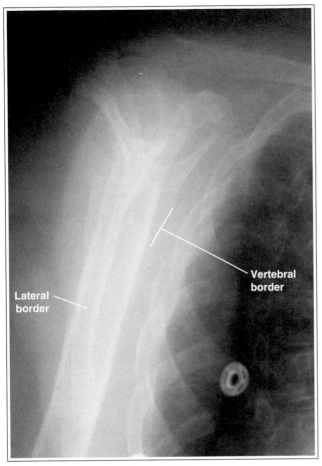

Image 27.

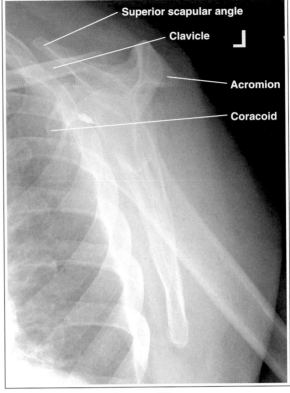

Image 28.

Analysis. The lateral and vertebral borders of the scapula are demonstrated without superimposition, and the humeral shaft and scapular body are superimposed. The vertebral scapular border is demonstrated next to the ribs, whereas the lateral border is visible laterally. The patient was not rotated enough to superimpose the borders of the scapular body. The proximal humerus is fractured.

Correction. Increase the patient obliquity.

Analysis. The scapular body, acromion, and coracoid processes are accurately aligned, but the superior scapular angle is demonstrated superior to the clavicle. The scapula is foreshortened. The patient's upper midcoronal plane and shoulder were leaning toward the IR.

Correction. Position the patient with the shoulders on the same transverse plane and tilt the upper midcoronal plane away from the IR until the midcoronal plane is vertical.

SHOULDER: ANTEROPOSTERIOR AXIAL PROJECTION (STRYKER "NOTCH" METHOD)

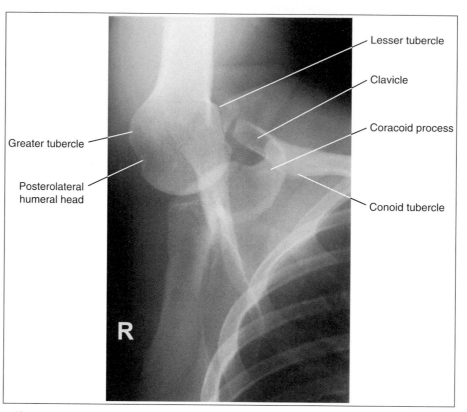

Lesser tubercle

Clavicle

Coracoid process

Greater tubercle

Posterolateral humeral head

Conoid tubercle

R

Figure 4-18. Anteroposterior axial (Stryker) shoulder image with accurate positioning.

Image Analysis

The patient's shoulder is in an AP projection. The coracoid process is situated directly lateral to the conoid tubercle of the clavicle.

- An AP projection of the patient's shoulder is obtained by placing the patient in a supine position with the shoulders at equal distances from the imaging table (Figure 4-19).
- *Detecting rotation:* Rotation on a Stryker notch image is detected by evaluating the relationship of the coracoid process with the conoid tubercle (an eminence on the inferior surface of the clavicle to which the conoid ligament is attached). The coracoid process is situated just lateral to the conoid tubercle on a nonrotated image. If the patient is rotated away from the affected shoulder, the coracoid process is situated medial to this position, and if the patient is rotated toward the affected shoulder, the coracoid process is situated lateral to this position.

The posterolateral aspect of the humeral head is demonstrated in profile laterally, and the greater and lesser tubercles are demonstrated in partial profile.

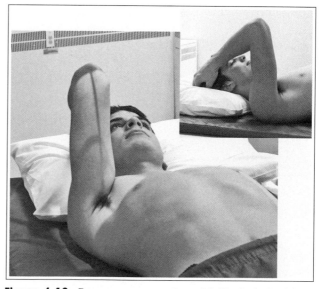

Figure 4-19. Proper anteroposterior axial (Stryker) shoulder image positioning.

The coracoid process is superimposed over the lateral clavicle.

- *Accurate Stryker notch positioning:* The Stryker notch image is obtained to diagnose Hill-Sachs defect of the shoulder. The Hill-Sachs defect is a posterolateral notch defect in the humeral head that is created by impingement of the articular surface of the humeral head against the anteroinferior rim of the glenoid cavity. The Stryker notch image of the shoulder is obtained by placing the patient supine on the imaging table in an AP projection with the affected arm elevated until the humerus is vertical (90-degree angle with torso). The elbow is then flexed, and the palm of the hand is placed on the top of the patient's head. The central ray is then angled 10 degrees cephalad.

- *Poor humeral positioning and central ray angulation:* Accurate humeral positioning with the 10 degrees of cephalic central ray angulation places the posterolateral aspect of the humeral head in profile laterally and demonstrates the greater and lesser tubercles in partial profile. Poor humeral positioning and central ray angulation result in the posterolateral aspect of the humeral head being obscured. Distinguish poor humeral positioning from poor central ray angulation by evaluating the coracoid process and lateral clavicle relationship. When the central ray is angled 10 degrees cephalad the coracoid process is superimposed over the lateral clavicle. If less than a 10-degree cephalad angle is used, the coracoid process will be demonstrated inferior to the clavicle and the humeral shaft will demonstrate increased foreshortening (see Image 29). If more than a 10-degree cephalad angle is used, the coracoid process will be demonstrated superior to the clavicle and the humeral shaft will demonstrate decreased foreshortening.

- *Humeral abduction and posterolateral humeral head visualization:* When the central ray is angled accurately but the humerus is inadequately abducted, the coracoid process is superimposed over the lateral clavicle and the posterolateral aspect of the humeral head will be obscured. If the humerus is elevated beyond vertical, the humeral shaft will be demonstrated with decreased foreshortening (see Image 30) and the humeral head will be demonstrated more on end. If the humerus is elevated to a position less than vertical, the humeral shaft will demonstrate increased foreshortening and a decrease in density (see Image 31).

- *Distal humeral tilting and posterolateral humeral head visibility:* Visibility of the posterolateral aspect of the humeral head is also dependent on the degree of medial and lateral tilt of the distal humerus. When the humerus is positioned vertically and parallel with the midsagittal plane, the posterolateral humeral head is demonstrated. If the distal humerus is allowed to tilt laterally, the humerus is rotated, the lesser tubercle appears in profile medially, and the greater tubercle and posterolateral humeral head are obscured (see Image 30). If the distal humerus is allowed to tilt medially, the lesser tubercle is obscured and the greater tubercle is demonstrated in profile laterally (see Image 32).

The coracoid process is centered within the collimated field. The humeral head, coracoid process, lateral clavicle, and glenoid cavity are included within the field.

- Center a 10-degree cephalic central ray to the coracoid process to place it at the center of the collimated field. The coracoid process can be palpated ¾ inch (2 cm) inferior to the midpoint of the lateral half of the clavicle and medial to the humeral head. Even on very muscular patients the concave pocket formed inferior to the lateral half of the clavicle and medial to the humeral head can be used to center the central ray. The coracoid process should be palpated before the arm is elevated.

- Center the IR to the central ray, open the longitudinal collimated field enough to include the shoulder, and transversely collimate to within ½ inch (1.25 cm) of the lateral humeral skinline.

- An 8- × 10-inch (18- × 24-cm) IR placed lengthwise should be adequate to include all the required anatomical structures.

Anteroposterior Axial (Stryker Notch) Shoulder Image Analysis

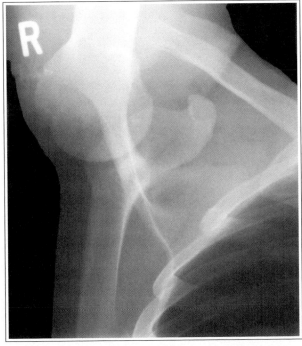

Image 29.

Analysis. The coracoid process appears inferior to the clavicle, and the humeral shaft demonstrates increased foreshortening. The central ray was angled less than the required 10 degrees cephalad.

Correction. Place a 10-degree cephalic angle on the central ray.

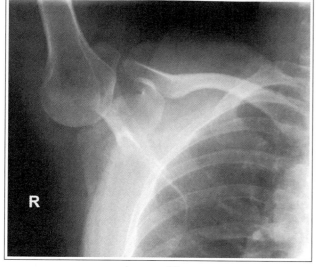

Image 30.

Analysis. The coracoid process is superimposed over the lateral clavicle, and the humeral shaft demonstrates decreased foreshortening. The posterolateral humeral head and greater tubercle are obscured, and the lesser tubercle is demonstrated in profile. The humerus was elevated beyond a vertical position, and the distal humerus was tilted laterally.

Correction. Adduct the humerus until it is in a vertical position, and tilt the distal humerus medially until the humerus is aligned parallel with the midsagittal plane.

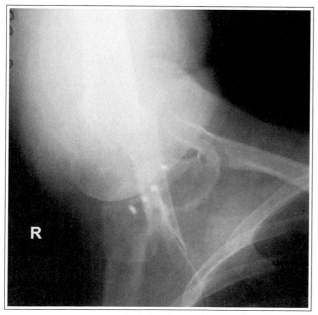

Image 31.

Analysis. The posterolateral humeral head is obscured, and the humeral shaft demonstrates increased foreshortening and a decrease in density. The humerus was elevated less than vertically.

Correction. Elevate the humerus until it is placed at a 90-degree position with the patient's torso.

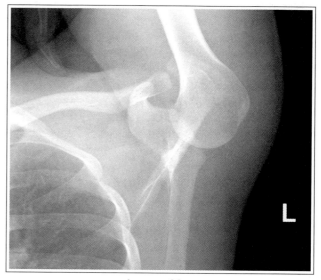

Image 32.

Analysis. The posterolateral humeral head and lesser tubercle are obscured. The greater tubercle is in profile laterally. The distal humerus was tilted medially.

Correction. Tilt the distal humerus laterally until it is parallel with the midsagittal plane.

SHOULDER: TANGENTIAL PROJECTION (SUPRASPINATUS "OUTLET")

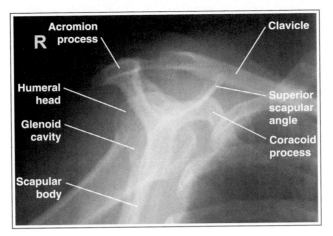

Figure 4-20. Tangential (outlet) shoulder image with accurate positioning.

Image Analysis

The lateral and vertebral scapular borders are superimposed, demonstrating a lateral scapula. The scapular body and acromion and coracoid processes form a Y, with the scapular body as the leg and the acromion and coracoid processes as the arms. The glenoid cavity is demonstrated on end at the converging point of the arms and leg of the Y.

- To place the scapular body in a lateral position, begin by placing the patient in an upright PA projection, with the affected arm abducted slightly or hanging freely. The arm position aligns the vertebral border of the scapula parallel with the IR when the scapula is in a lateral position, allowing the coracoid and acromion processes to be demonstrated in profile. From this PA projection, rotate the patient's body toward the affected scapula until the midcoronal plane is approximately 45 degrees for the nonabducted arm position (Figure 4-21) and 60 degrees for the abducted arm position or until the lateral and vertebral scapular borders are superimposed (Figure 4-22). Also see Figure 4-20.
- **Amount of body obliquity required:** The degree of body obliquity required to obtain a lateral scapula varies with the degree of arm abducted. When the tangential outlet image is obtained with the patient's arm abducted (see Figure 4-22), the shoulder is retracted (drawn backward) as the patient is rotated because the humerus does not rotate with the body. This shoulder retraction causes the scapula to glide around the thoracic cavity, moving toward the spinal column. When the scapula is in this posterior position, the patient's body needs to be rotated more to bring the scapular body lateral. When the patient's arm is allowed to hang freely for the image, the shoulder is not retracted, resulting in the scapular body being positioned more anteriorly and therefore

requiring less obliquity to bring it into a lateral position (see Figure 4-21).

- **Using scapular palpation to determine accurate degree of body obliquity:** The proper degree of body rotation for any arm position is determined by palpating the lateral and vertebral scapular borders. Because the superior portions of the lateral and vertebral borders are heavily covered with muscles, it is best to palpate them just superior to the inferior scapular angle. Once these anatomical structures are located, rotate the patient's body until the vertebral border of the scapula is superimposed over the lateral border and the inferior scapular angle is positioned in profile.
- **Detecting mispositioning:** If the patient obliquity is not accurate for the tangential outlet image, the Y formation of the scapula is not attained, the medial and lateral

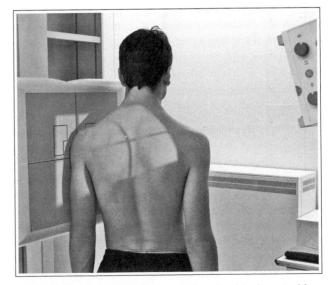

Figure 4-21. Proper tangential (outlet) shoulder image with arm dangling (nonabducted).

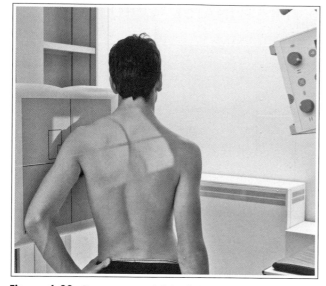

Figure 4-22. Proper tangential (outlet) shoulder image with arm abducted.

borders of the scapular body are not superimposed but are demonstrated next to each other, and the glenoid cavity is not demonstrated on end.

- To determine whether patient obliquity needs to be increased or decreased to superimpose the scapular body and position the glenoid cavity on end, identify the borders of the scapula. The lateral border is thick, with two cortical outlines that are separated by approximately ¼ inch (0.6 cm), whereas the cortical outline of the vertebral border demonstrates a single thin line. If the vertebral border is demonstrated next to the ribs and the lateral border is visible laterally, patient obliquity was insufficient to superimpose the borders (see Image 33). If the lateral border is demonstrated next to the ribs and the vertebral border is visible laterally, patient obliquity was excessive (see Image 34).

The lateral clavicle and acromion process are demonstrated approximately ½ inch (1.25 cm) superior to the humeral head and supraspinous fossa, and the superior scapular angle is at the level of the inferior aspect of the clavicle.

- The tangential outlet image is taken to identify osteophyte formation on the inferior surfaces of the lateral clavicle and acromion process angle. For these inferior surfaces to best be visualized, the central ray must transverse the area at a 10- to 15-degree angle. This alignment is accomplished by positioning the midcoronal plane vertically and angling the central ray 10 to 15 degrees caudally and is demonstrated on a tangential outlet image when the lateral clavicle and acromion process are visible approximately ½ inch (1.25 cm) superior to the humeral head and supraspinous fossa and when the superior scapular angle is shown at the same level as the inferior clavicle.

- If the tangential outlet image is taken without the 10- to 15-degree angle or with the patient's upper midcoronal plane tilted toward the IR, the lateral clavicle and acromion process will be demonstrated less than ½ inch (1.25 cm) superior to the humeral head and supraspinous fossa, and the superior scapular spine will be visible superior to the clavicle (see Image 35).

The AC joint is at the center of the collimated field. The acromion process, lateral clavicle, superior scapular spine, coracoid process, and half of the scapular body should be included within the field.

- To place the AC joint in the center of the collimated field, center the central ray to the superior aspect of the humeral head.
- Center the IR to the central ray, and open the longitudinal collimation enough to include the acromion process and lateral clavicle. Transverse collimate to within ½ inch (1.25 cm) of the lateral humeral skinline.
- An 8- × 10-inch (18- × 24-cm) IR placed lengthwise should be adequate to include all the required anatomical structures.

Tangential (Outlet) Image Analysis

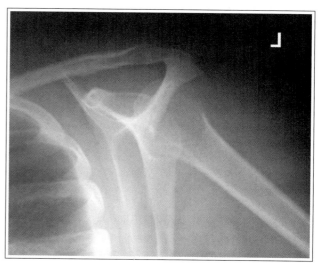

Image 33.

Analysis. The lateral and vertebral borders of the scapula are demonstrated without superimposition, and the glenoid cavity is not demonstrated on end but is demonstrated laterally. The vertebral scapular border is demonstrated next to the ribs, whereas the lateral border is demonstrated laterally. The patient was not rotated enough to superimpose the scapular body. The lateral clavicle and acromion process is demonstrated less than ½ inch (1.25 cm) superior to the humeral head and supraspinous fossa, and the superior scapular spine is visible superior to the clavicle. The upper midcoronal plane was tilted toward the IR, and/or the central ray was not angled 10 to 15 degrees caudally.

Correction. Increase the patient obliquity, position the midcoronal plane vertically, and place a 10- to 15-degree caudal angle on the central ray.

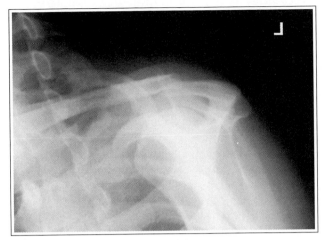

Image 34.

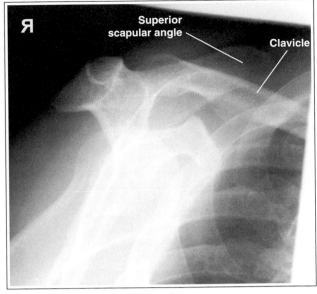

Image 35.

Analysis. The lateral and vertebral borders of the scapula are demonstrated without superimposition, and the glenoid cavity is not demonstrated on end but appears medially. The lateral scapular border is demonstrated next to the ribs, and the vertebral border is demonstrated laterally. The patient was rotated more than necessary to superimpose the borders of the scapular body.

Correction. Decrease the patient obliquity.

Analysis. The lateral clavicle and acromion process are demonstrated less than ½ inch (1.25 cm) superior to the humeral head and supraspinous fossa, and the superior scapular spine is demonstrated superior to the clavicle. The upper midcoronal plane was tilted toward the IR, and/or the central ray was not angled 10 to 15 degrees caudally.

Correction. Position the midcoronal plane vertically, and place a 10- to 15-degree caudal angle on the central ray.

CLAVICLE: ANTEROPOSTERIOR PROJECTION

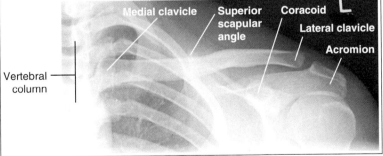

Figure 4-23. Anteroposterior clavicular image with accurate positioning.

Image Analysis

The clavicle is demonstrated in an AP projection without longitudinal foreshortening. The medial clavicular end lies next to the lateral edge of the vertebral column.

- An AP projection of the clavicle is obtained by placing the patient in either a supine or upright position with

the shoulders at equal distances from the imaging table or upright IR holder (Figure 4-24).

- *Positioning for kyphosis:* The kyphotic patient will have less discomfort if the image is taken with the patient in an upright position. If it is not possible to place the kyphotic patient in an upright position, use angled sponges under the shoulders and thorax to place

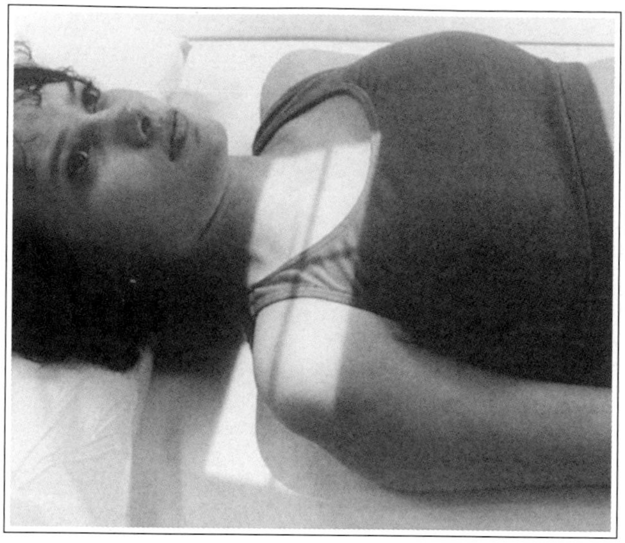

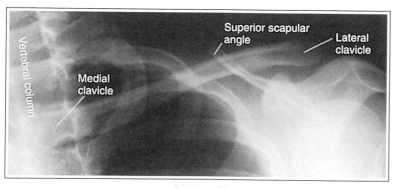

Figure 4-24. Proper anteroposterior clavicular positioning.

the shoulders at equal distances from the imaging table. An imaging table sponge also helps with patient comfort.

- *Detecting clavicular rotation:* Rotation and therefore longitudinal foreshortening on an AP clavicle image is detected by evaluating the relationships of the medial clavicular end with the vertebral column. If the patient is rotated away from the affected clavicle, the medial end of the clavicle is superimposed over the vertebral column (see Image 36). If the patient is rotated toward the affected clavicle, the medial end of the clavicle draws away from the vertebral column and the clavicle is longitudinally foreshortened (see Image 37).
- Although a PA projection would position the clavicle closer to the IR, resulting in less magnification and greater image detail, the AP projection is the more

commonly performed because it causes less patient discomfort during positioning and allows the clavicle to be easily palpated.

The clavicle is demonstrated without inferosuperior foreshortening. The midclavicle is superimposed on the superior scapular angle.

- Inferosuperior foreshortening of the clavicle results when the patient's upper midcoronal plane is allowed to tilt anteriorly or posteriorly. This tilting can often be avoided by instructing the patient to arch the upper thorax and shoulders backward, straightening the vertebral column.
- *Detecting inferosuperior foreshortening:* Inferosuperior foreshortening of the clavicle is demonstrated when the superior scapular angle is visible superiorly or inferiorly to the midclavicle. If the upper midcoronal plane is tilted anteriorly (forward), the superior scapular angle will be demonstrated superior to the midclavicle (see Image 38). If the upper midcoronal plane is tilted posteriorly (backward), the superior scapular angle is shown inferior to the midclavicle (see Image 39).

The midclavicle is at the center of the collimated field. The entire clavicle and the acromion process are included within the field.

- The midclavicle is located by palpating the medial and lateral ends of the clavicle and centering the central ray halfway between them.
- Center the IR to the central ray and open the longitudinal and transverse collimation enough to include all aspects of the medial and lateral clavicular ends.
- A 10- × 12-inch (24- × 30-cm) IR placed crosswise should be adequate to include all the required anatomical structures.

Anteroposterior Clavicle Image Analysis

Superior scapular angle

Lateral clavicle

Medial clavicle

Vertebral column

Image 36.

Analysis. The medial end of the clavicle is superimposed over the vertebral column. The patient was rotated away from the affected clavicle for this image.

Correction. Place the patient in an AP projection by rotating the patient toward the affected clavicle. The shoulders should be placed at equal distances from the IR.

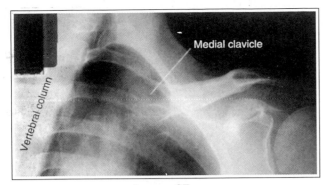

Image 37.

Analysis. The medial end of the clavicle is drawn away from the vertebral column, and the clavicle is longitudinally foreshortened. The patient was rotated toward the affected shoulder for this image.

Correction. Place the patient in an AP projection by rotating the patient away from the affected clavicle. The shoulders should be placed at equal distances from the IR.

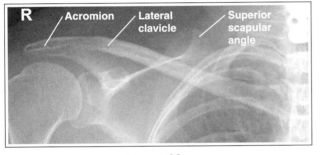

Image 38.

Analysis. The superior scapular angle is projected superior to the midclavicle. The clavicle has been inferosuperiorly foreshortened. The upper midcoronal plane was tilted anteriorly.

Correction. Instruct the patient to arch the upper thorax and shoulders backward, straightening the upper vertebral column and midcoronal plane.

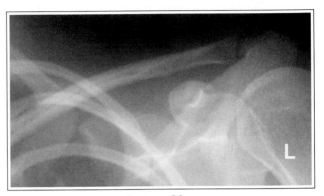

Image 39.

Analysis. The superior scapular angle is projected inferiorly to the midclavicle. The clavicle has been transversely foreshortened. The upper midcoronal plane was tilted posteriorly. The medial end of the clavicle is not included on the image. The central ray was positioned too laterally.

Correction. Instruct the patient to arch the upper thorax and shoulders forward, straightening the upper vertebral column and midcoronal plane. Center the central ray approximately 1 inch (2.5 cm) medially, and open collimation enough to include the medial end of the clavicle.

CLAVICLE: ANTEROPOSTERIOR AXIAL POSITION

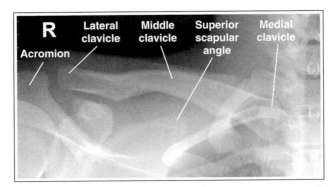

Figure 4-25. Anteroposterior axial clavicular image with accurate positioning.

Image Analysis

The clavicle is demonstrated in an AP axial projection without body rotation. The medial end of the clavicle lies next to the lateral edge of the vertebral column.

- An AP axial projection of the clavicle is accomplished by placing the patient in either a supine or upright position with shoulders positioned at equal distances from the imaging table or upright IR holder (Figure 4-26).
- *Detecting clavicular rotation:* Rotation on an AP axial clavicle image is detected by evaluating the relationships of the medial clavicular end with the vertebral column. If the patient is rotated away from the affected clavicle, the medial end of the clavicle is superimposed over the vertebral column. If the patient is rotated toward the affected clavicle, the medial end of the clavicle is drawn away from the vertebral column and the clavicle is longitudinally foreshortened. (See Images 36 and 37; rotation on the AP and AP axial clavicle images are similar, but the clavicle on the AP axial image would be situated more superiorly on the thorax.)

The medial end of the clavicle is superimposed over the first, second, or third rib; the middle and lateral thirds of the clavicle are demonstrated superior to the acromion process; and the clavicle bows slightly upward.

- A 15- to 30-degree cephalic angle is used on the axial projection of the clavicle to project more of the clavicle superior to the thorax region and to demonstrate the degree of fracture displacement when present. Even though the amount of angulation used may vary among radiology departments, all images result in superior projection of the clavicle. The larger the angle, the more superiorly the clavicle is projected. Ideally, because 80% of clavicle fractures occur at the middle

third and 15% at the lateral third, the central ray should be angled enough to project the lateral and middle thirds of the clavicle superior to the thorax and scapula.

- Compare Images 40 and 41, and note how an increase in cephalic angulation has projected the lateral and middle thirds of the clavicle above the scapula. The clavicle fracture demonstrated on these images is quite obvious, but a subtle nondisplaced fracture could be obscured by the scapular structures if an AP axial projection were not included in the exam.

The midclavicle is at the center of the collimated field. The entire clavicle and the acromion process are included within the field.

- The midclavicle is located by palpating the lateral and medial ends of the clavicle and centering the central ray halfway between the ends.
- Center the IR to the central ray and open the longitudinal and transverse collimation enough to include all aspects of the lateral and medial clavicular ends.
- An 8- × 10-inch (18- × 24-cm) or 10- × 12-inch (24- × 30-cm) IR placed crosswise should be adequate to include all the required anatomical structures.

Axial Clavicle Image Analysis

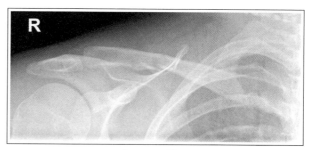

Image 40.

Analysis. The lateral and middle thirds of the clavicle are superimposed by the scapula. The cephalic central ray angulation was not adequate to project the lateral and middle thirds of the clavicle superior to the scapula. A midclavicular fracture is present.

Correction. Increase the cephalic central ray angulation enough to project the clavicle above the scapula.

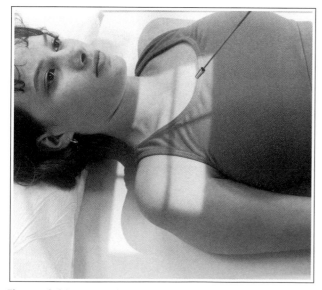

Figure 4-26. Proper anteroposterior axial clavicular positioning.

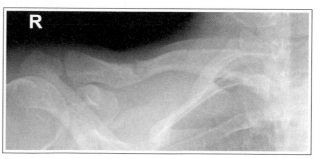

Image 41.

Analysis. The lateral and middle thirds of the clavicle are projected above the scapula. A nondisplaced fracture of the middle third of the clavicle is evident.

Correction. No corrective movement is necessary.

ACROMIOCLAVICULAR JOINT: ANTEROPOSTERIOR PROJECTION

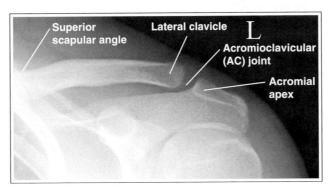

Figure 4-27. Anteroposterior acromioclavicular joint image (without weights) with accurate positioning.

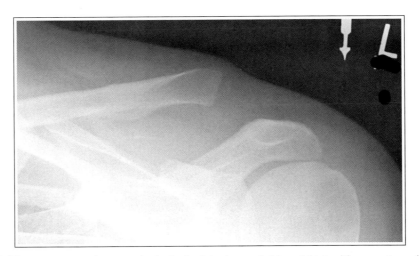

Figure 4-28. Anteroposterior acromioclavicular joint image (with weights) with accurate positioning.

Image Analysis

The weight-bearing image displays a word or arrow marker, pointing downward, to indicate that it is the weight-bearing image.

The lateral clavicle and acromion process are demonstrated in an AP projection. The lateral clavicle is nearly horizontal, and approximately ⅛ inch (0.3 cm) of space is present between the lateral clavicle and the acromial apex.

- An AP projection of the AC joint is obtained by placing the patient in an upright position with both shoulders

positioned at equal distances from the upright IR holder (Figure 4-29).

- *Weight-bearing AC joint images:* To evaluate the AC joint for possible injury to the AC ligament, which extends between the lateral clavicular end and the acromion process, the AP projection should be taken first without weights. Then a second AP projection should be taken with the patient holding 5- to 8-lb weights (Figure 4-30). If injury to the AC ligament has occurred, the AC joint space is wider on the weight-bearing image than on the image taken without weights.

- For the weight-bearing image, equal weights should be attached to the arms regardless of whether the examination

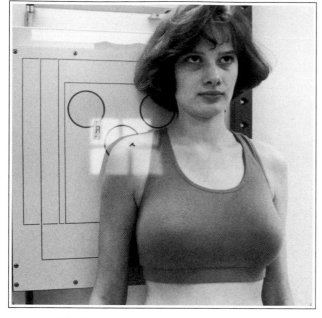

Figure 4-29. Proper anteroposterior acromioclavicular joint positioning (without weights).

is unilateral (one side) or bilateral (both sides), keeping the shoulders on the same transverse plane. Attach the weights to the patient's wrists or slide them onto the patient's forearms after the elbows are flexed to 90 degrees, and instruct the patient to allow the weights to depress the shoulders.

- *Detecting rotation:* Rotation on an anteroposterior AC joint image is detected by evaluating the relationships of the lateral clavicle with the acromion apex and of the

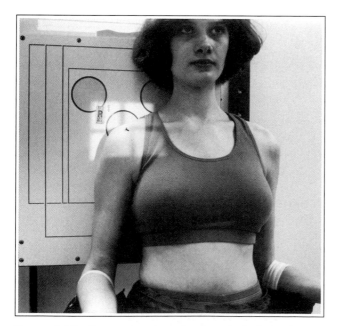

Figure 4-30. Proper anteroposterior acromioclavicular joint positioning (with weights).

scapular body with the thoracic cavity. If the patient was rotated toward the affected AC joint, the lateral end of the clavicle and the acromion apex are rotated out of profile, resulting in a narrowed or closed AC joint. The thoracic cavity also moves toward the scapular body, increasing the amount of scapular body superimposition (see Image 42, right shoulder). If the patient is rotated away from the affected AC joint, the lateral end of the clavicle and the acromion apex demonstrate a slightly greater AC joint space with only a small amount of rotation and may be closed with a greater degree of rotation. The scapular body demonstrates decreased thoracic cavity superimposition (see Image 42, left shoulder).

The lateral clavicle demonstrates minimal acromion process superimposition, and the midclavicle is superimposed over the scapular spine. The lateral clavicle and acromion process are demonstrated without transverse foreshortening.

- Inferosuperior foreshortening of the clavicle and acromion process results when the patient's upper midcoronal plane is allowed to tilt anteriorly or posteriorly. This tilting can often be avoided by instructing the patient to arch the upper thorax and shoulders backward, straightening the vertebral column.

- *Detecting inferosuperior foreshortening:* Inferosuperior foreshortening of the clavicle and acromion process is demonstrated when the lateral clavicle demonstrates greater or less than minimal superimposition of the acromion process and the superior scapular angle appears superiorly or inferiorly to the midclavicle. If the upper midcoronal plane is tilted anteriorly (forward), the lateral clavicle will demonstrate increased acromion process superimposition and the superior scapular angle will be demonstrated superior to the midclavicle (see Image 43). If the upper midcoronal plane is tilted posteriorly (backward), the lateral clavicle will demonstrate decreased acromion process superimposition and the superior scapular angle will be visible inferior to the midclavicle (see Image 44).

- *Positioning for kyphosis:* For the kyphotic patient little can be done to improve patient positioning, but a cephalic central ray angulation can be used to offset the forward angle of the scapula. The central ray should be angled enough to align it perpendicular to the scapular body.

The AC joint of interest is at the center of the collimated field, and the lateral clavicle and acromion process are included within the field.

- *Unilateral AC joint images:* Center a perpendicular central ray to the AC joint of interest. The AC joint is located by palpating along the clavicle until the most lateral tip is reached, then moving approximately ½ inch (1 cm) inferiorly. Center the IR to the central ray, and open the longitudinally and transversely collimated

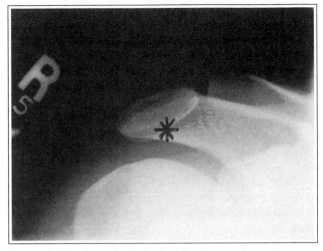

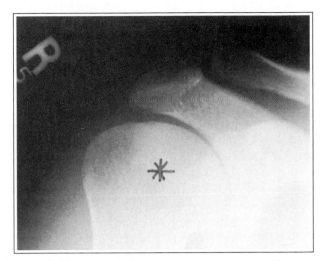

Figure 4-31. Acromioclavicular joint image taken without weights and showing good centering. Star indicates location of central ray.

Figure 4-32. Acromioclavicular joint image taken with weights and showing poor centering. Star indicates location of central ray.

field to approximately a 4-inch (10-cm) field size. An 8- × 10-inch (18- × 24-cm) IR placed crosswise should be adequate to include all the anatomical structures.

- **Bilateral AC joint image:** Center a perpendicular central ray to the midsagittal plane at a level 1 inch (2.5 cm) superior to the jugular notch. Center the IR to the central ray, and open the longitudinally collimated field to approximately a 4-inch (10-cm) field size. Transverse collimate should be left open the full IR length. A 14- × 17-inch (35- × 43-cm) or 7- × 17-inch (14- × 43-cm) IR placed crosswise should be adequate to include both AC joints. This method is not recommended, because it unnecessarily exposes the thyroid and uses diverged x-rays to record the AC joints.
- **Alternate central ray:** An AP axial projection of the AC joint is taken with a 15-degree cephalic central ray

angle centered at the level of the AC joint. This projection demonstrates the AC joint superior to the acromion process.

- **Ensuring identical central ray alignment with and without weights:** Repalpate for the AC joint to ensure that the same centering is obtained when the patient is given weights. Because the shoulders are depressed when weights are used, the AC joint moves inferiorly. If the central ray is not centered the same for both images, x-ray beam divergence may result in a false reading. Compare Figures 4-31 and 4-32, images of the same patient, taken without weights and with weights, respectively. Because the central ray was not centered in the same location it is uncertain whether the separation demonstrated on the weight-bearing image is a result of ligament injury or poor central ray centering.

Acromioclavicular Joint Image Analysis

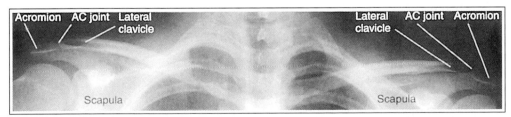

Image 42.

Analysis. This image was taken with the central ray centered on the vertebral column to position both AC joints on one receptor. This method is not recommended, because it unnecessarily exposes the thyroid and uses diverged x-rays to record the AC joints. When bilateral AC joint images are

ordered, each AC joint should be imaged separately, as described previously. The right AC joint is closed, and the right scapular body demonstrates greater thoracic superimposition than the left; the left AC joint is open. The patient was rotated toward the right shoulder.

Correction. Take the image of each AC joint on a separate receptor. Rotate the patient toward the left shoulder until the shoulders are at equal distances from the IR.

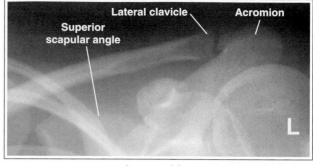

Image 44.

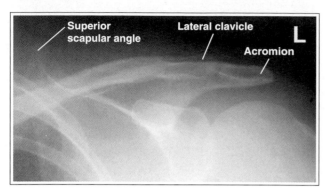

Image 43.

Analysis. The lateral end of the clavicle is completely superimposed on the acromion process, and the superior scapular angle appears superior to the midclavicle. The upper midcoronal plane was tilted anteriorly, transversely foreshortening the clavicle and acromion process.

Correction. Instruct the patient to arch the upper thorax and shoulders backward, straightening the upper vertebral column and midcoronal plane.

Analysis. The acromion process is demonstrated without clavicular superimposition, and the superior scapular angle appears inferior to the midclavicle. The upper midcoronal plane was tilted posteriorly, inferosuperiorly foreshortening the clavicle and acromion process.

Correction. Instruct the patient to arch the upper thorax and shoulders forward, straightening the upper vertebral column and midcoronal plane.

SCAPULA: ANTEROPOSTERIOR PROJECTION

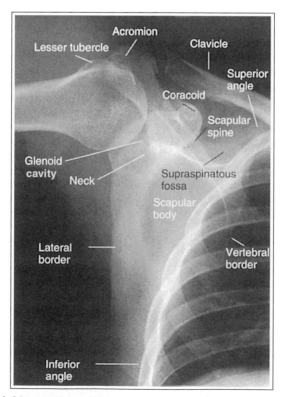

Figure 4-33. Anteroposterior scapular image with accurate positioning.

Image Analysis

Density is uniform across the scapular body.

- *Image density of shoulder girdle and thoracic cavity:* Although the anteroposterior thickness is approximately the same across the entire scapula, the overall image density is not uniform. On AP scapular images the medial portion of the scapula, which is superimposed by the thoracic cavity, demonstrates darker density than the lateral scapula, which is superimposed by the soft tissue of the shoulder girdle. This image density difference is a result of the difference in density (number of atoms per given area) that exists between the thoracic cavity and the shoulder soft tissue.

- The thoracic cavity is largely composed of air, which contains very few atoms in a given area, whereas the same area of soft tissue contains many compacted atoms. As the radiation goes through the patient's body, fewer photons are absorbed in the thoracic cavity than in the shoulder girdle, because fewer atoms with which the photons can interact are present in the thoracic cavity. Consequently, more photons penetrate the thoracic cavity to expose the IR than penetrate the shoulder girdle.

- Taking the exposure on expiration can help to decrease the image density of the portion of the scapula that is superimposed by the thoracic cavity by reducing the air and slightly compressing the tissue in this area. If the AP scapular image is taken on inspiration, the medial scapular body demonstrates increased density (see Image 45).

The bony trabecular patterns and cortical outlines of the scapula are sharply defined.

- Patient respiration also determines how well the scapular details are demonstrated. Some positioning textbooks suggest that a breathing technique be used to better visualize the vertebral border and medial scapular body through the air-filled lungs. Although visualization of this anatomy would be improved with such a technique, it is difficult to obtain a long enough exposure time (3 seconds) to adequately blur the ribs and vascular lung markings when the overall exposure (mAs) necessary for an AP scapula image is so small. If an adequate exposure time cannot be set to use breathing technique, the exposure should be taken on expiration.

The scapula is demonstrated in an AP projection without transverse foreshortening. The anterior and posterior margins of the glenoid cavity are nearly superimposed.

- When the patient's body is positioned in a true AP projection with the arms against the sides, the scapular body is placed at a 35- to 45-degree angle with the IR, with the lateral scapula situated more anteriorly than the medial scapula. This positioning results in transverse foreshortening of the scapular body.

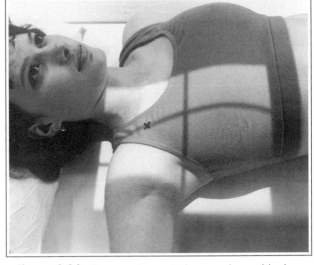

Figure 4-34. Proper anteroposterior scapular positioning.

- *Positioning for an AP scapular projection:* An AP scapular image is obtained by abducting the humerus, then supinating the hand and flexing the elbow to externally rotate the arm (Figure 4-34). Each of these arm movements, with the sternoclavicular and AC joints, works to retract the shoulder (force it backward). Humeral abduction causes the scapula to glide around the thoracic surface, moving the scapula laterally, and shoulder retraction reduces transverse scapular foreshortening as it forces the lateral aspect of the scapula posteriorly. This movement of the scapula places it very close to an AP projection. To take advantage of gravity and obtain maximum shoulder retraction, take the image with the patient in a supine position.

- *Detecting poor shoulder retraction:* Poor retraction of the scapula can be identified by evaluating the image of the scapular body and glenoid cavity. If the patient's arm is not sufficiently externally rotated and abducted, and the shoulder sufficiently retracted, the transverse scapular body is foreshortened, and the glenoid cavity is demonstrated somewhat on end (see Image 46).

The scapula is demonstrated in an AP projection without longitudinal foreshortening. The superior scapular angle is approximately $1/4$ inch (0.6 cm) inferior to the clavicle.

- Longitudinal foreshortening of the scapular body is caused by poor midcoronal plane positioning and could result when the AP scapular image is taken with the patient in the upright position or when the patient is kyphotic. To prevent such foreshortening, position the patient's midcoronal plane vertically when the patient is upright. A longitudinally foreshortened scapula can be identified on a scapular image that has the arm adequately abducted when the superior scapular angle is more or less than $1/4$ inch (0.6 cm) inferior to the clavicle. When the superior scapular angle is demonstrated less than $\frac{1}{4}$ inch (0.6 cm) from the clavicle, the upper mid-coronal plane was tilted anteriorly. When the superior scapular angle appears more than $\frac{1}{4}$ inch (0.6 cm) inferior to the clavicle, the upper midcoronal plane was tilted posteriorly.

- *Angulation for kyphosis:* Longitudinal foreshortening of the scapular body on the kyphotic patient cannot be improved with patient positioning, but a cephalic central ray angulation can be used to offset the forward angle of the scapula. Angle the central ray to align it perpendicular to the scapular body.

The lateral border of the scapula is demonstrated without thoracic cavity superimposition, and the supraspinatous fossa and the superior angle of the scapula are demonstrated without superimposition of the clavicle. The thoracic cavity is superimposed over the vertebral border of the scapula. The humeral shaft demonstrates at least 90 degrees of abduction.

- Demonstrating the lateral portion of the scapula with adequate density often causes the medial scapula, which is superimposed by the thoracic cavity, to demonstrate excessive density. To increase the proportion of scapular body demonstrated without thoracic cavity superimposition, the humerus is abducted.
- *Effect of humeral abduction:* Abduction of the humerus is accomplished by combined movements of the shoulder joint and rotation of the scapula around the thoracic cage. The ratio of movement in these two articulations is two parts glenohumeral to one part scapulothoracic. When the arm is abducted, the lateral scapula is drawn from beneath the thoracic cavity and the glenoid cavity moves superiorly. Because the first 60 degrees of humeral abduction involves primarily movement of the glenohumeral joint without accompanying scapular movement, it takes at least 90 degrees of humeral abduction to demonstrate the lateral border of the scapula without thoracic cavity superimposition, and the supraspinatous fossa and superior angle without clavicle superimposition. The farther the arm is abducted, the more of the lateral scapular body is demonstrated without thoracic cavity superimposition. With 0 to 60 degrees of humeral abduction, the inferolateral border of the scapula is superimposed by the thoracic cavity and the clavicle is superimposed over the supraspinatous fossa and superior scapular angle. Image 45 demonstrates an image taken with 60 degrees of abduction, and Image 47 was taken without humeral abduction.
- *Positioning for trauma:* Trauma patients often experience great pain with arm abduction. Because of this pain, the abduction movement may take place almost entirely at the glenohumeral articulation, instead of involving the combined movements of the glenohumeral and scapulothoracic articulations. When the scapulothoracic articulation is not involved with the movement of humeral abduction, the inferolateral border and inferior angle of the scapula remain superimposed by the thoracic cavity, and the supraspinatous fossa and superior border remain superimposed by the clavicle. In this situation little can be done to draw the scapula away from the thoracic cavity, although the exposure can be taken on expiration and a technique used that better demonstrates the parts of the scapula superimposed by the thorax. An AP scapular body image can be obtained in a trauma situation by using the posterior oblique (Grashey) shoulder position as discussed earlier in this chapter (p. 227). In this position the patient is rotated toward the affected shoulder, bringing the scapula AP. The central ray should be centered 2 inches (5 cm) inferior to the coracoid process, and the kVp and exposure reduced to prevent the dark density caused by the air-filled lungs.

The midscapular body is at the center of the collimated field. The entire scapula, consisting of the inferior and superior angles, the coracoid and acromion processes, and glenoid cavity, is included within the field.

- To ensure that the entire scapula, from the coracoid process to the inferior angle, is included on the image, center a perpendicular central ray approximately 2 inches (5 cm) inferior to the palpable coracoid process. The coracoid process can be palpated $\frac{3}{4}$ inch (2 cm) inferior to the midpoint of the lateral half of the clavicle and medial to the humeral head. Even for very muscular patients the concave pocket formed inferior to the lateral half of the clavicle and the medial humeral head can be used to center the central ray. The coracoid process should be palpated before the arm is abducted. This positioning accurately aligns the longitudinal and transverse aspects of the scapula. If the arm cannot be adequately abducted, the transverse centering should be $\frac{1}{2}$ inch (1 cm) more medial.
- Center the IR to the central ray, and open the longitudinal collimation to the top shoulder skinline. Transversely collimate to within $\frac{1}{2}$ inch (1.25 cm) of the lateral body skinline.
- A 10- × 12-inch (24- × 30-cm) IR placed lengthwise should be adequate to include all the required anatomical structures.

Anteroposterior Scapular Image Analysis

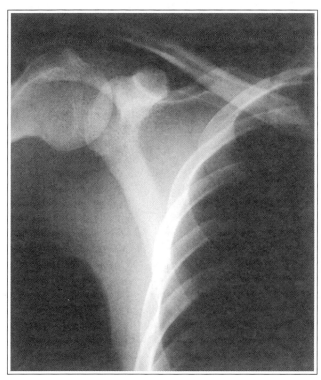

Image 45.

Analysis. The portion of the scapula superimposed by the thoracic cavity demonstrates excessive density. The examination was taken on inspiration. The inferolateral border of the scapula is superimposed by the thoracic cavity, and the superior angle is superimposed by the clavicle. The humeral shaft is inadequately abducted.

Correction. Take the exposure on expiration or use a breathing technique, and abduct the arm to 90 degrees.

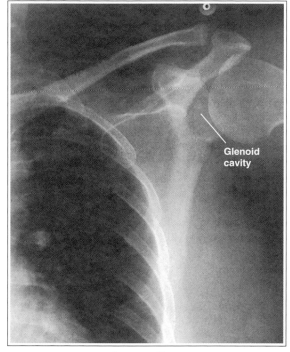

Image 46.

Analysis. The transverse axis of the scapular body is foreshortened, and the articulating surface of the glenoid cavity is demonstrated. This AP scapular image was taken with the patient in an upright position, resulting in insufficient shoulder retraction.

Correction. Place the patient supine to maximize shoulder retraction, or instruct the patient to retract the shoulder toward the IR.

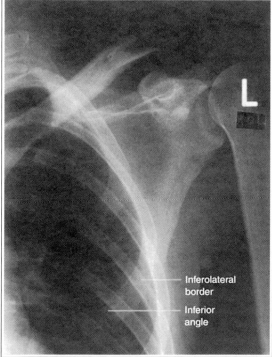

Image 47.

Analysis. The inferolateral border of the scapula is superimposed by the thoracic cavity, and the superior angle is superimposed by the clavicle. The humeral shaft is not abducted 90 degrees with the body.

Correction. Abduct the humerus 90 degrees from the body. This adjustment will draw the inferolateral border of the scapula away from the thoracic cavity and shift the superior angle away from the clavicle.

SCAPULA: LATERAL POSITION (LATEROMEDIAL OR MEDIOLATERAL PROJECTION)

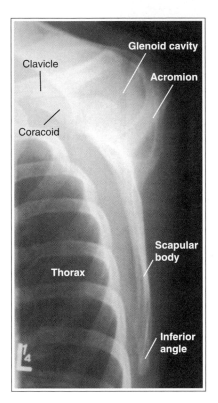

Figure 4-35. Lateral scapular image with accurate positioning.

Image Analysis

The scapular body is in a lateral position. The lateral and vertebral scapular borders are superimposed, and the scapular body is demonstrated without superimposing the thoracic cavity.

- The scapular body is placed in a lateral position by first placing the patient in an upright PA projection with the affected arm drawn across the chest so the hand can grasp the unaffected shoulder. From this position, rotate the patient's body toward the affected scapula until the lateral and vertebral scapular borders are superimposed (Figure 4-36).
- The degree of body obliquity required to superimpose the scapular borders depends on the degree of humeral elevation. As the humerus is elevated, the inferior angle of the scapula glides around the thoracic cage, moving the scapula more anteriorly. The more the scapula glides around the thorax, the less body obliquity is required to superimpose the vertebral and lateral scapular borders.

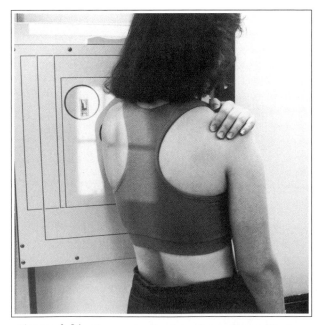

Figure 4-36. Proper standing lateral scapular positioning.

- To position the long axis of the scapular body parallel with the IR and demonstrate it with the least amount of foreshortening, elevate the arm to a 90-degree angle with the body.
- The proper degree of body rotation for any arm position is determined by palpating the lateral and vertebral scapular borders. Because the superior portions of the lateral and vertebral borders are heavily covered with muscles, it is best to palpate them just superior to the inferior scapular angle. Adjusting the arm position slightly while palpating can also help in locating the scapular borders and inferior angle. Once these anatomical structures are located, rotate the patient's body until the vertebral border of the scapula is superimposed over the lateral border and the inferior scapular angle is positioned in profile. Because abduction of the humerus shifts the scapula laterally, the amount of rotation is dependent on the amount of humerus elevation. When the humerus is elevated to 90 degrees, approximately 30 degrees of patient obliquity is necessary. If the arm is elevated less than 90 degrees, the amount of obliquity needs to be increased, and if the arm is elevated more than 90 degrees, the amount is decreased.
- ***Positioning the supine patient:*** For the supine patient a lateral scapula image is obtained by placing the patient in a posterior oblique position. The lateral and vertebral scapular borders and the inferior scapular angle should be palpated using the same method as described for the standing patient; however, the patient is rotated toward the unaffected shoulder to superimpose the vertebral and lateral scapular borders and place the inferior angle in profile (Figure 4-37).
- ***Detecting inaccurate rotation:*** If the body was not accurately rotated for a lateral scapular image, the borders of the scapula are not superimposed but are demonstrated next to each other. When such an image has been produced, one can determine whether patient obliquity was excessive or insufficient by identifying the scapular borders.

The lateral border is thick, being identified by two cortical outlines that are separated by approximately $\frac{1}{4}$ inch (0.6 cm), whereas the cortical outline of the vertebral border is a single thin line. If the lateral border is demonstrated next to the ribs and the vertebral border is demonstrated laterally, the patient has been rotated too much (see Image 48). If the vertebral border is demonstrated next to the ribs and the lateral border is demonstrated laterally, the patient was not rotated enough to superimpose the borders (see Image 49).

The humerus is drawn away from the superior scapular body, and the superior scapular angle is superimposed over the coracoid process base.

- Eighty percent of scapular fractures involve the body or neck of the scapula. The neck of the scapula is best visualized on the AP projection, because it is demonstrated on end in the lateral position. If a fracture of the scapular body is present or suspected, the lateral position should be taken to demonstrate the anteroposterior alignment of the fracture.
- ***Effect of humeral elevation on scapular visualization:*** To best demonstrate the scapular body, position its long axis parallel with the long axis of the IR by elevating the humerus to a 90-degree angle with the patient's body (Figures 4-38 and 4-39). This positioning causes the scapula to glide anteriorly around the thoracic cavity and tilts the glenoid fossa slightly upward, placing the long axis of the scapular body parallel with the IR (see Figure 4-35). The humerus is also drawn away from the superior scapular body, allowing it to be visualized without humeral superimposition.
- If humeral elevation is increased above 90 degrees with the patient still grasping the opposite shoulder, the lateral border of the scapula is placed parallel with the IR

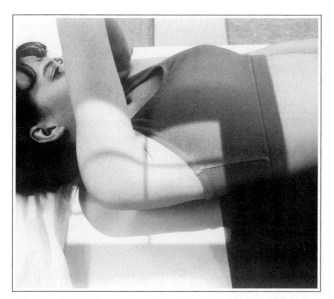

Figure 4-37. Proper recumbent lateral scapular positioning.

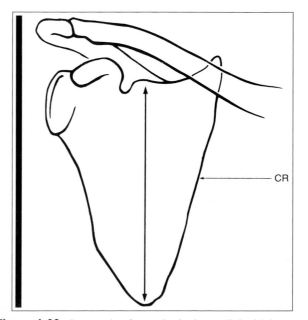

Figure 4-38. Long axis of scapular body parallel with image receptor. *CR*, Central ray.

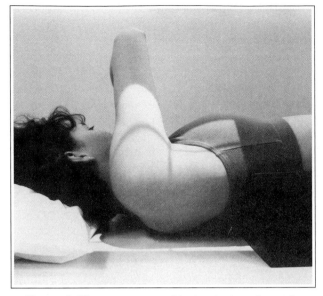

Figure 4-39. Proper arm positioning for lateral scapula.

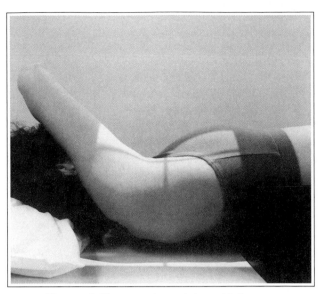

Figure 4-41. Arm elevated above 90 degrees.

(Figures 4-40 and 4-41). This positioning distorts the superior scapular body and demonstrates the superior scapular angle and scapular spine below the coracoid and acromion processes, respectively (see Image 4-50).

- If the humerus is not elevated but rests on the patient's chest with the patient still grasping the opposite shoulder, the vertebral border of the scapula is positioned parallel with the image (Figures 4-42 and 4-43). This arm positioning produces a shoulder image that is similar to that obtained for the scapular Y position: The superior scapular body is superimposed over the glenoid cavity

and the proximal humerus, the coracoid and acromion processes are visible in profile, and the anteroposterior relationship of the humeral head and glenoid cavity is demonstrated (see Image 51).

The midscapular body is at the center of the collimated field. The entire scapula, consisting of the inferior angle and the coracoid and acromion processes, is included within the field.

- To place the midscapular body in the center of the collimated field, center a perpendicular central ray to the midscapular body.

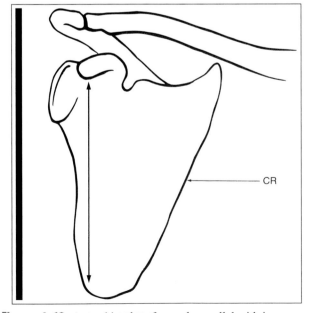

Figure 4-40. Lateral border of scapula parallel with image receptor. *CR*, Central ray.

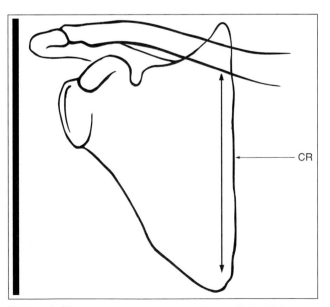

Figure 4-42. Vertebral border of scapula parallel with image receptor. *CR*, Central ray.

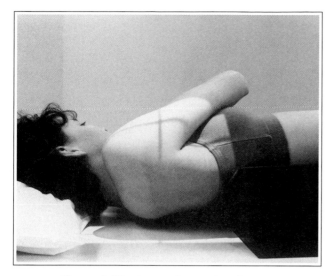

Figure 4-43. Arm resting against thorax.

- Center the IR to the central ray, and open the longitudinal collimation enough to include both the acromion and inferior scapular angles. Transversely collimate to within ½ inch (1.25 cm) of the closest lateral skinline.
- A 10- × 12-inch (24- × 30-cm) IR placed lengthwise should be adequate to include all the required anatomical structures.

Lateral Scapular Image Analysis

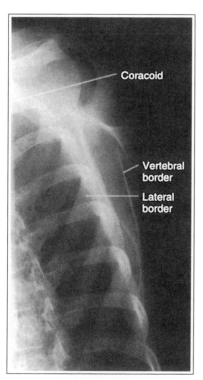

Image 48.

Analysis. The lateral and vertebral borders of the scapula are demonstrated without superimposition. The lateral

border is next to the ribs, and the vertebral border is demonstrated laterally. The patient was rotated more than required for this image.

Correction. Decrease the patient obliquity. The amount of change required is half of the distance demonstrated between the lateral and vertebral borders. When patient obliquity is decreased, the lateral border moves away from the thoracic cavity and the vertebral border moves closer to the thoracic cavity.

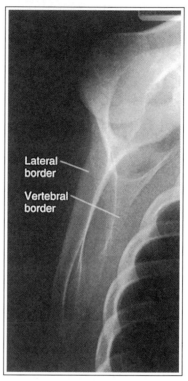

Image 49.

Analysis. The lateral and vertebral borders of the scapula are demonstrated without superimposition. The thick lateral border is demonstrated laterally, and the vertebral border is visible next to the ribs. The patient was not rotated enough for this image.

Correction. Increase the patient obliquity. The amount of change necessary is half the distance demonstrated between the lateral and vertebral borders.

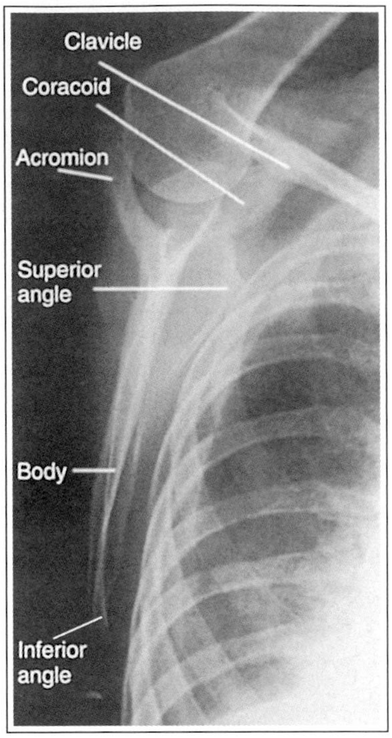

Image 50.

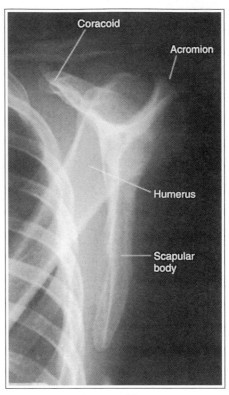

Image 51.

Analysis. The lateral and vertebral borders of the scapula are superimposed, indicating that patient obliquity was adequate. Note that the superior angle is demonstrated next to the thoracic cavity, inferior to the coracoid process. The patient's arm was elevated more than 90 degrees, positioning the lateral border of the scapula parallel with the IR (see Figures 4-40 and 4-41).

Correction. Depress the arm, positioning it at a 90-degree angle with the body. This depression causes the inferior angle to draw posteriorly around the thoracic cavity. Because of this posterior scapular movement, it is necessary to increase patient obliquity slightly to obtain a lateral scapula. It is suggested that the scapular borders and inferior angle be repalpated to obtain accurate patient obliquity.

Analysis. The superior scapular body is superimposed by the glenoid cavity, the proximal humeral head and the coracoid and acromion processes are clearly demonstrated, and the glenoid cavity is demonstrated "on end." The patient's arm was not elevated but rested on the patient's chest, positioning the vertebral border of the scapula parallel with the IR (see Figures 4-42 and 4-43).

Correction. For the scapular body to be best demonstrated, the arm should be elevated to approximately 90 degrees with the body. If the coracoid and acromion processes or the anteroposterior relationship between the glenoid fossa and humeral head is of interest, no corrective movement is necessary.

REFERENCES

1. Rubin SA, Gray RL, Green WR: The scapular "Y": a diagnostic aid in shoulder trauma, *Radiology* 110:725-726, 1974.
2. De Smet AA: Anterior oblique projection in radiography of the traumatized shoulder, *AJR Am J Roentgenol* 134:515-518, 1980.

Image Analysis of the Lower Extremity

The following image analysis criteria are used for all lower extremity images and should be considered when the analysis is completed.

Facility's identification requirements are demonstrated on image as identified in Chapter 1.

A right or left marker, identifying the side being imaged, is present and is not superimposed over anatomy of interest. Specific placement of marker is as described in Chapter 1.

No evidence of preventable artifacts is present.

- Consult with the ordering physician and the patient about whether bandages or splints can be removed.

The bony trabecular patterns and cortical outlines of the phalanges are sharply defined.

- Sharply defined recorded details are obtained when patient motion is controlled, a detail screen and a small focal spot are used, and a short object–image receptor distance (OID) is maintained. Increased spatial resolution is also obtained when the smallest IR is selected for digital images.

Contrast and density are adequate to demonstrate the surrounding soft tissue and bony structures. Penetration is sufficient to visualize the bony trabecular patterns and cortical outlines of the lower extremity.

- An optimal kilovolt-peak (kVp) technique, as demonstrated in Table 5-1, sufficiently penetrates the bony and soft-tissue structures of the lower extremity and provides a contrast scale necessary to visualize the bony details. To obtain optimal density, set a manual milliampere-seconds (mAs) value based on the part thickness.
- If the patient's lower extremity thickness measures less than 5 inches (13 cm), a grid is not required. If the patient's lower extremity thickness measures more than 5 inches (13 cm), a grid should be used because this thickness would produce enough scatter radiation to negatively affect image contrast. When a grid is used, increase the kVp to around 70 to penetrate the structure and to provide an adequate scale of contrast. Increase the exposure (mAs) by the standard density conversion factor for the grid ratio being used, to compensate for the scatter and the primary radiation the grid will absorb.

The long axis of the imaged structure is aligned with the long axis of the collimated field.

- Aligning the long axis of the imaged structure with the long axis of the collimator's longitudinal light line enables tight collimation without clipping needed anatomical structures.

TABLE 5-1 Lower Extremity Technical Data			
Part, Position, and Projection	**kVp**	**Grid**	**SID**
Toe	55-65		40-48 inches (100-120 cm)
Foot	55-65		40-48 inches (100-120 cm)
Plantodorsal (axial) projection, calcaneus	65-75		40-48 inches (100-120 cm)
Lateral position, calcaneus	55-65		40-48 inches (100-120 cm)
Ankle	55-65		40-48 inches (100-120 cm)
Lower leg	65-75		40-48 inches (100-120 cm)
AP projection, knee	Nongrid: 60-70		
Lateral position, knee			40-48 inches (100-120 cm)
AP oblique position, knee	Grid: 65-75	If measures over 13 cm	
PA axial (Holmblad) position, knee	60-70		40-48 inches (100-120 cm)
AP axial (Beclere) projection, knee	60-70		40-48 inches (100-120 cm)
Tangential (axial) projection knee	60-70		48-72 inches (120-180 cm)
Femur	70-80	Grid	40-48 inches (100-120 cm)

AP, Anteroposterior; *kVp,* kilovolt peak; *SID,* source–image receptor distance; *PA,* posteroanterior.

TOE: ANTEROPOSTERIOR PROJECTION

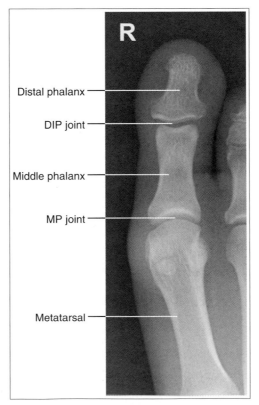

Distal phalanx
DIP joint
Middle phalanx
MP joint
Metatarsal

Figure 5-1. First anteroposterior toe image with accurate positioning.

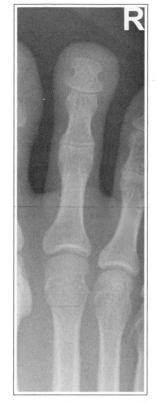

Figure 5-2. Second anteroposterior toe image with accurate positioning.

Image Analysis

The digit demonstrates no rotation. Soft-tissue width and midshaft concavity are equal on both sides of the phalanges.

- An anteroposterior (AP) projection of the toe is obtained by flexing the supine patient's knee until the plantar foot surface rests flat against the image receptor (IR). The lower leg, ankle, and foot should remain aligned, and equal pressure should be applied across the plantar surface (Figure 5-3).
- *Detecting toe rotation:* Toe rotation is controlled by the position of the foot. Take a few minutes to study a toe skeleton, and note that in an AP projection concavity of the midshaft of the proximal phalanx is equal on both sides. Also note that the posterior (plantar) surface of the proximal phalanx demonstrates more concavity than the anterior (dorsal) surface. As the skeleton is rotated medially or laterally, the amount of concavity increases on the side toward which the posterior surface is rotated, whereas the side toward which the anterior surface is rotated demonstrates less concavity. The same observations can be made about the soft tissue that surrounds the phalanges. More soft-tissue thickness is present on the posterior (plantar) surface than the anterior (dorsal) surface, so the side demonstrating the greatest soft-tissue width on an image will be the side toward which the posterior surface is rotated. Look for this midshaft concavity and soft-tissue width variation to indicate rotation on a toe image. With lateral toe rotation, phalangeal soft-tissue width and midshaft concavity are greater on the side positioned away from the lateral foot surface (see Image 1). With medial toe rotation, phalangeal soft-tissue width and midshaft concavity are greater on the side positioned away from the medial

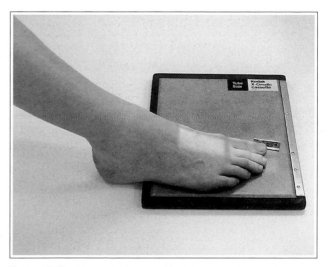

Figure 5-3. Proper patient positioning for anteroposterior toe image.

foot surface (see Image 2). If the patient's toenail is visualized, which is often the case with the first toe, it can also be used to determine the direction of toe rotation. The nail rotates in the same direction as the foot.

The interphalangeal (IP) and metatarsophalangeal (MP) joints appear as open spaces, and the phalanges are demonstrated without foreshortening.

- The IP and MP joint spaces are open and the phalanges are demonstrated without foreshortening when the toe was fully extended and a 10- to 15-degree proximal (toward the calcaneus) central ray was centered to the MP joint. This toe positioning and central ray placement align the joint spaces perpendicular to the IR and parallel with the central ray. They also prevent foreshortening of the phalanges, because the long axes of the phalanges are aligned perpendicular to the central ray.
- Failure to align the central ray and phalanges accurately will result in closed joint spaces and foreshortened phalanges (see Image 3).
- ***Central ray angulation for nonextendable toes:*** In patients who are unable to extend their toes, the toes may be elevated on a radiolucent sponge to bring the phalanges parallel with the IR or the central ray may be angled until it is perpendicular to the phalanx of interest or parallel with the joint space of interest.

No soft-tissue overlap from adjacent digits is present.

- Spreading the toes slightly prevents soft-tissue overlapping from adjacent toes. It is difficult to evaluate the soft tissue of an affected toe when it is superimposed by other soft tissue.

The MP joint is at the center of the collimated field. The distal and proximal phalanges and half of the metatarsal are included within the field.

- Centering the central ray to the MP joint places the joint in the center of the image.
- Open the longitudinal collimation to include the distal phalanx and the distal half of the metatarsal. To include half of the metatarsal, extend the light field 2 inches (5 cm) proximal to the between-toe interconnecting tissue. Transverse collimation should be to within ½ inch (1.25 cm) of the toe skinline.
- One third of an 8- × 10-inch (18- × 24-cm) detailed screen-film or computed radiography IR placed crosswise should be adequate to include all the required anatomical structures. Digital imaging requires tight collimation, lead masking, and no overlap of individual exposures to produce optimal images.

Anteroposterior Toe Image Analysis

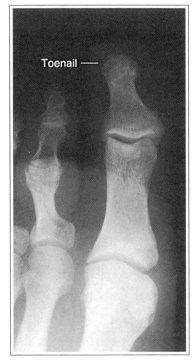

Image 1.

Analysis. The phalanges demonstrate greater soft-tissue width and midshaft concavity on the medial surface. The toe was laterally rotated.

Correction. Medially rotate the foot and toe until they are flat against the IR.

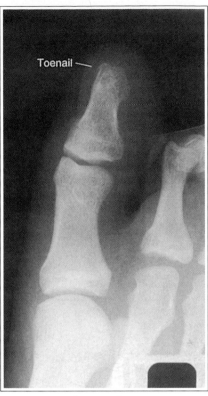

Image 2.

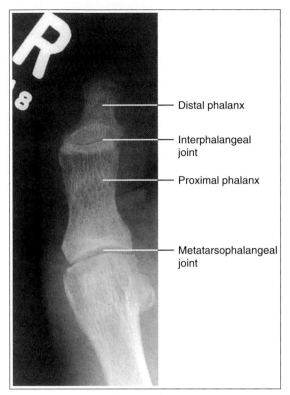

Image 3.

Analysis. The phalanges demonstrate greater soft-tissue width and midshaft concavity on the lateral surface. The outline of the toenail is visible on the medial surface. The foot was medially rotated.

Correction. Laterally rotate the foot and toe until they are flat against the IR.

Analysis. The IP and MP joint spaces are closed, and the phalanges are foreshortened. The patient's toe was flexed, and the central ray was not adequately angled to open these joints or to demonstrate the phalanges without foreshortening.

Correction. If the patient's condition allows, extend the toe, placing it flat against the IR. If the patient is unable to extend the toe, angle the central ray proximally until it is aligned perpendicular to the phalanx of interest or parallel with the joint space of interest.

TOE: ANTEROPOSTERIOR OBLIQUE PROJECTION

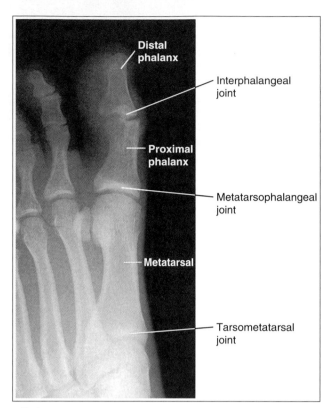

Distal phalanx

Interphalangeal joint

Proximal phalanx

Metatarsophalangeal joint

Metatarsal

Tarsometatarsal joint

Figure 5-4. Anteroposterior oblique toe image with accurate positioning.

Image Analysis

The digit is rotated 45 degrees. Twice as much soft-tissue width and more phalangeal and metatarsal concavity are present on the side of the digit rotated away from the IR.

- An AP oblique toe image is obtained by placing the affected foot on the IR and then rotating the foot until the affected toe is rotated 45 degrees from the AP projection (Figure 5-5). When the first through third toes

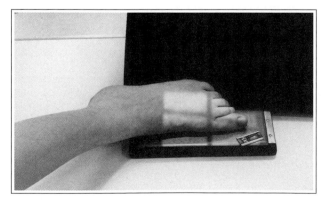

Figure 5-5. Proper patient positioning for anteroposterior oblique toe image.

are of interest, the foot should be rotated medially. When the fourth and fifth toes are of interest, the foot should be rotated laterally. The variation in rotation for the different toes is to obtain an oblique position with the least amount of OID.

- ***Toe midshaft concavity with various positions and projections:*** Examine a toe skeleton in an AP projection and in an oblique and a lateral position. Note how the midshaft concavity of the proximal phalanx varies as the digit is rotated. In an AP projection the midshaft concavity is equal on the two sides. In an oblique position the midshaft concavity is greater on the side toward which the posterior surface is rotated. In a lateral position the posterior aspect of the digit demonstrates more concavity than the anterior aspect. The same observations can be made about the soft tissue that surrounds the phalanges. More soft-tissue thickness is present on the posterior (plantar) surface than on the anterior (dorsal) surface, so the side demonstrating the greatest soft-tissue width on an image will be the side toward which the posterior surface is rotated.

- ***Verifying toe rotation on oblique image:*** To verify the accuracy of rotation on an oblique toe image and to determine the proper way to reposition the patient when digit obliquity was insufficient or excessive, study the midshaft concavity of the proximal phalanx and compare the soft-tissue width on both sides of the digit. A toe image taken at 45 degrees of obliquity demonstrates more phalangeal midshaft concavity and twice as much soft-tissue width on the side positioned farther from the IR. When the midshaft concavity of the proximal phalanx and soft-tissue width are closer to equal on both sides of the digit, the toe was not adequately rotated (see Image 4). When more than twice the width of soft tissue is present on one side of the digit than on the other and when the posterior aspect of the proximal phalanx's midshaft demonstrates more concavity than the anterior aspect, the toe was rotated more than 45 degrees for the image (see Image 5).

The IP and MP joints are visible as open spaces, and the phalanges are demonstrated without foreshortening.

- The IP and MP joint spaces are open and the phalanges are demonstrated without foreshortening when the toe was fully extended and a perpendicular central ray was centered to the MP joint. This toe positioning and central ray placement align the joint spaces perpendicular to the IR and parallel with the central ray. They also prevent foreshortening of the phalanges, because the long axes of the phalanges are aligned parallel with the IR and perpendicular to the central ray. If the toe was not extended, the resulting image demonstrates closed joint spaces and foreshortened phalanges (see Image 6).
- *Central ray angulation for nonextendable toes:* In patients who are unable to extend their toes, the central ray should be angled proximally (toward the calcaneus) until it is perpendicular to the phalanx of interest or parallel with the joint space of interest.

No soft-tissue or bony overlap from adjacent digits is present.

- The adjacent toes should be drawn away from the affected toe to prevent overlapping. It may be necessary to use tape or another immobilization device to maintain the unaffected toe's position. If the unaffected toes are not drawn away, they may be superimposed over the affected toe (see Image 7). It is difficult to evaluate the affected digit when it is superimposed by other digits.

The MP joint is at the center of the collimated field. The distal and proximal phalanges and half of the metatarsal are included within the field.

- Centering a perpendicular central ray to the MP joint places the joint in the center of the image.
- Open the longitudinal collimation to include the distal phalanx and the distal half of the metatarsal. To include half of the metatarsal extend the light field 2 inches (5 cm) proximal to the between-toe interconnecting tissue. Transverse collimation should be to within ½ inch (1.25 cm) of the toe.
- One third of an 8- × 10-inch (18- × 24-cm) detailed screen-film or computed radiography IR placed crosswise

should be adequate to include all the required anatomical structures. Digital imaging requires tight collimation, lead masking, and no overlap of individual exposures to produce optimal images.

Anteroposterior Oblique Toe Image Analysis

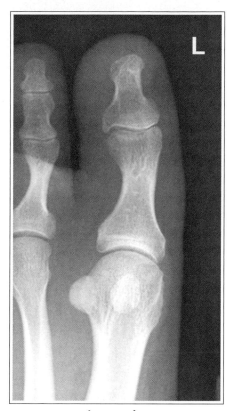

Image 4.

Analysis. Soft-tissue width and midshaft concavity on both sides of the phalanges are nearly equal. The toe was rotated less than 45 degrees.

Correction. Increase toe and foot obliquity until the affected toe is at a 45-degree angle with the IR.

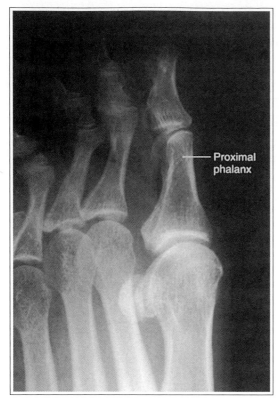

Image 5.

Analysis. The proximal phalanx demonstrates more concavity on the lateral aspect of the toe than the medial aspect. The toe has been rotated close to a lateral position.

Correction. Decrease toe and foot obliquity until the affected toe is at a 45-degree angle with the IR.

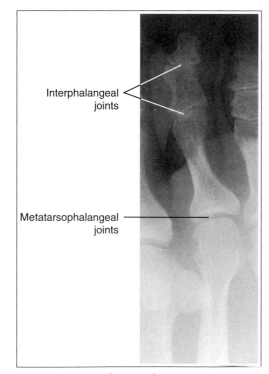

Image 6.

Analysis. The IP and MP joint spaces are obscured, and the phalanges are foreshortened. The patient's toe was flexed, and the central ray was not angled to open these joints or to demonstrate the phalanges without foreshortening.

Correction. If the patient's condition allows, extend the toe, placing it flat against the IR. If the patient's toe cannot be extended, angle the central ray until it is aligned perpendicular to the phalanx of interest or parallel with the joint space of interest.

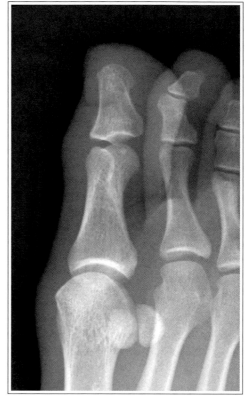

Image 7.

Analysis. Soft-tissue and bony overlap of the adjacent digit onto the affected digit is present. The toes were not spread apart.

Correction. Draw the unaffected toes away from the affected toe. It may be necessary to use tape or another immobilization device if the patient is unable to maintain the position.

TOE: LATERAL POSITION

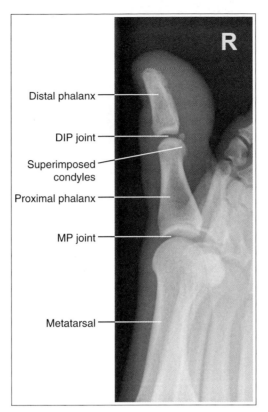

Figure 5-6. First lateral toe image with accurate positioning.

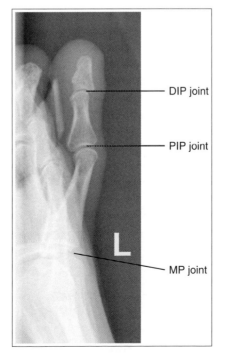

Figure 5-7. Second lateral toe image with accurate positioning.

Image Analysis

The digit is demonstrated in a lateral position. The posterior surface of the proximal phalanx demonstrates more concavity than the anterior surface, and the condyles are superimposed. The soft-tissue outline of the nail, when shown, is demonstrated in profile anteriorly.

- A lateral toe image is obtained by rotating the foot and toe until the affected toe is placed in a lateral position. Whether the foot is medially or laterally rotated to achieve this goal depends on which toe is being imaged. When the first, second, and third toes are imaged, rotate the foot medially (Figure 5-8). When the fourth and fifth toes are imaged, rotate the foot laterally (Figure 5-9).

- ***Inadequate toe rotations:*** In a lateral position the posterior (plantar) surface of the proximal phalanx demonstrates more concavity than the anterior (dorsal) surface and the condyles are superimposed. Inadequate rotation demonstrates nearly equal concavity on the posterior and anterior surfaces of the proximal phalanx and the condyles without superimposition (see Image 8). Evaluate the degree of metatarsal head superimposition to determine if the toe was rotated too much or not enough when a poor lateral toe image is produced. Compare Images 8 and 9. In Image 8 the metatarsal heads are shown without superimposition, indicating that the amount of foot and toe rotation should be increased. In Image 9 the metatarsal heads demonstrate slight superimposition, indicating that the amount of foot and toe rotation should be decreased.

No soft-tissue or bony overlap from adjacent toes is present.

- The adjacent toes should be drawn away from the affected toe to prevent overlapping. It may be necessary to use tape or another immobilization device to maintain

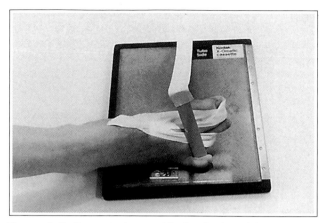

Figure 5-9. Proper patient positioning for lateral image of the fifth toe.

the unaffected toe's position. If the unaffected toes are not drawn away, they may be superimposed over the affected toe (see Image 10).

The proximal interphalangeal (PIP) joint is at the center of the collimated field. The distal and proximal phalanges and the MP joint space are included within the field.

- Centering a perpendicular central ray to the PIP joint places the joint in the center of the image.

- Open the longitudinal collimation to include the distal phalanx and MP joint space. The MP joint space is located approximately 1 inch (2.5 cm) proximal to the between-toe interconnecting tissue. Transverse collimation should be to within ½ inch (1.25 cm) of the toe skinline.

- One third of an 8- × 10-inch (18- × 24-cm) detailed screen-film or computed radiography IR placed crosswise should be adequate to include all the required anatomical structures. Digital imaging requires tight collimation, lead masking, and no overlap of individual exposures to produce optimal images.

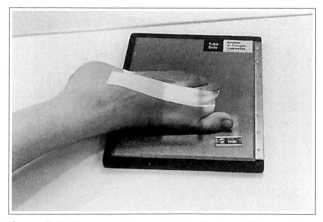

Figure 5-8. Proper patient positioning for lateral image of the first toe.

Lateral Position Toe Image Analysis

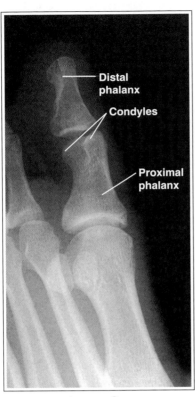

Image 8.

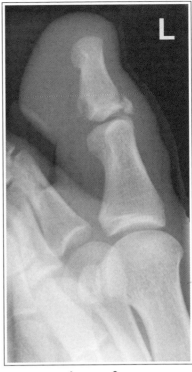

Image 9.

Analysis. The proximal phalanx demonstrates nearly equal midshaft concavity, the condyles are shown without superimposition, and the metatarsal heads are shown without superimposition. The foot and toe were not rotated enough for the toe to be placed in a lateral position.

Correction. Increase the patient's toe and foot obliquity until the affected toe is in a lateral position. For this patient it may also be necessary to draw the unaffected toes away from the affected toe to prevent superimposition.

Analysis. The proximal phalanx demonstrates nearly equal midshaft concavity, the condyles are shown without superimposition, and the metatarsal heads are slightly superimposed. The foot and toe were rotated too much for the toe to be placed in a lateral position.

Correction. Decrease the patient's toe and foot obliquity until the affected toe is in a lateral position.

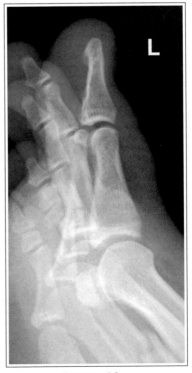

Image 10.

Analysis. Soft-tissue and bony overlap of digits is present. The adjacent unaffected digits were not drawn away from the affected digit.

Correction. The patient's unaffected toes should be drawn away from the affected toe. It may be necessary to use tape or another immobilization device to help the patient maintain this position.

FOOT: ANTEROPOSTERIOR PROJECTION (DORSOPLANTAR PROJECTION)

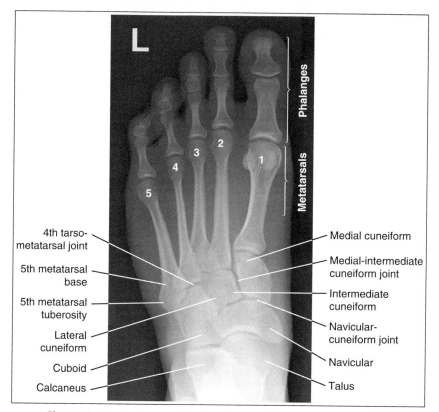

Figure 5-10. Anteroposterior foot image with accurate positioning.

Image Analysis

Foot demonstrates uniform density across the phalanges, metatarsals, and tarsals.

- When an exposure (mAs) is set that will adequately demonstrate the proximal metatarsals and tarsals, the distal metatarsals and phalanges are often overexposed because of the difference in AP foot thickness in these two regions (see Image 11). A compensating filter placed over the phalanges and MP joints can be used to absorb some of the photons that reach these areas, thereby obtaining more uniform foot density (Figure 5-11). The filter should be positioned so it extends 1 inch (2.5 cm) proximal to the between-toe interconnecting tissue in order to cover the MP joints.

The foot demonstrates an AP projection. The joint space between the medial (first) and intermediate (second) cuneiforms is open, approximately ¾ inch (2 cm) of

the calcaneus is demonstrated without talar superimposition, and concavity on both sides of the first metatarsal midshaft is equal.

- An AP projection of the foot is obtained by flexing the supine patient's knee and placing the plantar foot surface against the IR (Figure 5-12). The lower leg, ankle, and foot should remain aligned, and equal pressure should be applied across the plantar surface.
- *Effect of foot rotation:* If the lower leg, ankle, and foot are not aligned or if more pressure is placed on the medial or lateral plantar surface, foot rotation will result, and the medial and intermediate cuneiform joint space will be closed. When the foot is laterally rotated, the navicular tuberosity, which superimposes itself on an AP projection, is rolled into profile, and the talus moves over the calcaneus, resulting in less than ¾ inch (2 cm) of calcaneal demonstration without talar superimposition. An increase in metatarsal base superimposition also occurs (see Images 11 and 12).

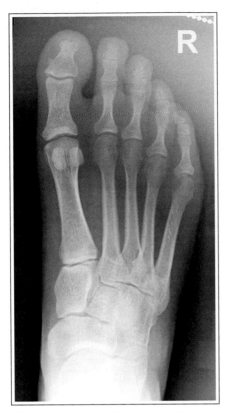

Figure 5-11. Anteroposterior foot image with compensating filter used on the toes.

- When the foot is medially rotated, the talus moves away from the calcaneus, resulting in more than ³/₄ inch (2 cm) calcaneal visualization without talar superimposition.
- A decrease in superimposition of the metatarsal bases also occurs (see Image 13).
- *Standing AP projection of the foot:* This image may also be obtained with the patient in a standing position. An AP standing foot image should meet the same evaluating criteria used for a nonstanding AP foot image.

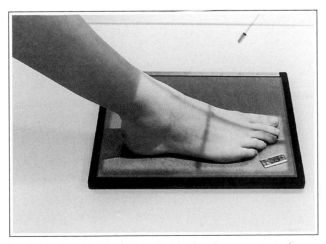

Figure 5-12. Proper patient positioning for anteroposterior foot image.

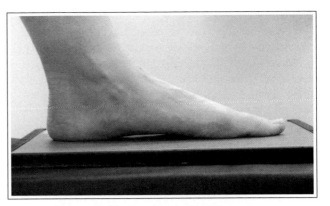

Figure 5-13. Low longitudinal foot arch.

The tarsometatarsal and navicular-cuneiform joint spaces are open.

- The bones of the foot with their ligament and muscular structures are arranged in a longitudinal arch that is visible on the medial foot surface. This arch places the tarsometatarsal and navicular-cuneiform joint spaces at a set angle with the IR. To demonstrate these joints as open spaces, angle the central ray until it is aligned parallel with them. This is accomplished in most patients by using a 10- to 15-degree proximal (toward the calcaneus) angle or aligning the central ray perpendicular with the dorsal surface. The exact degree of angulation needed depends on the height of the longitudinal arch. A 10-degree angle should be used when the patient's longitudinal arch is low, as demonstrated in Figure 5-13. A 15-degree angle is needed in a patient with a high arch, as demonstrated in Figure 5-14. Higher-arched patients require a slightly higher angle. Omitting or employing an inaccurate central ray angulation results in obstructed tarsometatarsal and navicular-cuneiform joint spaces (see Image 14).

The third metatarsal base is at the center of the collimated field. The proximal calcaneus, talar neck, tarsals, metatarsals, phalanges, and surrounding foot soft tissue are included within the field.

- To place the third metatarsal base in the center of the image, center the central ray to the midline of the foot

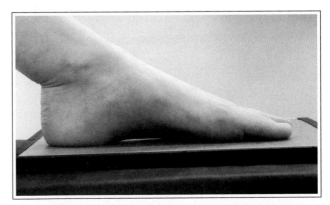

Figure 5-14. Average longitudinal foot arch.

at a level ½ inch (1.25 cm) distal to the fifth metatarsal tuberosity. The fifth metatarsal tuberosity can be palpated along the lateral foot surface, approximately halfway between the ball of the foot and the calcaneus.

- Open the longitudinal collimation enough to include the phalanges. Transverse collimation should be to within ½ inch (1.25 cm) of the foot skinline.
- Half of a 10- × 12-inch (24- × 30-cm) detailed screen-film or computed radiography IR placed lengthwise should be adequate to include all the required anatomical structures. Digital imaging requires tight collimation, lead masking, and no overlap of individual exposures to produce optimal images.

Anteroposterior Foot Image Analysis

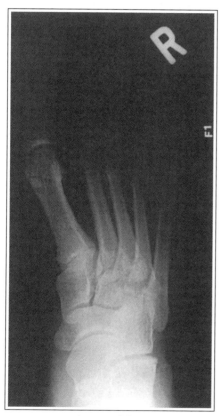

Image 11.

Analysis. The phalanges and distal metatarsals are overexposed. A compensating filter was not used on this portion of the foot. The joint space between the medial and intermediate cuneiforms is closed, the navicular tuberosity is demonstrated in profile, and less than ¾ inch (2 cm) of the calcaneus is demonstrated without talar superimposition. More pressure was placed on the patient's lateral plantar surface than on the medial surface, resulting in lateral foot rotation.

Correction. Position a compensating filter over the phalanges and distal metatarsal. Rotate the foot medially until the pressure over the entire plantar surface is equal. The lower leg, ankle, and foot should be aligned.

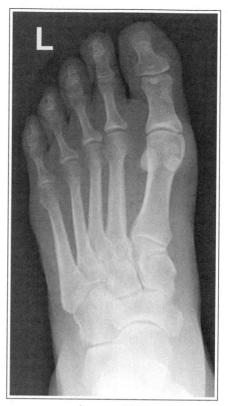

Image 12.

Analysis. The joint space between the medial and intermediate cuneiforms is closed, the navicular tuberosity is demonstrated in profile, and less than ¾ inch (2 cm) of the calcaneus is demonstrated without talar superimposition. More pressure was placed on the patient's lateral plantar surface than on the medial surface, resulting in lateral foot rotation.

Correction. Rotate the foot medially until the pressure over the entire plantar surface is equal. The lower leg, ankle, and foot should be aligned.

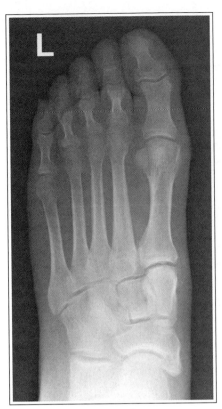

Image 13.

Analysis. The joint space between the medial and intermediate cuneiforms is closed, the calcaneus demonstrates no talar superimposition, and the metatarsal bases demonstrate decreased superimposition. More pressure was placed on the patient's medial plantar surface than on the lateral surface, resulting in medial foot rotation.

Correction. Rotate the foot laterally until the pressure over the entire plantar surface is equal. The lower leg, ankle, and foot should be aligned.

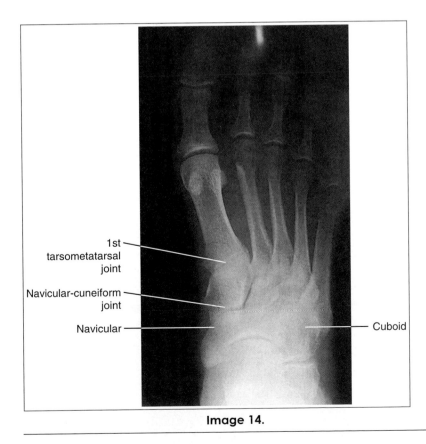

1st tarsometatarsal joint

Navicular-cuneiform joint

Navicular

Cuboid

Image 14.

Analysis. The tarsometatarsal and navicular-cuneiform joint spaces are obscured. The central ray was not aligned parallel with these joint spaces.

Correction. Direct the central ray 10 to 15 degrees proximally (toward the calcaneus), or angle the central ray until it is perpendicular with the dorsal surface. Less angulation is needed for patients with low longitudinal arches, whereas more angulation is required for patients with high arches.

FOOT: ANTEROPOSTERIOR OBLIQUE PROJECTION (MEDIAL ROTATION)

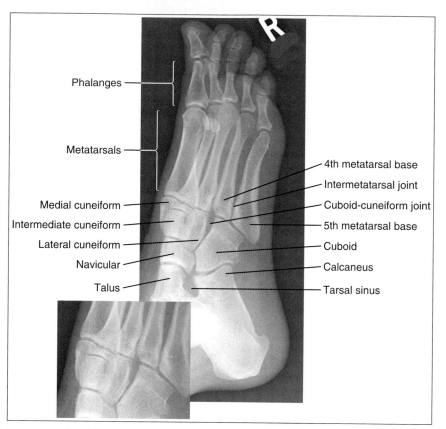

Figure 5-15. Anteroposterior oblique foot image with accurate positioning in a patient with a high longitudinal arch.

Image Analysis

Foot demonstrates uniform density across the phalanges, metatarsals, and tarsals.

- When an exposure (mAs) is set that will adequately demonstrate the proximal metatarsals and tarsals, the distal metatarsals and phalanges are often overexposed because of the difference in AP foot thickness in these two regions. A compensating filter placed over the patient's phalanges and distal metatarsals can be used to obtain uniform foot density. The filter should be positioned so it extends approximately 1 inch (2.5 cm) proximal to the between-toe interconnecting tissue in order to cover the metatarsal heads.

The foot demonstrates adequate obliquity. The cuboid-cuneiform joint space is open, the first and second intermetatarsal joints are closed but the second through fifth intermetatarsal joint spaces are open, and the tarsi sinus and fifth metatarsal tuberosity are well demonstrated.

- To obtain an AP oblique foot image, begin with the patient in a supine position with the knee flexed until the plantar foot surface rests against the receptor. Medially rotate the

patient's leg and foot until the foot forms a 30- to 60-degree angle with the IR (Figure 5-16).

- **Determining required obliquity:** To determine whether a 30- or 60-degree rotation is needed, view the medial aspect of the patient's foot in an AP projection to judge the height of the patient's longitudinal arch. Less obliquity is required in a patient with a low longitudinal arch than in a

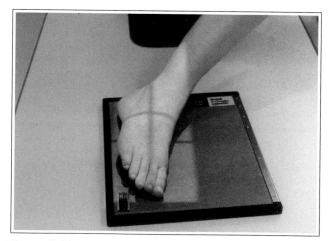

Figure 5-16. Proper patient positioning for an anteroposterior oblique foot image.

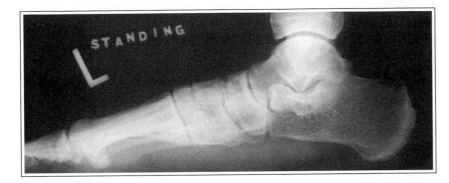

Figure 5-17. Lateral foot image of a patient with a low longitudinal arch.

patient with a high arch. If the patient has a low arch, such as that demonstrated in Figures 5-13 and 5-17, rotate the patient's foot approximately 30 degrees medially; if the patient's foot has an average arch, as demonstrated in Figures 5-14 and 5-18 and in Figure 5-20, rotate the foot approximately 45 degrees medially; and if the patient's arch is high, as demonstrated in Figures 5-15 and 5-19, rotate the foot approximately 60 degrees. The average arch requires 45 degrees of rotation. As the foot is rotated, keep the lower leg, ankle, and foot aligned to better judge the degree of foot obliquity.

- *Judging the degree of the rotation on oblique foot images:* On lateral foot images the height of the longitudinal arches can be compared by evaluating the amount of cuboid demonstrated posterior to the navicular bone. Note that more cuboid is visible posterior to the navicular

bone on the lateral foot image in Figure 5-19 than in Figure 5-17 and in Figure 5-20. A lateral foot image from a patient with an average longitudinal arch demonstrates approximately ½ inch (1.25 cm) of cuboid posterior to the navicular bone, whereas a patient with a high arch will demonstrate approximately ¾ inch (2 cm) and low arch approximately ¼ inch (0.6 cm). On oblique images, accurate obliquity has been obtained when the cuboid-cuneiform and second through fifth intermetatarsal joint spaces are open. This accuracy is demonstrated on the oblique images in Figures 5-15 and 5-18, even though they were taken with different degrees of obliquity. This can be confirmed by studying the amount of first and second metatarsal base superimposition, the amount of space demonstrated between the metatarsal heads, and the demonstration of the sinus tarsi. When the foot is rotated medially, the first metatarsal base rotates beneath the second metatarsal base, and the second through third metatarsal heads move closer together. The greater the foot obliquity, the greater the superimposition of the metatarsal heads.

- *Underrotation versus overrotation:* If the degree of foot obliquity is inadequate for an oblique foot image, the longitudinally running foot joints (cuneiform-cuboid, navicular-cuboid, and second through fifth intermetatarsal joint spaces) are closed. To determine whether the patient's foot has been underrotated or overrotated evaluate the intermetatarsal joint spaces between the fourth and fifth metatarsals. If this joint space is closed and the fourth metatarsal base is superimposed over the fifth metatarsal base, the foot was not rotated enough (see Image 15). If the fourth-fifth intermetatarsal joint space is closed and the fifth proximal metatarsal is superimposed over the fourth metatarsal tubercle, the foot was overrotated (see Image 16). The fourth metatarsal tubercle is a rounded, protruding surface located just distal to the fourth metatarsal base.

The third metatarsal base is at the center of the collimated field. The phalanges, metatarsals, tarsals, calcaneus, and surrounding foot soft tissue are included within the field.

- Centering a perpendicular central ray to the midline of the foot at the level of the fifth metatarsal tuberosity places the base of the proximal third metatarsal in the center of

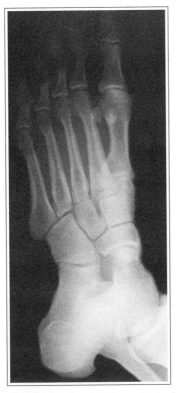

Figure 5-18. Oblique foot image of a patient with an average longitudinal arch.

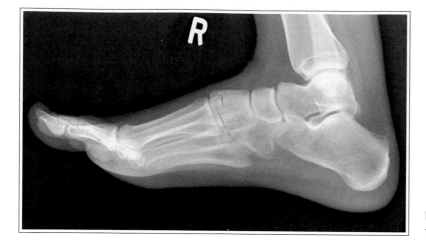

Figure 5-19. Lateral foot image of a patient with a high longitudinal arch.

the image. The fifth tuberosity can be palpated approximately halfway between the ball of the foot and the heel.

- Open the longitudinal collimation enough to include the phalanges and calcaneus. Transverse collimation should be to within ½ inch (1.25 cm) of the foot skinline.
- Half of a 10- × 12-inch (24- × 30-cm) detailed screen-film or computed radiography IR placed lengthwise should be adequate to include all the required anatomical structures. Digital imaging requires tight collimation, lead masking, and no overlap of individual exposures to produce optimal images.

Anteroposterior Oblique Foot Image Analysis

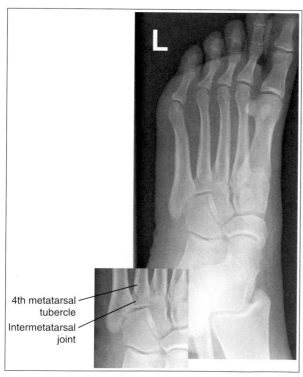

Image 15.

Analysis. The lateral cuneiform-cuboid, navicular-cuboid, and third through fifth intermetatarsal joint spaces are closed. The fourth metatarsal tubercle is demonstrated without superimposition of the fifth metatarsal. The foot was not medially rotated enough.

Correction. Increase the degree of medial foot rotation. The amount of increase needed is half the amount of fourth and fifth metatarsal base superimposition demonstrated on the image.

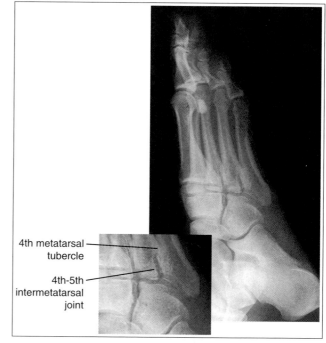

Image 16.

Analysis. The lateral cuneiform-cuboid, navicular-cuboid, and intermetatarsal joint spaces are closed, and the fifth proximal metatarsal is superimposed over the fourth metatarsal tubercle. The patient's foot was overrotated.

Correction. Decrease the lateral foot rotation.

FOOT: LATERAL POSITION (MEDIOLATERAL AND LATEROMEDIAL PROJECTIONS)

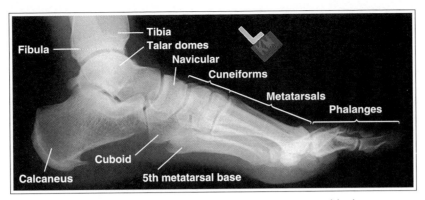

Figure 5-20. Mediolateral foot image with accurate positioning.

Image Analysis

Contrast and density are adequate to demonstrate the fat pads on the foot and ankle.

- *Fat pads on the foot and ankle:* Two soft-tissue structures located around the foot and ankle may indicate joint effusion and injury: the anterior pretalar fat pad and the posterior pericapsular fat pad. The anterior pretalar fat pad is visible anterior to the ankle joint and rests next to the neck of the talus (Figure 5-21). Surrounding the ankle joint is a fibrous, synovium-lined capsule that is attached to the borders of the tibia, fibula, and talus. On injury or disease invasion the synovial membrane secretes synovial fluid, resulting in distention of the fibrous capsule. Anterior fibrous capsule distention results in

displacement of the anterior pretalar fat pad. Because neither the fibrous capsule nor the ankle ligaments can be detected on plain radiography, displacement of this fat pad indicates joint effusion and the possibility of underlying injuries.

- The posterior fat pad is positioned within the indentation formed by the articulation of the posterior tibia and talar bones (see Figure 5-21). This fat pad is displaced in the same manner as the anterior pretalar fat pad, although it is less sensitive and requires more fluid evasion to be displaced.

The foot is in a lateral position. The domes of the talus are superimposed, the tibiotalar joint is open, and the distal fibula is superimposed by the posterior half of the distal tibia.

- To obtain a lateral foot image, begin with the patient in a supine position with the leg extended (Figure 5-22) and the foot dorsiflexed until its long axis forms a 90-degree angle with the lower leg. Rotate the patient toward the affected leg until the lateral foot surface is against the IR, then adjust the degree of rotation until this surface is aligned parallel with the IR (Figure 5-23). For most patients this positioning places the lower leg parallel with the imaging table. If this is not the case, as for a patient with a large upper thigh, the foot and IR should be elevated with an immobilization device until the lower leg is brought parallel with the imaging table.

- *Accurate longitudinal arch visualization:* This position may not bring the medial plantar foot surface perpendicular to the IR. If this is so, do not try to adjust the leg in an attempt to position this surface perpendicular to the IR. The true relationship of this surface to the IR and the metatarsals to one another depends on the height of the patient's longitudinal arch and the incline of the calcaneus. Adjusting the patient's plantar surface may result in poor talar dome positioning and an erroneous longitudinal arch height.

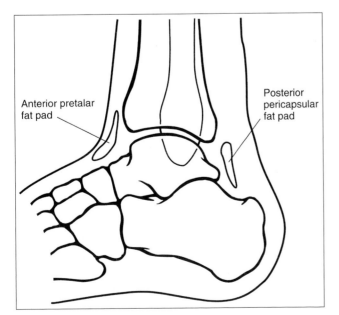

Figure 5-21. Location of fat pads.

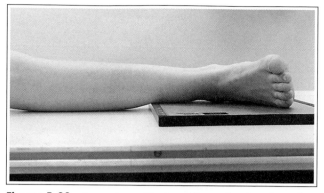

Figure 5-22. Accurate positioning of lower leg for a lateral foot image.

- The height of the longitudinal arch can be determined by measuring the amount of cuboid demonstrated posterior to the navicular bone. The average foot image demonstrates approximately ½ inch (1.25 cm) of the cuboid, as shown in Figure 5-20. Because the bones that form the foot arch are held in position by ligaments and tendons, weakening of these tissues may result in a decreased or low arch. On a lateral foot image this decrease in arch height is demonstrated as a decrease in the amount of cuboid demonstrated posterior to the navicular bone. Figure 5-17 shows a lateral foot image of a patient with a low longitudinal arch, and Figure 5-19 shows a patient with a high arch. A lateral foot image from a patient with a low longitudinal arch demonstrates approximately ¼ inch (0.6 cm) of cuboid posterior to the navicular bone, whereas approximately ¼ inch (0.6 cm) is demonstrated in an image from a patient with a low arch. When such an image is obtained, evaluate the talar domes to ensure that this cuboid-navicular relationship is a result of a low or high arch and not poor positioning. The talar domes should be superimposed.
- ***Talar domes:*** The domes of the talus are formed by the most medial and lateral aspects of the talar's trochlear surface. On a lateral foot image, they appear as domed structures that articulate with the tibia. On a properly

positioned lateral foot image, the talar domes should be superimposed and appear as one and the tibiotalar joint should be open. When the lateral foot is mispositioned, the domes are individually demonstrated, and they obscure the tibiotalar joint. Proximal-distal misalignment of the domes results from poor knee and lower leg positioning, and anteroposterior misalignment of the domes results from poor foot positioning.

- ***Effect of lower leg and knee positioning on proximal-distal talar dome superimposition:*** Often, if the knee is not fully extended (Figure 5-24) or if the distal tibia is not elevated to place the lower leg parallel with the IR in patients with large upper thighs, the proximal tibia is positioned farther from the imaging table than the distal tibia. The resulting image demonstrates the lateral talar dome proximal to the medial talar dome; the height of the longitudinal arch appears less than it actually is because the cuboid shifts anteriorly and the navicular bone moves posteriorly in this position; and the talocalcaneal joint will be narrowed (see Image 17). If the distal tibia is positioned farther from the table than the proximal tibia, the medial talar dome is demonstrated proximal to the lateral dome; the height of the longitudinal arch appears higher than it actually is because the cuboid shifts proximally and the navicular bone moves anteriorly in this position; and the talocalcaneal joint will be widened (see Image 18).
- When viewing a lateral foot image that demonstrates one of the talar domes proximal to the other, evaluate the height of the longitudinal arch and the degree of narrowing or widening of the talocalcaneal joint to determine which dome is the proximal dome. If the navicular bone is superimposed over more of the cuboid than expected and the talocalcaneal joint is narrowed, the lateral dome is the proximal dome; if the navicular bone is superimposed over less of the cuboid than expected and the talocalcaneal joint is wider, the medial dome is the proximal dome.

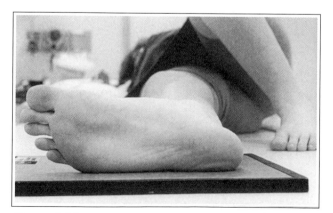

Figure 5-23. Accurate positioning of the lateral foot surface.

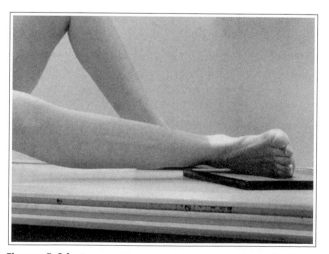

Figure 5-24. Poor positioning of the knee and lower leg for a lateral foot image.

- ***Effect of foot positioning on anteroposterior talar dome superimposition:*** To demonstrate accurate anteroposterior alignment of the talar domes, position the lateral surface of the foot parallel with the IR. If this surface is not parallel with the IR, one of the talar domes is demonstrated anterior to the other. When the leg is rotated more than needed to place the lateral foot surface parallel with the IR, as demonstrated in Figure 5-25, the medial talar dome is demonstrated anterior to the lateral talar dome (see Image 19). If the leg is not rotated enough to place the lateral foot surface parallel with the IR, as demonstrated in Figure 5-26, the medial talar dome is demonstrated posterior to the lateral talar dome (see Image 20).

- When viewing a lateral foot image that demonstrates one of the talar domes anterior to the other, evaluate the position of the fibula in relation to the tibia to determine how to reposition the patient. On most lateral foot images with accurate positioning the fibula is positioned in the posterior half of the tibia. If the fibula is demonstrated more posteriorly than this relationship on a foot image with poor positioning, the medial talar dome is anterior and the patient was positioned with the forefoot depressed and the heel elevated (leg externally rotated), as demonstrated in Figure 5-25. If the fibula is demonstrated more anteriorly than this relationship, the medial talar dome is posterior and the patient was positioned with the forefoot elevated and the heel depressed (leg internal rotation), as demonstrated in Figure 5-26.

- Carefully evaluate lateral foot images with poor positioning. Often, both knee and foot corrections are needed simultaneously to obtain accurate positioning.

The long axis of the foot is positioned at a 90-degree angle with the lower leg.

- In most cases, when a patient is relaxed, the foot rests in plantar flexion. Plantar flexion results in a forced

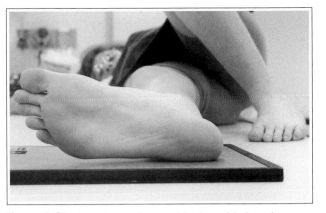

Figure 5-26. Poor lateral foot positioning with the calcaneus depressed (leg internally rotated).

flattening of the anterior pretalar fat pad, reducing its usefulness in the detection of joint effusion (see Image 21). Consequently, it is best to dorsiflex the foot, placing its long axis at a 90-degree angle with the lower leg. This positioning also places the tibiotalar joint in a neutral position and helps keep the leg and foot from rolling too far anteriorly. Anterior foot rotation elevates the heel and rotates the foot.

The proximal metatarsals are at the center of the collimated field. The phalanges, metatarsals, tarsals, talus, calcaneus, 1 inch (2.5 cm) of the distal lower leg, and surrounding foot soft tissue are included within the field.

- Centering a perpendicular central ray halfway between the distal toes and heel and the anteroposterior aspect of the foot places the bases of the metatarsals at the center of the collimated field.

- Open the longitudinal collimation enough to include the patient's toes and heel. Transverse collimation should be to a point 1 inch (2.5 cm) proximal to the medial malleolus (Figure 5-27).

- A diagonally placed 8- × 10-inch (18- × 24-cm) or a 10- × 12-inch (24- × 30-cm) detailed screen-film or computed radiography IR placed crosswise should be adequate to include all the required anatomical structures.

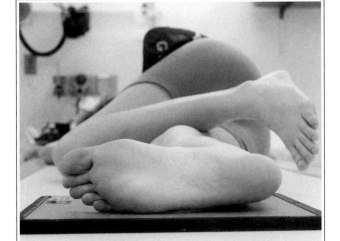

Figure 5-25. Poor lateral foot positioning with the calcaneus elevated (leg externally rotated).

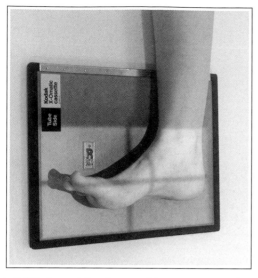

Figure 5-27. Lateral foot image with accurate central ray *(CR)* centering and collimation.

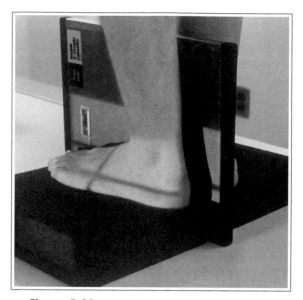

Figure 5-29. Poor lateromedial foot positioning.

WEIGHT-BEARING LATEROMEDIAL PROJECTION

A standing lateromedial foot projection is accomplished by placing the IR against the medial aspect of the foot and aligning the lateral foot surface parallel with the IR, as demonstrated in Figure 5-28. Even pressure should be applied to both feet. Notice that the patient's heel is situated slightly away from the IR when the lateral foot surface is parallel with the IR. The resulting image should meet all the analysis requirements listed for the mediolateral projection.

The most common misposition for the standing lateromedial projection of the foot shows the medial talar dome positioned anterior to the lateral talar dome and the distal fibula positioned too posteriorly on the tibia (see Image 19).

This misposition is a result of aligning the medial foot surface parallel with the IR, as demonstrated in Figure 5-29, rather than the lateral surface. When such an image is obtained, move the patient's heel away from the IR (leg internally rotated).

Lateral Foot Position Image Analysis

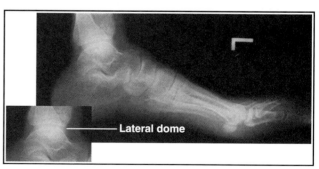

Image 17.

Analysis. The tibiotalar joint space is obscured, and one talar dome is demonstrated proximal to the other dome. Because the navicular bone is superimposed over most of the cuboid and the talocalcaneal joint is narrowed, the lateral talar dome is the proximal dome. The proximal tibia was elevated, as demonstrated in Figure 5-25.

Correction. Extend the knee, positioning the lower leg parallel with the IR, as demonstrated in Figure 5-22. If the knee was extended for this image, elevate the lower leg until it is positioned parallel with the IR.

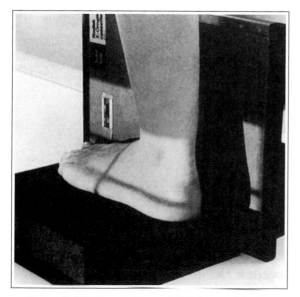

Figure 5-28. Proper lateromedial foot positioning.

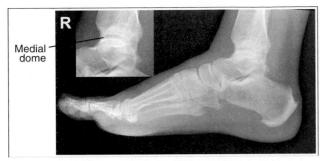

Image 18.

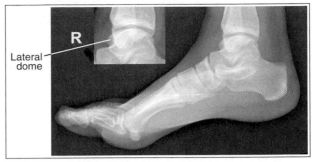

Image 20.

Analysis. The tibiotalar joint space is obscured, and one talar dome is demonstrated proximal to the other dome. Because more than ½ inch (1.25 cm) of cuboid is visible distal to the navicular bone and the talocalcaneal joint is widened, the medial dome is the proximal dome. The distal tibia was elevated.

Correction. Position the lower leg parallel with the IR.

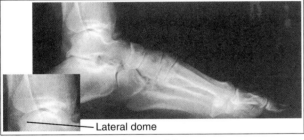

Image 19.

Analysis. The medial talar dome is positioned anterior to the lateral dome, as indicated by the posterior position of the fibula on the tibia. The lateral foot surface was not positioned parallel with the IR. If this is a mediolateral projection, the forefoot was depressed and heel was elevated (leg externally rotated), as demonstrated in Figure 5-25. If this is a standing lateromedial projection, the medial surface of the patient's heel was placed next to the IR, as demonstrated in Figure 5-29.

Correction. For a mediolateral projection, elevate the patient's forefoot and depress the patient's heel (internally rotate the leg) until the lateral foot surface is positioned parallel with the IR, as demonstrated in Figure 5-23. For a standing lateromedial projection, draw the patient's heel away from the IR until the lateral foot surface is positioned parallel with the IR, as demonstrated in Figure 5-28.

Analysis. The medial talar dome is positioned posterior to the lateral dome, as indicated by the anterior position of the distal fibula on the tibia. The lateral foot surface was not positioned parallel with the IR but was positioned with the forefoot elevated and heel depressed (leg internally rotated), as demonstrated in Figure 5-26.

Correction. Depress the patient's forefoot and elevate the heel (externally rotated leg) until the lateral foot surface is positioned parallel with the IR, as demonstrated in Figure 5-23.

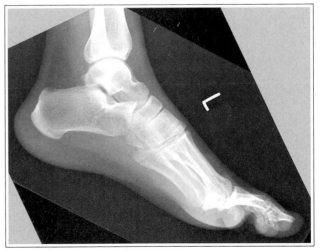

Image 21.

Analysis. The lower leg and long axis of the foot do not form a 90-degree angle. The patient's foot was in plantar flexion. A small amount of foot rotation is also present.

Correction. Dorsiflex the foot until the lower leg and long axis of the foot form a 90-degree angle.

CALCANEUS: PLANTODORSAL (AXIAL) PROJECTION

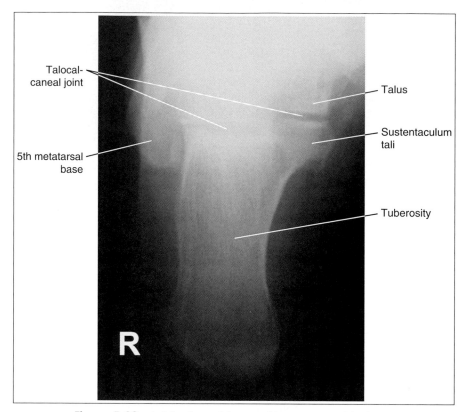

Figure 5-30. Axial calcaneal image with accurate positioning.

Image Analysis

The talocalcaneal joint is demonstrated as an open space, and the calcaneal tuberosity is demonstrated without distortion.

- The talocalcaneal joint space is demonstrated as an open space, and the calcaneal tuberosity appears without distortion, when the correct central ray angulation and foot position are used. For a patient who has foot mobility, place the foot in a neutral, vertical position and direct a 40-degree central ray angulation toward the plantar foot surface (Figure 5-31). This positioning places the central ray parallel with the talocalcaneal joint space and perpendicular to the calcaneal tuberosity (Figure 5-32).
- *Compensating for plantar-flexed or dorsiflexed foot:* When the patient's foot is dorsiflexed beyond a 90-degree position with the lower leg or is plantar flexed, the central ray needs to be adjusted to maintain its accurate position with the calcaneal joint space and tuberosity. If the patient's foot is dorsiflexed beyond the vertical position and a 40-degree angulation is used, the calcaneal joint spaces would be obscured and the tuberosity elongated (Figure 5-33 and Image 22). For this

situation the central ray angulation should be decreased to maintain accurate central ray alignment. If the patient's foot is plantar flexed and a 40-degree central ray angulation is used, the calcaneal joint space is obscured and the tuberosity foreshortened (Image 23 and Figure 5-34). For this situation the central ray angulation should be increased to maintain accurate central ray alignment.

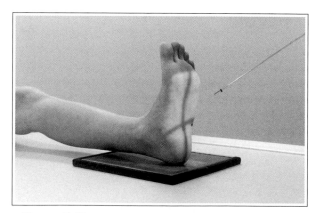

Figure 5-31. Proper axial calcaneal image positioning.

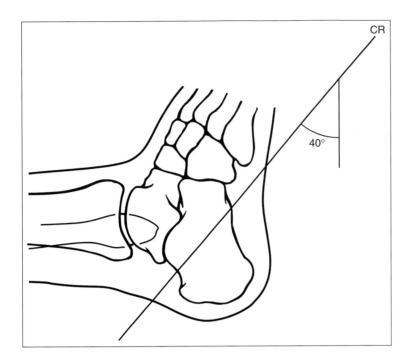

Figure 5-32. Central ray angled 40 degrees with foot in 90-degree position. *CR*, Central ray.

- The angulation that is required for each of these situations can be estimated by locating the base of the fifth metatarsal and the point of the fibula. The fifth metatarsal base is palpable on the lateral foot surface approximately halfway between the ball of the foot and the heel. Once these structures are located, angle the central ray parallel with an imaginary line drawn between them. When the axial calcaneal image is taken with the foot in plantar flexion and the central ray is angled as just discussed to demonstrate the talocalcaneal joint space, the calcaneal tuberosity will be elongated because

of the acute angle created between the central ray and IR (see Image 24).

The second through fourth distal metatarsals are not demonstrated on the medial or lateral aspect of the foot, respectively.

- To prevent calcaneal tilting, place the patient supine on the imaging table with the leg fully extended and the foot dorsiflexed until its long axis is placed in a vertical position, without medial or lateral rotation or foot inversion or eversion. If the ankle is internally rotated

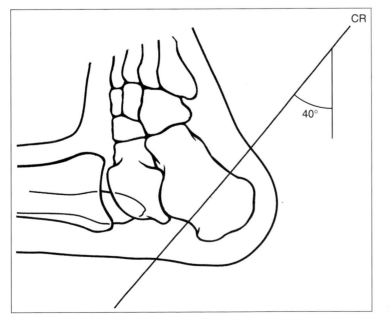

Figure 5-33. Central ray angled 40 degrees with foot in dorsiflexion. *CR*, Central ray.

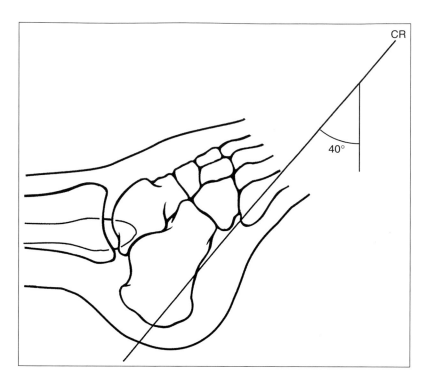

Figure 5-34. Central ray angled 40 degrees with foot in plantar flexion. *CR*, Central ray.

or the foot inverted, the first and second metatarsals are demonstrated medially. If the ankle is externally rotated or the foot everted, the fourth and fifth metatarsals are demonstrated laterally (see Images 24 and 25).

The proximal calcaneal tuberosity is at the center of the collimated field. The calcaneal tuberosity and the talocalcaneal joint space are included within the field.

- Centering the central ray to the midline of the foot at the level of the fifth metatarsal base places the proximal tuberosity in the center of the collimated field.
- Open the longitudinal collimation enough to include the patient's entire heel. Transverse collimation should be to within ½ inch (1.25 cm) of the heel skinline.
- Half of an 8- × 10-inch (18- × 24-cm) IR detailed screen-film or computed radiography IR placed crosswise should be adequate to include all the required anatomical structures. Digital imaging requires tight collimation, lead masking, and no overlap of individual exposures to produce optimal images.

Plantodorsal (Axial) Calcaneal Image Analysis

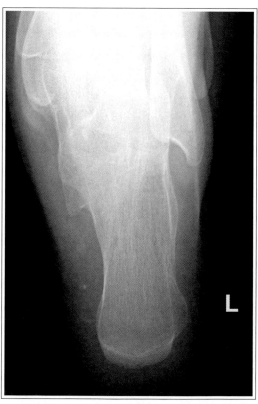

Image 22.

Analysis. The talocalcaneal joint space is obscured, and the calcaneal tuberosity is elongated. The foot was dorsiflexed beyond the vertical position, and a 40-degree central ray angulation was used.

Correction. Plantar flex the foot to a vertical position, and use a 40-degree angulation. If the patient cannot plantar flex the foot, decrease the degree of central ray angulation, aligning the central ray with the fifth metatarsal base and the distal point of the fibula.

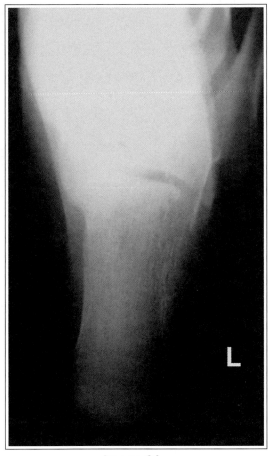

Image 24.

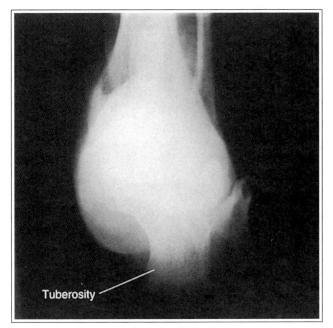

Image 23.

Analysis. The talocalcaneal joint space is obscured, and the calcaneal tuberosity is foreshortened. The foot was in plantar flexion, and the standard 40-degree central ray angulation was used.

Correction. If patient condition allows, dorsiflex the foot to a vertical, neutral position. If the patient cannot dorsiflex the foot, increase the central ray angulation, aligning the central ray with the fifth metatarsal base and the distal point of the fibula. Because of the acute angle that will be set up between the central ray and IR with this method, the calcaneal tuberosity will be elongated (see Image 24).

Analysis. The talocalcaneal joint space is shown as an open space, and the calcaneal tuberosity demonstrates elongation. The foot was in plantar flexion, and the central ray was angled so it was aligned with an imaginary line that connects the fifth metatarsal tuberosity and the distal point of the fibula. The fourth and fifth metatarsals are demonstrated on the lateral aspect of the foot. The ankle was externally rotated, and/or the foot was everted.

Correction. Elongation is not preventable if the patient's foot cannot be dorsiflexed because of the acute angle that is created between the central ray and IR. Internally rotate the leg until the ankle is in an AP projection, and/or bring the foot to a neutral position without eversion.

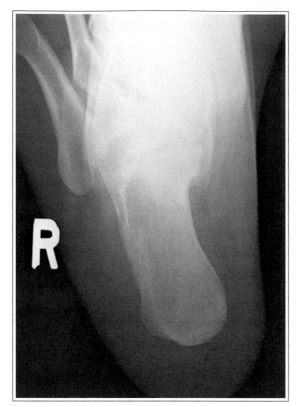

Image 25.

Analysis. The fourth and fifth metatarsals are demonstrated on the lateral aspect of the foot. The ankle was externally rotated, and/or the foot was everted.

Correction. Internally rotate the leg until the ankle is in an AP projection, and/or bring the foot to a neutral position without eversion.

CALCANEUS: LATERAL POSITION (MEDIOLATERAL PROJECTION)

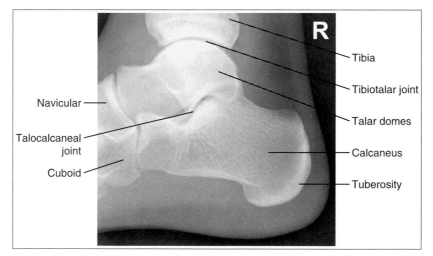

Figure 5-35. Lateral calcaneal image with accurate positioning.

Image Analysis

The calcaneus and distal tibia and fibula are in a lateral position: The domes of the talus are superimposed, the tibiotalar joint space is open, and the distal fibula is superimposed by the posterior half of the distal tibia.

- To obtain a lateral calcaneal image, begin with the patient in a supine position, with the leg extended (Figure 5-36) and the foot dorsiflexed until its long axis

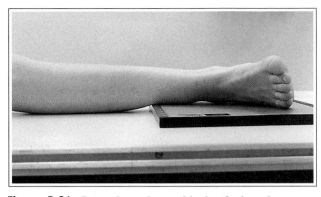

Figure 5-36. Proper lower leg positioning for lateral calcaneal image.

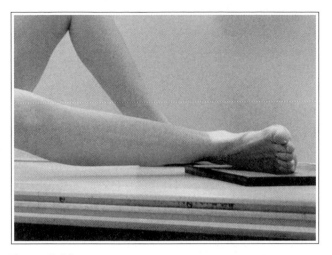

Figure 5-38. Poor knee and lower leg positioning for lateral calcaneal image.

forms a 90-degree angle with the lower leg. Rotate the patient toward the affected leg until the lateral foot surface is against the IR; then adjust the degree of rotation until the surface is aligned parallel with the IR (Figure 5-37). For most patients this positioning places the lower leg parallel with the imaging table. If this is not the case, as with a patient with a large upper thigh, the foot and IR should be elevated to place the lower leg parallel with the imaging table.

- **Talar domes:** The domes of the talus are formed by the most medial and lateral aspects of the talar's trochlear surface. They are visible on a lateral calcaneal image as domed structures that articulate with the tibia. When a lateral calcaneus image has been obtained, the talar domes should be superimposed and appear as one, and the tibiotalar joint should be open. If the lateral calcaneus is mispositioned, the domes are individually demonstrated and they obscure the tibiotalar joint. Misalignment of the domes will result from poor knee and foot positioning.

- **Effect of lower leg positioning on talar dome superimposition:** Often, if the knee is not fully extended (Figure 5-38) or if the distal tibia is not elevated to place the lower leg parallel with the IR (in a patient

with a large upper thigh), the proximal tibia is positioned farther from the imaging table than the distal tibia. The resulting image demonstrates the lateral talar dome proximal to the medial talar dome, and the height of the longitudinal arch appears less than it actually is, because the cuboid shifts anteriorly and the navicular bone moves posteriorly in this position, and the talocalcaneal joint will be narrowed (see Image 26). If the distal tibia is positioned farther from the imaging table than the proximal tibia, the medial talar dome is demonstrated proximal to the lateral dome, and the height of the longitudinal arch appears higher than it actually is, because the cuboid shifts posteriorly and the navicular bone moves anteriorly, and the talocalcaneal joint will be wider (see Image 27).

- When viewing a lateral calcaneal image that demonstrates one of the talar domes proximal to the other, evaluate the height of the longitudinal arch and the degree of narrowing or widening of the talocalcaneal joint to determine which dome is the proximal dome. If the navicular bone is superimposed over more of the cuboid than expected and the talocalcaneal joint is narrowed, the lateral dome is the proximal dome; if the navicular bone is superimposed over less of the cuboid than expected and the talocalcaneal joint is wider, the medial dome is the proximal dome.

- **Effect of foot positioning on talar dome superimposition:** To demonstrate accurate anteroposterior alignment of the talar domes, the lateral surface of the foot should be positioned parallel with the IR. If this surface is not parallel with the IR, the talar domes are demonstrated with one anterior to the other. When the leg is rotated more than needed to place the lateral foot surface parallel with the IR, as demonstrated in Figure 5-39, the medial talar dome is demonstrated anterior to the lateral talar dome (see Image 28). If the leg is not rotated enough to place the lateral foot surface parallel with the IR, as demonstrated in Figure 5-40, the medial talar dome

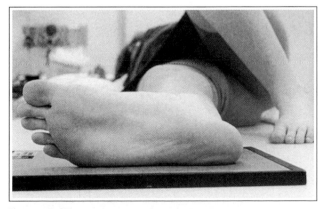

Figure 5-37. Proper lateral foot surface positioning for lateral calcaneal image.

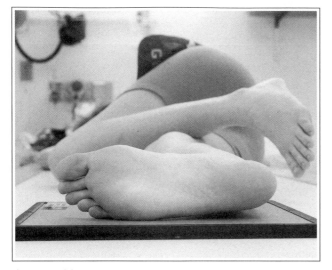

Figure 5-39. Poor lateral foot positioning with the calcaneus elevated (leg internally rotated).

is demonstrated posterior to the lateral talar dome (see Image 29).

- When imaging a lateral calcaneus image that demonstrates one of the talar domes anterior to the other, image the position of the fibula in relationship to the tibia to determine how the patient should be repositioned. On most lateral calcaneus images with accurate positioning, the fibula is positioned in the posterior half of the tibia. On a calcaneus image with poor positioning, if the fibula is demonstrated more posteriorly, the medial talar dome is anterior and the patient was positioned with the forefoot depressed and the heel elevated (leg externally rotated), as demonstrated in Figure 5-39. If the fibula is demonstrated more anteriorly (leg internally rotated), the medial domes are posterior and the patient was positioned with the forefoot elevated and the heel depressed, as demonstrated in Figure 5-40.
- Carefully evaluate lateral calcaneal images with poor positioning. Often, both knee and foot corrections are needed simultaneously to obtain accurate positioning.

The long axis of the foot is positioned at a 90-degree angle with the lower leg.

- In most cases, when a patient is relaxed the foot rests in plantar flexion, making it difficult for the patient to maintain a lateral position. Often the patient rotates the foot too far anteriorly, elevating the heel and rotating the foot (see Image 30). Consequently, it is best to dorsiflex the patient's foot, placing its long axis at a 90-degree angle with the lower leg.

The midcalcaneus is at the center of the collimated field. The tibiotalar joint, talus, calcaneus, and calcaneus-articulating tarsal bones are included within the field.

- Center a perpendicular central ray 1 inch (2.5 cm) distal to the medial malleolus to place the calcaneus in the center of the collimated field. Centering to the midcalcaneus better demonstrates the calcaneus and the surrounding calcaneotarsal and talocalcaneal articulations, allowing for accurate calcaneal inclination measurements and for visualization of calcaneal tuberosity displacement.
- Open the longitudinal collimation enough to include the calcaneus and tibiotalar joint, which is located at the level of the palpable medial malleolus. Including the tibiotalar joint on all lateral calcaneal images provides a method of judging rotation and determining how to reposition when a rotated lateral calcaneal image has been obtained. Transverse collimation should be to the calcaneal tuberosity and the calcaneotarsal joint spaces. Ensure that the calcaneotarsal joint spaces are included by extending the transverse collimation at least 2 inches (5 cm) anterior to the medial malleolus (Figure 5-41).
- Half of an 8- × 10-inch (18- × 24-cm) detailed screen-film or computed radiography IR placed crosswise should be adequate to include all the required anatomical structures. Digital imaging requires tight collimation, lead masking, and no overlap of individual exposures to produce optimal images.

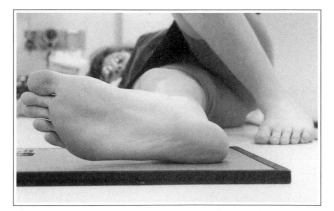

Figure 5-40. Poor lateral foot positioning with the calcaneus depressed (leg externally rotated).

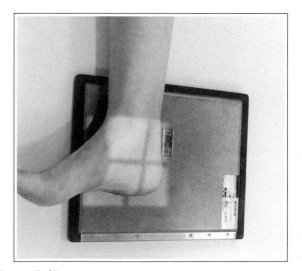

Figure 5-41. Accurate lateral calcaneal image with central ray *(CR)* centering and collimation.

Lateral Calcaneal Image Analysis

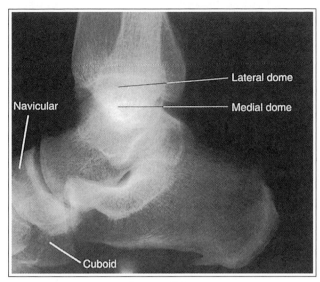

Image 26.

Analysis. The tibiotalar joint space is obscured, and one talar dome is demonstrated proximal to the other dome. Because the navicular bone is superimposed over most of the cuboid and the talocalcaneal joint is narrowed, the lateral dome is the proximal dome. The proximal tibia was elevated, as demonstrated in Figure 5-38.

Correction. Extend the knee to position the lower leg parallel with the IR, as demonstrated in Figure 5-36. If the knee was extended for this image, elevate the lower leg until it is positioned parallel with the IR.

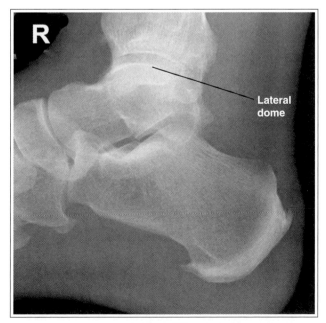

Image 27.

Analysis. The tibiotalar joint space is obscured, and one talar dome is demonstrated proximal to the other dome.

Because more than ½ inch (1.25 cm) of cuboid is demonstrated distal to the navicular bone and the talocalcaneal joint is widened, the medial dome is the proximal dome. The distal tibia was elevated.

Correction. Position the lower leg parallel with the IR.

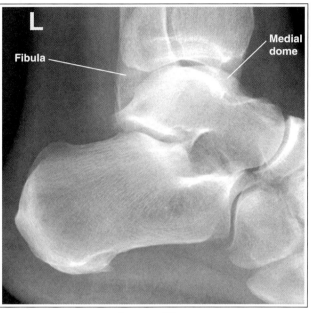

Image 28.

Analysis. The medial talar dome is positioned anterior to the lateral talar dome, as indicated by the posterior position of the fibula on the tibia. The lateral foot surface was not positioned parallel with the IR. The patient's forefoot was depressed and the heel was elevated (leg externally rotated), as demonstrated in Figure 5-39.

Correction. Elevate the patient's forefoot and depress the heel (internally rotate the leg) until the lateral foot surface is parallel with the IR, as demonstrated in Figure 5-37.

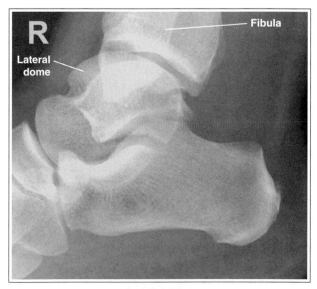

Image 29.

Analysis. The medial talar dome is positioned posterior to the lateral dome, as indicated by the anterior position of the distal fibula on the tibia. The lateral foot surface was positioned not parallel with the IR but with the forefoot elevated and the heel depressed, as demonstrated in Figure 5-40.

Correction. Depress the patient's forefoot and elevate the heel until the lateral foot surface is positioned parallel with the IR, as demonstrated in Figure 5-37.

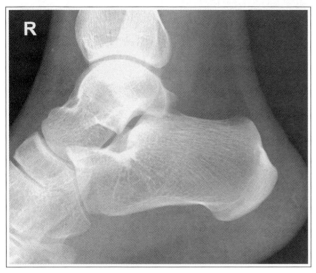

Image 30.

Analysis. The lower leg and the long axis of the foot do not form a 90-degree angle. The patient's foot was in plantar flexion.

Correction. Dorsiflex the foot until the lower leg and the long axis of the foot form a 90-degree angle.

ANKLE: ANTEROPOSTERIOR PROJECTION

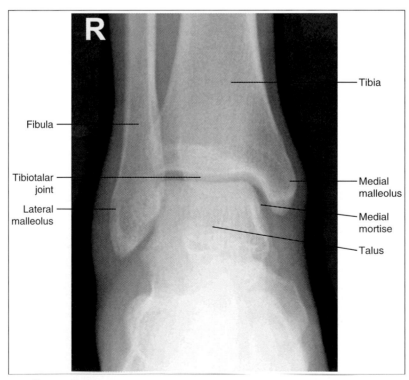

Figure 5-42. Anteroposterior ankle image with accurate positioning.

Image Analysis

The ankle is demonstrated in an AP projection. The medial mortise (tibiotalar articulation) is open, and the distal tibia and talus are superimposed over the distal fibula by a small amount (¹/₈ inch), closing the lateral mortise (fibulotalar articulation).

- An AP projection of the ankle is obtained by positioning the patient supine on the image table, with the leg fully extended and the foot dorsiflexed until its long axis is placed in a vertical position (Figure 5-43). In this position, the intermalleolar line (imaginary line drawn between the medial and lateral malleoli) is at a 15- to 20-degree angle with the IR. The medial malleolus is positioned farther from the IR than the lateral malleolus.
- ***Detecting direction of ankle rotation:*** If the ankle was not positioned in an AP projection but is rotated laterally or medially, the medial mortise is obscured. When an AP ankle image demonstrates a closed medial mortise, one can determine which way the patient's leg was rotated by evaluating the amount of tibia and talar superimposition of the fibula and the position of the medial malleolus. In external rotation, the tibia and talus demonstrate greater superimposition of the fibula and the posterior aspect of the medial malleolus (Figure 5-44) is situated medial to the anterior aspect (see Image 31). In internal rotation the fibula is demonstrated without talar superimposition (see Image 32).

The tibiotalar joint space is open, and the tibia is demonstrated without foreshortening.

- The tibiotalar joint is open and the tibia is demonstrated without foreshortening if the patient's lower leg was positioned parallel with the IR and the central ray was centered at the level of the tibiotalar joint.
- ***Evaluating the openness of the tibiotalar joint:*** On an AP ankle image, determine whether an open joint was

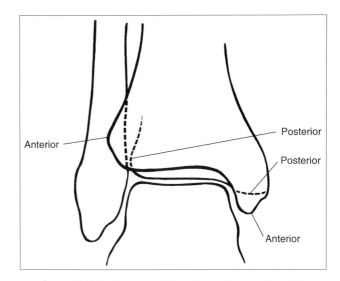

Figure 5-44. Anatomy of anterior and posterior ankle.

obtained and whether the tibia is demonstrated without foreshortening by evaluating the anterior and posterior margins of the distal tibia. On an AP ankle image with accurate positioning, the anterior margin is demonstrated approximately ¹/₈ inch (3 mm) proximal to the posterior margin (Figure 5-44). If the proximal lower leg was elevated or the central ray was centered proximal to the tibiotalar joint, the anterior tibial margin is projected distally, resulting in a narrowed or obscured tibiotalar joint space (see Image 33). If the distal lower leg was elevated or the central ray was centered distal to the tibiotalar joint, the anterior tibial margin is projected more proximal to the posterior margin than on an AP ankle image, expanding the tibiotalar joint space and demonstrating the tibial articulating surface (see Image 34).

- ***Effect of foot positioning on tibiotalar joint visualization:*** The position of the foot also determines how well the tibiotalar joint space is demonstrated. The patient's foot should be placed vertically, with its long axis positioned at a 90-degree angle with the lower leg. When the ankle image is taken with the foot dorsiflexed, the trochlear surface of the talus is wedged into the anterior tibial region, resulting in a narrower-appearing joint space. If the foot is plantar-flexed, the calcaneus is moved proximally, beneath the body of the talus, resulting in talocalcaneal superimposition and possibly hindering visualization of the talar trochlear surface.

The tibiotalar joint space is at the center of the collimated field. The distal fourth of the tibia and fibula, the talus, and the surrounding ankle soft tissue are included within the field.

- To place the tibiotalar joint in the center of the image, center a perpendicular central ray to the ankle midway between the malleoli. The medial malleolus is located at the same level as the tibiotalar joint space. Open the

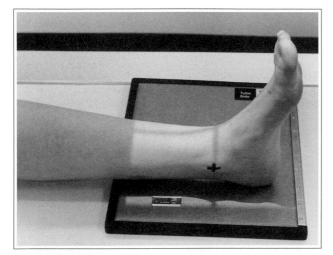

Figure 5-43. Proper patient positioning for anteroposterior ankle image.

longitudinal collimation to include the calcaneus and one fourth of distal lower leg. Transverse collimation should be to within ½ inch (1.25 cm) of the ankle skinline.

- Either one half of a 10- × 12-inch (24- × 30-cm) detailed screen-film IR placed crosswise or a single 8- × 10-inch (18- × 24-cm) digital IR placed lengthwise should be adequate to include all the required anatomical structures.

Anteroposterior Ankle Image Analysis

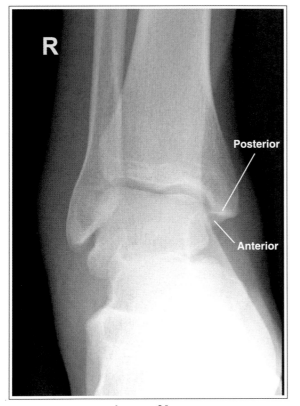

Image 31.

Analysis. The ankle was not placed in an AP projection. The medial mortise is obscured, the tibia and talus demonstrate increased superimposition of the fibula, and the posterior aspect of the medial malleolus is situated medial to the anterior aspect. The ankle was externally rotated.

Correction. Rotate the leg internally, placing the long axis of the foot in a vertical position.

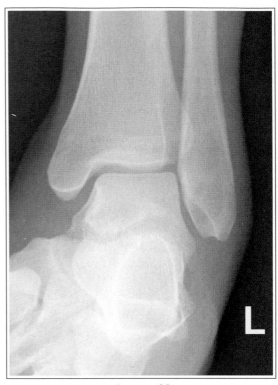

Image 32.

Analysis. The ankle was not placed in an AP projection. The fibula is demonstrated without talar superimposition. The ankle was internally rotated.

Correction. Rotate the leg externally, placing the long axis of the foot in a vertical position.

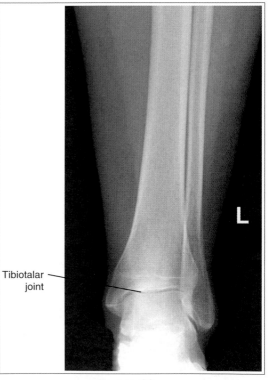

Image 33.

Analysis. The tibiotalar joint is closed. The anterior tibial margin has been projected into the joint space. Either the proximal tibia was elevated owing to knee flexion, or the central ray was centered superior to the tibiotalar joint.

Correction. Extend the knee, lowering the proximal tibia until the lower leg is parallel with the IR, or center the central ray to the tibiotalar joint (located at the level of the medial malleolus).

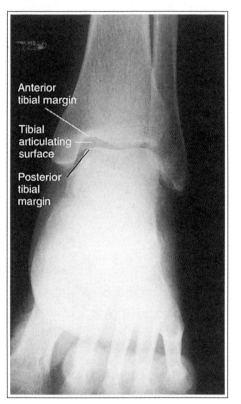

Image 34.

Analysis. The tibiotalar joint is distorted. The anterior tibial margin is projected superior to the posterior margin, and the tibial articulating surface is demonstrated. Either the distal tibia was elevated or the central ray was centered inferior to the tibiotalar joint.

Correction. Depress the distal tibia or elevate the proximal tibia until the lower leg is parallel with the IR, or center the central ray to the tibiotalar joint at the level of the medial malleolus.

ANKLE: ANTEROPOSTERIOR OBLIQUE PROJECTION (INTERNAL ROTATION—15- TO 20-DEGREE MORTISE AND 45-DEGREE OBLIQUE)

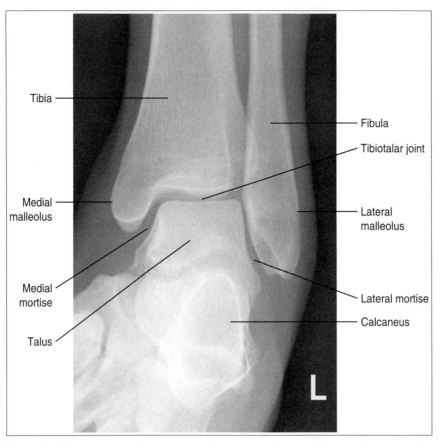

Figure 5-45. Anteroposterior (mortise) oblique ankle image with accurate positioning.

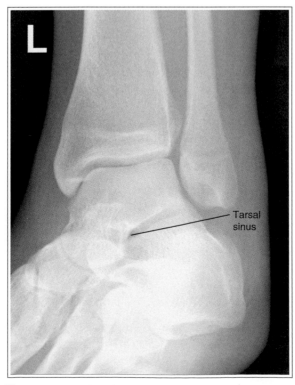

Figure 5-46. Anteroposterior (45-degree) oblique ankle image with accurate positioning.

Image Analysis

Mortise oblique: The ankle demonstrates 15 to 20 degrees of obliquity. The distal fibula is demonstrated without talar superimposition, demonstrating an open lateral mortise (talofibular joint), and the lateral and medial malleoli are demonstrated in profile. The tibia demonstrates slight fibular superimposition.

45-degree oblique: The ankle demonstrates 45-degrees of obliquity: The medial mortise is closed and the lateral mortise is partially closed, the fibula is demonstrated without tibial superimposition, and the tarsi sinus (opening between the calcaneus and talus) is shown but not clearly identifiable as an open space.

- To obtain an AP oblique ankle image with accurate positioning, place the patient in a supine AP projection with the leg extended and the foot positioned vertically (Figure 5-47). The leg and foot are then rotated the desired amount. Make certain the foot does not invert during rotation.

  Mortise oblique: While viewing the plantar surface of the foot, place your index fingers on the most prominent aspects of the lateral and the medial malleoli. Rotate the patient's entire leg internally (medially) 15 to 20 degrees, until your index fingers and the malleoli are positioned at equal distances from the IR (Figure 5-48). An imaginary line drawn between the malleoli (intermalleolar plane) is then aligned parallel with the IR. This rotation moves the fibula away from the talus to demonstrate an open lateral mortise.

  45-degree oblique: For the 45-degree AP oblique ankle projection, internally rotate the leg and foot until the long axis of the foot is aligned 45 degrees with the IR (Figure 5-49).

Detecting degree of ankle and leg rotation when inadequate:

  Mortise oblique: If the ankle and leg are internally rotated less than the needed 15 to 20 degrees, the medial

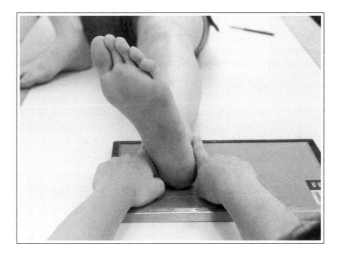

Figure 5-48. Aligning the intermalleolar line parallel with IR for oblique ankle image.

mortise will be open while the lateral mortise will be closed (Image 35). If the ankle was internally rotated more than 15 to 20 degrees, the image will demonstrate a closed medial mortise and an open tibiofibular joint and the tarsi sinus as shown in Figure 5-46.

45-degree oblique: If the ankle and leg are internally rotated less than 45 degrees, the distal fibula is demonstrated without talar superimposition, demonstrating an open lateral mortise, and the malleoli will be shown in profile (Figure 5-45). If the ankle and leg are internally rotated slightly more than 45 degrees, the medial and lateral mortise will be closed, the fibula will be demonstrated with very little if any talar superimposition, and the tarsi sinus will be demonstrated (Images 36 and 37).

The tibiotalar joint space is open, and the tibia is demonstrated without foreshortening.

- The tibiotalar joint space is open and the tibia is demonstrated without foreshortening when the patient's lower

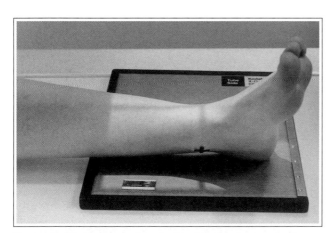

Figure 5-47. Proper patient positioning for anteroposterior oblique ankle image.

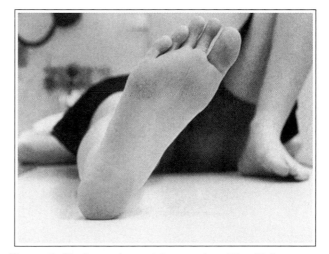

Figure 5-49. Proper internal foot rotation: 15 to 20 degrees from vertical.

leg was positioned parallel with the IR and the central ray was centered at the level of the tibiotalar joint (see Figure 5-47).

- ***Evaluating the openness of the tibiotalar joint:*** On an oblique ankle image, you can determine whether the positioning and central ray alignment goals have been met by evaluating the anterior and posterior margins of the distal tibia. On an oblique ankle image with accurate positioning, the anterior margin should be visualized approximately ⅛ inch (3 mm) proximal to the posterior margin. If the proximal lower leg was elevated or the central ray was centered proximal to the tibiotalar joint, the anterior tibial margin is projected distally, resulting in a narrowed or obscured tibiotalar joint. If the patient's distal lower leg was elevated or the central ray was centered distal to the tibiotalar joint, the anterior tibial margin is projected too far superior to the posterior margin, expanding the tibiotalar joint space and demonstrating the tibial articulating surface (see Image 38).

The calcaneus is demonstrated distal to the lateral mortise and fibula.

- To position the calcaneus distal to the lateral mortise and fibula, place the foot in a neutral position by positioning its long axis at a 90-degree angle with the lower leg. If the foot was plantar-flexed for an oblique image, the calcaneus obscures the distal aspect of the lateral mortise and the distal fibula (see Image 39).

The tibiotalar joint space is at the center of the collimated field. The distal fourth of the fibula and tibia, the talus, and the surrounding ankle soft tissue are included within the field.

- To place the tibiotalar joint in the center of the image, center a perpendicular central ray to the ankle midway between the malleoli. The medial malleolus is located at the same level as the tibiotalar joint space. Open the longitudinal collimation to include the calcaneus and one fourth of the distal lower leg. Transverse collimation should be to within ½ inch (1.25 cm) of the ankle skinline.
- Either one half of a 10- × 12-inch (24- × 30-cm) detailed screen-film IR placed crosswise or a single 8- × 10-inch (18- × 24-cm) digital IR placed lengthwise should be adequate to include all the required anatomical structures.

Anteroposterior Oblique Ankle Image Analysis

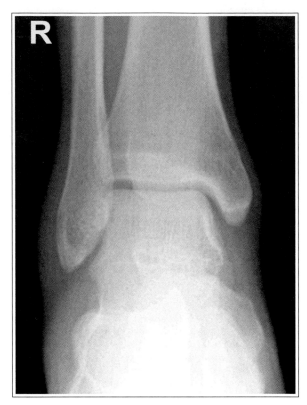

Image 35. Mortise oblique.

Analysis. The lateral mortise (talofibular joint) is closed, and the medial mortise is demonstrated as an open space. The tarsal sinus is not visible. The patient's leg and ankle were not internally rotated enough.

Correction. Rotate the entire leg internally until the most prominent aspects of the lateral and medial malleoli are positioned at equal distances from the IR, as demonstrated in Figure 5-48.

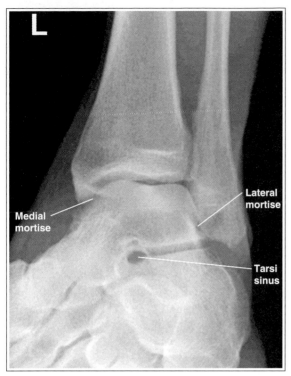

Image 36. 45-degree oblique.

Analysis. The lateral and medial mortises are closed, the fibula is demonstrated without tibial superimposition, and the tarsi sinus is demonstrated. The patient's leg and ankle were internally rotated more than 45 degrees.

Correction. Rotate the leg and foot externally until the long axis of the foot is at a 45-degree angle with the IR as demonstrated in Figure 5-49.

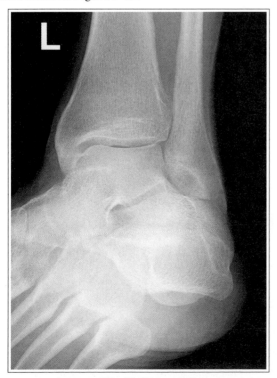

Image 37. 45-degree oblique.

Analysis. The lateral and medial mortises are closed, the fibula is demonstrated without tibial superimposition, and the tarsi sinus is faintly evident. The patient's leg and ankle were internally rotated more than 45 degrees.

Correction. Rotate the leg and foot externally until the long axis of the foot is at a 45-degree angle with the IR as demonstrated in Figure 5-49.

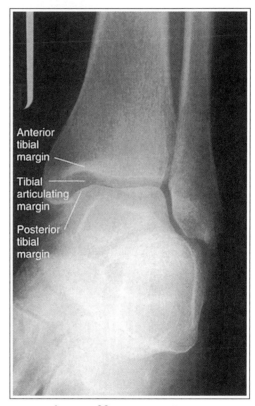

Image 38. Mortise oblique.

Analysis. The tibiotalar joint space is expanded. The anterior tibial margin has been projected superior to the posterior margin, and the tibial articulating surface is demonstrated. Either the distal tibia was elevated or the central ray was centered distal to the tibiotalar joint.

Correction. Depress the distal tibia or elevate the proximal tibia until the lower leg is placed parallel with the IR, or center the central ray to the tibiotalar joint at the level of the medial malleolus.

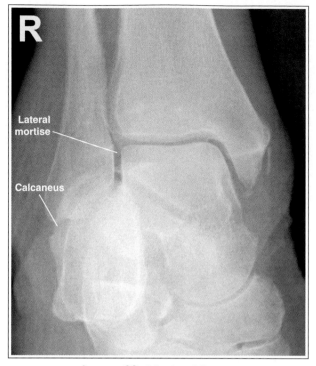

Image 39. Mortise oblique.

Analysis. The calcaneus is obscuring the distal aspect of the lateral mortise and distal fibula. The foot was in plantar flexion when the image was taken.

Correction. Dorsiflex the foot until its long axis forms a 90-degree angle with the lower leg.

ANKLE: LATERAL POSITION (MEDIOLATERAL PROJECTION)

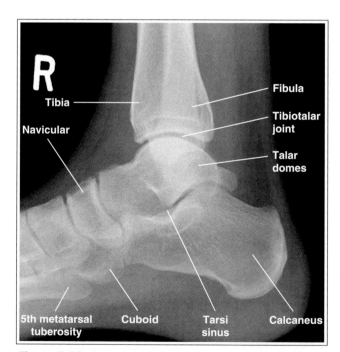

Figure 5-50. Lateral ankle image with accurate positioning.

Image Analysis

Contrast and density are adequate to demonstrate the fat pads on the foot and ankle.

• *Fat pads on the ankle:* Two soft-tissue structures located around the ankle may indicate joint effusion

and injury: the anterior pretalar fat pad and the posterior pericapsular fat pad. The anterior pretalar fat pad is demonstrated anterior to the ankle joint and rests next to the neck of the talus (Figure 5-51). Surrounding the ankle joint is a fibrous, synovium-lined capsule attached to the borders of the tibia, fibula, and talus. On injury or disease invasion, the synovium membrane secretes

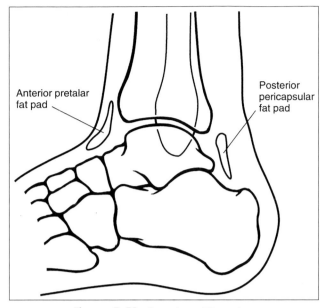

Figure 5-51. Location of fat pads.

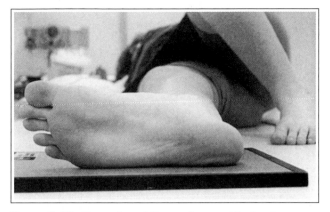

Figure 5-53. Proper lateral foot surface positioning for lateral ankle image.

synovial fluid, resulting in distention of the fibrous capsule. Distention of the anterior fibrous capsule results in displacement of the anterior pretalar fat pad. Because neither the fibrous capsule nor the ankle ligaments can be demonstrated on plain radiography, displacement of this fat pad indicates joint effusion and the possibility of underlying injuries.

- The posterior fat pad, positioned within the indentation formed by the articulation of the posterior tibia and talar bones (see Figure 5-51), is displaced in the same manner as the anterior pretalar fat pad, although it is less sensitive and requires more fluid evasion to be displaced.

The ankle is in a lateral position. The domes of the talus are superimposed, the tibiotalar joint is open, and the distal fibula is superimposed by the posterior half of the distal tibia.

- To obtain a lateral ankle image, begin with the patient in a supine position, with the leg extended (Figure 5-52) and the foot dorsiflexed until its long axis forms a 90-degree angle with the lower leg. Rotate the patient and affected leg until the lateral foot surface is against the IR, then

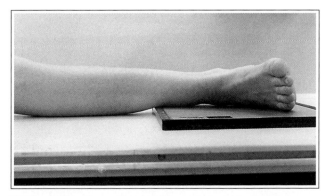

Figure 5-52. Proper knee and lower leg positioning for lateral ankle image.

adjust the degree of rotation until the surface is aligned parallel with the IR (Figure 5-53). For most patients this positioning places the lower leg parallel with the imaging table. If this is not the case, as with a patient with a large upper thigh, the foot and IR should be elevated until the lower leg is parallel with the imaging table.

- ***Importance of proper positioning:*** This positioning may not bring the medial plantar foot surface perpendicular to the IR. If this is so, do not try to adjust the leg in an attempt to position this surface perpendicular to the IR. The true relationship of the surface to the IR and the metatarsals to one another depends on the height of the patient's longitudinal arch and the incline of the calcaneus. Adjusting the patient's plantar surface may result in poor talar dome positioning and an erroneous longitudinal arch height.

- ***Talar domes:*** The domes of the talus are formed by the most medial and lateral aspects of the talar's trochlear surface. On a lateral ankle image, they are visualized as domed structures that articulate with the tibia and appear as one and the tibiotalar joint is open. Proximal-distal misalignment of the domes results from poor knee and lower leg positioning, and anteroposterior misalignment of the domes results from poor foot positioning.

- ***Effect of lower leg positioning on talar dome superimposition:*** Often, if the knee is not fully extended (Figure 5-54) or if the distal tibia is not elevated to place the lower leg parallel with the IR in a patient with large upper thighs, the proximal tibia is positioned farther from the imaging table than the distal tibia. The resulting image demonstrates the lateral talar dome proximal to the medial talar dome; and the height of the longitudinal arch appears less than it actually is, because the cuboid shifts anteriorly and the navicular bone moves posteriorly in this position and the talocalcaneal joint will be narrowed (see Image 40). If the distal tibia is positioned farther from the table than the proximal tibia, the medial talar dome is demonstrated proximal to the lateral dome, and the height of the longitudinal arch appears greater than it actually is, because the cuboid shifts proximally and the navicular bone moves anteriorly in this position and the talocalcaneal joint will be widened (see Image 41).

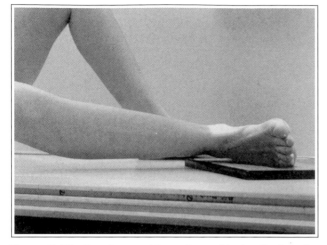

Figure 5-54. Poor knee and lower leg positioning for lateral ankle image.

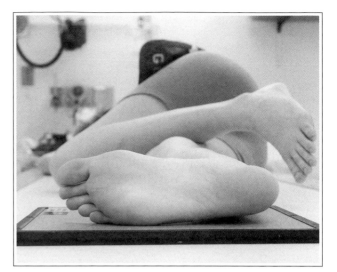

Figure 5-55. Poor foot positioning with the calcaneus elevated (leg externally rotated).

- When viewing a lateral calcaneal image that demonstrates one of the talar domes proximal to the other, evaluate the height of the longitudinal arch and the degree talocalcaneal joint visualization to determine which dome is the proximal dome. If the navicular bone is superimposed over more of the cuboid than expected and a narrowed talocalcaneal joint is seen, the lateral dome is the proximal dome. If the navicular bone is superimposed over less of the cuboid than expected and a wider talocalcaneal joint is seen, the medial dome is the proximal dome.
- ***Effect of foot positioning on talar dome superimposition:*** To demonstrate accurate anteroposterior alignment of the talar domes, position the lateral surface of the foot parallel with the IR. If this surface is not parallel with the IR, the talar domes are demonstrated one anterior to the other. When the leg is rotated more than needed to place the lateral foot surface parallel with the IR (leg externally rotated), as demonstrated in Figure 5-55, the medial talar dome is demonstrated anterior to the lateral talar dome (see Image 42). If the leg is not rotated enough to place the lateral foot surface parallel with the IR (leg internally rotated), as demonstrated in Figure 5-56, the medial talar dome is demonstrated posterior to the lateral talar dome (see Image 43).
- When taking a lateral ankle image that demonstrates one of the talar domes anterior to the other, observe the position of the fibula in relation to the tibia to determine how the patient should be repositioned. On most lateral ankle images with accurate positioning, the fibula is positioned in the posterior half of the tibia. On an image with poor positioning, if the fibula is demonstrated more posteriorly, the medial dome is anterior and the patient was positioned with the forefoot depressed and the heel elevated (leg externally rotated), as demonstrated in Figure 5-55. If the fibula is demonstrated more anteriorly, the medial domes are posterior and the patient was positioned with the forefoot elevated and the heel depressed (leg internally rotated), as demonstrated in Figure 5-56.

- Carefully evaluate lateral ankle images with poor positioning. Often, both knee and foot corrections are needed simultaneously to obtain accurate positioning.

The long axis of the foot is positioned at a 90-degree angle with the lower leg.

- In most cases, when the patient is relaxed, the foot rests in plantar flexion. Plantar flexion results in a forced flattening of the anterior pretalar fat pad, reducing its usefulness in the detection of joint effusion (see Image 44). Consequently, it is best to dorsiflex the patient's foot, placing its long axis at a 90-degree angle with the lower leg. This positioning also places the tibiotalar joint in a neutral position and helps prevent the leg from rolling too far anteriorly. Anterior foot rotation elevates the heel and rotates the foot.

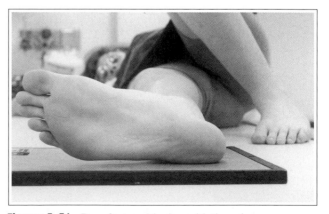

Figure 5-56. Poor foot positioning with the calcaneus depressed (leg internally rotated).

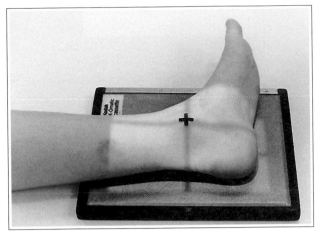

Figure 5-57. Lateral ankle image with proper central ray *(CR)* centering and collimation.

The tibiotalar joint is at the center of the collimated field. The talus, 1 inch (2.5 cm) of the fifth metatarsal base, the surrounding ankle soft tissue, and the distal fourth of the fibula and tibia are included within the field.

- Centering a perpendicular central ray to the ankle midline at the level of the palpable medial malleolus places the tibiotalar joint in the center of the collimated field (Figure 5-57).
- Open the longitudinal collimation enough to include the calcaneus and one fourth of the distal tibia and fibula. Transversely collimate to include 3 inches (7.5 cm) of the proximal forefoot, ensuring that approximately 1 inch (2.5 cm) of the fifth metatarsal base is included on the image. An inversion injury of the foot and ankle may result in a fracture of the fifth metatarsal base, known as a *Jones fracture* (Figure 5-58). Including the fifth

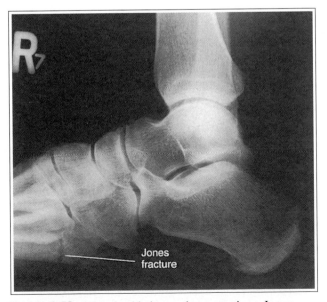

Figure 5-58. Lateral ankle image demonstrating a Jones fracture.

metatarsal base on the lateral ankle image allows it to be evaluated for a Jones fracture.

- Either one half of a 10- × 12-inch (24- × 30-cm) detailed screen-film IR placed crosswise or a single 8- × 10-inch (18- × 24-cm) computed radiography IR placed lengthwise should be adequate to include all the required anatomical structures.

Lateral Ankle Image Analysis

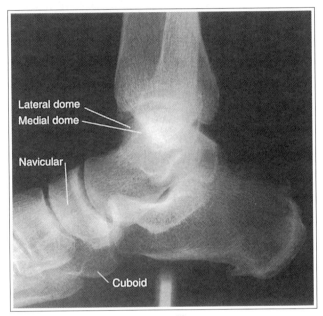

Image 40.

Analysis. The tibiotalar joint space is obscured, and one talar dome is demonstrated proximal to the other dome. Because the navicular bone is superimposed over most of the cuboid, and the talocalcaneal joint will be narrowed, the lateral dome is the proximal dome. The proximal tibia was elevated, as demonstrated in Figure 5-54.

Correction. Extend the knee to position the lower leg parallel with the IR, as demonstrated in Figure 5-52. If the knee was extended for this image, elevate the lower leg until it is positioned parallel with the IR.

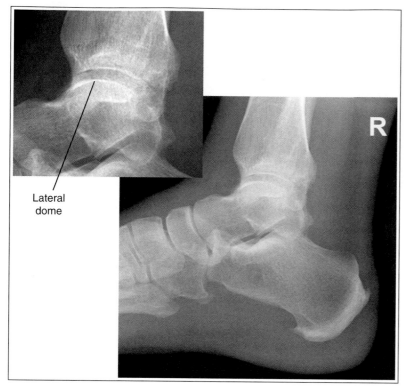

Lateral dome

Image 41.

Analysis. The tibiotalar joint space is obscured, and one talar dome is demonstrated proximal to the other dome. Because more than ½ inch (1.25 cm) of cuboid is visible posterior to the navicular bone and the talocalcaneal joint is widened, the medial dome is the proximal dome. The distal tibia was elevated.

Correction. Depress the distal lower leg until the lower leg is aligned parallel with the IR.

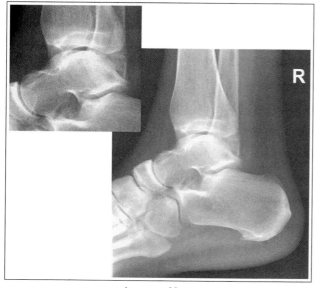

Image 42.

Analysis. The medial talar dome is positioned anterior to the lateral talar dome, as indicated by the posterior position of the fibula on the tibia. The lateral foot surface was not positioned parallel with the IR. The patient's forefoot was depressed and the heel elevated (leg externally rotated), as demonstrated in Figure 5-55.

Correction. Elevate the patient's forefoot, and depress the heel (internally rotate the leg) until the lateral foot surface is parallel with the IR, as demonstrated in Figure 5-53.

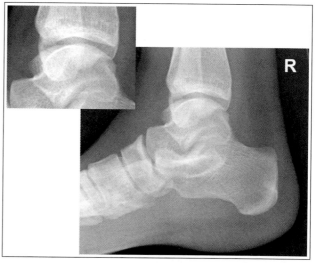

Image 43.

Analysis. The medial talar dome is positioned posterior to the lateral dome, as indicated by the anterior position of the distal fibula on the tibia. The lateral foot surface was positioned not parallel with the IR, but with the forefoot elevated and the heel depressed (leg internally rotate), as demonstrated in Figure 5-56.

Correction. Depress the forefoot and elevate the heel (externally rotate the leg) until the lateral foot surface is positioned parallel with the IR, as demonstrated in Figure 5-53.

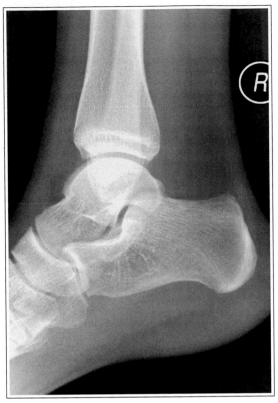

Image 44.

Analysis. The lower leg and long axis of the foot do not form a 90-degree angle. The patient's foot was in plantar flexion.

Correction. Dorsiflex the foot until the lower leg and long axis of the foot form a 90-degree angle with the lower leg.

LOWER LEG: ANTEROPOSTERIOR PROJECTION

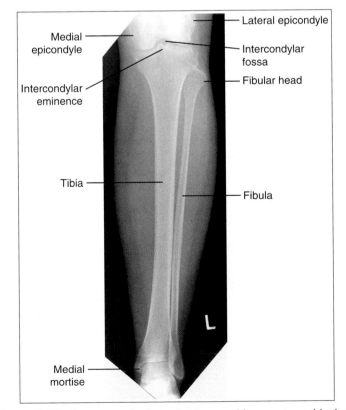

Figure 5-59. Anteroposterior lower leg image with accurate positioning.

Image Analysis

Image density is uniform across the lower leg.

- *Anode-heel effect:* A factor that should be considered when positioning the lower leg is the anode-heel effect. Because a long (17-inch [43-cm]) field is used for the length of the adult lower leg, a difference in intensity of the beam is present between the cathode and anode ends of the IR. This noticeable intensity variation is a result of increased photon absorption at the thicker, "heel" portion of the anode compared with the thinner, "toe" portion when a long field is used. Consequently, image density at the anode end of the tube is less than that at the cathode end.

- Using this knowledge to your advantage can help you produce images of the lower leg that demonstrate uniform density at both ends. Position the thicker proximal lower leg at the cathode end of the tube and the thinner distal lower leg at the anode end. Then set an exposure (mAs) that adequately demonstrates the proximal lower leg. Because the anode will absorb some of the photons aimed at the anode end of the IR, the distal lower leg, which requires less exposure than the proximal lower leg, will not be overexposed.

The lower leg demonstrates an AP projection.
The tibia demonstrates only minimal superimposition of the proximal and distal fibula, and the fibular midshaft is demonstrated free of tibial superimposition.

- To obtain an AP projection of the lower leg, place the patient in a supine position with the knee fully extended and the foot placed vertically. Dorsiflex the foot to a 90-degree angle with the lower leg (Figure 5-60).

- *Detecting lower leg rotation:* Rotation of the lower leg can be identified on an AP lower leg image by evaluating the relationship of the fibula to the tibia. When the patient's leg is externally (laterally) rotated, the fibula shifts toward and eventually beneath the tibia, obscuring the medial mortise (see Image 45). When the patient's leg is internally (medially) rotated, the head of the fibula draws from beneath the tibia (see Image 46).

- *Positioning for fracture:* For a patient with a known or suspected fracture who is unable to position both the ankle and knee into an AP projection simultaneously, position the joint closer to the fracture in the truer position. When the fracture is situated closer to the ankle, the ankle should meet the preceding requirements for a true distal lower leg AP projection (see Image 47). When the fracture is situated closer to the knee, the knee should meet the requirements for accurate positioning for a proximal lower leg AP projection. Depending on the degree of tibial and fibular rotation at the fracture site, the other joint may or may not be accurately positioned for an AP projection.

The knee and tibiotalar joint spaces are closed.

- The proximal tibia slopes distally from the anterior condylar margin to the posterior condylar margin by approximately 5 degrees. When the lower leg is placed parallel with the IR and the central ray is centered to the midshaft of the lower leg, x-rays that diverge in the opposite direction are used to record the image of the proximal tibia (Figure 5-61). The distal lower leg also slopes distally from the anterior tibial margin to the posterior margin by approximately 3 degrees. Although the x-rays diverge in the same direction as the slope of the distal tibia, they diverge at a greater angle. Because the angle of x-ray divergence is not aligned parallel with either the proximal or distal tibia, the knee and ankle joints are demonstrated as closed spaces on an AP lower leg image.

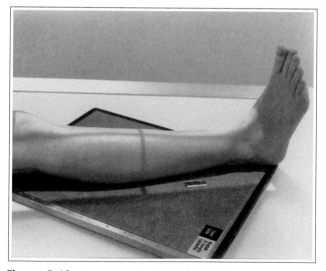

Figure 5-60. Proper patient positioning for anteroposterior lower leg image.

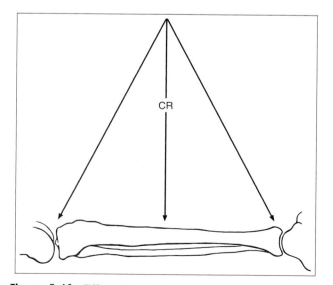

Figure 5-61. Effect of x-ray divergence on anteroposterior lower leg image. *CR*, Central ray.

The tibial midshaft is at the center of the collimated field. The tibia, fibula, ankle, knee, and surrounding lower leg soft tissue are included within the field.

- A perpendicular central ray is centered to the midpoint of the lower leg to place it in the center of the image.
- To include the ankle and knee joints on the image, you must consider the degree of x-ray beam divergence that occurs when a long body part is imaged (see Figure 5-61). A 14- × 17-inch (35- × 43-cm) detailed screen-film or computed radiography IR, placed diagonally, should be adequate to include both the ankle and the knee. To ensure that both joints are included, the film should extend 1 to 1½ inches (2.5 to 4 cm) beyond each joint space. The ankle is located at the level of the medial malleolus, and the knee joint is located 1 inch (2.5 cm) distal to the palpable medial epicondyle.
- Once the lower leg is accurately positioned with the IR, center the central ray to the midpoint of the lower leg and open the longitudinal collimation field until it extends just beyond both the knee and the ankle. For patients with long lower legs, it may be necessary to raise the source-image receptor distance (SID) above the standard 40 inches (102 cm) to obtain a longitudinally collimated field long enough to include both joints on the same IR. Transverse collimation should be to within ½ inch (1.25 cm) of the lower leg skinline.

Anteroposterior Lower Leg Image Analysis

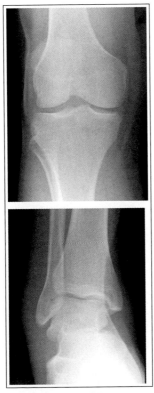

Image 45.

Analysis. This is an externally rotated AP knee and ankle image to simulate the way an externally rotated AP tibial image would appear.

Correction. Internally (medially) rotate the leg until the foot is vertical.

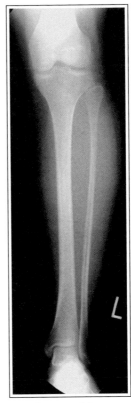

Image 46.

Analysis. The proximal and distal fibula demonstrate minimal tibial superimposition. The leg was medially (internally) rotated.

Correction. Laterally (externally) rotate the leg until the foot is vertical.

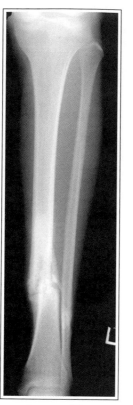

Image 47.

Analysis. A distal tibial and fibular fracture is present. The ankle joint is positioned in a true AP projection, but the knee joint demonstrates medial rotation. This rotation is caused by rotation at the fracture site.

Correction. No corrective movement is required.

LOWER LEG: LATERAL POSITION (MEDIOLATERAL PROJECTION)

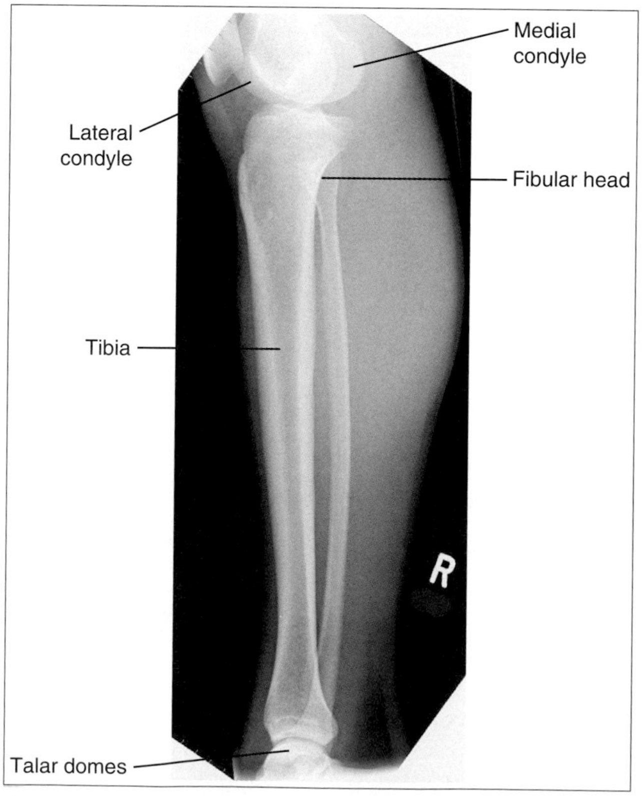

Figure 5-62. Lateral lower leg image with accurate positioning.

Image Analysis

Image density is uniform across the lower leg.

- *Anode-heel effect:* To take advantage of the anode-heel effect, position the thicker proximal lower leg at the cathode end of the tube and the thinner distal lower leg at the anode end. Then set an exposure (mAs) that will adequately demonstrate the midpoint of the lower leg. Because the anode absorbs some of the photons aimed at the anode end of the IR, the distal lower leg, which requires less exposure than the proximal lower leg, will not be overexposed.

The lower leg demonstrates a lateral position. The distal fibula is superimposed by the posterior half of the distal tibia. The fibular midshaft is free of tibial superimposition. The tibia is partially superimposed over the fibular head, and the medial femoral condyle is demonstrated posterior to the lateral condyle if the leg is extended; the condyles are superimposed if the knee is flexed at least 30 degrees (compare Figure 5-62 and Image 48).

- To obtain a lateral lower leg image, begin by placing the patient in a supine position with the leg extended and the foot dorsiflexed until it forms a 90-degree angle with the lower leg. Next, rotate the leg, positioning the lateral foot surface against the IR and the femoral epicondyles perpendicular to the IR (Figure 5-63).
- *Detecting leg rotation:* If the distal lower leg was not placed in a lateral position, the tibiofibular relationship is altered. If the patient's leg was externally rotated (patella positioned too close to the IR and heel elevated off the IR), the distal fibula is situated too far posterior on the tibia, and the fibular head is demonstrated free of tibial superimposition (see Image 49). If the patient's leg was internally rotated (patella positioned too far away from IR and forefoot elevated off the IR), the distal fibula is situated too far anterior on the tibia and the fibular head and neck, and possibly the midshaft is superimposed by the tibia (see Image 50).

- Superimposition of the femoral condyles is not a good indication of rotation on a lateral lower leg image. The amount of their superimposition depends on the degree of knee flexion and the way in which the diverged x-ray beams are aligned with the medial condyle. See p. 317 (lateral knee) for a discussion of central ray alignment and the superimposition of the femoral condyles.
- *Positioning for fracture:* For a patient with a known or suspected fracture who is unable to position both the ankle and knee into a lateral position simultaneously, position the joint closer to the fracture in the truer position. If the fracture is situated closer to the distal lower leg, the distal lower leg should meet the preceding requirements for a true lateral position. If the fracture is situated closer to the proximal lower leg, the proximal lower leg should meet the preceding requirements for a lateral position. Depending on the degree of tibial and fibular rotation at the fracture site, the other end of the lower leg may or may not be in a lateral position.

The tibial midshaft is at the center of the collimated field. The tibia, fibula, ankle, knee, and surrounding lower leg soft tissue are included within the field.

- A perpendicular central ray is centered to the midpoint of the lower leg to demonstrate the tibial midshaft in the center of the image.
- To include the ankle and knee joints on the image, you must consider the degree of x-ray beam divergence that occurs while imaging of a long body part. A 14- × 17-inch (35- × 43-cm) detailed screen-film or computed radiography IR, placed diagonally, should be adequate to include both the ankle and the knee. To ensure that both joints are included, the IR should extend 1 inch (2.5 cm) beyond each joint space. The ankle is located at the level of the medial malleolus, and the knee is located 1 inch (2.5 cm) distal to the palpable medial epicondyle.

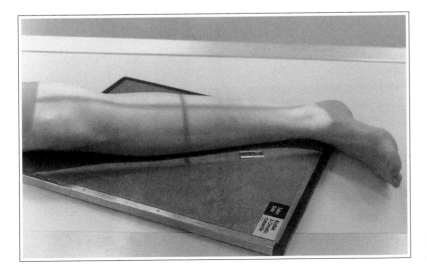

Figure 5-63. Proper patient positioning for lateral lower leg image.

- Once the lower leg is accurately positioned with the IR, center the central ray to the midshaft of the tibia, and open the longitudinal collimation until it extends just beyond both the knee and the ankle. For patients with long lower legs that have to be placed diagonally on the IR, it may be necessary to raise the SID above the standard 40 inches (102 cm) to obtain a longitudinally collimated field long enough to include both joints on the same image. Transverse collimation should be to within ½ inch (1.25 cm) of the lower leg skinline.

Lateral Lower Leg Image Analysis

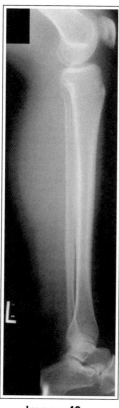

Image 48.

Analysis. The distal and proximal ends of the fibula are superimposed by the tibia, whereas the fibular midshaft is free of superimposition. The knee is flexed approximately 45 degrees, and the femoral condyles are superimposed.

Correction. No corrective movement is required, although knee flexion may result in elevation of the proximal lower leg and foreshortening of the tibia and fibula.

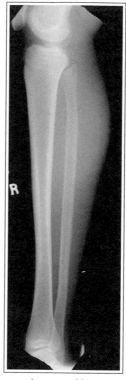

Image 49.

Analysis. The distal fibula is situated too far posterior on the tibia, and the fibular head is free of tibial superimposition. The leg was externally rotated.

Correction. Internally rotate the leg until the lateral foot surface is positioned parallel with the IR.

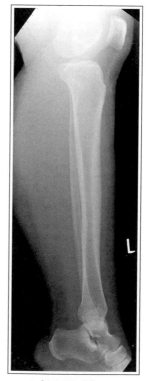

Image 50.

Analysis. The distal fibula is situated too far anterior on the tibia and the fibular head and midshaft are superimposed by the tibia. The leg was internally rotated.

Correction. Externally rotate the leg until the lateral foot surface is positioned parallel with the IR.

KNEE: ANTEROPOSTERIOR PROJECTION

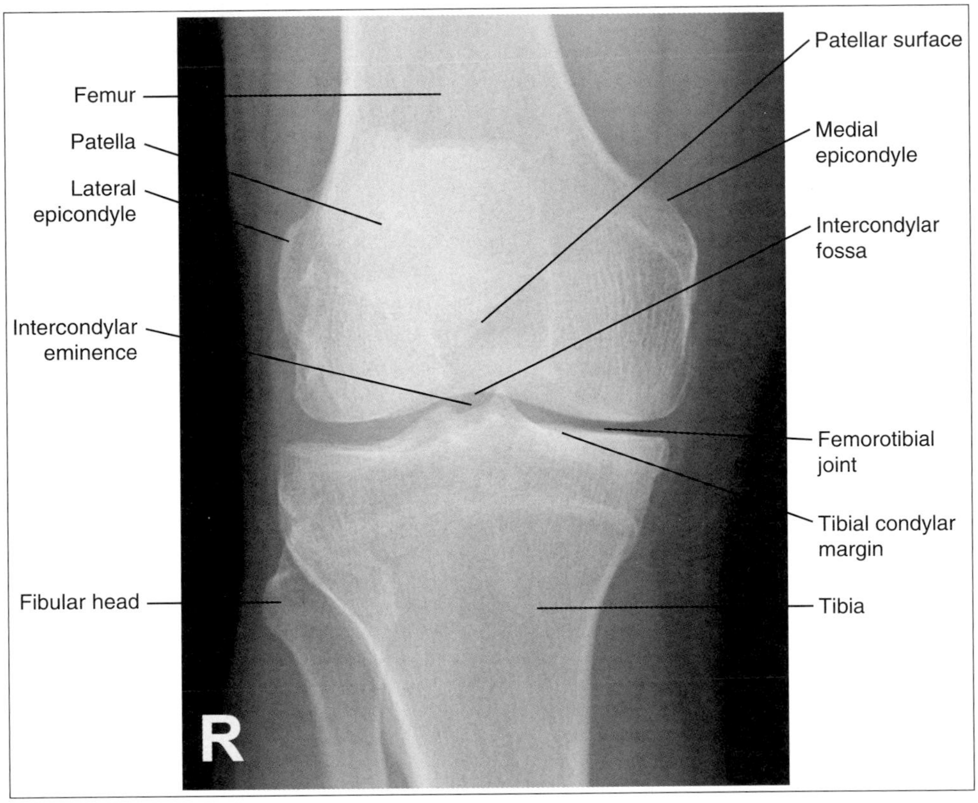

Femur

Patella

Lateral epicondyle

Intercondylar eminence

Fibular head

Patellar surface

Medial epicondyle

Intercondylar fossa

Femorotibial joint

Tibial condylar margin

Tibia

R

Figure 5-64. Anteroposterior knee image with accurate positioning.

Image Analysis

The knee demonstrates an AP projection. The medial and lateral femoral epicondyles are demonstrated in profile, the femoral condyles are symmetrical, the intercondylar eminence is centered within the intercondylar fossa, and the tibia is superimposed over $1/4$ inch (0.6 cm) of the fibular head.

- To obtain an AP knee image, place the patient in a supine position with the knee fully extended. Internally rotate the leg until an imaginary line drawn between the medial and lateral femoral epicondyles is positioned parallel with the IR (Figure 5-65). This positioning places the medial and lateral femoral epicondyles at equal distances from the IR as well as medially and laterally in profile, respectively. It also centers the intercondylar eminence within the intercondylar fossa and draws the fibular neck and a portion of the fibular head from beneath the tibia.

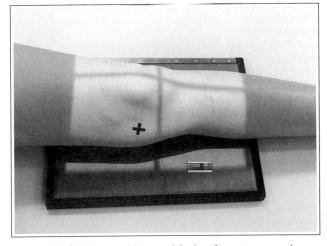

Figure 5-65. Proper patient positioning for anteroposterior knee image.

- **Effect of rotation:** If the femoral epicondyles are not positioned parallel with the IR, an AP projection has not been obtained. If the patient's leg was not internally rotated enough to place the epicondyles at equal distances from the IR, they are not in profile, the medial femoral condyle appears larger than the lateral condyle, and the tibia is superimposed over more than ¼ inch (0.6 cm) of the fibular head (see Image 51). If the patient's leg was internally rotated more than needed to place the femoral epicondyles at equal distances from the IR, the epicondyles are not demonstrated in profile, the lateral femoral condyle appears larger than the medial condyle, and the tibia is superimposed over less than ¼ inch (0.6 cm) of the fibular head (see Image 52).

The knee joint space is open, the anterior and posterior condylar margins of the tibia are superimposed, the intercondylar eminence and tubercles are demonstrated in profile, and the fibular head is demonstrated approximately ½ inch (1.25 cm) distal to the tibial plateau.

- The anterior and posterior condylar margins of the tibia are superimposed if the correct central ray angulation, as determined by the patient's upper thigh and buttocks thickness, is used. By studying the tibial plateau region, you will see that the tibial plateau slopes distally approximately 5 degrees from the anterior condylar margin to the posterior condylar margin on both the medial and lateral aspects (Figure 5-66). Only if the

central ray is aligned parallel with the tibial plateau slope is an open knee joint space obtained.

- **Determining the central ray angulation:** When a patient is placed in a supine position, the degree and direction of the central ray angulation required depends on the thickness of the patient's upper thigh and buttocks. This thickness determines how the lower leg and the tibial plateau align with the IR. Figure 5-67 shows a guideline that can be used to determine the central ray angulation for different body sizes; it illustrates the relationship of the tibial plateau to the imaging table as the patient's upper thigh thickness increases. Note that a decrease occurs in femoral decline, and a shift occurs in the direction of the tibial plateau slope as the thickness of the thigh decreases. Because of this plateau shift, the central ray angulation must also be adjusted to keep it parallel with the plateau and to achieve an open knee joint.

- For optimal AP knee images, measure from the patient's anterior superior iliac spine (ASIS) to the imaging table on either side to determine the central ray angulation to use for each knee examination. When measuring this distance, do not include the patient's abdominal tissue. Keep the calipers situated laterally next to the ASIS. If the measurement is less than 18 cm, a 5-degree caudal angle should be used. If the measurement is 19 to 24 cm, a perpendicular beam should be used. If the measurement is greater than 24 cm, a 5-degree cephalad angle should be used. Using the correct central ray angulation not only

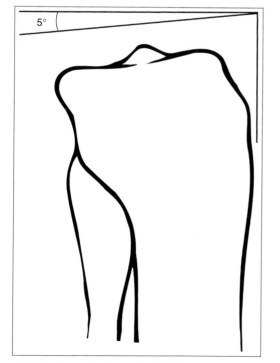

Figure 5-66. Slope of the proximal tibia. *(Reproduced with permission from Martensen K: Alternative AP knee method assures open joint space,* Radiol Technol *64:19-23, 1992. Courtesy* Radiologic Technology, *published by the American Society of Radiologic Technologists.)*

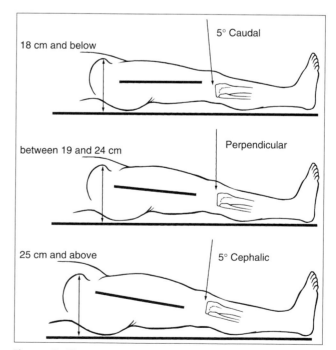

Figure 5-67. Determining central ray *(CR)* angle from the patient's thigh thickness. *(Reproduced with permission from Martensen K: Alternative AP knee method assures open joint space,* Radiol Technol *64:19-23, 1992. Courtesy* Radiologic Technology, *published by the American Society of Radiologic Technologists.)*

results in an open knee joint space but also provides optimal demonstration of the intercondylar eminence and tubercles without foreshortening.

- *Analysis of joint space narrowing:* On an AP knee image with adequate positioning, joint space narrowing is evaluated by measuring the medial and the lateral aspects of the knee joint, which are also referred to as *compartments*. The measurement of each of these compartments is obtained by determining the distance between the most distal femoral condylar surface and the posterior condylar margin of the tibia on each side. Comparison of these measurements with each other, with measurements from previous images, or with measurements of the other knee determines joint space narrowing or a valgus or varus deformity. In a *valgus deformity* the lateral compartment is narrower than the medial compartment; in a *varus deformity* the medial compartment is narrower (see Images 53 and 54).

- Precise measurements of the compartments are necessary to ensure early detection of joint space narrowing and are best obtained when the knee joint space is completely open. If an inaccurate central ray angulation was used for an AP knee image, the knee joint is narrowed or obscured, the intercondylar eminence and tubercles are foreshortened, and the tibial plateau is demonstrated.

- *Effect of poor central ray angulation:* When examining an AP knee image for which an inaccurate central ray angulation was used, you can determine how to adjust the angulation by judging the shape of the fibular head and its proximity to the tibial plateau. If the fibular head is foreshortened and demonstrated more than ½ inch (1.25 cm) distal to the tibial plateau, the cephalad angle was too great (see Image 55). If the fibular head is elongated and demonstrated less than ½ inch (1.25 cm) distal to the tibial plateau, the caudad angle was too great (see Image 56).

- *Compensating for the nonextendable knee:* If the patient is unable to fully extend the knee, an open knee joint can be obtained by doing the following:
    1. Aligning the central ray perpendicular with the anterior lower leg surface
    2. Decreasing the angulation 5 degrees; placing the central ray parallel with the tibial plateau

- For example, if the central ray is perpendicular to the anterior lower leg surface when a 15-degree cephalic angulation is used, the angle should be decreased to 10 degrees if the knee cannot be extended (see Image 57). This setup demonstrates an open knee joint space, a foreshortened distal femur and proximal lower leg, and an elongated intercondylar fossa.

The patella lies just superior to the patellar surface of the femur and is situated slightly lateral to the knee midline. The intercondylar fossa is partially demonstrated.

- The position of the patella and the degree of intercondylar fossa demonstration are determined by the amount of knee flexion. To visualize the patella and fossa as required,

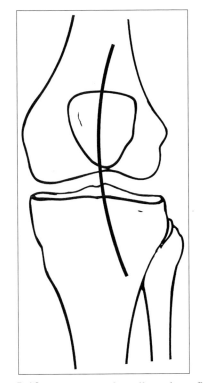

Figure 5-68. Movement of patella on knee flexion.

the leg must be in full extension. As the knee is flexed, the patella shifts distally and medially onto the patellar surface of the femur and then laterally into the intercondylar fossa, duplicating a C-shaped path that is open laterally (Figure 5-68). Thus, the patella is demonstrated at different locations depending on the degree of knee flexion. Generally, when the knee is flexed 20 degrees, the patella is demonstrated on the patellar surface. With 30 to 70 degrees of knee flexion, the patella is demonstrated between the patellar surface and the intercondylar fossa. At 90 degrees to full knee flexion, the patella is demonstrated within the intercondylar fossa.

- The extent of intercondylar fossa demonstration also changes with knee flexion. In full extension, only a slight indentation between the distal medial and lateral femoral condyles indicates the location of the intercondylar fossa. As the knee is flexed, the amount of intercondylar fossa that is demonstrated increases. When the knee is flexed to between 50 and 60 degrees, the intercondylar fossa is shown in profile (see Image 57). When the knee is flexed less than 50 degrees or more than 60 degrees, demonstration of the fossa will decrease.

- *Patellar subluxation:* With patellar subluxation (partial patellar dislocation), the patella may be situated more laterally than normal on an AP knee image (see Image 58). When an image demonstrates a laterally situated patella, evaluate the symmetry of the femoral condyles and the relationship of the tibia and fibular head to rule out external rotation before assuming that the patella is subluxed. External rotation also results in a laterally located patella.

The knee joint is at the center of the collimated field. One fourth of the distal femur and proximal lower leg and the surrounding soft tissue are included within the field.

- Center the central ray to the midline of the knee at a level 1 inch (2.5 cm) distal to the palpable medial epicondyle to place the knee joint in the center of the collimated field. (As long as the knee remains extended, an alternative central ray placement is ½ inch (1.25 cm) distal to the patellar apex.) Open the longitudinal collimation enough to include one fourth of the distal femur and proximal lower leg. Transverse collimation should be to within ½ inch (1.25 cm) of the knee skinline.

- An 8- × 10-inch (18- × 24-cm) or 10- × 12-inch (24- × 30-cm) screen-film or computed radiography IR placed lengthwise should be adequate to include all the required anatomical structures.

Anteroposterior Knee Image Analysis

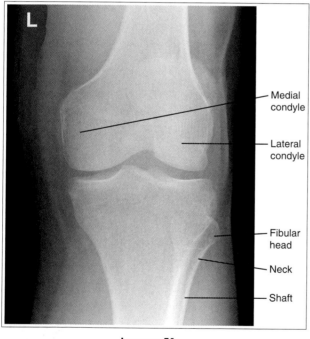

Image 51.

Analysis. The femoral epicondyles are not in profile, the medial femoral condyle appears larger than the lateral condyle, and the fibular head demonstrates more than ¼ inch (0.6 cm) of tibial superimposition. The leg was externally rotated.

Correction. Internally rotate the leg until the femoral epicondyles are at equal distances from the IR.

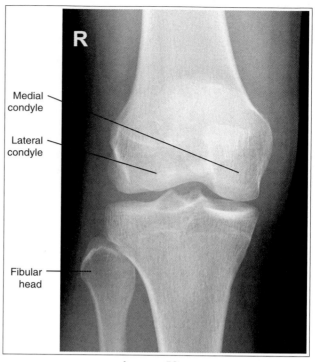

Image 52.

Analysis. The femoral epicondyles are not in profile, the lateral femoral condyle appears larger than the medial condyle, and the fibular head demonstrates less than ¼ inch (0.6 cm) of tibial superimposition. The leg was internally rotated.

Correction. Externally rotate the leg until the femoral epicondyles are at equal distances from the film.

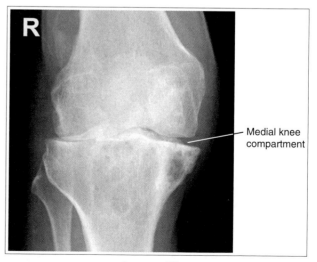

Image 53.

Analysis. The lateral knee compartment is narrower than the medial knee compartment. The patient's knee demonstrates a valgus deformity.

Correction. No corrective movement is required.

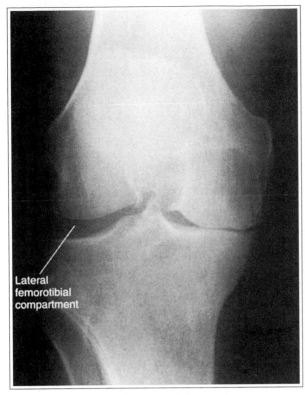

Image 54.

Analysis. The medial knee compartment is narrower than the lateral knee compartment. The patient's knee demonstrates a varus deformity.

Correction. No corrective movement is required.

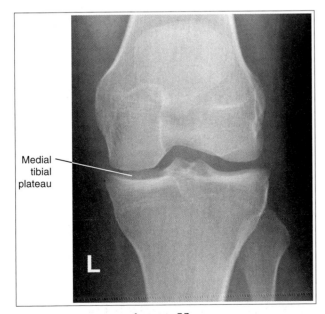

Image 55.

Analysis. The knee joint space is obscured, the medial tibial plateau is demonstrated, the fibular head is foreshortened and demonstrated more than ½ inch (1.25 cm)

distal to the tibial plateau. Excessive cephalad angulation is indicated.

Correction. Angle the central ray caudally approximately 5 degrees for every ¼ inch (0.6 cm) of tibial plateau demonstrated. For this image, approximately ½ inch (1.25 cm) of the tibial plateau is demonstrated between the anterior and posterior tibial margins. The central ray should be adjusted approximately 10 degrees, because a 5-degree cephalad angle was used. When the image is retaken, a 5-degree caudal angle should be used.

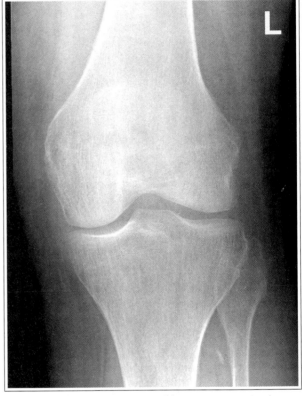

Image 56.

Analysis. The medial knee joint space is closed, the proximal ridges of the femoral condyles are convex, and the fibular head is elongated and demonstrated less than ½ inch (1.25 cm) distal to the tibial plateau. Excessive caudal angulation is indicated.

Correction. If an open medial knee joint space is desired, the central ray should be adjusted cephalically.

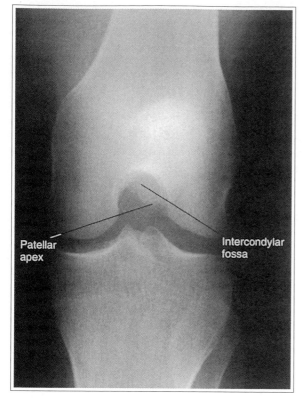

Image 57.

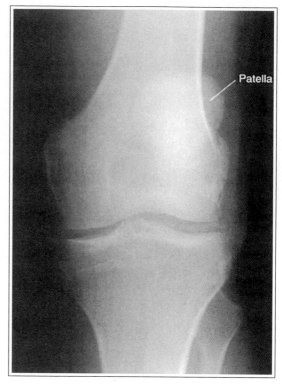

Image 58.

Analysis. This is an AP knee image taken with the knee flexed approximately 50 to 60 degrees and the central ray aligned parallel with the tibial plateau. The knee joint space is open, the intercondylar fossa is demonstrated in profile, and the patellar apex is superimposed over the intercondylar fossa. Because of the acute angle of the lower leg and femur with the IR, the distal femur and proximal lower leg are foreshortened and the intercondylar fossa is slightly elongated.

Correction. If the patient's condition allows, fully extend the knee. If the patient is unable to extend the knee, no corrective movement is required.

Analysis. The knee demonstrates no signs of rotation even though the patella is superimposed over the lateral aspect of the knee. The patient has a subluxed patella.

Correction. No corrective movement is required.

KNEE: ANTEROPOSTERIOR OBLIQUE PROJECTION (INTERNAL AND EXTERNAL ROTATION)

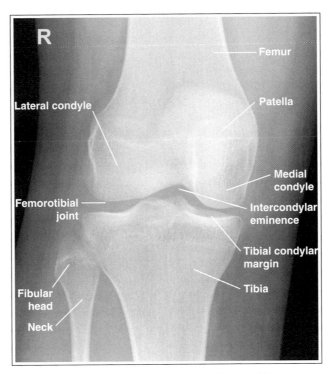

Figure 5-69. Anteroposterior (internal) oblique knee image with accurate positioning.

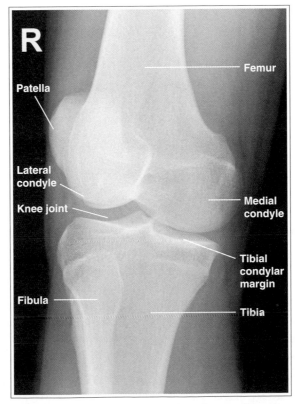

Figure 5-70. Anteroposterior (external) oblique knee image with accurate positioning.

Image Analysis

The knee joint space is open. The anterior and posterior condylar margins of the tibia are superimposed, and the fibular head is approximately ½ inch (1.25 cm) distal to the tibial plateau.

- The anterior and posterior condylar margins of the tibia are superimposed by the use of the correct central ray angulation as determined by the patient's upper thigh and buttocks thickness. By studying the tibial plateau region, you will see that the tibial plateau slopes distally approximately 5 degrees from the anterior condylar margin to the posterior condylar margin on both the medial and lateral aspects. Only if the central ray is aligned parallel with this slope is a truly open joint space obtained.

- ***Determining the central ray angulation:*** When a patient is placed in a supine position, the degree and direction of the central ray angulation required depends on the thickness of the patient's upper thigh and buttocks, because it is this thickness that will determine the central ray angulation that should be used for different body sizes. Figure 5-71 demonstrates how the relationship of the tibial plateau varies as the patient's upper thigh thickness changes.

- For optimal oblique knee images, measure each patient from the ASIS to the imaging table, after the patient has

been accurately positioned, to determine the correct central ray angulation to use for each examination. When measuring this distance, do not include the patient's abdominal tissue in the measurement. Keep the calipers situated laterally, next to the ASIS. If the measurement is 18 cm or below, a 5-degree caudal angle should be used. If the measurement is 19 to 24 cm, a perpendicular beam should be used. If the measurement is above 24 cm, a 5-degree cephalad angle should be used. It is not uncommon to require a cephalic angle for the medial oblique knee image, because the patient's hip is often elevated to accomplish the needed degree of internal obliquity, or to need a caudal angle for the lateral oblique knee image, because the patient's hip is placed closer to the imaging table to obtain the needed external obliquity.

- If an inaccurate central ray angulation was used for an oblique knee image, the knee joint space is narrowed or obscured and the anterior and posterior margins of the tibial plateau are not superimposed.

- ***Effect of poor central ray angulation:*** When evaluating an oblique knee image for which an inaccurate central ray angulation was used, you can determine how to adjust the angulation by judging the shape of the fibular head and its proximity to the tibial plateau. If the fibular head is foreshortened and demonstrated more than ½ inch (1.25 cm) distal to the tibial plateau (Image 59), the cephalad angle was too great and if the fibular head is elongated and demonstrated less than ½ inch (1.25 cm) distal to the tibial plateau, the caudad angle was too great (Image 60).

The knee joint is at the center of the collimated field. One fourth of the distal femur and the proximal lower leg are included within the field.

- The central ray should be centered to the midline of the knee at the level of the knee joint, which is located 1 inch (2.5 cm) distal to the palpable medial femoral epicondyle, to place the knee joint in the center of the collimated field. Open the longitudinal collimation to include one fourth of the distal femur and the proximal lower leg. Transverse collimation should be within ½ inch (1.25 cm) of the knee skinline.

- An 8- × 10-inch (18- × 24-cm) or 10- × 12-inch (24- × 30-cm) screen-film or computed radiography IR placed lengthwise should be adequate to include all the required anatomical structures.

INTERNAL (MEDIAL) OBLIQUE POSITION

The knee has been rotated 45 degrees internally. The fibular head is demonstrated free of tibial superimposition, and the lateral femoral condyle is visible in profile without medial condyle superimposition.

- An AP (internal) oblique knee image with accurate positioning is obtained by placing the patient in an AP knee projection, then internally rotating the leg until an

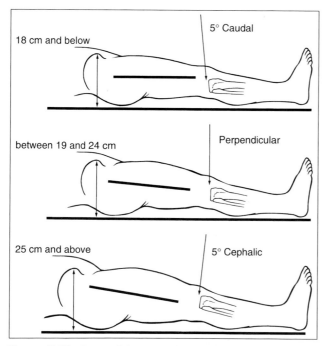

Figure 5-71. Determining central ray (*CR*) angle from the patient's thigh thickness. (*Reproduced with permission from Martensen K: Alternative AP knee method assures open joint space,* Radiol Technol *64:19-23, 1992. Courtesy Radiologic Technology, published by the American Society of Radiologic Technologists.*)

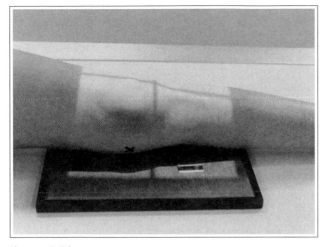

Figure 5-72. Proper patient positioning for anteroposterior (internal) oblique knee image.

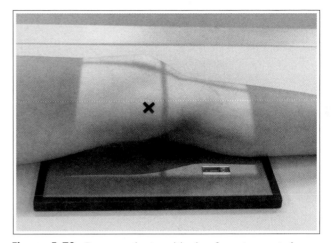

Figure 5-73. Proper patient positioning for anteroposterior (external) oblique knee image. X indicates medial femoral epicondyle.

imaginary line drawn between the medial and lateral femoral epicondyles is positioned at a 45-degree angle with the IR (Figure 5-72). This position places the lateral condyle in profile and rotates the fibular head from beneath the tibia, opening the proximal tibiofibular articulation. If the femoral epicondyles are rotated less than 45 degrees with the IR, the tibia is partially superimposed over the fibular head (see Image 60). If the femoral epicondyles are rotated more than 45 degrees with the IR, the femoral condyles are nearly superimposed (see Image 61).

EXTERNAL (LATERAL) OBLIQUE POSITION
The knee has been rotated 45 degrees externally. The fibular head, neck, and shaft are superimposed by the tibia, and the fibular head is aligned with the anterior edge of the tibia. The external femoral condyle is demonstrated in profile without lateral condyle superimposition.

- An AP (external) oblique knee image with accurate positioning is obtained by placing the patient in an AP knee projection, then externally rotating the leg until an imaginary line drawn between the medial and lateral femoral epicondyles is positioned at a 45-degree angle with the IR (Figure 5-73). This position places the medial condyle in profile and rotates the tibia onto the fibula, demonstrating superimposition of the tibia and fibula on the image. If the femoral epicondyles are rotated less than 45 degrees with the IR, the fibular head demonstrates decreased tibial superimposition or will be positioned more toward the center of the tibia (see Image 62). If the femoral epicondyles are rotated more than 45 degrees with the IR, the fibular head is not aligned with the anterior edge of the tibia but is posterior to the placement. The more posteriorly situated the fibula is, the farther away from 45 degrees the patient was positioned (see Image 63).

Anteroposterior Oblique Knee Image Analysis

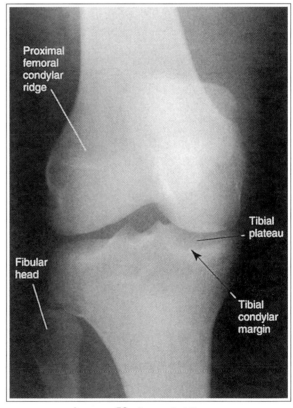

Image 59. Internal oblique.

Analysis. The fibular head is demonstrated without tibial superimposition, and the lateral femoral condyle is demonstrated in profile, indicating accurate obliquity. The knee joint space is obscured, the fibular head is foreshortened and demonstrated more than ½ inch (1.25 cm) distal to the tibial plateau. The central ray angulation was too cephalad.

Correction. Decrease the degree of central ray angulation approximately 5 degrees for every ¼ inch (0.6 cm) of tibial plateau demonstrated. For this image, approximately ¼ inch of the tibial plateau is demonstrated between the anterior and posterior tibial margins; therefore the central ray should be adjusted approximately 5 degrees.

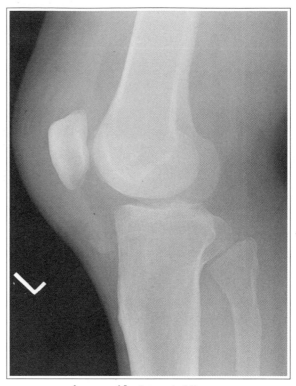

Image 61. Internal oblique.

Analysis. The medial femoral condyle is superimposed over most of the lateral condyle. The patient's knee was rotated more than 45 degrees.

Correction. Decrease the medial knee obliquity until the femoral epicondyles are aligned at a 45-degree angle with the IR.

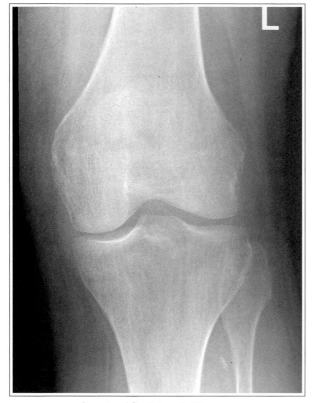

Image 60. Internal oblique.

Analysis. The tibia is partially superimposed over the fibular head. The patient's knee was rotated less than 45 degrees. The joint space is closed, and the fibular head is elongated and demonstrated less than ½ inch (1.25 cm) from the tibial plateau. The central ray angulation was too caudal.

Correction. Increase the medial knee obliquity until the femoral epicondyles are aligned at a 45-degree angle with the IR. Increase the degree of central ray angulation approximately 5 degrees for every ¼ inch (0.6 cm) of tibial plateau demonstrated.

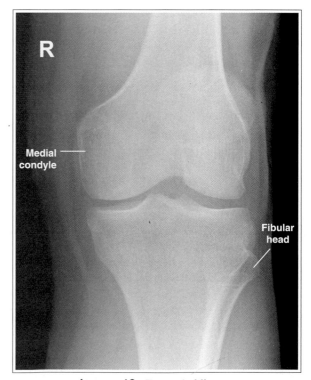

Image 62. External oblique.

Analysis. The fibular head, neck, and shaft are not super-imposed by the tibia. The patient's knee was rotated less than 45 degrees.

Correction. Increase the lateral knee obliquity until the femoral epicondyles are aligned at a 45-degree angle with the IR.

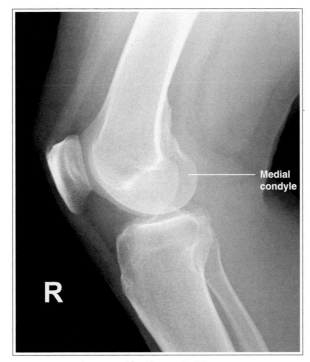

Image 63. External oblique.

Analysis. The fibular head is not aligned with the anterior edge of the tibia but is demonstrated posterior to this placement, and the femoral condyles and the medial condyle are nearly superimposed; the medial condyle is posterior. The patient's knee was rotated more than 45 degrees.

Correction. Decrease the lateral knee obliquity until the femoral epicondyles are aligned at a 45-degree angle with the IR.

KNEE: LATERAL POSITION (MEDIOLATERAL PROJECTION)

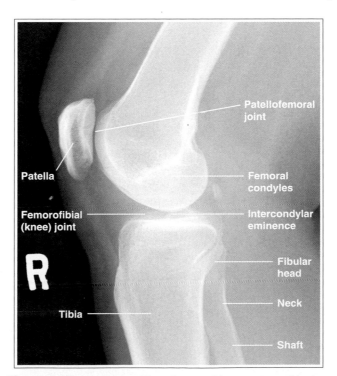

Figure 5-74. Mediolateral knee image with accurate positioning.

Image Analysis

Contrast and density are adequate to demonstrate the suprapatellar fat pads.

- *Suprapatellar fat pads:* Two soft-tissue structures of interest at the knee are used to diagnose joint effusion and knee injury. They are the posterior and anterior suprapatellar fat pads. Both are located anterior to the patellar surface of the distal femur and are separated by the suprapatellar bursa (Figure 5-75). Fluid that collects in the suprapatellar bursa causes the anterior and posterior suprapatellar fat pads to separate. It is a widening of this space that indicates a diagnosis of joint effusion.

The patella is situated proximal to the patellar surface of the femur, and the patellofemoral joint is open.

- The knee should be flexed 10 to 15 degrees. With less than 20 degrees of knee flexion, the patella is situated proximal to the patellar surface of the femur, the quadriceps are relaxed, and the patella is fairly mobile. In this patellar position the anterior and posterior suprapatellar fat pads can be easily used to evaluate knee joint effusion. Conversely, when the knee is flexed 20 degrees or more, a tightening of the surrounding knee muscles and tendons is present, the patella comes into contact with the patellar surface of the femur, and the anterior and posterior suprapatellar fat pads are obscured, eliminating their usefulness in diagnosing joint effusion (see Image 64).
- Some authors indicate that 20 to 30 degrees of knee flexion should be used on a lateral knee. Facility routines dictate the actual number of degrees that should be used.

- *Positioning for fracture:* If a patellar or other knee fracture is suspected, the knee should remain extended to prevent displacement of bony fragments or vascular injury.

The distal articulating surfaces of the medial and lateral femoral condyles are superimposed, and the knee joint space is open.

- Take a few minutes to study a femoral bone. Place it upright with the distal femoral condylar surfaces resting against a flat surface. Notice how the femoral shaft inclines medially approximately 10 to 15 degrees. When a patient is in an erect position, this is how the femurs are positioned. This femoral incline gives the body stability (Figure 5-76). The amount of inclination a person displays depends on pelvic width and femoral shaft length. The wider the pelvis and the shorter the femoral shaft length, the more medially the femora incline.
- When the patient is placed in a recumbent lateral position for a lateral knee image (Figure 5-77), some of the

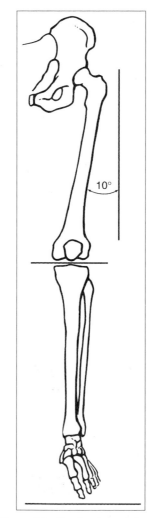

Figure 5-76. Femoral inclination in upright position. *(Reproduced with permission from Martensen K: The knee, In-Service Reviews in Radiologic Technology, vol 14, no 7, Birmingham, Ala, 1991, In-Service Reviews.)*

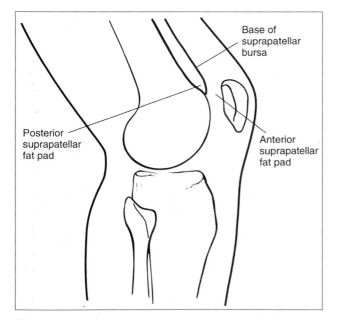

Figure 5-75. Location of suprapatellar fat pads. *(Reproduced with permission from Martensen K: The knee, In-Service Reviews in Radiologic Technology, vol 14, no 7, Birmingham, Ala, 1991, In-Service Reviews.)*

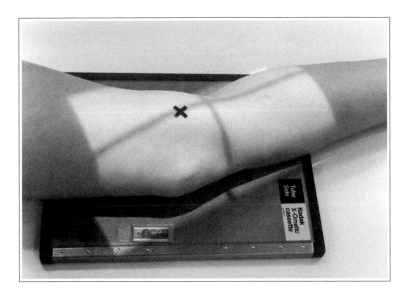

Figure 5-77. Proper patient positioning for lateral knee image. X indicates medial femoral epicondyle.

medial femoral inclination is reduced, resulting in projection of the medial condyle distal to the lateral condyle and into the knee joint space (Figure 5-78). This can be demonstrated by laying the femoral bone on its lateral side. Note how the distal condylar surfaces are no longer on the same plane. The medial condyle is situated distal to the lateral condyle. The amount of distance demonstrated between these two condyles depends on the amount of medial femoral incline the femur displayed in the upright position, the length of the femur, and the width of the pelvis from which the femur originated. If the medial condyle remains in this distal position, it obscures the knee joint space on the image. This is why a cephalic angle is needed for most lateral knee images.

- **Determining central ray angulation:** Because the degree of femoral inclination varies among patients, so must the degree of central ray angulation. For a patient with a wide pelvis and short femora, a 5- to 7-degree cephalad angle is the most reliable angulation to use. For a patient with a narrow pelvis and long femora, very little if any angulation is required. Although females commonly demonstrate greater pelvic width and femoral inclination and males demonstrate narrower pelvic width and femoral inclination, variations occur in both sexes. Each patient's pelvic width and femoral length should be evaluated to determine the degree of angulation to use.

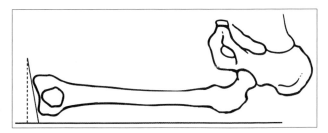

Figure 5-78. Reduction in femoral inclination in supine position.

- **Effect of central ray angulation on femoral condylar superimposition:** If an inaccurate central ray angulation is used on a lateral knee image, the distal articulating surfaces of the femoral condyles are not superimposed on the image. Whenever this occurs, the knee joint space is narrowed or closed. If a patient required a cephalic angulation to project the medial condyle proximally, but no angle was used, the image demonstrates the distal articulating surface of the medial condyle distal to the distal articulating surface of the lateral condyle (see Image 65). If a patient did not require a cephalic angulation but one was used, or if the cephalad angle was too great, the distal surface of the medial condyle is projected proximal to the distal surface of the lateral condyle (see Image 66). It should also be noted that the tibiofibular joint is better visualized on this image because the proximal tibia is moved proximally, somewhat off the fibular head.

- **Distinguishing lateral and medial condyles:** The first step you should take when evaluating an image on which the distal condylar surfaces are not aligned is to determine which condyle is the lateral and which is the medial. The most reliable method for identifying the medial condyle is to locate the rounded bony tubercle known as the *adductor tubercle.* It is located posteriorly on the medial aspect of the femur, just superior to the medial condyle. The size and shape of the tubercle are not identical on every patient, although this surface is considerably different from the same surface on the lateral condyle, which is smooth. Once the adductor tubercle is located, the medial condyle is also identified. Another difference between the medial and lateral condyles is evident on their distal articulating surfaces. The distal surface of the medial condyle is convex, and the distal surface of the lateral condyle is flat.

- **Supine (cross-table) lateral knee image:** When a lateral knee image is taken with the patient supine, with the IR placed against the medial or lateral aspect of the knee, and with a horizontal central ray, the cephalad central ray angulation is not required, as long as the patient's femoral inclination is not reduced by shifting the distal femur laterally.

The anterior and posterior surfaces of the medial and lateral femoral condyles are superimposed, and the tibia is partially superimposed over the fibular head.

- How the central ray is aligned with the femur determines the relationship between the tibia and fibula, especially when a cephalic angulation is used. Study a femoral bone that is positioned in a mediolateral projection with the femoral epicondyles placed directly on top of each other. Note that in this position the medial condyle is situated not only distal but also posterior to the lateral condyle, indicating that the medial condyle must be projected proximally and anteriorly for it to be super-imposed over the lateral condyle.

- ***Positioning to superimpose the anterior and posterior aspects of the femoral condyles:*** Two positioning methods can be used to accomplish this goal. For the first and easier method, position the femoral epicondyles directly on top of each other, so that an imaginary line drawn between them is perpendicular to the IR. Then, direct the central ray across the femur, as indicated in Figure 5-79. With this method the central ray projects the medial

condyle anteriorly and proximally. This method also demonstrates the fibular head partially superimposed by the tibia, which is an accurate lateral tibiofibular relationship (see Figure 5-74).

- For the second method, align the femoral epicondyles perpendicular to the IR, then roll the patient's patella toward the IR approximately ¼ inch (0.6 cm) to move the medial condyle anteriorly onto the lateral condyle. Finally, align the central ray with the femur as demonstrated in Figure 5-80, projecting the medial condyle proximally. This method produces an image on which the condyles are superimposed but the fibular head is demonstrated without tibial superimposition (see Image 67). Regardless of the method your facility prefers, a true lateral knee image has not been obtained unless the condyles are superimposed.

- ***Effect of knee rotation on femoral condylar superimposition:*** When an image is obtained that demonstrates one femoral condyle anterior to the other, the patella must be rolled closer to (leg externally rotated) or farther away from (leg internally rotated) the IR for superimposed condyles to be obtained. The first step in determining which way to roll the knee is to distinguish one condyle from the other. As described previously, the most reliable method is to locate the adductor tubercle of the medial condyle. When a lateral knee image is obtained that demonstrates the adductor tubercle and

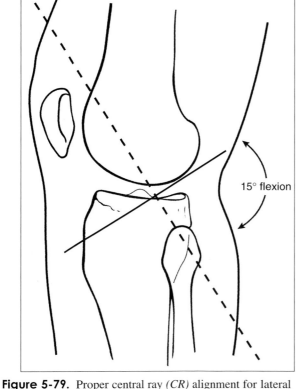

Figure 5-79. Proper central ray *(CR)* alignment for lateral knee image. *(Reproduced with permission from Martensen K: The knee, In-Service Reviews in Radiologic Technology, vol 14, no 7, Birmingham, Ala, 1991, In-Service Reviews.)*

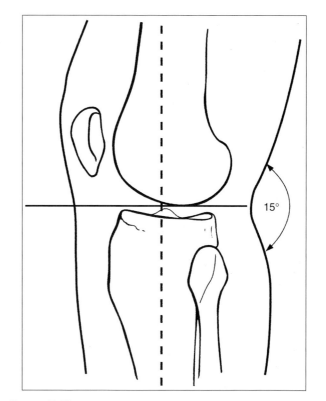

Figure 5-80. Central ray *(CR)* aligned with femur for lateral knee image. *(Reproduced with permission from Martensen K: The knee, In-Service Reviews in Radiologic Technology, vol 14, no 7, Birmingham, Ala, 1991, In-Service Reviews.)*

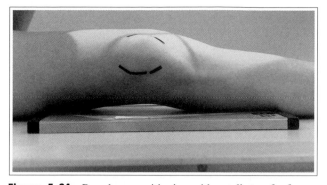

Figure 5-81. Poor knee positioning with patella too far from image receptor (leg internally rotated).

medial condyle posterior to the lateral condyle, the patella was situated too far from the IR (leg internally rotated) (Figure 5-81 and Image 68). When a lateral knee image is obtained that demonstrates the medial condyle anterior to the lateral condyle, the patella was situated too close to the IR (leg externally rotated) (Figure 5-82 and Image 69).

- Another method used to determine knee rotation is to view the tibiofibular relationship to determine how to reposition for poorly superimposed condyles. If the tibia is superimposed over the fibular head, the patella was positioned too far from the IR. If the fibular head is free of tibial superimposition, the patella was positioned too close to the IR. Although this relationship is reliable for most patients, the alignment of the central ray affects the results. Image 70 demonstrates such a case. Those using the adductor tubercle and medial condyle to determine how this patient should be repositioned would roll the patient's patella toward the IR (externally rotated leg). Those using the tibiofibular relationship would roll the patient's patella away from the IR (internally rotated leg). The adductor tubercle method is more reliable. This patient's patella needed to be rolled toward the IR to superimpose the condyles. It should also be noted that the tibiofibular relationship should not be used when the patient's knee is flexed

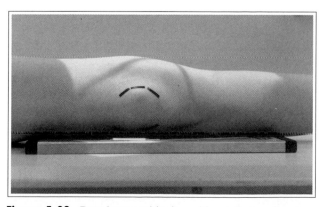

Figure 5-82. Poor knee positioning with patella too close to image receptor (leg externally rotated).

approximately 90 degrees (see Image 5-71). When the patient's knee is flexed to this degree, it is femoral elevation and depression that determine the tibiofibular relationship, not leg rotation. To best understand this change, view the skeletal leg in a lateral position with 90 degrees of leg flexion. Observe how the tibiofibular relationship results in increased tibial superimposition of the fibula when the proximal femur is elevated and a decreased tibial superimposition of the fibula as the proximal femur is depressed.

The knee joint is at the center of the collimated field. One fourth of the distal femur and proximal lower leg are included within the field.

- Center the central ray to the midline of the knee at the level of the knee joint space, which is located 1 inch (2.5 cm) distal to the palpable medial epicondyle, to center the knee joint in the collimated field. Open the longitudinal collimation enough to include one fourth of the distal femur and proximal lower leg. Transverse collimation should be to within ½ inch (1.25 cm) of the knee skinline.
- An 8- × 10-inch (18- × 24-cm) or 10- × 12-inch (24- × 30-cm) screen-film or computed radiography IR placed lengthwise should be adequate to include all the required anatomical structures.

Lateral Knee Image Analysis

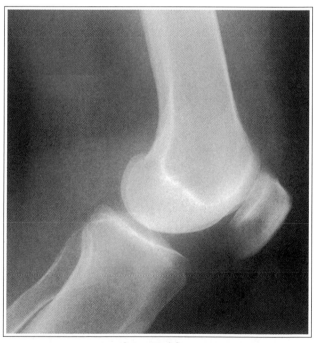

Image 64.

Analysis. The patient's knee is overflexed, the patella is in contact with the patellar surface of the femur, and the suprapatellar fat pads are obscured.

Correction. Decrease the amount of knee flexion.

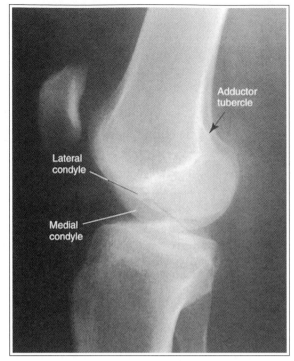

Image 65.

Analysis. The distal articulating surfaces of the femoral condyles are not superimposed. The medial condyle is distal to the lateral condyle.

Correction. A cephalic angulation should be used to project the medial condyle proximally. Adjust the angle approximately 5 degrees for every ¼ inch (0.6 cm) of distance demonstrated between the medial and lateral distal surfaces.

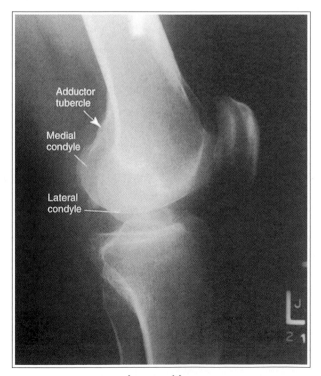

Image 66.

Analysis. The distal articulating surfaces of the femoral condyles are not superimposed. The medial condyle has been projected proximally to the lateral condyle. An excessively cephalad angle was used.

Correction. Decrease the central ray angulation approximately 5 degrees for every ¼ inch (0.6 cm) of distance demonstrated between the medial and lateral distal surfaces.

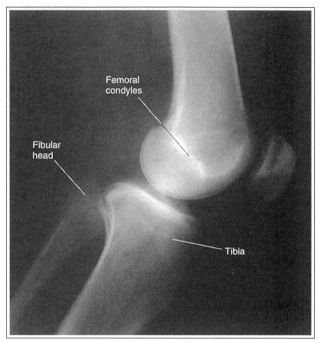

Image 67.

Analysis. The femoral condyles are superimposed, and the tibiofibular articulation is demonstrated. The image was taken with the femoral epicondyles aligned perpendicular to the IR, then rolled toward the IR approximately ¼ inch (0.6 cm) to move the medial condyle anteriorly onto the lateral condyle. The central ray was then aligned with the femur, as demonstrated in Figure 5-80.

Correction. For a more accurate demonstration of the tibia and fibula relationship, position the femoral epicondyles perpendicular to the IR and align the central ray across the femur, as demonstrated in Figure 5-79.

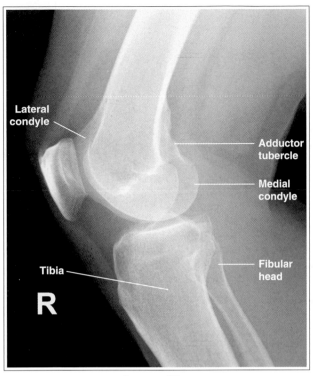

Image 68.

Analysis. The anterior and the posterior aspects of the femoral condyles are not superimposed. The medial condyle is situated posteriorly. The patient's patella was positioned too far from the IR (leg internally rotated).

Correction. Roll the patella closer to the IR (externally rotate the leg). Because both condyles will move simultaneously, the amount of adjustment required is only half of the distance demonstrated between the posterior surfaces.

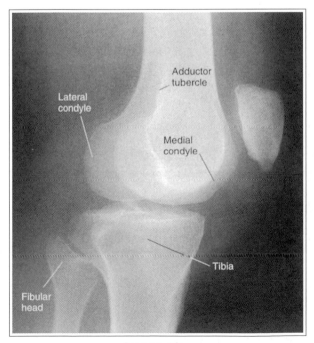

Image 69.

Analysis. The anterior and the posterior aspects of the femoral condyles are not superimposed. The medial condyle is situated anteriorly. The patella was positioned too close to the IR (leg externally rotated).

Correction. Roll the patella farther away from the IR (internally rotate the leg). Because both condyles will move simultaneously, the amount of adjustment required is only half the distance demonstrated between the posterior surfaces.

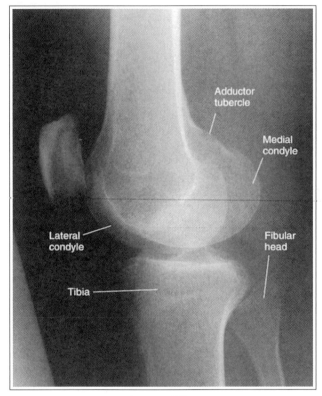

Image 70.

Analysis. The anteroposterior aspects of the femoral condyles are not superimposed. The medial condyle is situated posteriorly. The patella was positioned too far from the IR (leg internally rotated).

Correction. Roll the patella closer to the IR (externally rotate the leg). Because both condyles move simultaneously, the amount of adjustment required is only half the distance demonstrated between the posterior surfaces.

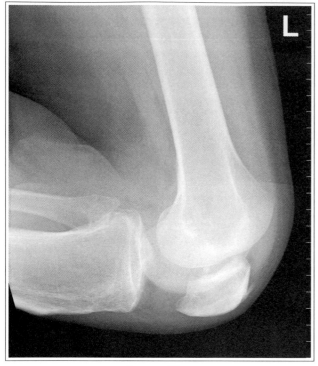

Image 71.

Analysis. The knee is flexed 90 degrees, and the medial condyle is demonstrated distal and posterior to the lateral condyle. The fibula is demonstrated without tibial superimposition. The proximal femur was elevated because the patient had a thick proximal thigh, and the patella was positioned too far from the IR.

Correction. Unflex the knee to 10 to 15 degrees of flexion, elevate the distal femur or adjust the central ray angulation cephalically, and rotate the patella closer to the IR.

KNEE: INTERCONDYLAR FOSSA (POSTEROANTERIOR AXIAL PROJECTION) (HOLMBLAD METHOD)

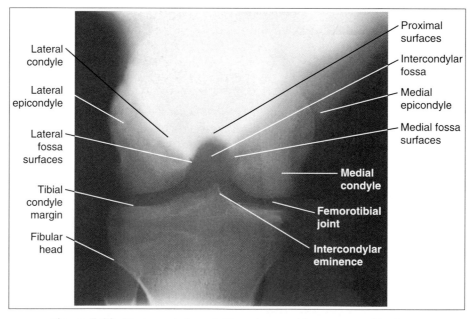

Figure 5-83. Posteroanterior axial knee image with accurate positioning.

Image Analysis

The medial and the lateral surfaces of the intercondylar fossa and the femoral epicondyles are demonstrated in profile, and the fibular head is partially superimposed over the proximal tibia.

- The posteroanterior (PA) axial projection is performed by positioning the patient on hands and knees on the imaging table and then requesting the patient to lean forward until the femur and the central ray form a 20- to 30-degree angle (femur-imaging table angle is 60 to 70 degrees) (Figures 5-84 and 5-85). The IR is positioned under the affected knee.

- ***Mechanics of PA axial projection:*** To understand the way in which the femur is positioned for this image, study a femoral skeletal bone. Place the femoral bone upright with the distal femoral condylar surfaces resting against a flat surface. While imaging the posterior femoral surface, lean the femur anteriorly until the intercondylar fossa is positioned in profile. In this PA axial projection, note how the femoral shaft inclines medially approximately 10 to 15 degrees. The amount of inclination the femoral bone displays depends on the length of the femoral shaft and the width of the pelvis from which the femur originated. The longer the femur and the wider the pelvis, the more femoral inclination is demonstrated.

- To obtain an intercondylar fossa image with superimposed medial and superimposed lateral surfaces, this inclination should not offset. If the inclination is offset by shifting the distal femur laterally or the proximal femur medially and positioning the femur vertically, the medial and the lateral aspects of the intercondylar fossa are not superimposed and the patella is situated laterally (see Image 72). This fact can be demonstrated by placing the femoral skeleton bone vertically and imaging the change in the demonstration of the intercondylar fossa.

- ***Effect of foot mispositioning:*** Mispositioning of the patient's foot may also result in rotation of the femur

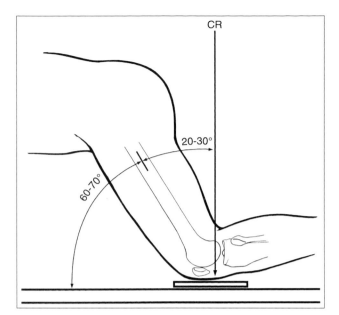

Figure 5-85. Posteroanterior axial knee position. *CR,* Central ray.

and demonstrate the medial and the lateral aspects of the intercondylar fossa without superimposition. The long axis of the patient's foot should be positioned perpendicular to the imaging table. If the heel was allowed to rotate medially (internally), the medial and lateral aspects of the intercondylar fossa are not superimposed, and the patella is rotated laterally (Image 72). If the heel was rotated laterally (externally), the medial and lateral aspects of the intercondylar fossa are not superimposed, the patella is demonstrated medially, and the tibia is demonstrated without fibular head superimposition (see Image 73).

The proximal surfaces of the intercondylar fossa are superimposed, and the patellar apex is demonstrated proximal to the intercondylar fossa.

- The proximal surfaces of the intercondylar fossa are superimposed when the femoral shaft is placed at a 60- to 70-degree angle with the imaging table (see Figure 5-84). To better study this relationship, place a femoral skeleton bone in the PA axial position. While viewing the posterior intercondylar fossa, move the proximal femur closer to and farther away from the imaging table. Note how the proximal surfaces of the fossa are in profile and superimposed only when the femur is at a 60- to 70-degree angle with the imaging table. The position of the femur with respect to the imaging table also determines the position of the patella (see AP knee discussion and Figure 5-68, p. 309). As the knee is flexed (the proximal femur is brought away from the imaging table), the patella moves distally onto the patellar surface of the femur and into the intercondylar fossa. The degree of knee flexion used for the PA axial projection situates the patella just proximal to the fossa.

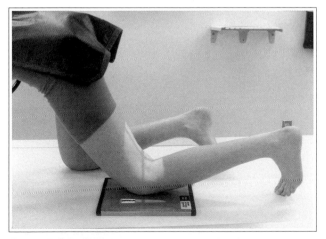

Figure 5-84. Proper patient positioning for posteroanterior axial knee image.

- *Effect of femur positioning:* If a PA axial image is obtained that demonstrates the proximal intercondylar fossa's surfaces without superimposition, view the patella's position to determine whether the patient's proximal femur was positioned too close to or too far from the imaging table. If the patellar apex is demonstrated within the fossa, the knee was overflexed (proximal femur positioned too far away from the imaging table) (see Image 74). If the patella is demonstrated laterally and proximal to the fossa, the knee was underflexed (proximal femur position too close to the table) (see Image 75).

The knee joint space is open and the tibia plateau and intercondylar eminence and tubercles are demonstrated in profile. The fibular head is demonstrated approximately ½ inch (1.25 cm) distal to the tibial plateau.

- To obtain an open knee joint space and demonstrate the tibial plateau and intercondylar eminence and tubercles in profile, dorsiflex the patient's foot and rest the foot on the toes. Because the tibial plateau slopes downward from the anterior tibial margin to the posterior margin, this positioning is necessary to elevate the distal tibia and align the anterior and posterior tibial margins perpendicular to the IR. If the foot is not dorsiflexed and resting on the toes, the knee joint space is narrowed or closed and the tibial plateau is demonstrated (see Images 73 and 75).

- *Determining repositioning for closed knee joint*: If a PA axial knee image is obtained that demonstrates a closed or narrowed knee joint space and the tibial plateau surface, evaluate the proximity of the fibular head to the tibial plateau to determine the needed adjustment. If the fibular is head is less than ½ inch (1.25 cm) from the tibial plateau (see Image 73), the distal lower leg needs to be depressed. If the fibular head is more than ½ inch (1.25 cm) from the tibial plateau (see Image 75), the distal lower leg needs to be elevated. The amount of lower leg adjustment required would be half of the distance needed to bring the fibular head to within ½ inch (1.25 cm) of the tibial plateau. The small amount of lower leg adjustment that would be needed can be accomplished by varying the degree of foot dorsiflexion or plantar-flexion.

The intercondylar fossa is at the center of the collimated field. The distal femur, proximal tibia, and intercondylar fossa eminence and tubercles are included within the field.

- Center a perpendicular central ray to the midline of the knee, at a level 1 inch (2.5 cm) distal to the palpable medial femoral epicondyle, to place the intercondylar fossa in the center of the collimated field. Open the longitudinal collimation enough to include the femoral epicondyles. Transverse collimation should be to within ½ inch (1.25 cm) of the knee skinline.

- An 8- × 10-inch (18- × 24-cm) screen-film or computed radiography IR placed lengthwise should be adequate to include all the required anatomical structures.

Posteroanterior Axial Knee Image Analysis

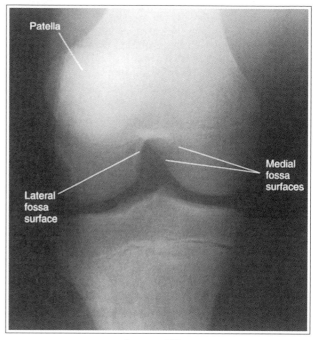

Image 72.

Analysis. The medial and the lateral aspects of the intercondylar fossa are not superimposed, and the patella is situated laterally. Either the femur was too vertical or the heel was rotated medially.

Correction. Position the distal femur medially or the proximal femur laterally, allowing the femur to incline medially, and align the long axis of the patient's foot perpendicular to the imaging table.

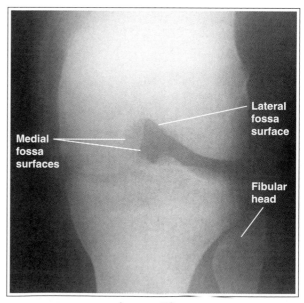

Image 73.

Analysis. The medial and the lateral aspects of the inter-condylar fossa are not superimposed, the patella is situated medially, and the tibia is demonstrated without fibular head superimposition. The heel was laterally rotated. The knee joint is obscured, the tibial plateau is demonstrated, and the fibula is positioned closer than $\frac{1}{2}$ inch (1.25 cm) to the tibial plateau.

Correction. Rotate the heel medially until the foot's long axis is aligned perpendicular to the imaging table and depress the distal lower leg by decreasing the amount of foot dorsiflexion.

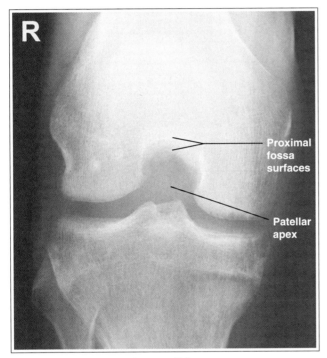

Image 74.

Analysis. The proximal surfaces of the intercondylar fossa are demonstrated without superimposition, and the patella is positioned within the intercondylar fossa. The knee was overflexed (femur positioned too far away from the imaging table).

Correction. Extend the knee (position the proximal femur closer to the imaging table). The amount of movement needed is half the distance demonstrated between the anterior and posterior proximal intercondylar fossa's surfaces.

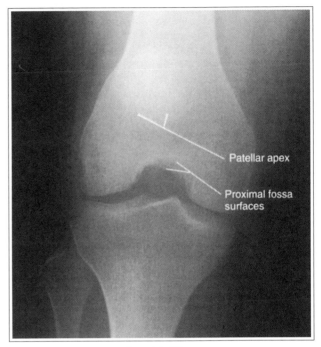

Image 75.

Analysis. The proximal intercondylar fossa's surfaces are demonstrated without superimposition, and the patella is positioned too far proximal to the fossa. The knee was underflexed (femur positioned too close to the imaging table). The knee joint is obscured, the tibial plateau is demonstrated, and the fibular head is shown more than $\frac{1}{2}$ inch (1.25 cm) from the tibial plateau.

Correction. Flex the knee (position the femur farther away from the imaging table) and elevate the distal lower leg by increasing the amount of foot dorsiflexion.

KNEE: INTERCONDYLAR FOSSA (ANTEROPOSTERIOR AXIAL PROJECTION) (BÉCLERE METHOD)

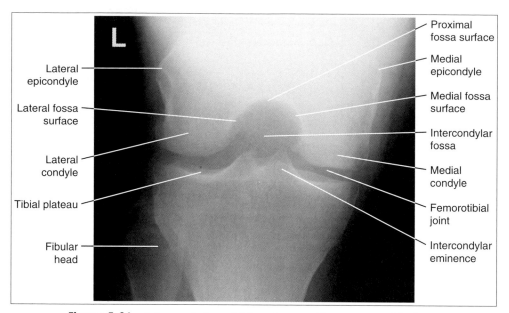

Figure 5-86. Anteroposterior axial knee image with accurate positioning.

Image Analysis

The intercondylar fossa is shown in its entirety, the medial and lateral surfaces of the intercondylar fossa and the femoral epicondyles are demonstrated in profile, and the tibia is partially superimposed over the fibular head.

- The AP axial projection (Béclere method) is performed by placing the patient on the imaging table in a supine position with the affected hip and knee in an AP projection and flexed until the long axis of the femur is at a 60-degree angle with the imaging table. Then adjust the lower leg until the knee is flexed approximately 45 degrees (Figure 5-87). A curved or regular IR is positioned under the knee and is elevated on an immobilization device until it is as close to the posterior knee as possible and the central ray is aligned parallel with the tibial plateau.

- To demonstrate the intercondylar fossa in its entirety, with superimposed medial and lateral surfaces, the patient's knee needs to be in an AP projection. This is accomplished by internally rotating the leg until an imaginary line connecting the medial and lateral femoral epicondyles is positioned parallel with the imaging table.

- ***Effect of rotation:*** If the femoral epicondyles are not positioned parallel with the IR, the medial and lateral surfaces of the intercondylar fossa will not be superimposed

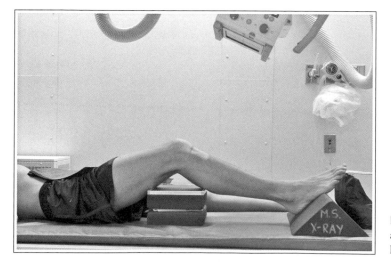

Figure 5-87. Proper patient positioning for anteroposterior axial projection (Béclere method) knee image.

and in profile, and the intercondylar fossa will not be fully demonstrated. The direction of poor knee rotation can be detected by evaluating the degree of tibial and fibular superimposition and the difference in femoral condylar width. It the patient's leg is not internally rotated enough, the medial femoral condyle appears larger than the lateral condyle and the tibia demonstrates increased fibular superimposition (see Image 76). If the patient's leg is internally rotated more than the amount needed to align the femoral epicondyles parallel with the IR, the lateral femoral condyle will appear larger than the medial condyle, and the tibia will demonstrate decreased superimposition (see Image 77).

The proximal surface of the intercondylar fossa is in profile, and the patellar apex is demonstrated superior to the fossa.

- The proximal surface of the intercondylar fossa is in profile when the central ray is aligned parallel with it. This is accomplished when the long axis of the femur is flexed at a 60-degree angle with the imaging table.
- *Adjusting for poor proximal intercondylar fossa visualization:* With a set central ray, poor alignment of the proximal surface occurs when the femur is aligned more or less than 60 degrees with the imaging table. If an AP axial position is achieved and the proximal intercondylar fossa surfaces are demonstrated without superimposition, view the patella apex's position to determine how femoral flexion would need to be adjusted to obtain accurate positioning and demonstrate the entire intercondylar fossa. As the knee is flexed, the patella shifts distally onto the patellar surface of the femur and then into the intercondylar fossa. Therefore if the long axis of the femur is aligned more than 60 degrees with the imaging table, resulting in increased knee flexion, the patellar apex will be demonstrated within the intercondylar fossa (see Image 78). If the long axis of the femur is aligned less than 60 degrees with the imaging table, resulting in less knee flexion, the proximal intercondylar fossa surfaces will not be aligned and the patellar apex will be shown above the intercondylar fossa (see Image 79).

The knee joint space is open, the anterior and posterior condylar margins of the tibia are superimposed, the intercondylar eminence and tubercles are demonstrated in profile, and the fibular head is demonstrated approximately 1/2 inch (1.25 cm) distal to the tibial plateau.

- To obtain an open knee joint space and demonstrate the intercondylar eminence and tubercles in profile, the central ray must be aligned parallel with the tibial plateau. This alignment is obtained by first positioning the central ray perpendicular with the anterior lower leg surface and then decreasing the obtained angulation by 5 degrees. The 5-degree decrease is needed because the tibial plateau slopes distally by 5 degrees from the anterior condylar margin to the posterior condylar margin.

- *Effect of poor lower leg positioning:* If an AP axial image demonstrates a closed or narrowed knee joint space and the tibial plateau, evaluate the proximity of the fibular head to the tibial plateau. If the fibular head is demonstrated more than 1/2 inch (1.25 cm) distal to the tibial plateau, the distal lower leg was elevated too high or the central ray was too cephalically angled (see Image 80). If the fibular head is demonstrated less than 1/2 inch (1.25 cm) distal to the tibial plateau, the distal lower leg was too depressed or the central ray was too caudally angled (see Image 81).

The intercondylar fossa is at the center of the collimated field. The distal femur, proximal tibia, and intercondylar fossa eminence and tubercles are included within the field.

- Center the central ray to the midline of the knee, at a level 1 inch (2.5 cm) distal to the palpable medial femoral epicondyle, to place the intercondylar fossa in the center of the collimated field. Open the longitudinal collimation enough to include the femoral epicondyles. Transverse collimation should be to within 1/2 inch (1.25 cm) of the knee skinline.

- An 8- × 10-inch (18- × 24-cm) IR placed crosswise or a curved IR should be adequate to include all the required anatomical structures. A curved IR that is built up on an immobilization device enough to place the IR adjacent to the affected knee will demonstrate the least amount of magnification and distortion of the image. If a curved IR is unavailable, an 8- × 10-inch (18- × 24-cm) screen-film or computed radiography IR should be positioned crosswise and built up on an immobilization device, bringing it as close as possible to the affected knee.

Anteroposterior Axial Knee Image Analysis

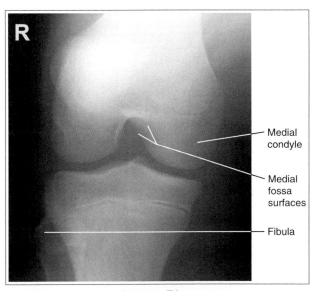

R

Medial condyle

Medial fossa surfaces

Fibula

Image 76.

Analysis. The medial and the lateral aspects of the inter-condylar fossa are not superimposed, the medial femoral condyle is wider than the lateral condyle, and the fibular head demonstrates increased tibial superimposition. The patient's leg was externally rotated.

Correction. Internally rotate the leg until an imaginary line connecting the femoral epicondyles is aligned parallel with the imaging table.

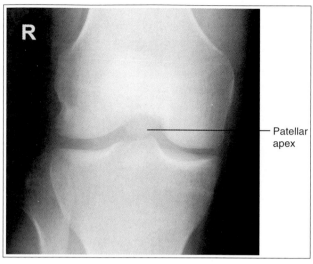

Image 78.

Analysis. The proximal surfaces of the intercondylar fossa are not superimposed and the patellar apex is demonstrated within the intercondylar fossa. The long axis of the femur was aligned at more than a 60-degree angle with the imaging table.

Correction. Decrease the degree of hip and knee flexion until the long axis of the femur is aligned 60 degrees with the imaging table.

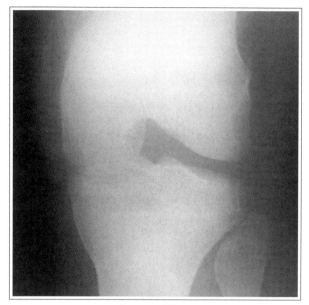

Image 77.

Analysis. The medial and lateral aspects of the intercondy-lar fossa are not superimposed, the lateral femoral condyle is wider than the medial condyle, and the fibular head demonstrates no tibial superimposition. The patient's leg was internally rotated. The knee joint space is closed, and the fibular head is shown less than ½ inch (1.25 cm) distal to the tibial plateau. The distal lower leg was too depressed.

Correction. Externally rotate the leg until an imaginary line connecting the femoral epicondyles is aligned parallel with the imaging table, and elevate the distal lower leg until the knee is flexed 45 degrees or adjust the central ray angle cephalically.

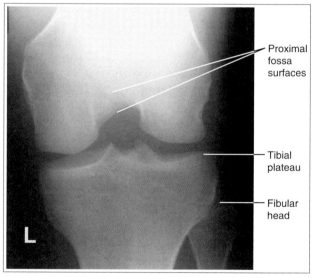

Image 79.

Analysis. The proximal surfaces of the intercondylar fossa are not superimposed, and the patellar apex is demon-strated proximal to the intercondylar fossa. The long axis of the femur was aligned at less than a 60-degree angle with the imaging table. The knee joint is closed, and the fibular head is demonstrated more than ½ inch (1.25 cm) distal to the tibial plateau. The distal lower leg was elevated too high, or the central ray was angled too cephalically.

Correction. Increase the degree of hip and knee flexion until the long axis of the femur is aligned 60 degrees with the imaging table. Elevate the distal lower leg until the knee is flexed 45 degrees, or adjust the central ray caudally.

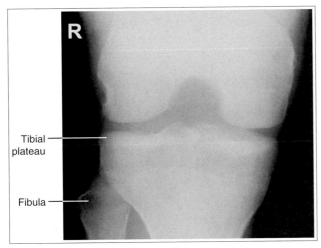

Image 80.

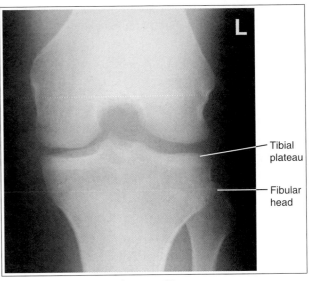

Image 81.

Analysis. The knee joint is closed, and the fibular head is demonstrated more than ½ inch (1.25 cm) distal to the tibial plateau. The distal lower leg was elevated too high, or the central ray was angled too cephalically.

Correction. Depress the distal lower leg until the knee is flexed 45 degrees, or adjust the central ray caudally.

Analysis. The knee joint is closed, and the fibular head is demonstrated less than ½ inch (1.25 cm) distal to the tibial plateau. The distal lower leg was depressed, or the central ray was angled too caudally.

Correction. Elevate the distal lower leg until the knee is flexed 45 degrees, or adjust the central ray cephalically.

PATELLA: TANGENTIAL (AXIAL) PROJECTION (MERCHANT METHOD)

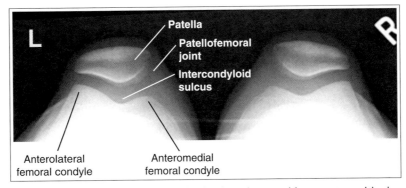

Figure 5-88. Tangential (axial) projection knee image with accurate positioning.

Image Analysis

Scatter radiation is controlled.

- An optimal 60 to 70 kVp technique sufficiently penetrates the bony and soft-tissue structures of the knee and provides high image contrast. If it is necessary to increase the kilovoltage above 70 to penetrate a thicker knee, a grid is not needed as described previously for this

examination, because of the long OID. When a long OID is used, scatter radiation that would expose the IR when a short OID is used is scattered at a direction away from the IR. Because scatter radiation is not being directed toward the IR, a grid is not needed to absorb the scatter. This is also referred to as the *air-gap technique.*

The knee demonstrates no rotation. The patellae, anterior femoral condyles, and intercondylar sulci are

demonstrated superiorly, and the lateral femoral condyle demonstrates slightly more height than the medial condyle.

- The tangential (axial) projection method uses an axial viewer knee-supporting device, as demonstrated in Figure 5-89. This freestanding device maintains the knees at a set degree of flexion, provides straps that restrain the patient's legs, and contains an IR holder that keeps the receptor at the proper angle with the central ray. To obtain a tangential (axial) projection image of the patellae, place the patient supine on the imaging table with the legs dangling off the end of the table. Set the axial viewer at a standard 45-degree angle, and position it at the end of the imaging table beneath the patient's knees and calves. Situate the patient's ankles between the viewer's receptor holder, and place the receptor on the ankles so that it rests against the viewer's receptor holder (see Figure 5-89).

- To demonstrate the knees without rotation and to position the patellae, anterior femoral condyles, and intercondylar sulci superiorly, internally rotate the patient's legs until the palpable femoral epicondyles are aligned parallel with the imaging table. Then secure the legs in this position by wrapping the axial viewer's Velcro straps around the patient's calves. This positioning places the distal femora in an AP projection with the imaging table. Because the lateral condyles are situated anterior to the medial condyles, the lateral condyles demonstrate more height on a tangential (axial) projection image if the legs are adequately rotated. If the legs are not sufficiently rotated, the patellae are situated laterally, and either the anterior femoral condyles demonstrate equal height or the medial condyles demonstrate greater height than the lateral condyles (see Image 82). Both knees may not be rotated equally; often only one knee is rotated.

- ***Patellar position on a tangential (axial) projection image:*** Because this image is taken to demonstrate subluxation (partial dislocation) of the patella, the position of the patellae above the intercondylar sulci on a tangential (axial) projection image may vary. In a normal knee the patella is directly above the intercondylar sulcus on a tangential (axial) projection image, as shown in Figure 5-88. With patellar subluxation, the patella is lateral to the intercondylar sulcus, as demonstrated in Image 83.

- Do not mistake a subluxed patella for knee rotation. Although both conditions result in a laterally positioned patella, the rotated knee demonstrates the femoral condyles at the same height, whereas with a subluxed patella the lateral condyle is higher than the medial condyle.

- ***Positioning to demonstrate patellar subluxation:*** To demonstrate patellar subluxation, the quadriceps femoris (four muscles that surround the femoral bone) must be in a relaxed position. This is accomplished by instructing the patient to relax the leg muscles, allowing the calf straps to maintain the internal leg rotation. If the patient does not relax the quadriceps muscles, a patella that would be subluxed on relaxation of the muscles will appear normal.

The patellofemoral joint spaces are open with no superimposition of the upper anterior thigh soft tissue, patellae, or tibial tuberosities.

- ***Accurate femur positioning:*** The position of the patient's legs on the axial viewer must be precise for an open patellofemoral joint space to be obtained. The height of the axial viewer is adjustable. It should be set to a height that positions the long axis of the patient's femurs parallel with the table. If the distal femurs are positioned closer to the table than the proximal femurs, the angled central ray traverses the anterior thigh soft

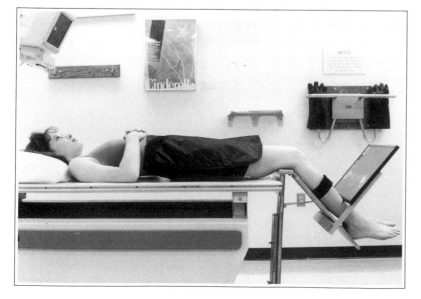

Figure 5-89. Proper patient positioning for tangential (axial) projection knee image.

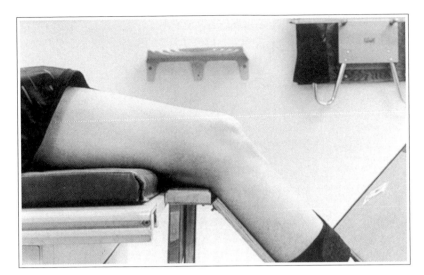

Figure 5-90. Poor femur positioning.

tissue, projecting it into the patellofemoral joint space (Figure 5-90 and Image 84). Although the patellofemoral joint space remains open on such an image, the space is underexposed.

- *Knee relationship to axial viewer:* The relationship of the patient's posterior knee curves to the bend of the axial viewer determines whether the central ray will be parallel with the patellofemoral joint spaces. To demonstrate open patellofemoral joint spaces, position the posterior curves of the knees directly above the bend in the axial viewer, as demonstrated in Figure 5-91. If the posterior curves of the knees are situated at or below the bend of the axial viewer (causing the knees to be flexed more than the degree that is set on the axial viewer), the central ray is not parallel with the patellofemoral joint space, and the patellae are resting against the intercondylar sulci (Figure 5-92 and Image 85). If the posterior curves of the knees are situated too far above the bend of the axial viewer (causing the

knees to be extended more than the degree set on the axial viewer), the tibial tuberosities are demonstrated within the patellofemoral joint space (Figure 5-93 and Image 86).

- *Positioning and central ray angulation for large calves:* The tibial tuberosities may also be demonstrated within the patellofemoral joint spaces in a patient with large posterior calves, even when the posterior knee curves have been accurately positioned to the bend of the axial viewer. The knees of a patient with large calves are not flexed as much as the axial viewer degree is set. For such patients the central ray angulation should be increased (5 to 10 degrees) or the axial viewer's angulation should be decreased until the knees are flexed 45 degrees.

- *Determining central ray angulation:* The angle of the central ray and angle placed on the axial viewer also determine how well the patellofemoral joint space is demonstrated. Although 45 degrees is the standard

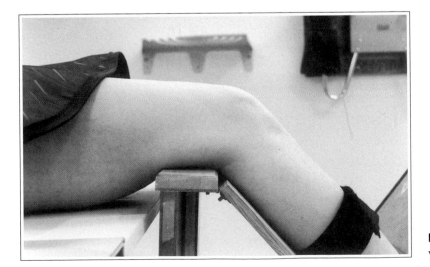

Figure 5-91. Proper posterior knee and axial viewer positioning.

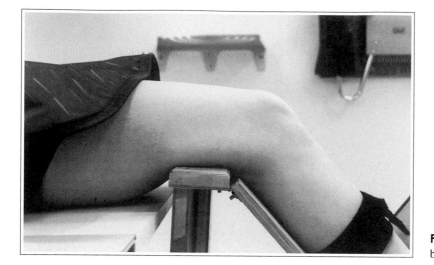

Figure 5-92. Posterior knee curve situated below bend in axial viewer.

angle, the reviewer is capable of supporting the leg at 30-, 60-, or 75-degree angles as well. Each of these angles requires a predetermined central ray angulation if an open patellofemoral joint is to be obtained.

- The easiest way to determine the central ray angle to use for the different axial viewer angles is to know that the sum of the central ray angle and the axial viewer's angle must equal 105 degrees. For example, if the axial viewer is set at 30 degrees, the central ray angulation must be set at 75 degrees (30 + 75 = 105).
- Evaluate the shadow of the knees that is created on the receptor when the centering light is on, before exposing the IR. When the patient has been accurately positioned, these shadows will display oval silhouettes with indentations on each side that outline the patellae (Figure 5-94).

A point midway between the patellofemoral joint spaces is at the center of the collimated field.

The patellae, anterior femoral condyles, and intercondylar sulci are included within the field.

- A standard 60-degree caudally angled central ray is centered between the knees at the level of the patellofemoral joint spaces, to place the patellofemoral joint spaces in the center of the collimated field (see Figure 5-94). An SID of 72 inches (183 cm) is generally used to offset the magnification caused by the long OID.
- Open the longitudinal collimated field to include the patellae and the distal femurs. Transverse collimation should be to within ½ inch (1.25 cm) of the lateral knee skinline.
- A 10- × 12-inch (24- × 30-cm) or 11- × 14-inch (28- × 35-cm) screen-film or computed radiography IR placed crosswise should be adequate to include all the required anatomical structures.

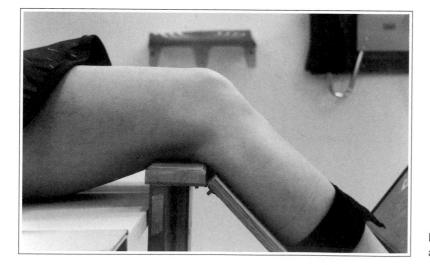

Figure 5-93. Posterior knee curve situated above bend in axial viewer.

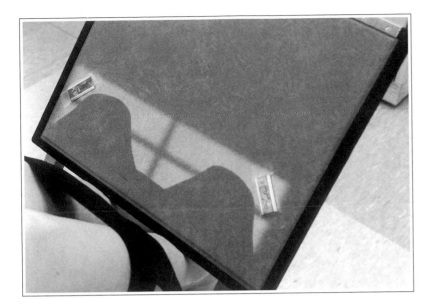

Figure 5-94. Proper knee shadows and central ray centering.

Tangential (Axial) Patella Image Analysis

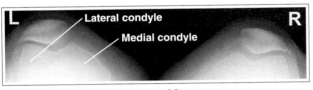

Image 82.

Analysis. The patellae are demonstrated directly above the intercondylar sulci and are rotated laterally. The medial femoral condyles demonstrate more height than the lateral condyles. The legs were externally rotated.

Correction. Internally rotate the patient's legs until the patellae are situated superiorly, then restrain the legs by wrapping the axial viewer's Velcro straps around the calves.

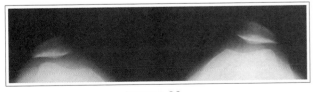

Image 83.

Analysis. The femoral condyles are visible superiorly, with the lateral femoral condyles demonstrating more height than the medial condyles. The patellae appear lateral to the intercondylar sulci and demonstrate subluxation.

Correction. No positioning movement is needed.

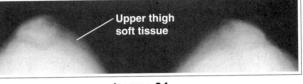

Image 84.

Analysis. Soft tissue from the patient's anterior thighs has been projected onto the patellae and patellofemoral joint spaces. The height of the axial viewer was not set high enough to position the femurs parallel with the table. The distal femurs were positioned closer to the table than the proximal femurs, as demonstrated in Figure 5-90.

Correction. Increase the height of the axial viewer until the long axes of the femurs are positioned parallel with the table, as demonstrated in Figure 5-89.

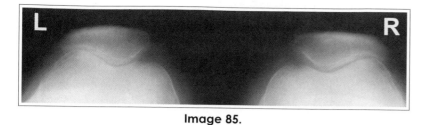

Image 85.

Analysis. The patellae are resting against the intercondylar sulci, obscuring the patellofemoral joint spaces. The patient's posterior knee curve was positioned at or below the bend on the axial viewer, as demonstrated in Figure 5-92.

Correction. Slide the patient's knees away from the axial viewer until the patient's posterior knee curvature is just superior to the bend of the reviewer, as demonstrated in Figure 5-91.

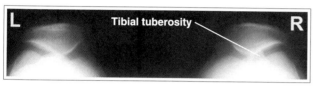

Image 86.

Analysis. The tibial tuberosities are demonstrated within the patellofemoral joint spaces. Either the posterior knee curve was positioned too far above the axial viewer's bend, as demonstrated in Figure 5-94, or the patient has large posterior calves.

Correction. Slide the knees toward the axial viewer until the posterior knee curvature is just superior to the bend on the viewer, as demonstrated in Figure 5-92. If the patient was accurately positioned but the calves are large, increase (5 to 10 degrees) the central ray angulation or decrease the axial viewer's angulation until the knees are flexed 45 degrees. The total sum of the axial viewer's angle and the central ray angulation will be less than 105 degrees.

FEMUR: ANTEROPOSTERIOR PROJECTION

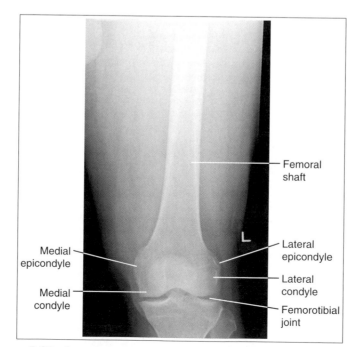

Figure 5-95. Anteroposterior distal femur image with accurate positioning.

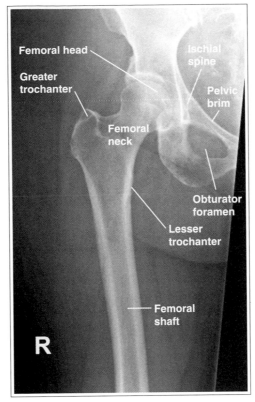

Figure 5-96. Anteroposterior proximal femur image with accurate positioning.

Image Analysis

Image density is uniform across the lower leg.

- *Anode-heel effect:* To take advantage of the anode-heel effect, position the thicker proximal lower leg at the cathode end of the tube and the thinner distal lower leg at the anode end. Then set an exposure (mAs) that will adequately demonstrate the midpoint of the lower leg. Because the anode absorbs some of the photons aimed at the anode end of the IR, the distal lower leg, which requires less exposure than the proximal lower leg, will not be overexposed.

DISTAL FEMUR
The distal femur demonstrates an AP projection. The medial and lateral femoral epicondyles are demonstrated in profile, the femoral condyles are symmetrical in shape, and the tibia is superimposed over 1/4 inch (0.6 cm) of the fibular head.

- To obtain an AP distal femoral image, place the patient in a supine position with the knee fully extended. Internally rotate the leg until the foot is rotated to a 15- to 20-degree angle and an imaginary line drawn between the medial and lateral femoral epicondyles is positioned parallel with the IR (Figures 5-97 and 5-98). This positioning places the medial and lateral femoral epicondyles

at equal distances from the IR, as well as medially and laterally in profile, respectively. It also centers the intercondylar eminence within the intercondylar fossa.

- *Effect of mispositioning:* If the femoral epicondyles are not positioned parallel with the IR, an AP projection has not been obtained. If the leg was not externally (laterally) rotated enough to place the epicondyles at equal distances from the IR, the epicondyles are not in profile, the medial femoral condyle is larger than the lateral condyle, and the tibia is superimposed over more

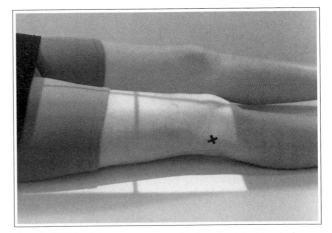

Figure 5-97. Proper patient positioning for anteroposterior distal femur image. X indicates lateral femoral epicondyle.

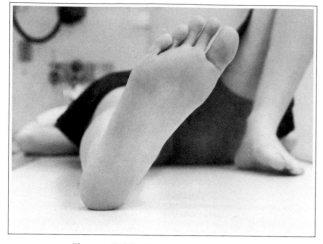

Figure 5-98. Proper foot rotation.

than ¼ inch (0.6 cm) of the fibular head (see Image 87). If the leg was internally (medially) rotated more than needed to place the femoral epicondyles at equal distances from the IR, the epicondyles are not demonstrated in profile, the lateral femoral condyle is larger than the medial condyle, and the tibia is superimposed over less than ¼ inch (0.6 cm) of the fibular head (see Image 88).

- *Positioning for femoral fracture:* When a patient has a fractured femur, the leg should not be internally rotated, but left as is. Forced internal rotation of a fractured femur may injure the blood vessels and nerves that surround the injured area. Because the leg is not internally rotated when a fracture is in question, the distal femur demonstrates external rotation.

The knee joint space is open but narrowed, and the anterior and posterior margins of the proximal tibia are superimposed.

- An open knee joint space is obtained when the anterior and posterior margins of the proximal tibia are superimposed. Because these margins slope distally from the anterior condylar margin to the posterior condylar margin, and the central ray is centered proximal to the knee joint, x-rays that diverge toward the proximal tibia are aligned close enough to parallel with the slope of the tibia to result in an open joint space. The joint space is narrower because the diverged x-rays project the distal femur partially into the joint space.

The distal femoral shaft is at the center of the collimated field. The distal femoral shaft and surrounding femoral soft tissue, the knee joint, and 1 inch (2.5 cm) of the lower leg are included within the field. Any orthopedic appliances located at the knee are included in their entirety.

- A perpendicular central ray is centered to the distal femoral shaft to place the shaft in the center of the image. This is accomplished by positioning the lower edge of the receptor approximately 2 inches (5 cm)

below the knee joint; the knee joint is located 1 inch (2.5 cm) distal to the medial epicondyle. This lower positioning is needed to prevent the diverged x-ray beams from projecting the knee joint off the IR.

- The longitudinal collimation should be left open the full length of the IR used. Transverse collimation should be to within ½ inch (1.25 cm) of the lateral femoral skinline.

- A 14- × 17-inch (35- × 43-cm) screen-film or computed radiography IR placed lengthwise should be adequate to include all the required anatomical structures.

- *Examination of the entire femur:* If the entire femur is of interest and images are taken of the distal and proximal ends of the femur, the images should demonstrate at least 2 inches (5 cm) of femoral shaft overlap. Any orthopedic appliance, such as an intramedullary rod, should be included in its entirety.

The pelvis demonstrates an AP projection. The ischial spine is aligned with the pelvic brim, and the obturator foramen is open.

- An AP projection of the pelvis is obtained by placing the patient supine on the imaging table with the legs extended (Figure 5-99). To ensure that the pelvis is not rotated, judge the distance from the ASIS to the imaging table on both sides of the patient. The distances should be equal.

- *Detecting pelvic rotation:* Rotation of the pelvis on a femoral image is detected by evaluating the relationship of the ischial spine and the pelvic brim and visualization of the obturator foramen. When the pelvis has been rotated toward the affected femur, the ischial spine is demonstrated without pelvic brim superimposition, and visualization of the obturator foramen is decreased (see Chapter 6, Image 1). When the pelvis has been rotated away from the affected femur, the ischial spine is not aligned with the pelvic brim but is demonstrated closer to the acetabulum, and demonstration of the obturator foramen is increased (see Chapter 6, Image 2).

The femoral neck is demonstrated without foreshortening, the greater trochanter is demonstrated in

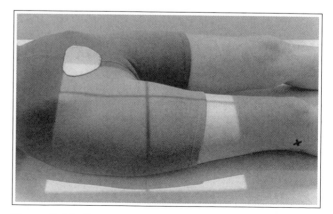

Figure 5-99. Proper patient positioning for anteroposterior proximal femur image.

profile laterally, and the lesser trochanter is superimposed by the femoral neck.

- The positions of the patient's foot and femoral epicondyle with respect to the imaging table determine how the femoral neck and trochanters appear on an AP femoral image.
- *Effect of leg and foot rotation:* Generally, when a patient is relaxed, the legs and feet are externally (laterally) rotated. On external rotation, the femoral neck inclines posteriorly (toward the imaging table) and is foreshortened on an AP femoral image. Increased external rotation increases the degree of posterior decline and foreshortening of the femoral neck on the image. If the patient's leg was externally (laterally) rotated enough to position the foot at a 45-degree angle and an imaginary line connecting the femoral epicondyles at a 60- to 65-degree angle with the imaging table, the femoral neck is demonstrated "on end," and the lesser trochanter is demonstrated in profile (Figure 5-100). If the patient's leg is positioned with the foot placed vertically and an imaginary line connecting the femoral epicondyles at approximately a 15- to 20-degree angle with the imaging table, the lesser trochanter is demonstrated in partial profile and the femoral neck is only partially foreshortened (see Image 89).
- For an AP femur image, which shows the femoral neck without foreshortening and the greater trochanter in profile, the patient's leg should be internally rotated until the foot is tilted 15 to 20 degrees from vertical and the femoral epicondyles are positioned parallel with the imaging table (see Figures 5-98 and 5-99).
- *Positioning for fracture:* When a patient has a fractured proximal femur, the leg should not be internally rotated, but left as is. Forced internal rotation of a fractured proximal femur may injure the blood vessels and nerves that surround the injured area. Because the patient's leg is not internally rotated when a fracture is in question, such an AP femoral image demonstrates the femoral neck with some degree of foreshortening and the lesser trochanter without femoral shaft superimposition (see Image 90).

The proximal femoral shaft is at the center of the collimated field. The proximal femoral shaft, hip, and surrounding femoral soft tissue are included within the field. Any orthopedic appliances located at the hip are included in their entirety.

- A perpendicular central ray is centered to the proximal femoral shaft to place it in the center of the image. This is accomplished by positioning the upper edge of the receptor at the level of the ASIS. If the collimated head can be moved, turn it until one of its axes is aligned with the long axis of the femur.
- The longitudinal collimation should be left open the full length of the IR. Transverse collimation should be to within ½ inch (1.25 cm) of the lateral femoral skinline. The surrounding femoral soft tissue should be included to allow detection of subcutaneous air or hematomas.
- A 14- × 17-inch (35- × 43-cm) screen-film or computed radiography IR placed lengthwise should be adequate to include all the required anatomical structures.
- *Gonadal shielding:* Gonadal shielding should be used on all male and female patients, although it is important that no pelvic anatomy that is next to the affected femur be covered with a shield. It is not uncommon for a patient with a proximal femur fracture to have an associated pelvic fracture. Remember that the shield placed on top of the patient will greatly magnify.

Anteroposterior Femur Image Analysis

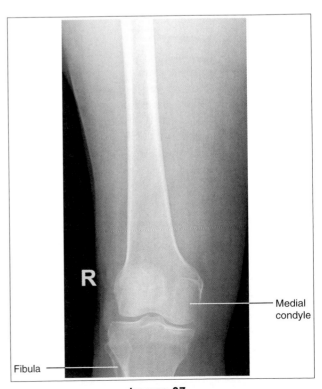

Image 87.

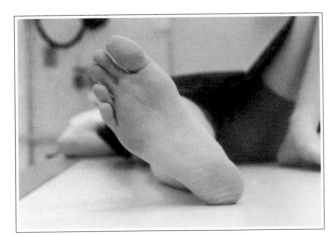

Figure 5-100. Poor foot rotation.

Analysis. The femoral epicondyles are not in profile, the medial femoral condyle appears larger than the lateral condyle, and the intercondylar eminence is not centered within the intercondylar fossa. The leg was externally rotated.

Correction. Internally rotate the leg until the femoral epicondyles are at equal distances from the IR.

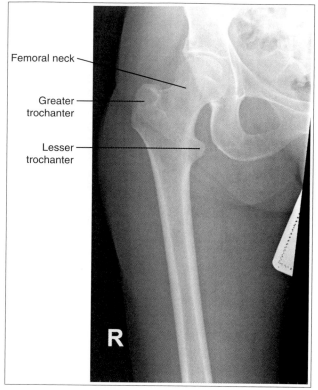

Image 89.

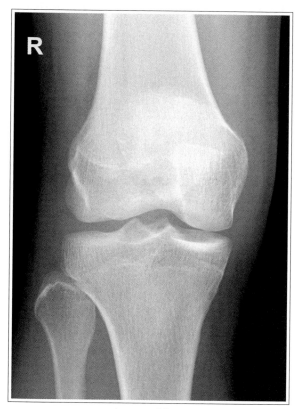

Image 88.

Analysis. This is a knee image but can be evaluated as if a distal femur. The femoral epicondyles are not in profile, the lateral femoral condyle appears larger than the medial condyle, and the tibia is superimposed over more than ¼ inch (0.6 cm) of the fibular head. The leg was internally rotated.

Correction. Externally rotate the leg until the femoral epicondyles are at equal distances from the IR.

Analysis. The femoral neck is partially foreshortened, and the lesser trochanter is demonstrated in profile. The leg was in external rotation, with the femoral epicondyles positioned at approximately a 30-degree angle with the imaging table.

Correction. Internally rotate the patient's entire leg until the foot is tilted 15 to 20 degrees from vertical and the femoral epicondyles are positioned parallel with the imaging table, as demonstrated in Figures 5-98 and 5-99.

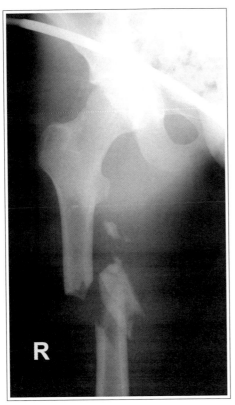

Image 90.

Analysis. The femoral neck is partially foreshortened, the lesser trochanter is demonstrated in profile, and the proximal femur demonstrates a fracture. The patient's leg was in external rotation.

Correction. Do not attempt to adjust the patient's leg position if a fracture of the proximal femur is suspected. No corrective movement is needed.

FEMUR: LATERAL POSITION (MEDIOLATERAL PROJECTION)

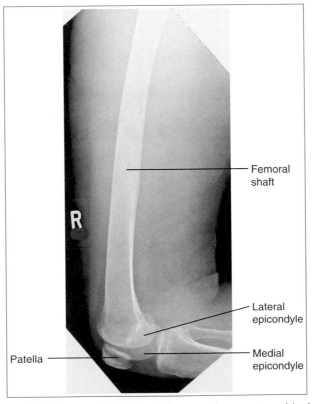

Figure 5-101. Lateral distal femur image with accurate positioning.

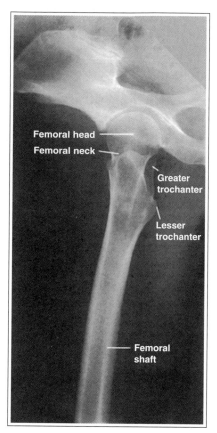

Figure 5-102. Lateral proximal femur image with accurate positioning.

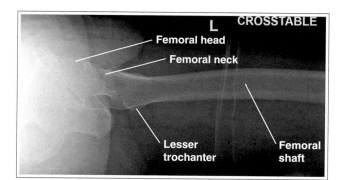

Figure 5-103. Cross-table lateral proximal femur image with accurate positioning.

Image Analysis

Image density is uniform across the lower leg.

- *Anode-heel effect:* To take advantage of the anode-heel effect, position the thicker proximal lower leg at the cathode end of the tube, and the thinner distal lower leg at the anode end. Then set an exposure (mAs) that will adequately demonstrate the midpoint of the lower leg. Because the anode absorbs some of the photons aimed at the anode end of the IR, the distal lower leg, which

requires less exposure than the proximal lower leg, will not be overexposed.

DISTAL FEMUR
The anterior and posterior margins of the medial and lateral femoral condyles are aligned, and the tibia is partially superimposed over the fibular head.

- To obtain a lateral distal femur image, place the patient in a supine position with the leg extended. Then rotate the patient onto the lateral aspect of the affected femur

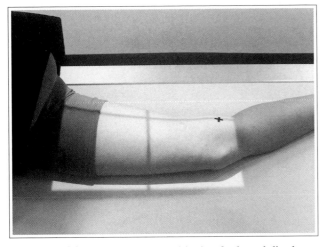

Figure 5-104. Proper patient positioning for lateral distal femur image. X indicates medial femoral epicondyle.

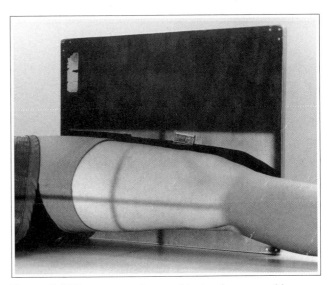

Figure 5-105. Proper patient positioning for cross-table lateral distal femur image.

until the femoral epicondyles are aligned perpendicular to the IR, and flex affected knee approximately 45 degrees (Figure 5-104). The unaffected leg can be drawn posteriorly and supported or flexed and drawn anteriorly across the proximal femur of the affected leg and supported at hip level. This positioning aligns the anterior and posterior margins of the medial and lateral femoral condyles and places a portion of the fibular head beneath the tibia.

- ***Effect of mispositioning:*** If the femoral epicondyles are not positioned perpendicular to the IR, the image demonstrates one femoral condyle anterior to the other condyle. The patient's patella must be rolled closer to or farther from the IR by adjusting patient rotation to align the condylar margins.
- The first step in determining which way to roll the patient's knee is to distinguish one condyle from the other. Because the central ray is centered proximal to the knee joint for a lateral femoral image, x-ray divergence will cause the medial condyle to project distally to the lateral condyle. Consequently, the distal condyle will be the medial condyle. If a lateral distal femur image is obtained that demonstrates the medial condyle posterior to the lateral condyle, the patient's patella was situated too far away from the IR (leg internally rotated) (see Image 5-91). If a lateral distal knee image is obtained that demonstrates the medial condyle anterior to the lateral condyle, the patient's patella was situated too close to the IR (leg externally rotated) (see Image 92).
- ***Supine femur image:*** In patients with a suspected or known fracture, rolling onto the side may cause further soft-tissue and bony injury. Consequently, a cross-table distal femur image should be taken (Figure 5-105). For this position, the patient remains in a supine position, the IR is placed against the medial aspect of the femur, and a horizontal beam is directed perpendicular to the IR.

The medial femoral condyle is projected distal to the lateral femoral condyle, closing the knee joint space.

- This image appearance is a result of central ray placement and x-ray divergence. Because the central ray is centered proximal to the femoral condyles, the x-rays that are used to record the images of the femoral condyles are diverged just as if a caudal angle were used. The divergence projects the medial condyle more distally than the lateral condyle because the medial condyle is situated farther from the IR.

The distal femoral shaft is at the center of the collimated field. The distal femoral shaft, the surrounding femoral soft tissue, the knee joint, and 1 inch (2.5 cm) of the lower leg are included within the field. Any orthopedic appliances located at the knee are included in their entirety.

- A perpendicular central ray is centered to the distal femoral shaft to place it in the center of the image. This is accomplished by positioning the lower edge of the receptor approximately 2 inches (5 cm) below the knee joint; the knee joint is located 1 inch (2.5 cm) distal to the medial epicondyle. The lower positioning is needed to prevent the diverged x-ray beams from projecting the knee joint off the IR.
- The longitudinal collimation should be left open the full length of the IR. Transverse collimation should be to within ½ inch (1.25 cm) of the lateral femoral skinline.
- A 14- × 17-inch (35- × 43-cm) screen-film or computed radiography IR placed lengthwise should be adequate to include all the required anatomical structures.
- ***Examination of the entire femur:*** If the entire femur is of interest and images are taken of the distal and the proximal ends of the femur, the images should demonstrate at least 2 inches (5 cm) of femoral shaft overlap.

Any orthopedic appliance, such as an intramedullary rod, should be included in its entirety.

PROXIMAL FEMUR

The lesser trochanter is demonstrated in profile medially, and the femoral neck and head are superimposed over the greater trochanter.

- To accomplish a lateral proximal femur position, begin by placing the patient supine on the imaging table. Roll the patient's pelvis toward the affected leg until the femur rests against the imaging table and the femoral epicondyles are aligned perpendicular to the imaging table (Figure 5-106). Adjust the pelvis so that it is rolled posteriorly just enough to prevent superimposition; 15 degrees from lateral position is sufficient. This femoral position accurately places the greater trochanter beneath the femoral neck and puts the lesser trochanter in profile medially.

- ***Effect of poor pelvis and leg rotation:*** If the pelvis is not rotated enough to place the femoral epicondyles perpendicular, the greater trochanter is demonstrated laterally (see Image 93). If the pelvis and leg are rotated too much, positioning the medial epicondyles anterior to the lateral, the greater trochanter is demonstrated medially (see Image 94).

The femoral shaft is demonstrated without foreshortening, the femoral neck is demonstrated "on-end," and the greater trochanter is demonstrated at the same transverse level as the femoral head.

- The femoral shaft is demonstrated without foreshortening and the femoral neck is demonstrated "on end" when the femur is positioned flat against the imaging table.

- ***Effect of femur abduction:*** To understand the relationship between the femoral shaft and neck, study a

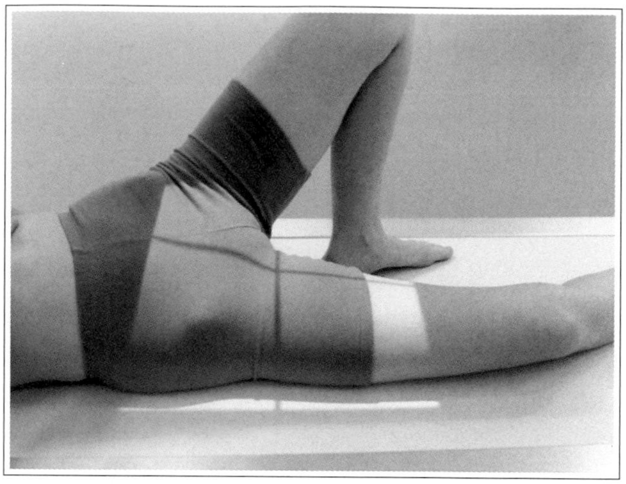

Figure 5-106. Proper patient positioning for lateral proximal femur image.

femoral skeletal bone placed in a lateral position. Notice that when the proximal femur rests against a flat surface in a lateral position, the femoral neck is on end. With this position, the femoral neck is completely foreshortened. Because of this foreshortening, the femoral neck cannot be evaluated on such a lateral image. If the femur is not positioned flat against the imaging table, the femoral neck is shown with decreased foreshortening and the femoral shaft with increased foreshortening (Image 95).

- ***Positioning for fracture:*** For a patient with a suspected or known fracture, flexing or abducting the affected leg or rolling the patient onto the affected side may cause further soft-tissue and bony injury. Therefore, an axiolateral position of the proximal femur should be used (Figures 5-103 and 5-107). Consult p. 359 for positioning instructions and evaluating criteria for this position.

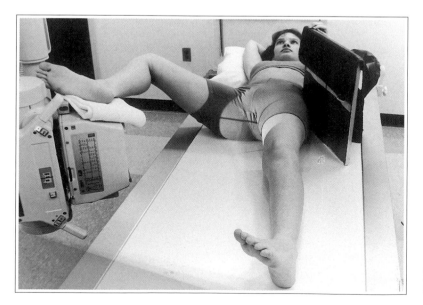

Figure 5-107. Proper patient positioning for cross-table lateral proximal femur image.

The long axis of the femoral shaft is aligned with the long axis of the collimated field.

- Aligning the long axis of the femoral shaft with the long axis of the collimated field allows tight collimation without clipping any portion of the femur or surrounding soft tissue.
- Because the femoral shaft lies across the table when it is abducted, the patient must be rotated on the imaging table until the femur is placed as close to the long axis of the collimation field as possible.

The proximal femoral shaft is at the center of the collimated field. The proximal femoral shaft, hip joint, and surrounding femoral soft tissue are included within the field. Any orthopedic appliances located at the hip are included in their entirety.

- A perpendicular central ray is centered to the proximal femoral shaft to place it in the center of the image. This is accomplished by positioning the upper edge of the receptor at the level of the ASIS (Figure 5-108). If the collimator head can be moved, turn it until one of its axes is aligned with the long axis of the femur.
- Leave the longitudinal collimation open the full length of the IR. Transverse collimation should be to within ½ inch (1.25 cm) of the lateral femoral skinline. The surrounding

femoral soft tissue should be included to detect subcutaneous air or hematomas.

- A 14- × 17-inch (35- × 43-cm) screen-film or computed radiography IR placed lengthwise should be adequate to include all the required anatomical structures.
- **Gonadal shielding:** Gonadal shielding should be used on all male patients. Because the patient is rotated for this image, it is difficult to place a shield on female patients without superimposing anatomy of interest.

Lateral Femur Image Analysis

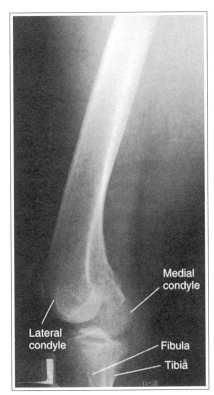

Image 91. Distal femur.

Analysis. The anterior and the posterior margins of the medial and lateral femoral condyles are not aligned. The medial condyle is posterior to the lateral condyle. The patella was too far from the IR (leg internally rotated).

Correction. Roll the patient anteriorly, positioning the patella closer to the IR (externally rotate the leg) and the femoral epicondyles perpendicular to the IR. The amount of movement needed is half of the distance demonstrated between either the anterior surfaces or the posterior surfaces of the femoral condyles.

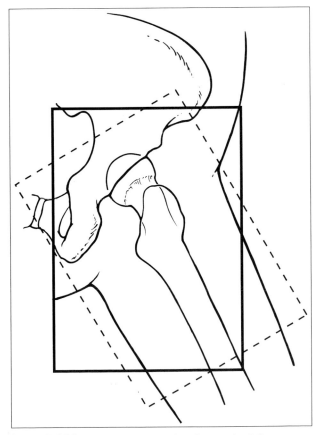

Figure 5-108. Central ray centering for proximal femur image. Dotted line rectangle indicates area covered if collimator head is turned.

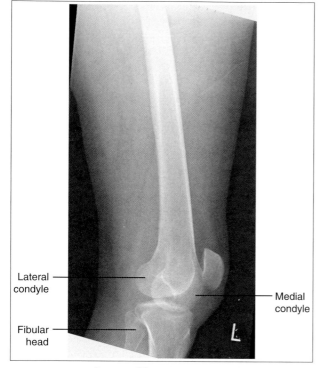

Image 92. Distal femur.

Analysis. The anterior and the posterior margins of the medial and lateral femoral condyles are not aligned. The medial condyle is positioned anterior to the lateral condyle. The patella was too close to the IR (leg externally rotated).

Correction. Roll the patient posteriorly, positioning the patella farther from the IR (internally rotate the leg) and the femoral epicondyles perpendicular to the IR. The amount of movement needed is half of the distance demonstrated between the anterior or the posterior surfaces of the femoral condyles.

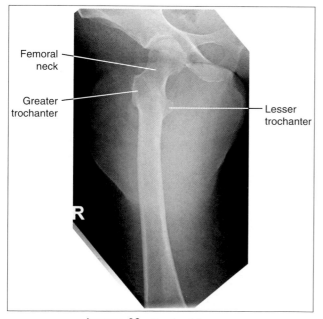

Image 93. Proximal femur.

Analysis. The greater trochanter is positioned laterally. The patient's leg was not rotated enough to position the femoral epicondyles perpendicular to the IR.

Correction. Increase the degree of external leg rotation until the femoral epicondyles are aligned perpendicular to the IR.

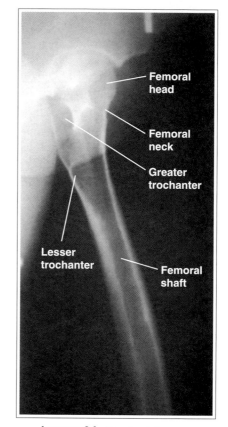

Image 94. Proximal femur.

Analysis. The greater trochanter is demonstrated medially next to the ischial tuberosity, and the lesser trochanter is not demonstrated in profile. The leg was rotated more than needed to position the femoral epicondyles perpendicular to the IR.

Correction. Decrease the amount of external leg rotation until the femoral epicondyles are aligned perpendicular to the IR.

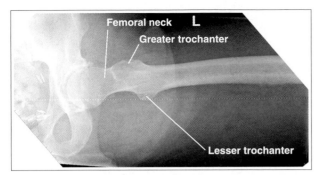

Image 95. Proximal femur.

Analysis. The femoral neck is demonstrated with decreased foreshortening, and the femoral shaft with increased foreshortening. The patient's femur was placed at a 45-degree angle with the imaging table.

Correction. The patient's pelvis should be rotated and the leg abducted as needed to place the femur against the imaging table.

Image Analysis of the Hip and Pelvis

HIP

The following image analysis criteria are used for all **hip and pelvic images** and should be considered when completing the analysis. Position- and projection-specific criteria relating to these topics are discussed with the other accompanying criteria for that position or projection.

Facility's identification requirements are visible on image as identified in Chapter 1.

A right or left marker, identifying correct side of patient, is present on the image and is not superimposed over anatomy of interest. Specific placement of marker is as described in Chapter 1.

No evidence of preventable artifacts, such as snaps, zippers, and objects in patient's pockets, is present. Patient's hand is not demonstrated beneath the hip.

- Patients often are asked to change into a gown before the hip is imaged, and their clothes are then locked in a locker. Make certain that the locker key is not left in the patient's gown pocket. Drawing the patient's arm and hand away from the affected hip ensures that the patient will not place the hand beneath the hip in an attempt to ease the hip discomfort that results from lying on the imaging table.

- Consult with the ordering physician and the patient about whether bandages or splints can be removed.

The bony trabecular patterns and the cortical outlines of the proximal femur and pelvic girdle are sharply defined.

- Sharply defined recorded details are obtained when patient motion is controlled, respiration is halted, and a short object–image receptor distance (OID) is maintained. Increased spatial resolution is also obtained when the smallest image receptor (IR) is selected for digital images.

Contrast and density are adequate to demonstrate the surrounding soft tissue and bony structures of the hip. Penetration is sufficient to visualize the bony trabecular patterns and the cortical outlines of the proximal femur and pelvic girdle.

- An optimal kilovolt-peak (kVp) technique, as shown in Table 6-1, sufficiently penetrates the proximal femur,

TABLE 6-1   Hip and Pelvic Technical Data

Position or Projection	kVp	Grid	AEC Chamber(s)	SID
AP projection, hip	70-85	Grid	Center	40-48 inches (100-120 cm)
Mediolateral (frog-leg) projection, hip	70-85	Grid	Center	40-48 inches (100-120 cm)
Axiolateral (inferosuperior) projection, hip	75-85	Grid		40-48 inches (100-120 cm)
AP projection, pelvis	65-85	Grid	Both outside	40-48 inches (100-120 cm)
AP oblique (frog-leg) projection, pelvis	65-85	Grid	Both outside	40-48 inches (100-120 cm)
AP axial projection, sacroiliac joints	80-85	Grid	Center	40-48 inches (100-120 cm)
AP oblique projection, sacroiliac joints	75-85	Grid	Center	40-48 inches (100-120 cm)

AEC, Automatic exposure control; *AP*, anteroposterior; *kVp*, kilovolt peak; *SID*, source–image receptor distance.

hip, and pelvic structures and provides a contrast scale necessary to visualize the pelvic and femoral details. Use a grid to absorb the scatter radiation produced by the proximal femur, hip, and pelvis, providing a higher-contrast image. To obtain optimal density, set a manual milliampere-seconds (mAs) level based on the patient's part thickness or choose the appropriate automatic exposure control (AEC) chamber when recommended (see Table 6-1). AEC is contraindicated if patient has hip or pelvic hardware or a prosthesis.

HIP: ANTEROPOSTERIOR PROJECTION

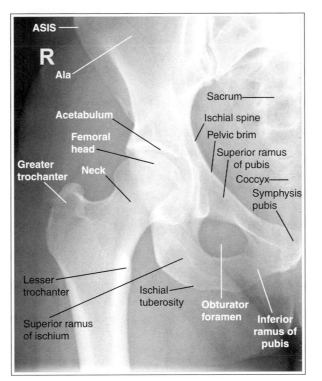

Figure 6-1. Anteroposterior hip image with accurate positioning.

Image Analysis

Contrast and density are adequate to demonstrate the fat planes of the hip.

- *Fat planes on anteroposterior (AP) hip and pelvic images:* When evaluating pelvic images, the reviewer not only analyzes the bony structures but also studies the placement of the soft-tissue fat planes. Four fat planes are of interest on AP hip images, and their visualization aids in the detection of intraarticular and periarticular disease: obturator internus fat plane, which lies within the pelvic inlet next to the medial brim; the iliopsoas fat plane, which lies medial to the lesser trochanter; the pericapsular fat plane, which is found superior to the femoral neck; and the gluteal fat plane, which lies superior to the pericapsular fat plane (Figure 6-2).

The pelvis demonstrates an AP projection. The ischial spine is aligned with the pelvic brim, the sacrum and coccyx are aligned with the symphysis pubis, and the obturator foramen is open.

- An AP projection of the hip is obtained by placing the patient supine on the imaging table with the legs extended (Figure 6-3). To ensure that the pelvis is not rotated, judge the distance from the anterior superior iliac spine (ASIS) to the imaging table on each side. The distances should be equal.

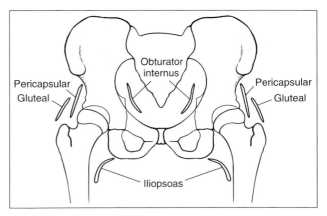

Figure 6-2. Location of fat planes.

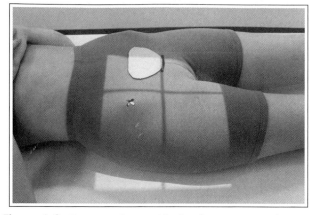

Figure 6-3. Proper patient positioning for anteroposterior hip image.

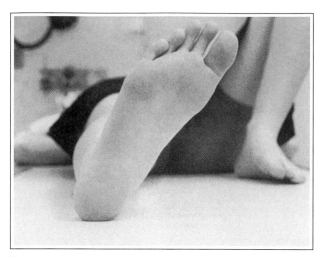

Figure 6-4. Proper internal foot rotation: 15 to 20 degrees from vertical.

- ***Detecting hip rotation:*** Rotation on an AP hip image is initially detected by evaluating the relationship of the ischial spine and the pelvic brim, the alignment of the sacrum and coccyx with the symphysis pubis, and the degree of obturator foramen demonstration. If the patient was rotated toward the affected hip, the ischial spine is demonstrated without pelvic brim superimposition; the sacrum and coccyx are not aligned with the symphysis pubis but are rotated away from the affected hip; and the obturator foramen is narrowed (see Image 1). If the patient has been rotated away from the affected hip, the ischial spine is not aligned with the pelvic brim but is demonstrated closer to the acetabulum; the sacrum and coccyx are not aligned with the symphysis pubis, but are rotated toward the affected hip; and the obturator foramen is widened (see Image 2).

The femoral neck is demonstrated without foreshortening, the greater trochanter is demonstrated in profile laterally, and the lesser trochanter is super-imposed by the femoral neck.

- ***Accurate leg positioning:*** To demonstrate an AP hip on an image, in which the femoral neck should be shown without foreshortening and the greater trochanter in profile, the patient's leg should be internally rotated until the foot is angled 15 to 20 degrees from vertical and the femoral epicondyles are positioned parallel with the imaging table (Figure 6-4). (See also Figure 6-2 and Image 2). A sandbag or tape may be needed to help the patient maintain this internal leg rotation.
- ***Poor leg positioning:*** The relationship of the patient's leg to the imaging table determines how the femoral neck and trochanters are shown on an AP hip image. Generally, when patients are relaxed, their legs and feet are externally (laterally) rotated. On external rotation the femoral neck declines posteriorly (toward the table) and is foreshortened on an AP hip image. Increased external rotation increases the degree of posterior decline and foreshortening of the femoral neck on the image. If the patient's leg is externally (laterally) rotated

enough to position the foot at a 45-degree angle and an imaginary line connecting the femoral epicondyles at a 60- to 65-degree angle with the imaging table, the femoral neck is demonstrated "on end" and the lesser trochanter is demonstrated in profile (Figure 6-5 and Image 3). If the patient's leg is positioned with the foot placed vertically and an imaginary line connecting the femoral epicondyles at approximately a 15- to 20-degree angle with the imaging table, the lesser trochanter is demonstrated in partial profile and the femoral neck is only partially foreshortened (see Image 4).

- ***Positioning for a fractured or dislocated proximal femur:*** When a patient has a dislocated or fractured proximal femur, the leg should not be internally rotated but left "as is." Forced internal rotation of a dislocated or fractured proximal femur may injure the blood supply and nerves that surround the injured area. Because the patient's leg is not internally rotated when a fracture is suspected, the resulting AP hip image may demonstrate the femoral neck with some degree of foreshortening

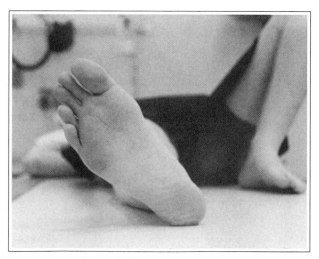

Figure 6-5. Poor foot rotation.

and the lesser trochanter without femoral shaft superimposition (see Image 5).

The femoral head and acetabulum are at the center of the collimated field if the hip joint is of greatest interest, and the femoral neck is at the center of the field if it is of greatest interest. The acetabulum, greater and lesser trochanters, femoral head and neck, and half of the sacrum, coccyx, and symphysis pubis are included within the field. Any orthopedic appliances located at the hip are included in their entirety.

- A perpendicular central ray should be centered 1½ inches (4 cm) distal to the midpoint of a line connecting the ASIS and superior symphysis pubis, to center the hip joint in the center of the collimated field, and 2½ inches (6.25 cm) distal to the midpoint of a line connecting the ASIS and superior symphysis pubis, to center the femoral neck in the center of the collimated field (Figure 6-6). Center the IR to the central ray and open the longitudinal collimation enough to include the ASIS and any hip orthopedic appliances. Transversely collimate to the patient's midsagittal plane and within ½ inch (1.25 cm) of the lateral hip skinline. Including half of the sacrum, coccyx, and symphysis pubis within the collimated field provides a way to evaluate pelvic rotation.
- A 10- × 12-inch (24- × 30-cm) IR placed lengthwise should be adequate to include all the required anatomical structures. A larger IR and lower centering point may be necessary to include hip orthopedic appliances.

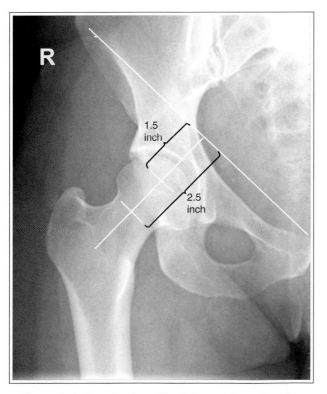

Figure 6-6. Localization of hip joint and femoral neck.

- **Gonadal shielding:** Use gonadal shielding on all male patients. Female patients should be shielded, although it is important that no pelvic anatomy be covered by the shield. It is not uncommon for patients with hip fractures to have an associated pelvic fracture. Remember that a shield placed on top of the patient will be greatly magnified.

Anteroposterior Hip Image Analysis

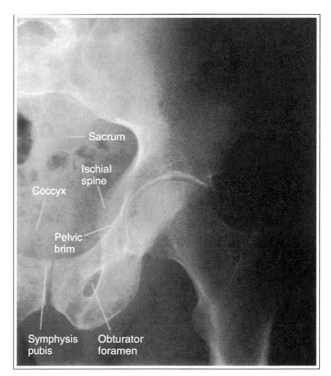

Image 1.

Analysis. The ischial spine is demonstrated without pelvic brim superimposition, the sacrum and coccyx are not aligned with the symphysis pubis but are rotated away from the affected hip, and the obturator foramen is narrowed. The patient was rotated toward the affected hip. The femoral neck is partially foreshortened, and the lesser trochanter is demonstrated in profile. The patient's leg was externally rotated.

Correction. Rotate the patient away from the affected hip until the ASISs are positioned at equal distances from the imaging table. Internally rotate the patient's leg until the foot is angled 15 to 20 degrees from vertical and the femoral epicondyles are positioned parallel with the imaging table, as demonstrated in Figure 6-4.

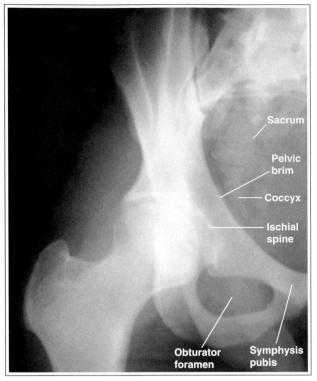

Image 2.

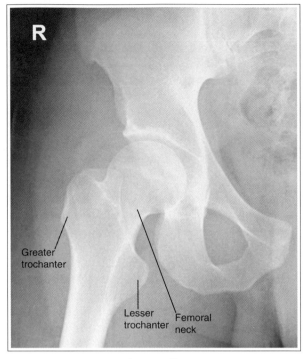

Image 3.

Analysis. The ischial spine is not aligned with the pelvic brim but is demonstrated closer to the acetabulum, the sacrum and coccyx are not aligned with the symphysis pubis but are rotated toward the affected hip, and the obturator foramen is clearly demonstrated. The patient was rotated away from the affected hip.

Correction. Rotate the patient toward the affected hip until the ASISs are positioned at equal distances from the imaging table.

Analysis. The femoral neck is completely foreshortened, and the lesser trochanter is demonstrated in profile. The patient's leg was in external rotation with the foot positioned at a 45-degree angle and the femoral epicondyles at a 25- to 30-degree angle with the imaging table, as demonstrated in Figure 6-5.

Correction. Internally rotate the patient's leg until the foot is angled 15 to 20 degrees from vertical and the femoral epicondyles are positioned parallel with the imaging table, as demonstrated in Figure 6-4.

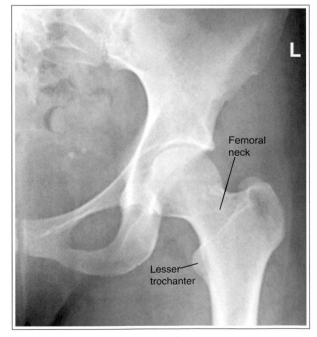

Image 4.

Analysis. The femoral neck is partially foreshortened, and the lesser trochanter is demonstrated in profile. The patient's leg was externally rotated, bringing the foot vertical and the femoral epicondyles to approximately a 15- to 20-degree angle with the imaging table.

Correction. Internally rotate the patient's leg until the foot is angled 15 to 20 degrees from vertical and the femoral epicondyles are positioned parallel with the imaging table, as demonstrated in Figure 6-4.

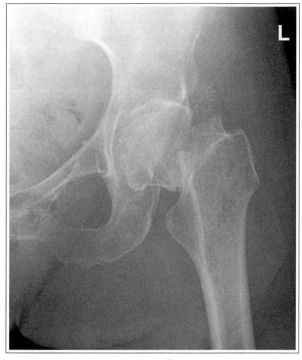

Image 5.

Analysis. The femoral neck is partially foreshortened and demonstrates a fracture. The lesser trochanter is demonstrated in profile. The patient's leg was in external rotation.

Correction. Do not attempt to adjust the patient's leg position if a fracture of the proximal femur is suspected. No corrective movement is needed.

HIP: MEDIOLATERAL (FROG-LEG) PROJECTION (MODIFIED CLEAVES METHOD)

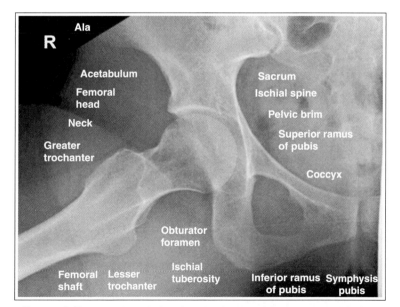

Figure 6-7. Mediolateral (frog-leg) hip image with accurate positioning.

Image Analysis

The pelvis demonstrates an AP projection. The ischial spine is aligned with the pelvic brim, the sacrum and coccyx are aligned with the symphysis pubis, and the obturator foramen is open.

- A frog-leg image of the hip is obtained by placing the patient supine on the imaging table with the unaffected leg extended and the affected leg flexed and abducted (Figure 6-8). To ensure that the pelvis is not rotated, judge the distance from the ASIS to the imaging table on each side. The distances should be equal.

- *Detecting hip rotation:* Rotation on a frog-leg hip image is detected by evaluating the relationship of the ischial spine and the pelvic brim, the alignment of the sacrum and coccyx with the symphysis pubis, and the demonstration of the obturator foramen. If the patient was rotated toward the affected hip, the ischial spine is demonstrated without pelvic brim superimposition, the sacrum and coccyx are not aligned with the symphysis pubis but are rotated away from the affected hip, and demonstration of the obturator foramen is decreased (see Image 6). If the patient was rotated away from the affected hip, the ischial spine is not aligned with the pelvic brim but is demonstrated closer to the acetabulum, the sacrum and coccyx are not aligned with the symphysis pubis but are rotated toward the affected hip, and demonstration of the obturator foramen is increased (see Image 7).
- *Lauenstein and Hickey methods, lateral hip:* The Lauenstein-Hickey method is a modification of the frog-leg position. For this method the patient is positioned as described for the frog-leg hip image with the femur flexed and abducted, except the pelvis is rotated toward the affected hip as needed to position the femur against the imaging table. Image 6 demonstrates how the rotated pelvis in this image would appear, and Image 11 demonstrates how the proximal femur would appear.

The lesser trochanter is demonstrated in profile medially, and the femoral neck is superimposed over the greater trochanter.

- *Accurate femur positioning:* To accurately position the greater trochanter beneath the proximal femur and position the lesser trochanter in profile, flex the patient's knee and hip until the femur is angled at 60 to 70 degrees with the imaging table (20 to 30 degrees from vertical) (Figure 6-9). If the knee and hip are not flexed enough to place the femur at this angle with the imaging table, the greater trochanter is demonstrated laterally, as it is on an AP projection (see Image 8). If the knee and hip are flexed too much, placing the femur at an angle greater than 60 to 70 degrees with the imaging table, the greater trochanter is demonstrated medially (see Image 9).
- The greater trochanter is also demonstrated medially, as demonstrated in Image 8, when the foot and ankle of the affected leg are elevated and placed on top of the unaffected leg. This positioning causes the femur to rotate externally. The foot of the affected leg should remain resting on the imaging table.
- *Effect of distal femur elevation on proximal femur visualization:* For a frog-leg hip image, the position of the greater and lesser trochanters in relationship to the proximal femur is determined when the patient flexes the knee and hip.
- Use a femoral skeletal bone to better understand how the relationship of the greater and lesser trochanters to the proximal femur changes as the distal femur is elevated with knee and hip flexion. Begin by placing the femoral bone on a flat surface in an AP position. While slowly elevating the distal femur, observe how the greater trochanter rotates around the proximal femur. First, the greater trochanter moves beneath the proximal femur; then, as elevation of the distal femur continues, it moves from beneath the proximal femur and is demonstrated on the medial side of the femur.

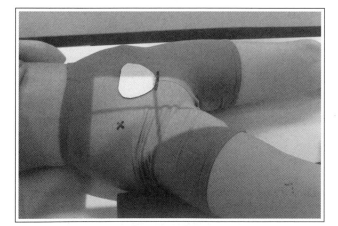

Figure 6-8. Proper patient positioning for mediolateral (frog-leg) hip image.

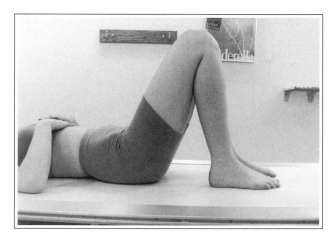

Figure 6-9. Proper knee and hip flexion: 60 to 70 degrees from imaging table.

The femoral neck is partially foreshortened, and the greater trochanter is demonstrated at a transverse level halfway between the femoral head and the lesser trochanter.

- *Accurate leg positioning:* To demonstrate the femoral neck and proximal femur with only partial foreshortening and the greater trochanter at a transverse level halfway between the femoral head and lesser trochanter on a pelvis image, abduct the femoral shafts to a 45-degree angle from vertical (Figure 6-10) (see also Figure 6-7).

- *Effect of leg abduction:* The degree of femoral abduction determines the amount of femoral neck foreshortening and the transverse level at which the greater trochanters are demonstrated between the femoral heads and lesser trochanters.

- Use a femoral skeleton bone to understand how leg abduction determines the visualization of the femoral neck and the position of the greater trochanter. Place the femoral bone on a flat surface in an AP position with the distal femur elevated until the greater trochanter is positioned beneath the proximal femur and the lesser trochanter is in profile (20 to 30 degrees from vertical or 60 to 70 degrees from flat surface). From this position, abduct the femoral bone (move the lateral surface of the femoral bone toward the flat surface). As the bone moves toward the flat surface, observe how the femoral neck is positioned more on end and the greater trochanter moves proximally (toward the femoral head).

- *Poor leg abduction:* If the femoral neck is demonstrated without foreshortening and the greater trochanter is at the same transverse level as the lesser trochanter on a frog-leg hip image, the femoral shaft was abducted 20 to 30 degrees from vertical (60- to 70-degree angle from the imaging table) (see Image 10 and Figure 6-11).

- If the proximal femoral shaft is demonstrated without foreshortening, the greater trochanter is at the same transverse level as the femoral head, and the femoral

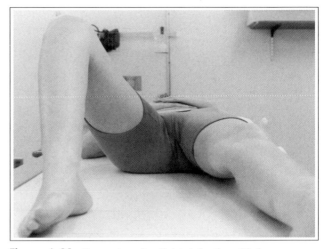

Figure 6-11. Femur in only slight abduction: 20 degrees from vertical (70 degrees from imaging table).

neck is demonstrated "on end" on a frog-leg hip image, the femoral shaft was abducted next to the imaging table (Image 11 and Figure 6-12).

The femoral head and acetabulum are at the center of the collimated field if the hip joint is of greatest interest, and the femoral neck is at the center of the field if it is of greatest interest. The acetabulum, greater and lesser trochanters, and femoral head and neck, as well as half of the sacrum, coccyx, and symphysis pubis are included within the field.

- Center a perpendicular central ray 1½ inches (4 cm) distal to the midpoint of a line connecting the ASIS and superior symphysis pubis, to center the hip joint in the center of the collimated field, and 2½ inches (6.25 cm) distal to the midpoint of a line connecting the ASIS and superior symphysis pubis, to center the femoral neck in the center of the collimated field. Center the IR to the central ray and open longitudinal collimation to include the ASIS. Transversely collimate to the patient's midsagittal plane and transversely collimate to within ½ inch (1.25 cm) of the lateral hip skinline.

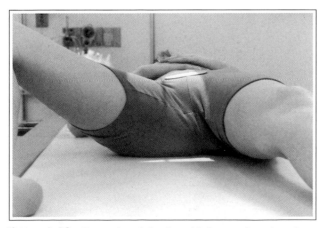

Figure 6-10. Proper leg abduction: 45 degrees from imaging table.

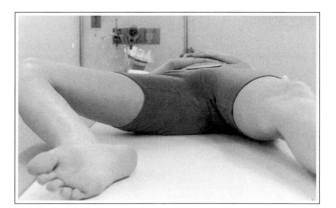

Figure 6-12. Femur in maximum abduction: 20 degrees from imaging table.

- Including half of the sacrum, coccyx, and symphysis pubis within the collimated field provides a way to evaluate pelvic rotation.
- A 10- × 12-inch (24- × 30-cm) IR placed lengthwise should be adequate to include all the required anatomical structures.
- *Gonadal shielding:* Use gonadal shielding on all male patients. Female patients should be shielded, although it is important that no pelvic anatomy be covered with the shield. Remember that the shield placed on top of the patient will be greatly magnified.

Mediolateral (Frog-Leg) Hip Image Analysis

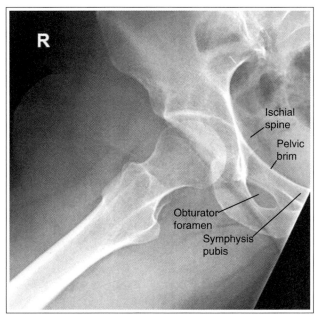

Image 6.

Analysis. The ischial spine is demonstrated without pelvic brim superimposition, the sacrum and coccyx are not aligned with the symphysis pubis but are rotated away from the affected hip, and the obturator foramen is not well demonstrated. The patient was rotated toward the affected hip.

Correction. Rotate the patient away from the affected hip until the ASISs are positioned at equal distances from the imaging table.

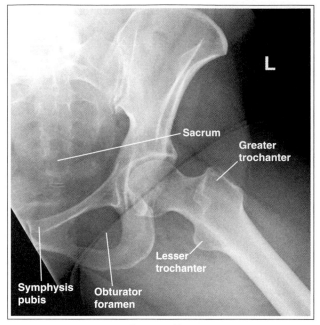

Image 7.

Analysis. The ischial spine is not aligned with the pelvic brim but is demonstrated closer to the acetabulum, the sacrum and coccyx are not aligned with the symphysis pubis but are rotated toward the affected hip, and obturator foramen is well demonstrated. The patient was rotated away from the affected hip.

Correction. Rotate the patient toward the affected hip until the ASISs are positioned at equal distances from the imaging table.

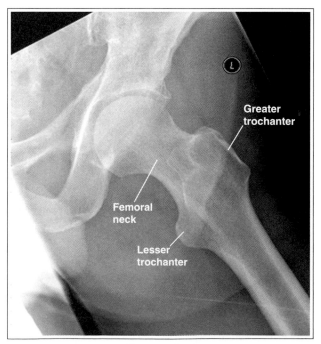

Image 8.

Analysis. The greater trochanter is positioned laterally. The patient's knee was not flexed enough to align the femur at a 60- to 70-degree angle with the imaging table (20 to 30 degrees from vertical), or the affected leg's foot and ankle were resting on top of the unaffected leg, elevating them off the imaging table. The femoral neck is demonstrated on end. The greater trochanter is visible at about the same transverse level as the femoral head. The femur was positioned close to the imaging table. If the femoral neck is of interest, decrease the degree of femoral abduction until the femur is at a 45-degree angle with the imaging table.

Correction. Increase the knee flexion until the femur is aligned at a 60- to 70-degree angle with the imaging table, as demonstrated in Figure 6-9, or lower the affected leg's foot to the imaging table.

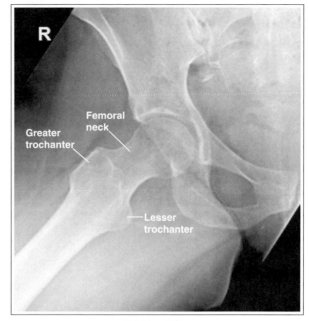

Image 10.

Analysis. The femoral neck is demonstrated without foreshortening, and the greater and lesser trochanters are demonstrated at approximately the same transverse level. The femur was in only slight abduction, at approximately a 70-degree angle with the imaging table (20 degrees from vertical), as demonstrated in Figure 6-11. The greater trochanter is partially demonstrated laterally, indicating that the leg was flexed less than the needed 60 to 70 degrees from the imaging table.

Correction. If the proximal femoral shaft demonstrates too much foreshortening for your facility standards, have the patient abduct the femur to a 45-degree angle with the imaging table. Increase the knee and hip flexion until the femur is positioned at a 60- to 70-degree angle with the imaging table, as demonstrated in Figure 6-9.

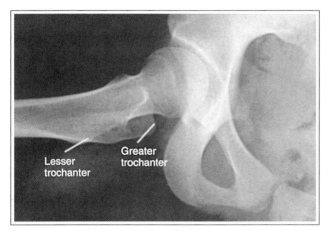

Image 9.

Analysis. The greater trochanter is positioned medially. The patient's knee was flexed more than needed, positioning the femur at an angle greater than 60 to 70 degrees with the imaging table (20 to 30 degrees from vertical).

Correction. Decrease the knee flexion until the femur is aligned at a 60- to 70-degree angle with the imaging table, as demonstrated in Figure 6-9.

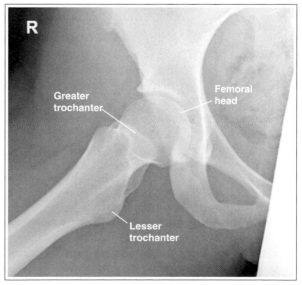

Image 11.

Analysis. The femoral neck is demonstrated on end. The greater trochanter is demonstrated on the same transverse level as the femoral head. The femur was positioned next to the imaging table, as demonstrated in Figure 6-12.

Correction. Decrease the degree of femoral abduction until the femur is at a 45-degree angle with the imaging table, as shown in Figure 6-10.

HIP: AXIOLATERAL (INFEROSUPERIOR) PROJECTION (DANELIUS-MILLER METHOD)

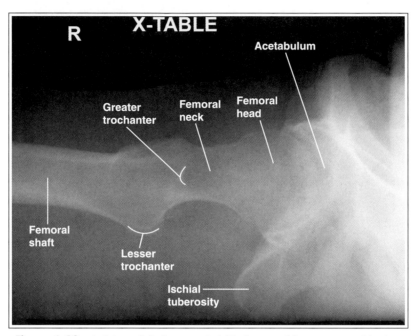

Figure 6-13. Axiolateral (inferosuperior) hip image with accurate positioning.

Image Analysis

Scatter radiation is controlled. Proximal femur demonstrates even density.

- Tight collimation and placement of a flat lead contact strip or the straight edge of a lead apron over the top, unused half of the IR, as demonstrated in Figure 6-14, also prevent scatter radiation from reaching the IR.
- *Compensating filter:* Frequently, when an exposure (mAs) is set that adequately demonstrates the hip joint, the proximal femur is overexposed because of the difference in body thickness in these two regions. A wedge-type compensating filter attached to the x-ray tube can be used to obtain uniform image density of the hip joint and proximal femur. Align the thin end of the filter with the femoral neck and the thicker end with the proximal femur.

The femoral neck is demonstrated without foreshortening, and the greater and lesser trochanters are demonstrated at approximately the same transverse level.

- An axiolateral image of the hip is obtained by placing the patient on the imaging table in an AP projection,

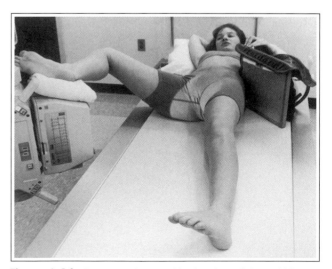

Figure 6-14. Proper patient positioning for axiolateral hip image.

with the unaffected hip positioned next to the lateral edge of the table. Flex the patient's unaffected leg until the femur is as close to a vertical position as the patient can tolerate, then abduct the leg as far as the patient will allow. Support this leg position by using a specially designed leg holder or suitable support.

- Flexion and abduction of the unaffected leg move its bony and soft-tissue structures away from the affected hip. Inadequate flexion or abduction of the unaffected leg results in superimposition of soft tissue onto the affected hip, preventing visualization of the affected hip (see Image 12).

- *IR placement:* Once the patient's unaffected leg has been positioned, place the grid-IR against the patient's affected side at the level of the iliac crest (see Figure 6-14). To demonstrate the affected femoral neck without fore-shortening, align the x-ray tube horizontally with the central ray perpendicular to the femoral neck and adjust the distal end of the IR until the receptor's long axis is perpendicular to the central ray and parallel with the femoral neck.

- *Localizing the femoral neck for central ray alignment:* To localize the affected femoral neck, first find the center of an imaginary line drawn between the superior symphysis pubis and the ASIS. Then bisect that line by drawing a perpendicular line distally (Figure 6-15). This imaginary

line parallels the long axis of the femoral neck as long as the leg is not abducted.

- Once the long axis of the femoral neck has been located, align the central ray perpendicular to it and the IR parallel with it.

- *Effect of central ray and femoral neck misalignment:* Misalignment of the central ray with the femoral neck results in femoral neck foreshortening and a shift in the transverse level at which the greater trochanter is located. If the angle formed between the femur and the central ray is too large, the greater trochanter is demonstrated proximal to the transverse level of the lesser trochanter and is superimposed by a portion of the femoral neck (see Image 13). If the angle between the femur and the central ray is too small, the greater trochanter is demonstrated distal to the transverse level of the lesser trochanter. This mispositioning seldom occurs, because the imaging table and tube position prevent such a small angle.

The lesser trochanter is demonstrated in profile posteriorly, and the greater trochanter is superimposed by the femoral shaft.

- Rotation of the patient's affected leg determines the relationship of the lesser and greater trochanter to the proximal femur on an axiolateral hip image. Generally, when a patient is placed on the imaging table and the affected leg is allowed to rotate freely, it is laterally (externally) rotated.

- *Effect of leg rotation on proximal femur visualization:* To position the proximal femur in a lateral position (90 degrees from the AP projection), demonstrating the lesser trochanter in profile posteriorly and superimposing the greater trochanter by the femoral shaft, the affected leg must be internally rotated until an imaginary line drawn between the femoral epicondyles is positioned parallel with the imaging table. The patient's foot is angled internally 15 to 20 degrees from a vertical position (Figure 6-16). If the affected leg is not rotated

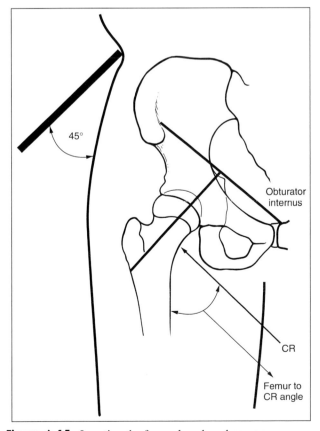

Figure 6-15. Locating the femoral neck and proper image receptor placement for small and average patients. *CR*, Central ray.

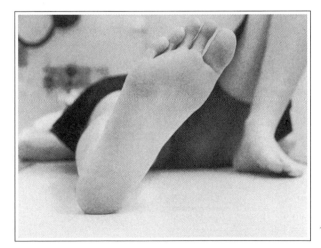

Figure 6-16. Proper foot position: 15 to 20 degrees from vertical.

internally, the greater trochanter is demonstrated posteriorly and the lesser trochanter is superimposed over
the femoral shaft (see Image 14). How much greater
trochanter is demonstrated without femoral shaft superimposition depends on the degree of external rotation.
Greater external rotation increases the amount of
greater trochanter shown.

- ***Positioning for a proximal femoral fracture or dislocation:*** When a patient has a dislocated hip or a suspected
  or known proximal femoral fracture, the leg should not
  be internally rotated, but left "as is." Forced internal
  rotation of a dislocated hip or fractured proximal femur
  may injure the blood supply and nerves that surround the
  injured area. Because the patient's leg is not internally
  rotated in such cases, it is acceptable for the greater
  trochanter to be demonstrated posteriorly and the lesser
  trochanter to be superimposed over the femoral shaft
  (see Image 15).

**The femoral neck is at the center of the collimated
field. The acetabulum, femoral head and neck, greater
and lesser trochanters, and ischial tuberosity are
included within the field. Any orthopedic appliance
should be included in its entirety.**

- Center a perpendicular central ray to the patient's
  midthigh, at the level of the femoral neck, to place it in the
  center of the collimated field. The center of the femoral
  neck is located at a level 2½ inches (6.25 cm) distal to the
  midpoint of a line connecting the ASIS and superior symphysis pubis. Open the longitudinal collimation the full
  length of the IR. Transversely collimate to within ½ inch
  (1.25 cm) of the proximal femoral skinline.
- A 10- × 12-inch (24- × 30-cm) IR placed lengthwise
  should be adequate to include all the required anatomical structures.
- ***IR placement alternative:*** The level at which the IR is
  placed along the patient's lateral body surface determines whether the acetabulum and femoral head are
  included on the IR. For patients with minimal lateral
  soft-tissue thickness, the upper IR edge should be firmly
  placed in the crease formed at the patient's waist, just
  superior to the iliac crest (see Figure 6-15). For patients
  with ample lateral soft-tissue thickness, the IR needs to
  be positioned superior to the iliac crest (Figure 6-17).
  This superior positioning will result in magnification
  because of the increase in the OID but is necessary if
  the acetabulum and femoral head are to be included on
  the axiolateral hip image.

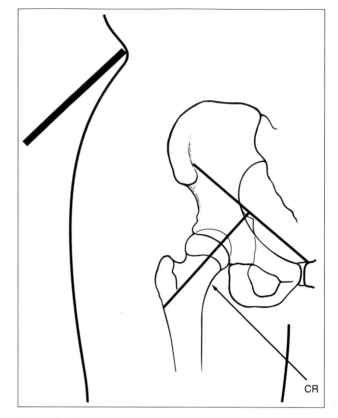

Figure 6-17. Proper image receptor placement for large
patients. *CR,* Central ray.

Axiolateral Hip Image Analysis

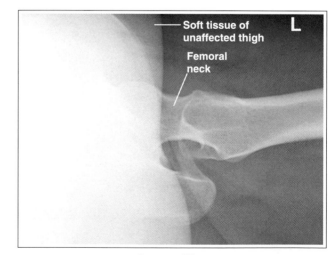

Image 12.

Analysis. Soft tissue from the unaffected thigh is superimposing the acetabulum and femoral head of the affected
hip. The unaffected leg was not adequately flexed or
abducted.

Correction. Flex and abduct the unaffected leg, drawing it away from the affected acetabulum and femoral head. If the patient is unable to further adjust the unaffected leg, the kVp and mAs can be increased to demonstrate this area. A wedge-type compensating filter may also be added to prevent overpenetration of the femoral neck and shaft.

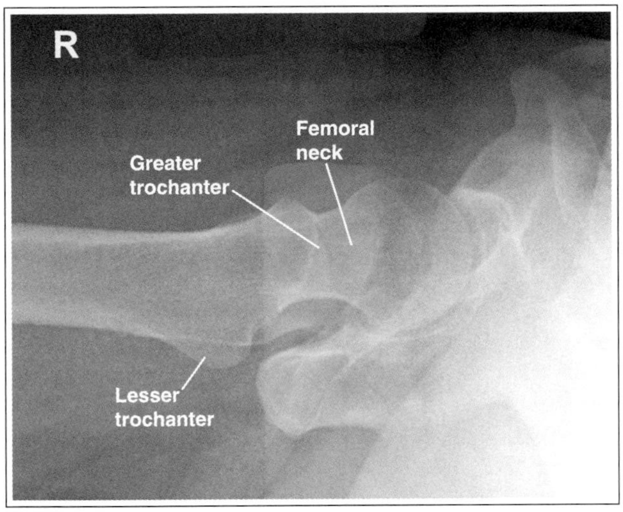

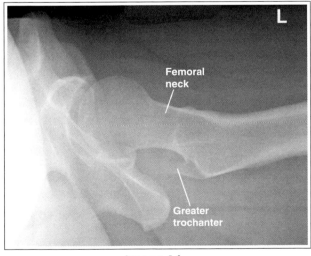

Image 13.

Analysis. The greater trochanter is demonstrated at a transverse level proximal to the lesser trochanter, and the femoral neck is partially foreshortened. The angle between the central ray and femur was too large.

Correction. Localize the femoral neck. Position the IR parallel with the femoral neck and the central ray perpendicular to the IR and femoral neck, as demonstrated in Figure 6-15.

Image 14.

Analysis. The greater trochanter is demonstrated posteriorly, and the lesser trochanter is superimposed over the femoral shaft. The patient's affected leg was in external rotation.

Correction. Internally rotate the patient's leg until the femoral epicondyles are aligned parallel with the imaging table and the foot is angled internally 15 to 20 degrees from vertical, as demonstrated in Figure 6-16.

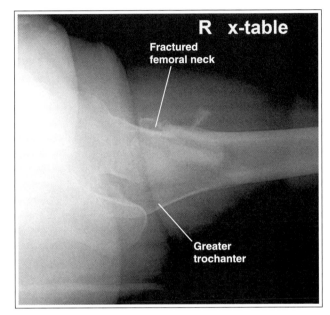

Image 15.

Analysis. A fracture of the femoral neck is present. The greater trochanter is demonstrated posteriorly, and the lesser trochanter is superimposed over the femoral shaft. The patient's leg was in external rotation.

Correction. Do not attempt to adjust the patient's leg position if a fracture of the proximal femur is suspected. No corrective movement is needed.

PELVIS

See page 348 for image analysis criteria for all hip and pelvic images.

PELVIS: ANTEROPOSTERIOR PROJECTION

Regarding the male and female pelves: Be aware of the bony architectural differences that exist between the male and female pelves (Table 6-2). These differences are the result of the need for the female pelvis to accommodate fetal growth during pregnancy and fetal passage during delivery.

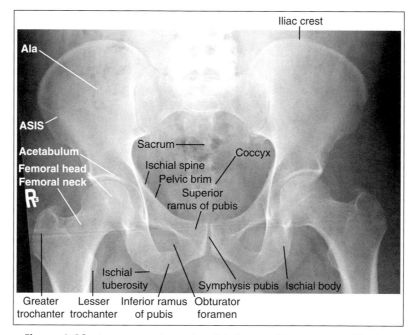

Figure 6-18. Anteroposterior male pelvis image with accurate positioning.

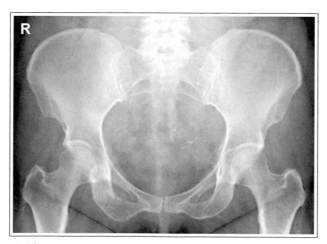

Figure 6-19. Anteroposterior female pelvis image with accurate positioning.

TABLE 6-2	Male and Female Pelvic Differences	
	Male	**Female**
Overall shape	Bulkier, deeper, narrower	Smaller, shallower, and wider
Ala	Narrower, nonflared	Wider, flared
Pubic arch angle	Acute angle	Obtuse angle
Inlet shape	Smaller, heart shaped	Larger, rounded shape
Obturator foramen	Larger	Smaller

Image Analysis

Contrast and density are adequate to demonstrate the fat planes of the pelvis.

- *Fat planes on AP pelvic images:* When evaluating pelvic images, the reviewer not only analyzes the bony structures but also studies the placement of the soft-tissue fat planes. Four fat planes of interest are present on AP pelvic images, and their visualization aids in the detection of intraarticular and periarticular disease: the obturator internus fat plane, which lies within the pelvic inlet next to the medial brim; the iliopsoas fat plane, which lies medial to the lesser trochanter; the pericapsular fat plane, which is found superior to the femoral neck; and the gluteal fat plane, which lies superior to the pericapsular fat plane (see Figure 6-29).

The pelvis demonstrates an AP projection. The ischial spines are aligned with the pelvic brim, the sacrum and coccyx are aligned with the symphysis pubis, and the ilia and the obturator foramina are uniform in size and shape.

- An AP projection of the pelvis is accomplished by placing the patient supine on the imaging table with the legs extended and the arms drawn away from the pelvic area (Figure 6-20). To ensure that the pelvis is not rotated, judge the distance from the ASIS to the imaging table on each side. The distances should be equal.
- *Detecting pelvic rotation:* A nonrotated pelvis image demonstrates symmetrical ilia and obturator foramina. Rotation is initially detected by evaluating the relationships of the ischial spines with the pelvic brim and of the sacrum and coccyx with the symphysis pubis. The ischial spines should be aligned with the pelvic brim, and the sacrum and coccyx should be in alignment with the symphysis pubis on a nonrotated pelvis.
- If the pelvis is rotated into a left posterior oblique (LPO) position, the left ilium is wider than the right, the left obturator foramen is narrower than the right, the left ischial spine is demonstrated without pelvic brim superimposition, and the sacrum and coccyx are not aligned with the symphysis pubis but are rotated toward the right hip (Image 16).

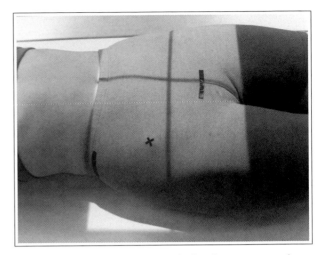

Figure 6-20. Proper patient positioning for anteroposterior pelvis image.

- If the patient was rotated into a right posterior oblique (RPO) position, the opposite is true. The right ilium is wider than the left, the right obturator foramen is narrower than the left, the right ischial spine is demonstrated without pelvic brim superimposition, and the sacrum and coccyx are rotated toward the left hip.

The femoral necks are demonstrated without foreshortening and the greater trochanters are demonstrated in profile laterally, whereas the lesser trochanters are superimposed by the femoral necks.

- *Accurate leg positioning:* To demonstrate the femoral necks without foreshortening and the greater trochanters in profile on an AP pelvis image, the patient's leg should be internally rotated until the feet are angled 15 to 20 degrees from vertical and the femoral epicondyles are positioned parallel with the imaging table (Figure 6-21) (see also Figure 6-18). Sandbags or tape may be needed to help maintain this internal leg rotation. A pelvic image may not demonstrate the proximal femurs with exactly

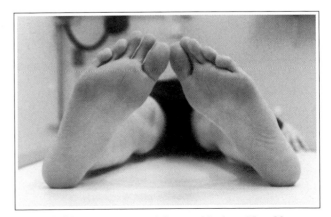

Figure 6-21. Proper internal foot positioning: 15 to 20 degrees from vertical.

the same degree of internal rotation. How each proximal femur will appear depends on the degree of internal rotation placed on that leg.

- **Poor leg positioning:** The relationship of the patient's entire leg to the imaging table determines how the femoral necks and trochanters are shown on an AP pelvis image. Generally when patients are relaxed, their legs and feet are externally (laterally) rotated. On external rotation the femoral necks decline posteriorly (toward the table) and are foreshortened on an AP pelvis image. Greater external rotation increases the posterior decline and foreshortening of the femoral necks. If the patient's legs are externally (laterally) rotated enough to position the feet at a 45-degree angle and an imaginary line connecting the femoral epicondyles at a 60- to 65-degree angle with the imaging table, the femoral necks are demonstrated "on end" and the lesser trochanters are demonstrated in profile (Figure 6-22 and Image 17). If the patient's legs are positioned with the feet placed vertically and an imaginary line connecting the femoral epicondyles at approximately a 15- to 20-degree angle with the imaging table, the lesser trochanter is demonstrated in partial profile and the femoral neck is only partially foreshortened (Image 18).
- **Positioning for a proximal femoral fracture:** Often, when a fracture of a proximal femur is suspected, a pelvic image is ordered instead of an image demonstrating just the affected hip. This is because pelvic fractures are frequently associated with proximal femur fractures. If a patient has a suspected fracture or a fractured proximal femur, the leg should not be internally rotated but should be left "as is." Forced internal rotation of a fractured proximal femur may injure the blood supply and nerves that surround the injured area. Because the patient's leg is not internally rotated when a fracture is in question, such a pelvic image demonstrates the affected femoral neck with some degree of foreshortening and the lesser trochanter without femoral shaft superimposition.

The inferior sacrum is at the center of the collimated field. The ilia, symphysis pubis, ischia, acetabula, femoral necks and heads, and greater and lesser trochanters are included within the field.

- Center a perpendicular central ray to the midsagittal plane at a level halfway between the symphysis pubis and the midpoint of an imaginary line connecting the ASIS, to place the inferior sacrum in the center of the collimated field. Center the IR to the central ray and open the longitudinal collimation the full 14-inch (35-cm) IR length for most adult patients. Transversely collimate to within ½ inch (1.25 cm) of the lateral skinline.
- A 14- × 17-inch (35- × 43-cm) IR placed crosswise should be adequate to include all the required anatomical structures.
- **Central ray centering for analysis of hip joint mobility:** When an AP pelvis image is being taken specifically to evaluate hip joint mobility, the central ray should be centered to the midsagittal plane at a level 1 inch (2.5 cm) superior to the symphysis pubis. Such positioning centers the hip joints on the image but may result in clipping of the superior ilia.
- **Gonadal shielding:** Use gonadal shielding on all male patients. Female patients should be shielded, although it is important that no pelvic anatomy be covered by the shield. Remember that a shield placed on top of the patient will be greatly magnified.

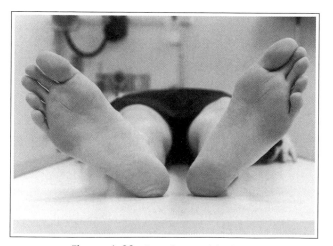

Figure 6-22. Poor foot positioning.

Anteroposterior Pelvis Image Analysis

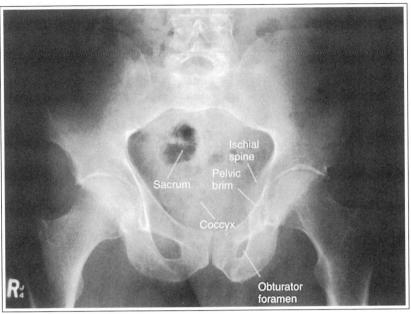

Image 16.

Analysis. The left obturator foramen is narrower than the right foramen, the left ischial spine is demonstrated without pelvic brim superimposition, and the sacrum and coccyx are rotated toward the right hip. The pelvis was rotated onto the left hip (LPO).

Correction. Rotate the patient toward the right hip until the ASISs are positioned at equal distances from the imaging table.

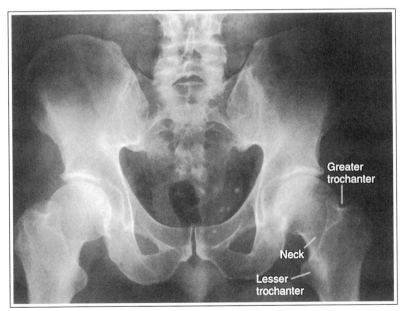

Image 17.

Analysis. The femoral necks are completely foreshortened, and the lesser trochanters are demonstrated in profile. The patient's legs were externally rotated, with the patient's feet at a 45-degree angle and the femoral epicondyles positioned at a 25- to 30-degree angle with the imaging table, as demonstrated in Figure 6-22.

Correction. Internally rotate the patient's legs until the feet are angled 15 to 20 degrees from vertical and the femoral epicondyles are positioned parallel with the imaging table, as demonstrated in Figure 6-21.

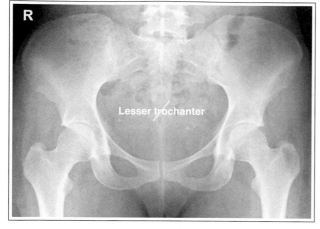

Image 18.

Analysis. The femoral necks are partially foreshortened, and the lesser trochanters are demonstrated in profile. The patient's legs were externally rotated, with the feet vertical and the femoral epicondyles at approximately a 15- to 20-degree angle with the imaging table.

Correction. Internally rotate the patient's legs until the feet are angled 15 to 20 degrees from vertical and the femoral epicondyles are positioned parallel with the imaging table, as demonstrated in Figure 6-21.

PELVIS: ANTEROPOSTERIOR OBLIQUE (FROG-LEG) PROJECTION (MODIFIED CLEAVES METHOD)

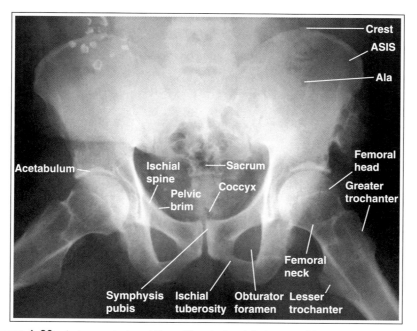

Figure 6-23. Anteroposterior oblique (frog-leg) pelvis image with accurate positioning.

Image Analysis

The pelvis demonstrates an AP projection. The ischial spines are aligned with the pelvic brim, the sacrum and coccyx are aligned with the symphysis pubis, and the ilia and the obturator foramina are uniform in size and shape.

- An AP projection of the pelvis is accomplished by placing the patient on the imaging table with the legs flexed and abducted (Figure 6-24). To ensure that the pelvis is

not rotated, judge the distance from the ASIS to the imaging table on each side. The distances should be equal.

- *Detecting pelvic rotation:* A nonrotated pelvis image will demonstrate symmetrical ilia and obturator foramina. Rotation can be detected by evaluating the relationships of the ischial spines with the pelvic brim and of the sacrum and coccyx with the symphysis pubis. The ischial spines should be aligned with the pelvic brim, and the sacrum and coccyx should align with the symphysis pubis on a nonrotated pelvis.

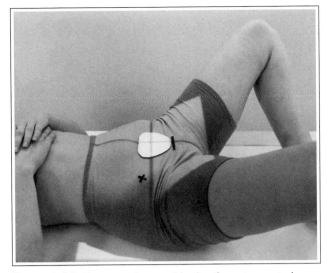

Figure 6-24. Proper patient positioning for anteroposterior oblique (frog-leg) pelvis image.

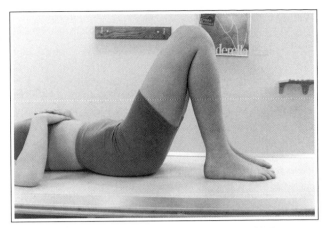

Figure 6-25. Proper knee and hip flexion: 60 to 70 degrees from imaging table.

- If the pelvis is rotated into an LPO position, the left ilium is wider than the right, the left obturator foramen is narrower than the right, the left ischial spine is demonstrated without pelvic brim superimposition, and the sacrum and coccyx are not aligned with the symphysis pubis but are rotated toward the right hip (see Image 19).

- If the patient is rotated into an RPO position, the opposite is true. The right ilium is wider than the left, the right obturator foramen is narrower than the left, the right ischial spine is demonstrated without pelvic brim superimposition, and the sacrum and coccyx are rotated toward the left hip.

The lesser trochanters are demonstrated in profile medially, and the femoral necks are superimposed over the adjacent greater trochanters.

- *Accurate femur positioning:* To accurately position the greater trochanters beneath the proximal femurs and position the lesser trochanters in profile, flex the patient's knees and hips until the femurs are angled 60 to 70 degrees with the imaging table (20 to 30 degrees from vertical) (Figure 6-25).

- ***Effect of distal femur elevation on proximal femur demonstration:*** For a frog-leg pelvis image, the relationship of the greater and the lesser trochanters with the proximal femurs is determined when the patient flexes the knees and hips.

- Use a femoral skeletal bone to better understand how the relationship of the greater and lesser trochanters with the proximal femur changes as the distal femur is elevated on knee and hip flexion. Begin by placing the femoral bone on a flat surface in an AP position. While slowly elevating the distal femur, observe how the greater trochanter rotates around the proximal femur. First, the greater trochanter moves beneath the proximal femur; then, as elevation of the distal femur continues,

it moves from beneath the proximal femur and is demonstrated on the medial side of the femur.

- ***Poor distal femur elevation:*** If the knees and hips are not flexed enough to place the femur at a 60- to 70-degree angle with the imaging table, the greater trochanters are demonstrated laterally, as with an AP projection (see Image 7, page 356). If the knees and hips are flexed too much, placing the femurs at an angle greater than 60 to 70 degrees with the imaging table, the greater trochanters are demonstrated medially (see Image 8, page 356).

The femoral necks are partially foreshortened, and the greater trochanters are demonstrated at a transverse level halfway between the femoral heads and lesser trochanters.

- *Accurate leg positioning:* To demonstrate the femoral necks and proximal femora with only partial foreshortening and the greater trochanters at a transverse level halfway between the femoral heads and lesser trochanters on a pelvis image, abduct the femoral shafts to a 45-degree angle from vertical (Figures 6-23 and 6-26).

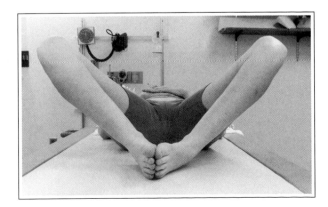

Figure 6-26. Proper femoral abduction: 45 degrees from imaging table.

- *Effect of leg abduction:* The degree of femoral abduction determines the amount of femoral neck foreshortening and the transverse level at which the greater trochanters are demonstrated between the femoral heads and lesser trochanters.

- Use a femoral skeleton bone to understand how leg abduction determines the demonstration of the femoral neck and the position of the greater trochanter. Place the femoral bone on a flat surface in an AP position with the distal femur elevated until the greater trochanter is positioned beneath the proximal femur and the lesser trochanter is in profile (20 to 30 degrees from vertical or 60 to 70 degrees with flat surface). From this position, abduct the femoral bone (move the lateral surface of the femoral bone toward the flat surface). As the bone moves toward the flat surface, observe how the femoral neck is positioned more on end and the greater trochanter moves proximally (toward the femoral head).

- *Poor leg abduction:* If the femoral necks are demonstrated without foreshortening and the greater trochanters are at the same transverse level as the lesser trochanters on a frog-leg pelvis image, the femoral shafts were abducted to 20 to 30 degrees from vertical (60- to 70-degree angle from the imaging table) (see Image 20 and Figure 6-27).

- If the proximal femoral shafts are demonstrated without foreshortening, the greater trochanters are at the same transverse level as the femoral heads, and the femoral necks are demonstrated "on end" on a frog-leg pelvis image, then the femoral shafts were abducted next to the imaging table (Image 21 and Figure 6-28).

- *Importance of Symmetrical Femoral Abduction:* A frog-leg pelvic image may not demonstrate the proximal femurs with exactly the same degree of femoral abduction. How each proximal femur appears depends on the degree of femoral abduction placed on that leg. As a standard, unless the image is ordered to evaluate hip mobility, both femurs should be abducted equally

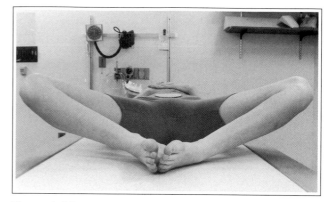

Figure 6-28. Femurs in maximum abduction: 20 degrees from imaging table.

for the image. This symmetrical abduction helps prevent pelvic rotation. It may be necessary to position an angled sponge beneath the patient's femurs to maintain the desired femoral abduction.

The inferior sacrum is at the center of the collimated field. The ilia, symphysis pubis, ischia, acetabula, femoral necks and heads, and greater and lesser trochanters are included within the field.

- Center a perpendicular central ray to the midsagittal plane at a level 1 inch (2.5 cm) superior to the symphysis pubis. Center the IR to the central ray and open the longitudinal collimation the full 14-inch (35-cm) length for most adult patients. Transversely collimate to within ½ inch (1.25 cm) of the lateral skinline.

- A 14- × 17-inch (35- × 43-cm) IR placed crosswise should be adequate to include all the required anatomical structures.

- *Gonadal shielding:* Use gonadal shielding on all male patients. Female patients should be shielded, although it is important that no pelvic anatomy be covered by the shield. Remember that the shield placed on top of the patient will greatly magnify.

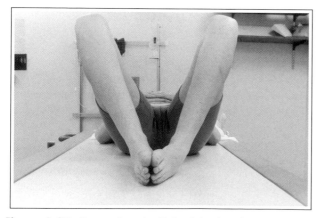

Figure 6-27. Femurs in only slight abduction: 20 degrees from vertical.

Anteroposterior Oblique (Frog-Leg) Pelvis Image Analysis

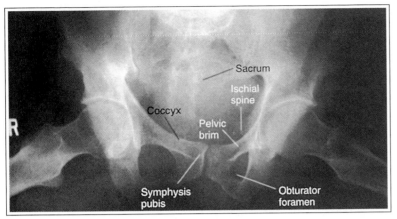

Image 19.

Analysis. The left obturator foramen is narrower than the right foramen, the left ischial spine is demonstrated without pelvic brim superimposition, and the sacrum and coccyx are rotated toward the right hip. The patient was rotated onto the left hip (LPO).

Correction. Rotate the patient toward the right hip until the ASISs are positioned at equal distances from the imaging table.

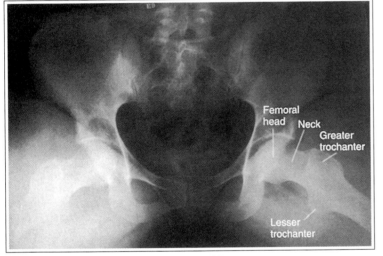

Image 20.

Analysis. The femoral necks are demonstrated without foreshortening, and the greater and lesser trochanters are demonstrated at approximately the same transverse level. The patient's femurs were in only slight abduction, at approximately a 70-degree angle with the imaging table (20 degrees from vertical), as demonstrated in Figure 6-27.

Correction. Consult with reviewers in your facility to determine whether this is an acceptable image. If the proximal femoral shafts demonstrate too much foreshortening, have the patient abduct the femurs to a 45-degree angle with the imaging table.

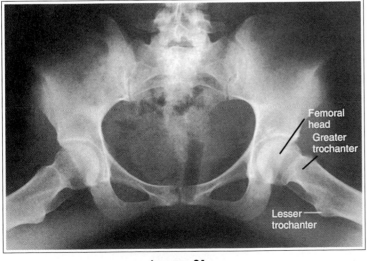

Image 21.

Analysis. The femoral necks are demonstrated "on end." The greater trochanters are demonstrated on the same transverse level as the femoral heads. The patient's femurs were positioned next to the imaging table, as demonstrated in Figure 6-28.

Correction. Consult with reviewers in your facility to determine whether this is an acceptable image. Because the femoral necks cannot be evaluated because of foreshortening, it may be necessary to have the patient position the femurs at a 45-degree angle with the imaging table.

SACROILIAC JOINTS: ANTEROPOSTERIOR AXIAL PROJECTION

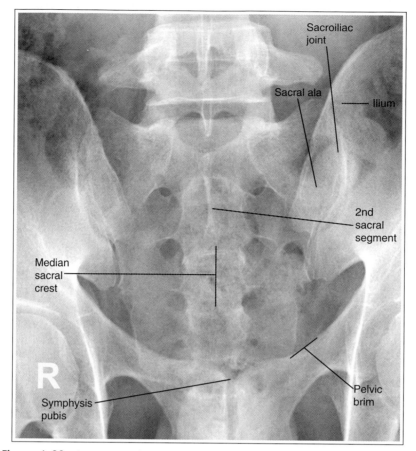

Figure 6-29. Anteroposterior axial sacroiliac joint image with accurate positioning.

Image Analysis

The sacroiliac joints are demonstrated in an AP axial projection. The median sacral crest is aligned with the symphysis pubis, and the sacrum is at an equal distance from the lateral wall of the pelvic brim on both sides.

- An AP axial projection of the sacroiliac joints is obtained by positioning the patient supine on the imaging table with the legs extended. Position the patient's shoulders and ASISs at equal distances from the imaging table to prevent rotation (Figure 6-30).
- *Detecting sacroiliac joint rotation:* Rotation is detected on an AP axial sacroiliac joint image by evaluating the alignment of the long axis of the median sacral crest with the symphysis pubis and the distance from the sacrum to the lateral pelvic brim. When the patient is rotated away from the supine position, the sacrum moves in a direction opposite from the movement of the symphysis pubis and is positioned next to the lateral pelvic brim situated farther from the imaging table. If the

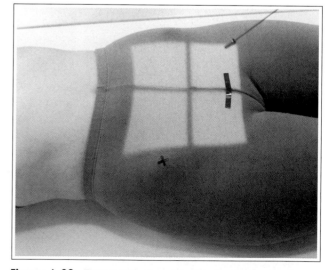

Figure 6-30. Proper patient positioning for anteroposterior axial sacroiliac joint image.

patient is rotated into an LPO position, the sacrum is rotated toward the patient's right pelvic brim. If the patient is rotated into an RPO position, the sacrum rotates toward the patient's left pelvic brim.

The sacroiliac joints are demonstrated without foreshortening, and the sacrum is elongated, with the symphysis pubis superimposed over the inferior sacral segments.

- The patient is positioned supine with the legs extended, and the lumbosacral curve causes the proximal sacrum and sacroiliac joints to be angled 30 to 35 degrees with the imaging table and IR. To demonstrate the sacroiliac joints without foreshortening, a 30-degree cephalic angle should be used for male patients and a 35-degree cephalic angle for female patients. Patients with less or greater lumbosacral curvature will require a decrease or increase, respectively, in cephalic angulation to maintain the 30- to 35-degree alignment of the central ray and sacroiliac joints. If an AP axial sacroiliac joint image is taken with a perpendicular central ray or without enough cephalad angulation, the sacroiliac joints and the first through third sacral segments are foreshortened (see Image 21). If the AP axial sacroiliac joint image is taken with too much cephalic angulation, the sacrum and sacroiliac joints demonstrate elongation and the symphysis pubis is superimposed the inferior aspects of the sacrum and sacroiliac joints (Image 23).

The long axis of the median sacral crest is aligned with the long axis of the collimated field.

- Aligning the long axis of the median sacral crest with the long axis of the collimated field allows for tight collimation and ensures that the central ray is angled directly into the sacroiliac joints. To obtain proper alignment, find the point halfway between the patient's palpable ASISs, then align this point and the palpable symphysis pubis with the center of the collimator's longitudinal light line.

The second sacral segment is at the center of the collimated field. The sacroiliac joints and the first through fourth sacral segments are included within the field.

- Center the central ray to the patient's midsagittal plane at a level 1½ inches (3 cm) superior to the symphysis pubis. Center the IR to the central ray, and open the longitudinally collimated field to the symphysis pubis. Transversely collimate to approximately a 9-inch (22-cm) field size.
- A 10- × 12-inch (24- × 30-cm) IR placed lengthwise should be adequate to include all the required anatomical structures.
- *Gonadal shielding:* Use gonadal shielding on all male patients. Female patients cannot be shielded, or sacral information will be obscured.

Anteroposterior Axial Sacroiliac Joint Image Analysis

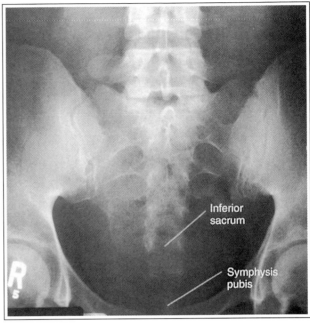

Inferior sacrum

Symphysis pubis

Image 22.

Analysis. The sacroiliac joints are foreshortened, and the inferior sacrum is demonstrated without symphysis pubis superimposition. The central ray was inadequately angled.

Correction. Angle the central ray 30 to 35 degrees cephalad.

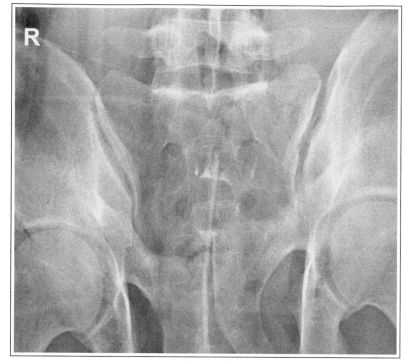

Image 23.

Analysis. The sacroiliac joints and sacrum are elongated, and the symphysis pubis is superimposed over the inferior aspects of the sacrum and sacroiliac joints. The central ray was angled too cephalically.

Correction. Angle the central ray 30 to 35 degrees cephalad.

SACROILIAC JOINTS: ANTEROPOSTERIOR OBLIQUE PROJECTION (LEFT POSTERIOR OBLIQUE AND RIGHT POSTERIOR OBLIQUE POSITIONS)

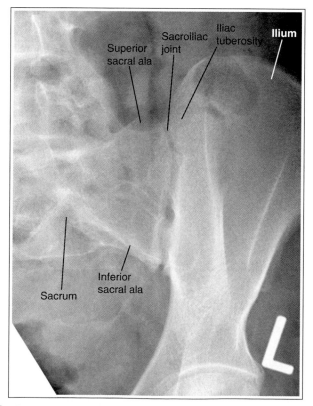

Figure 6-31. Anteroposterior oblique sacroiliac joint image with accurate positioning.

Image Analysis

A right or left marker identifying the sacroiliac joint positioned farther from the IR is present on the image and is not superimposed over anatomy of interest.

- Because the sacroiliac joint of interest is situated farther from the IR when posterior oblique images are taken, the marker used should identify the sacroiliac joint situated farther from the IR. This differs from the way most oblique images are marked; routinely, the side marked is the one positioned closer to the IR.

The ilium and sacrum are demonstrated without superimposition, and the sacroiliac joint is open.

- An AP oblique sacroiliac joint image is obtained by beginning with the patient positioned supine on the imaging table with the legs extended. From this position, rotate the patient toward the unaffected side until the midcoronal plane is at a 25- to 30-degree angle with the imaging table and IR. The sacral ala and ilium are positioned in profile. Place a radiolucent support beneath the patient's elevated hip and thorax to help maintain the position (Figure 6-32). Both posterior oblique positions (RPO and LPO) must be obtained to demonstrate the right and left sacroiliac joints. When posterior oblique images are taken, the elevated sacroiliac joint is the joint of interest.
- *Determining accuracy of obliquity:* The accuracy of an oblique sacroiliac joint can be determined by the lack of ilium and sacral superimposition. The degree of separation or cavity demonstrated between the ilium and sacrum, which represents the sacroiliac joint, varies from patient to patient. The ilia and sacrum fit very snugly together, and in older patients the joint spaces between them may be reduced in size or even nonexistent because of fibrous adhesions or synostosis. If the patient was not rotated enough to place the ilium and sacral ala in profile, the inferior and superior sacral aspects of the ala are demonstrated without ilium superimposition, whereas the lateral sacral ala is superimposed over the

iliac tuberosity (see Image 24). The lateral sacrum is also demonstrated without ilium superimposition. If the patient was rotated more than needed to position the ilium and sacral ala in profile, the ilium is superimposed over the lateral sacral ala and the inferior sacrum (see Image 25).

The long axis of the sacroiliac joint is aligned with the long axis of the collimated field.

- Aligning the long axis of the sacroiliac joint with the long axis of the collimated field allows for tight collimation without clipping any portion of the joint.

The sacroiliac joint of interest is at the center of the collimated field. The sacroiliac joint, sacral ala, and ilium are included within the field.

- Center the central ray 1 inch (2.5 cm) medial to the elevated ASIS to position the sacroiliac joint of interest in the center of the collimated field. Center the IR to the central ray and open the longitudinal collimation to the elevated iliac crest. Transverse collimation should be to the elevated ASIS.
- A 10- × 12-inch (24- × 30-cm) IR placed lengthwise should be adequate to include all the required anatomical structures.
- *Gonadal shielding:* Use gonadal shielding on all male patients. Female patients cannot be shielded, or sacral information will be obscured.

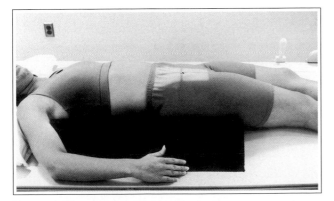

Figure 6-32. Proper patient positioning for anteroposterior oblique sacroiliac joint image.

Oblique Sacroiliac Joint Image Analysis

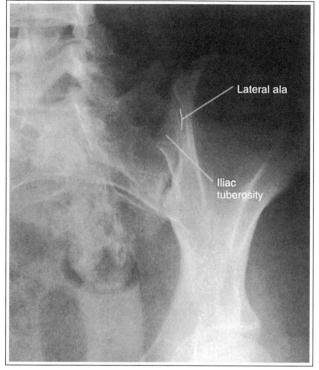

Image 24.

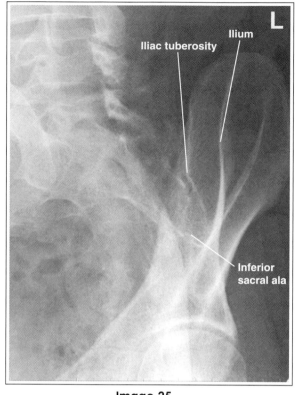

Image 25.

Analysis. The sacroiliac joint is closed. The superior and inferior sacral alae are demonstrated without iliac super-imposition, and the lateral sacral ala is superimposed over the iliac tuberosity. The patient was not rotated enough.

Correction. Increase the pelvic obliquity. Because both the sacral ala and the ilium move simultaneously, the adjustment made should be only half the amount of super-imposition of the sacral ala and iliac tuberosity.

Analysis. The sacroiliac joint is closed. The ilium is superimposed over the inferior sacral ala and the lateral sacrum. Pelvic obliquity was excessive.

Correction. Decrease the pelvic obliquity. Because both the sacral ala and the ilium move simultaneously, the amount of adjustment made should be only half the amount of ilial and sacral superimposition.

CHAPTER 7

Image Analysis of the Cervical and Thoracic Vertebrae

CERVICAL VERTEBRAE

The following image analysis criteria are used for all cervical and thoracic images and should be considered when completing the analysis. Position- and projection-specific criteria relating to these topics are discussed with the other accompanying criteria for that position or projection.

Facility's patient identification requirements are visible on image as identified in Chapter 1.

A right or left marker, identifying correct side of patient, is present on the image and is not superimposed over anatomy of interest. Specific placement of marker is as described in Chapter 1.

No evidence of preventable artifacts is present.

- Evaluate the patient's neck for any radiopaque objects that may obstruct visualization of the cervical and thoracic vertebrae, such as necklaces, earrings, body piercings, and lettering on clothing. It may be necessary to have a patient with a high-buttoned collar change into a snapless hospital gown.

The bony trabecular patterns and cortical outlines of the cervical vertebrae are sharply defined.

- Sharply defined recorded details are obtained when patient motion is controlled, respiration is halted, and a short object–image receptor distance (OID) is maintained. Increased spatial resolution is also obtained when the smallest image receptor (IR) is selected for digital images.

Contrast and density are adequate to demonstrate the surrounding soft tissue, air-filled trachea, and bony structures of the cervical and thoracic vertebrae. Penetration is sufficient to visualize the bony trabecular patterns and cortical outlines of the vertebral bodies, uncinate processes, spinous processes, and anterior tubercles of the cervical vertebrae, and the vertebral bodies, pedicles, spinous processes, and transverse processes of the thoracic vertebrae.

- An optimal kilovolt-peak (kVp) technique sufficiently penetrates the cervical and thoracic vertebral structures and provides the contrast scale necessary to visualize the vertebral details. A grid or air-gap technique is employed to absorb the scatter radiation produced by the shoulder, increasing detail visibility. To obtain optimal density, set a manual milliampere-seconds (mAs) level based on the patient's shoulder thickness or choose the appropriate automatic exposure control (AEC) chamber. Table 7-1 lists the technical data for the most common projections.

TABLE 7-1 Cervical and Thoracic Vertebrae Technical Data				
Position or Projection	kVp	Grid	AEC Chamber	SID
AP axial projection, cervical vertebrae	70-80	Grid	Center	40-48 inches (100-120 cm)
AP projection, "open mouth," C1 and C2	70-80	Grid		40-48 inches (100-120 cm)
Lateral position, cervical vertebrae	70-80	Optional air-gap technique	Center	72 inches (150-180 cm)
AP axial oblique projection, cervical vertebrae	70-80	Optional air-gap technique	Center	72 inches (150-180 cm)
Lateral "Twining" position, cervicothoracic vertebrae	65-85	Grid		40-48 inches (100-120 cm)
AP projection, thoracic vertebrae	75-85	Grid	Center	40-48 inches (100-120 cm)
Lateral position, thoracic vertebrae	80-90	Grid	Center	40-48 inches (100-120 cm)

AEC, Automatic exposure controls; *AP,* anteroposterior; *kVp,* kilovolt peak; *SID,* source–image receptor distance.

CERVICAL VERTEBRAE: ANTEROPOSTERIOR AXIAL PROJECTION

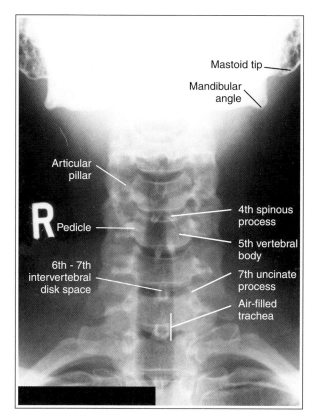

Figure 7-1. Anteroposterior axial cervical vertebral image with accurate positioning.

Image Analysis

The cervical vertebrae demonstrate an anteroposterior (AP) axial projection. The spinous processes are aligned with the midline of the cervical bodies, the mandibular angles and mastoid tips are at equal distances from the cervical vertebrae, the articular pillars and pedicles are symmetrically demonstrated lateral to the cervical bodies, and the distances from the vertebral column to the medial (sternal) ends of the clavicles are equal.

- An AP axial projection of the cervical vertebrae is obtained by placing the patient supine or upright, with the shoulders positioned at equal distances from the imaging table or upright IR (Figure 7-2). The patient's face should be positioned so it is forward, placing the mandibular angles and mastoid tips at equal distances from the imaging table or upright grid holder.

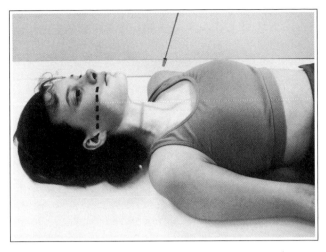

Figure 7-2. Proper patient positioning for anteroposterior cervical vertebral image.

- ***Effect of cervical rotation:*** When the patient and cervical vertebrae are rotated away from the AP axial projection, the vertebral bodies move toward the side positioned closer to the IR, and the spinous processes move toward the side positioned farther from the IR. The upper (C1 to C4) and lower (C5 to C7) cervical vertebrae can demonstrate rotation independently or simultaneously, depending on which part of the body is rotated. If the head is rotated but the thorax remains in an AP axial projection, the upper cervical vertebrae demonstrate rotation, as C1 rotates on C2, and the lower cervical vertebrae remain in an AP axial projection. If the thorax is rotated but the head remains in a forward position to match, the lower cervical vertebrae demonstrate rotation and the upper cervical vertebrae remain in an AP axial projection. If the patient's head and thorax are rotated simultaneously, the entire cervical column demonstrates rotation (see Image 1).
- ***Detecting rotation:*** Rotation is present on an AP image if (1) the mandibular angles and mastoid tips are not demonstrated at equal distances from the cervical vertebrae, (2) the spinous processes are not demonstrated in the midline of the cervical bodies, (3) the pedicles and articular pillars are not symmetrically demonstrated lateral to the vertebral bodies, and (4) the medial ends of the clavicles are not demonstrated at equal distances from the vertebral column (see Image 1). The side of the patient positioned closer to the imaging table or upright IR is the side the mandible is rotated toward and also the side that demonstrates less of the articular pillars and less clavicular and vertebral column superimposition.
- ***Positioning for trauma:*** When cervical vertebral images are exposed on a trauma patient with suspected subluxation or fracture, obtain the AP axial projection image with the patient positioned as is. *Do not* attempt to remove the cervical collar or adjust the head or body rotation, mandible position, or cervical column tilting. This might result in greater injury to the vertebrae or spinal cord.

Spinal cord injuries may occur from the mishandling of the patient after the initial injury has taken place.

The intervertebral disk spaces are open, the vertebral bodies are demonstrated without distortion, and each vertebra's spinous process is visualized at the level of its inferior intervertebral disk space.

- The cervical vertebral column demonstrates a lordotic curvature. This curvature and the shape of the vertebral bodies cause the disk articulating surfaces of the vertebral bodies to slant upward anteriorly to posteriorly.
- ***Importance of central ray angulation:*** To obtain open intervertebral disk spaces and undistorted vertebral bodies, the central ray must be angled in the same direction as the slope of the vertebral bodies. This can be easily discerned by viewing the lateral cervical image in Figure 7-3. Studying this lateral cervical image, you can see that when the correct central ray angulation is used, each vertebra's spinous process is located within its inferior intervertebral disk space. The degree of central ray angulation needed to obtain open intervertebral disk spaces and to accurately align the spinous processes within them depends on the degree of cervical lordotic curvature.
- If the AP cervical vertebrae examination is performed with the patient in an upright position, the cervical vertebrae demonstrate more lordotic curvature than if the examination is performed with the patient supine. In a supine position the gravitational pull placed on the middle cervical vertebrae results in straightening of the cervical curvature. Figure 7-3 demonstrates a lateral

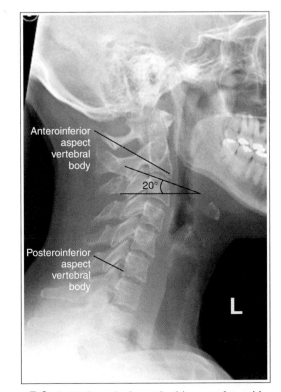

Figure 7-3. Lateral cervical vertebral image taken with patient upright.

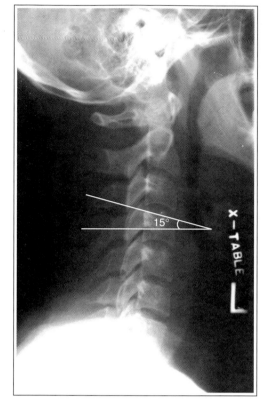

Figure 7-4. Lateral cervical vertebral image taken with patient supine.

cervical image taken with the patient in an upright position, and Figure 7-4 demonstrates a lateral cervical image taken with the patient supine. Notice the difference in lordotic curvature between these two images. Because of this difference the central ray angulation should be varied when an AP cervical vertebral image is taken with the patient erect rather than supine. In the erect position a 20-degree cephalad central ray angulation is needed to align the central ray parallel with the intervertebral disk spaces. In the supine position a 15-degree cephalad central ray angulation sufficiently aligns the central ray parallel with the intervertebral disk spaces.

- *Effect of central ray misalignment:* Misalignment of the central ray and the intervertebral disk spaces results in closed disk spaces, distorted vertebral bodies, and the projection of the spinous processes into the vertebral bodies. If the central ray angulation is not used or is insufficient, the resulting image demonstrates closed intervertebral disk spaces, and each vertebra's spinous process is demonstrated within its vertebral body (see Image 2). This anatomical relationship also results if the patient's head is tilted toward the x-ray tube for the examination, causing the cervical vertebrae to tilt anteriorly. If the central ray is angled more than needed to align the central ray parallel with the intervertebral disk spaces, or if the patient's cervical vertebral column was extended posteriorly for the examination, the

resulting image demonstrates closed intervertebral disk spaces, each vertebra's spinous process is demonstrated within the inferior adjoining vertebral body, and the uncinate processes are elongated (see Image 3).

The third cervical vertebra is demonstrated in its entirety, and the posterior occiput and mandibular mentum are superimposed.

- Accurate positioning of the occiput and mandibular mentum is achieved when an imaginary line connecting the upper occlusal plane (chewing surface of maxillary teeth) and the base of the skull is aligned perpendicular to the imaging table or upright IR. This positioning also aligns the acanthiomeatal line (an imaginary line connecting the point at which the upper lip and nose meet with the external ear opening) perpendicular to the imaging table or upright IR (see Figure 7-2). With this position you might expect the patient's mandible to be superimposed over the upper cervical vertebrae, but it will not be, because the cephalad central ray angulation used will project the mandible superiorly.
- *Effect of occiput-mentum mispositioning:* Mispositioning of the posterior occiput and the upper occlusal plane results in an obstructed image of the upper cervical vertebrae. If the occlusal plane is positioned superior to the base of the skull, the upper cervical vertebrae are superimposed over the occiput (see Image 4). If the upper occlusal plane is positioned inferior to the base of the skull, the mandibular mentum is superimposed over the superior cervical vertebrae (see Image 5).

The long axis of the cervical column is aligned with the long axis of the collimated field.

- Aligning the long axis of the cervical column with the long axis of the collimated field ensures that no lateral flexion of the cervical column is present (see Image 6) and allows for tight collimation (see Image 5). This alignment is obtained by aligning the midline of the patient's neck with the collimator's longitudinal light line.

The fourth cervical vertebra is centered within the collimated field. The third through seventh cervical vertebrae, the second thoracic vertebra, and the surrounding soft tissue are included within the field.

- Center the central ray to the patient's midsagittal plane at a level halfway between the external auditory meatus (EAM) and the jugular notch to center C4 to the collimated field.
- Open the longitudinal collimation to the EAM and the jugular notch. Transverse collimation should be to within ½ inch (1.25 cm) of the lateral neck skinline.
- An 8- × 10-inch (18- × 24-cm) IR placed lengthwise should be adequate to include all the required anatomical structures.

Anteroposterior Cervical Vertebrae Image Analysis

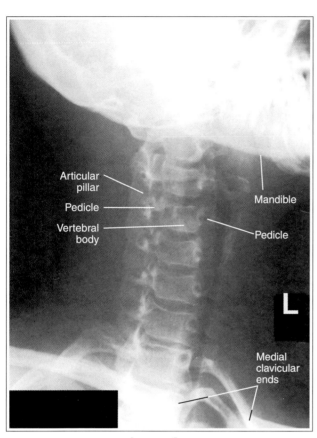

Image 1.

Analysis. The spinous processes are not aligned with the midline of the cervical bodies, and the pedicles and articular pillars are not symmetrically demonstrated lateral to the vertebral bodies. The mandible is rotated toward the patient's left side, and the medial end of the left clavicle demonstrates no vertebral column superimposition. The patient was rotated toward the left side (left posterior oblique [LPO] position).

Correction. Rotate the patient toward the right side until the shoulders are at equal distances from the imaging table or upright grid holder, and turn the patient's head toward the right side until the mandibular angles and mastoid tips are at equal distances from the imaging table or upright grid holder.

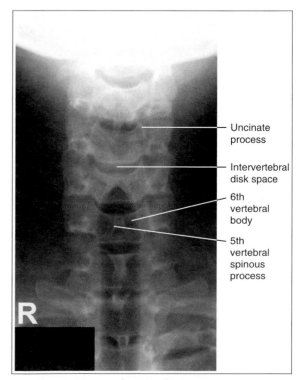

Image 2.

Analysis. The anteroinferior aspects of the cervical bodies (see Figure 7-3 for identification) are obscuring the intervertebral disk spaces, and each vertebra's spinous process is demonstrated within its vertebral body. The central ray angulation either was not used or was insufficient to align the central ray parallel with the intervertebral disk spaces.

Correction. Increase the amount of cephalic angulation.

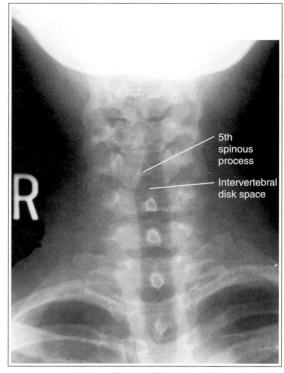

Image 3.

Analysis. The posteroinferior aspects of the cervical bodies (see Figure 7-3 for identification) are obscuring the intervertebral disk spaces, the uncinate processes are elongated, and each vertebra's spinous process is demonstrated within the inferior adjoining vertebral body. The central ray was angled too cephalically to align the central ray parallel with the intervertebral disk spaces.

Correction. Decrease the amount of cephalic central ray angulation.

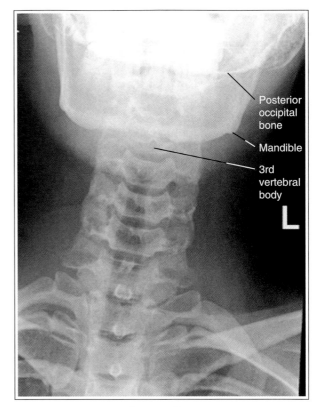

Image 5.

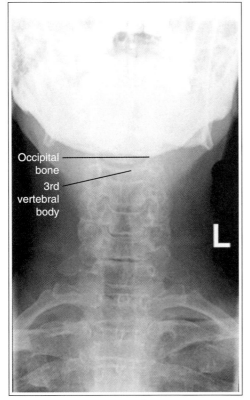

Image 4.

Analysis. A portion of the third cervical vertebra is superimposed over the posterior occipital bone, preventing a clear visualization of the third cervical vertebra. The upper occlusal plane was positioned superior to the base of the skull.

Correction. Tuck the chin half the distance demonstrated between the base of the skull and the mandibular mentum, or until an imaginary line connecting the upper occlusal plane and the base of the skull is aligned perpendicular to the imaging table or upright grid holder. For this patient the movement should be approximately 1 inch (2.5 cm).

Analysis. The mandible is superimposed over a portion of the third cervical vertebra. The upper occlusal plane was positioned inferior to the base of the occiput. The long axis of the cervical column is not aligned with the long axis of the collimated field, preventing tight collimation.

Correction. Raise the chin half the distance demonstrated between the base of the skull and the mandibular mentum, or until an imaginary line connecting the upper occlusal plane and the inferior base of the posterior occiput is aligned perpendicular to the imaging table or upright grid holder. Align the long axis of the cervical column with the long axis of the collimated field, and increase transverse collimation.

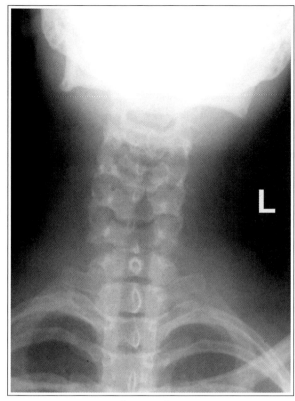

Image 6.

Analysis. The head is tilted toward the left side, causing the upper cervical vertebrae to flex laterally. The long axis of the cervical vertebral column was not aligned with the long axis of the collimated field.

Correction. Tilt the head toward the right side until the patient's upper neck midline and lower neck midline are aligned with the collimator's longitudinal light line.

CERVICAL ATLAS AND AXIS: ANTEROPOSTERIOR PROJECTION (OPEN-MOUTH POSITION)

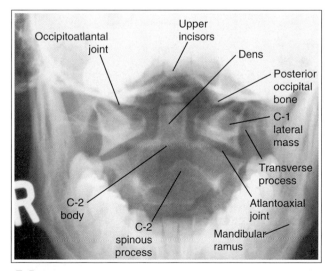

Figure 7-5. Anteroposterior atlas and axis image with accurate positioning.

Image Analysis

No evidence of preventable artifacts, such as hairpins, hair ornaments, and removable dental structures, is present.

- Instruct the patient to remove dental structures, such as false teeth or retainers, and any radiopaque objects located within the hair that may obstruct visualization of the atlas and axis.

The atlas and axis demonstrate an AP projection. The atlas is symmetrically seated on the axis, with the atlas's lateral masses at equal distances from the dens. The spinous process of the axis is aligned with the

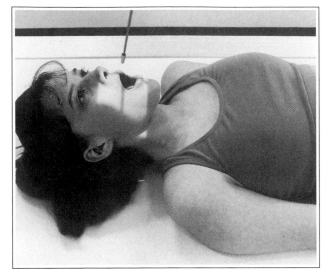

Figure 7-6. Proper patient positioning for anteroposterior atlas and axis image.

midline of the axis's body, and the mandibular rami are demonstrated at equal distances from the lateral masses.

- An AP projection of the atlas and axis is obtained by placing the patient in either a supine or an upright position with the shoulders, mandibular angles, and mastoid tips positioned at equal distances from the imaging table or upright IR (Figure 7-6).
- *Effect of rotation:* Rotation of the atlas and axis occurs when the head is turned away from an AP projection. On head rotation the atlas pivots around the dens, so the lateral mass located on the side from which the face is turned is displaced anteriorly, and the mass located on the side toward which the face is turned is displaced posteriorly. This displacement causes the space between the lateral mass and the dens to narrow on the side from which the face is turned and to enlarge on the side toward which the face is turned (see Image 7). As the amount of head rotation increases, the axis rotates in the same direction as the atlas, resulting in a shift in the position of its spinous process, in the direction opposite that in which the patient's face is turned.
- *Detecting direction of rotation:* To determine the way the patient's face was turned, judge the distance between the mandibular rami and the lateral masses. The side that demonstrates the greater distance is the side toward which the face was rotated.
- *Positioning for trauma:* When cervical vertebral images are taken on a trauma patient with suspected subluxation or fractures, obtain the AP projection with the patient's position left as is. *Do not* attempt to remove the cervical collar or to adjust head or body rotation, mandible position, or cervical vertebral column tilting. To do so might result in increased injury to the vertebrae or spinal cord.

The upper incisors and the base of the skull are demonstrated superior to the dens and the atlantoaxial joint.

- The dens and the atlantoaxial joint are located at the midsagittal plane, at a level $\frac{1}{2}$ inch (1.25 cm) inferior to an imaginary line connecting the mastoid tips. To demonstrate them without upper incisor (front teeth) or posterior occiput superimposition, instruct the patient to open the mouth as widely as possible. Then have the patient tuck the chin until an imaginary line connecting the upper occlusal plane (chewing surface of maxillary teeth) and the base of the skull is aligned perpendicular to the imaging table or upright grid holder. If the patient does not have upper teeth, one should imagine where the occlusal plane would be if the patient had teeth. This positioning also aligns the acanthiomeatal line (an imaginary line drawn between the point where the upper lip and nose meet the external ear opening) perpendicular with the imaging table or upright grid holder. It may be necessary to position a small angled sponge beneath the patient's head to maintain accurate head positioning, especially if the patient's chin has to be tucked so much that it is difficult to adequately open the mouth. The sponge causes the upper occlusal plane and base of the skull to align perpendicularly without requiring as much chin tucking.
- *Relationship of central ray angulation and patient position:* The lateral cervical image in Figure 7-7 demonstrates how the occlusal plane and the base of the

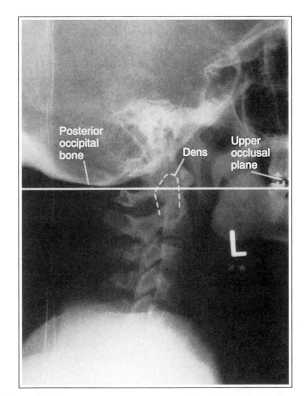

Figure 7-7. Lateral cervical vertebral image demonstrating upper incisor, dens, and posterior occiput relationship.

skull should be aligned for an accurate open-mouth image. After studying this image, you might conclude that the atlantoaxial joint will be free of upper incisor or occiput superimposition if the patient maintains this head position and simply drops the jaw. Because the upper incisors are positioned at a long OID, however, they are greatly magnified, causing them to be projected onto the dens and atlantoaxial joint. In most patients, when the upper occlusal plane and base of the skull are superimposed, magnification causes the upper incisors to be projected approximately 1 inch (2.5 cm) inferior to the base of the skull (see Image 8). For these incisors to be projected superiorly, a 5-degree cephalic angle should be placed on the central ray. The upper incisors will be projected approximately 1 inch (2.5 cm) for every 5 degrees of angulation. This angle adjustment is based on a 40-inch (102-cm) source–image receptor distance (SID); if a longer SID is used, the required angle adjustment would be less, whereas if a shorter SID is used, the angulation adjustment would be greater. If instead of an angle adjustment the patient's chin was tilted upward in an attempt to shift the upper incisors superiorly, the posterior occiput would simultaneously be shifted inferiorly.

- This inferior shift of the occiput would obscure the dens and possibly the atlantoaxial joint. The dens and atlantoaxial joint space may also be obscured if a 5-degree cephalad central ray angle was used but the occlusal plane and base of the skull were not superimposed. When the base of the skull is positioned inferior to the upper occlusal plane, the image demonstrates the dens and, depending on the degree of mispositioning, the atlantoaxial joint space superimposed onto the posterior occiput (see Image 9). When the occlusal plane is positioned inferior to the base of the skull, the posterior occiput is demonstrated superior to the dens, and the upper incisors are superimposed over a portion of the superior dens (see Image 10).

- ***Positioning for trauma:*** For the dens and atlantoaxial joint to be demonstrated without incisor or occiput superimposition in a trauma patient, the direction of the central ray must be changed from the standard position. A trauma patient's head and neck cannot be adjusted, so you must angle the central ray until it is aligned parallel with an imaginary line connecting the inferior orbital rim and the external ear opening (the IOML). This line is easily accessible in a patient wearing a cervical collar. The exact degree of angulation needed depends on the amount of chin elevation. Most patients in a cervical collar require approximately a 10-degree caudal angle. Once the angle is set, attempt to get the patient to drop the lower jaw. *Do not* adjust head rotation or tilting. If the cervical collar allows the lower jaw to move without elevating the upper jaw, instruct patient to drop the lower jaw. If the cervical collar prevents lower jaw movement without elevating the upper jaw, instruct the patient about the importance of holding the

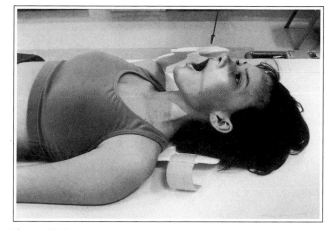

Figure 7-8. Proper patient positioning for anteroposterior atlas and axis image taken to evaluate trauma.

head and neck perfectly still, then have the ordering physician remove the front of the cervical collar so the patient can drop the jaw without adjusting the head or neck position (Figure 7-8). After the patient's jaw is dropped, align the central ray to the midsagittal plane at a level ½ inch (1.25 cm) inferior to the occlusal plane. Immediately after the image is taken, the physician should return the front of the cervical collar to its proper position. For trauma positioning, insufficient caudal angulation causes upper incisors to be demonstrated superior to the dens and the dens to be superimposed over the posterior occiput (see Image 11). If the central ray was angled too caudally, the posterior occiput is demonstrated superior to the dens, and the upper incisors are superimposed over the dens (see Image 12).

The atlantoaxial joint is open, and the axis's spinous process is demonstrated in the midline and slightly inferior to the dens.

- AP neck extension and flexion determine the alignment of the atlantoaxial joint with the imaging table and the position of the axis's spinous process to the dens. When the occlusal plane and base of the skull are aligned perpendicular to the imaging table, the atlantoaxial joint should be open.

- ***Effect of cervical column flexion and extension:*** If the cervical column is flexed, the atlantoaxial joint is closed and the spinous process of the axis is demonstrated closer to the dens (see Image 13). If the cervical column is extended, the atlantoaxial joint is closed and the spinous process of the axis is demonstrated more inferiorly to the dens.

The dens is centered within the collimated field.
The atlantoaxial and occipitoatlantal joints, the atlas's lateral masses and transverse processes, and the axis's dens and body are included within the field.

- Center the central ray through the open mouth to the midsagittal plane.

- Open the longitudinally collimated field to the patient's external ear opening. Transverse collimation should be to a 5-inch (12.5-cm) field size.
- An 8- × 10-inch (18- × 24-cm) IR placed lengthwise should be adequate to include all the required anatomical structures.

Anteroposterior Cervical Atlas and Axis Image Analysis

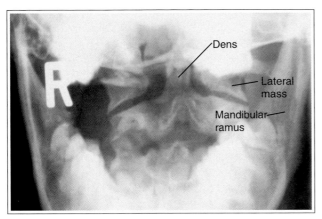

Image 7.

Analysis. The distances from the atlas's lateral masses to the dens and from the mandibular rami to the dens are narrower on the left side than on the right side, and the axis's spinous process is shifted from the midline toward the left. The face was rotated toward the right side.

Correction. Rotate the face toward the left side, until the mandibular angles and mastoid tips are positioned at equal distances from the imaging table or upright grid holder.

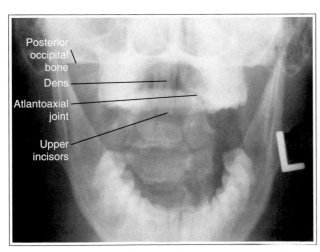

Image 8.

Analysis. The upper incisors are demonstrated approximately 1 inch (2.5 cm) inferior to the base of the skull, obscuring the dens and atlantoaxial articulation. The base of the skull is demonstrated directly superior to the dens.

Correction. If the upper occlusal plane and the base of the skull were aligned perpendicular to the imaging table and a perpendicular central ray was used for this image, do not adjust patient positioning; simply direct the central ray 5 degrees cephalad. If a 5-degree cephalad angulation was used for this image, do not adjust patient positioning; simply increase the cephalad angulation by 5 degrees. The incisors will shift approximately 1 inch (2.5 cm) for every 5 degrees of central ray angulation. (This angle adjustment is based on a 40-inch [102-cm] SID; if a longer SID is used, less angle adjustment is required, and if a shorter SID is used, more angle adjustment is required.)

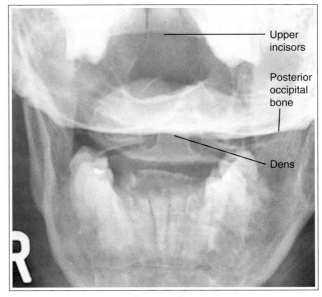

Image 9.

Analysis. The dens is superimposed over the posterior occiput. The upper incisors are demonstrated approximately 1½ inches (3.75 cm) superior to the base of the skull. The patient's head was not accurately positioned.

Correction. Tuck the chin toward the chest until an imaginary line connecting the upper occlusal plane with the base of the skull is aligned perpendicular to the IR. The needed movement is equal to half the distance demonstrated between the upper incisors and the base of the skull. For this patient, the chin should be tucked approximately ¾ inch (2 cm).

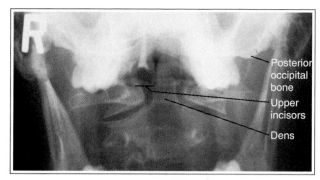

Image 10.

Analysis. The upper incisors are superimposed over the dens. The base of the skull is demonstrated approximately ½ inch (1.25 cm) superior to the upper incisors and ¼ inch (0.6 cm) superior to the dens. The upper occlusal plane was positioned inferior to the base of the skull.

Correction. Elevate the upper jaw until an imaginary line connecting the upper occlusal plane with the base of the skull is aligned perpendicular to the IR. The needed movement is equal to half of the distance demonstrated between the upper incisors and the base of the skull. For this patient the upper occlusal plane should be elevated approximately ¼ inch (0.6 cm).

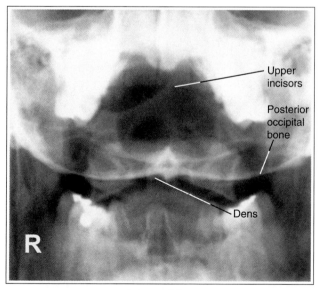

Image 11.

Analysis. This image displays trauma positioning. The upper incisors are demonstrated superior to the dens and the base of the skull, and the dens is superimposed over the posterior occiput. The central ray angulation was not directed enough caudally.

Correction. Angle the central ray approximately 5 degrees caudad for every 1 inch (2.5 cm) demonstrated between the upper incisors and the base of the skull. (This angle

adjustment is based on a 40-inch [102-cm] SID.) Because approximately 1 inch (2.5 cm) is demonstrated between the upper incisors and base of the skull on this image, the central ray angulation should be adjusted approximately 5 degrees caudally.

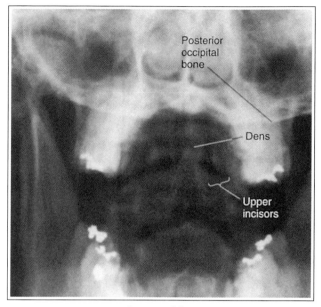

Image 12.

Analysis. This image displays trauma positioning. The upper incisors are superimposed over the dens, and the base of the skull is situated superior to the dens and upper incisors. The central ray was angled too caudally.

Correction. Angle the central ray approximately 5 degrees cephalically for every 1 inch (2.5 cm) demonstrated between the upper incisors and the base of the skull.

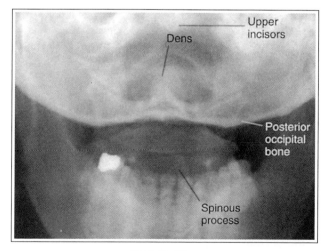

Image 13.

Analysis. The atlantoaxial joint is closed, the posterior occipital bone is superimposed over the dens, the upper incisors appear superior to the posterior occipital bone, and the axis's spinous process is demonstrated too inferior to the dens. The patient's head was not accurately positioned, and the cervical column was extended.

Correction. Tuck the chin toward the chest until an imaginary line connecting the upper occlusal plane with the base of the skull is aligned perpendicular to the IR

CERVICAL VERTEBRAE: LATERAL POSITION

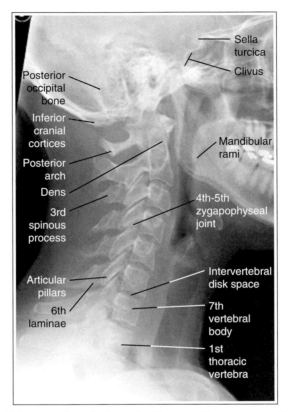

Figure 7-9. Lateral cervical vertebral image with accurate positioning.

Image Analysis

Contrast and density are adequate to demonstrate the prevertebral fat stripe. Scatter radiation is controlled.

- *Prevertebral fat stripe:* The soft-tissue structure of interest on a lateral cervical image is the prevertebral fat stripe. It is located in front of the anterior surfaces of the vertebrae and is visible on correctly exposed lateral cervical images with accurate positioning (Figure 7-10). The reviewer evaluates the distance between the anterior surface of the cervical vertebrae and the prevertebral fat stripe. Abnormal widening of this space is used for the detection and localization of fractures, masses, and inflammation.

- *Air-gap technique:* Because this examination uses a long OID, a grid is optional. When the OID is long, scatter radiation that would expose the IR at a short OID is scattered away from the IR. Because much of the scatter radiation is not being directed toward the IR,

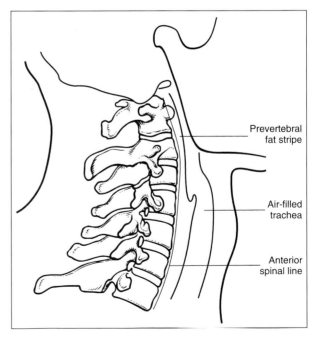

Figure 7-10. Location of prevertebral fat stripe.

a grid may not be needed to absorb the scatter. This is also referred to as the *air-gap technique*.

The bony trabecular patterns and cortical outlines of the cervical vertebrae are sharply defined.

- Sharply defined recorded details are obtained when patient motion is controlled, a detail screen and a small focal spot are used, a short OID is maintained, and the smallest possible IR is used (digital only).
- In the lateral position the patient's shoulder prevents the cervical vertebrae from being positioned close to the IR. A long OID will result in magnification and loss of recorded detail unless a 72-inch (183-cm) SID is used to offset the magnification. This decrease in image magnification provides an increase in recorded detail.

The cervical vertebrae demonstrate a lateral position. The anterior and posterior aspects of the right and left articular pillars and the right and left zygapophyseal joints of each cervical vertebra are superimposed, and the spinous processes are demonstrated in profile.

- A lateral cervical vertebral image is obtained by placing the patient in an upright position with the midcoronal plane positioned perpendicular to the IR (Figure 7-11). In this position the right and left sides of each cervical vertebra are superimposed, demonstrating the spinous processes and vertebral bodies in profile. To prevent rotation, superimpose the patient's shoulders, mastoid tips, and mandibular rami.
- *Effect of rotation:* The upper and lower cervical vertebrae can demonstrate rotation simultaneously or separately, depending on which part of the body is rotated. If the head was rotated and the thorax remained in a lateral position, the upper cervical vertebrae demonstrate rotation. If the thorax was rotated and the

head remained in a lateral position, the lower cervical vertebrae demonstrate rotation. If the patient's head and thorax were rotated simultaneously, the entire cervical column demonstrates rotation.

- *Detecting rotation:* Rotation can be detected on a lateral cervical image by evaluating each vertebra for anterior and posterior pillar superimposition and for zygapophyseal joint superimposition. When the patient is rotated, the pillars and zygapophyseal joints on one side of the vertebra move anterior to those on the other side (see Images 14 and 16). Because the two sides of the vertebrae are mirror images, it is very difficult to determine from a rotated lateral cervical image which side of the patient is rotated anteriorly and which is rotated posteriorly. The magnification of the side situated farther from the IR may give a moderately reliable clue at the articular pillar regions.
- *Positioning for trauma:* When cervical vertebral images are taken of a trauma patient with suspected subluxation or fracture, take the lateral projection with the patient's position left as is. *Do not* attempt to remove the cervical collar or to adjust head or body rotation, mandible position, or vertebral tilting. This might result in increased injury to the vertebrae or spinal cord. A trauma lateral cervical vertebral image is obtained by placing a lengthwise IR against the patient's shoulder and directing a horizontal beam to the cervical vertebrae (Figure 7-12). Such an image should meet as many of the analysis requirements listed for a nontrauma lateral image as possible without moving the patient. A 10- × 12-inch (24- × 30-cm) IR may be needed to include all of the required structures.

The posterior arch of C1 and the spinous process of C2 are demonstrated in profile without posterior occiput superimposition, and their bodies are demonstrated without mandibular superimposition. The cranial cortices and the mandibular rami are superimposed, the superior and inferior aspects of the right and left

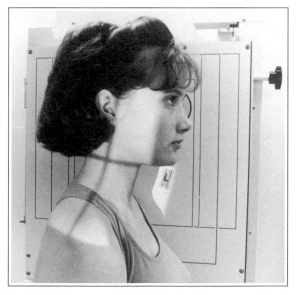

Figure 7-11. Proper patient positioning for lateral cervical vertebral image.

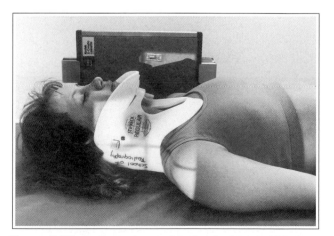

Figure 7-12. Proper patient positioning for lateral cervical vertebral image taken to evaluate trauma.

articular pillars and the zygapophyseal joints of each cervical vertebra are superimposed, and the intervertebral disk spaces are open.

- When the patient is positioned for a lateral cervical image, place the head in a lateral position with the midsagittal plane aligned parallel with the IR, and the chin elevated until the acanthiomeatal line (an imaginary line connecting the point where upper lip and nose meet with the external ear opening) is aligned parallel with the floor and the interpupillary line is aligned perpendicular to the IR. This positioning accomplishes five goals: alignment of the cervical vertebral column parallel with the IR; demonstration of C1 and C2 without occiput or mandibular superimposition; superimposition of the anterior and posterior, and superior and inferior aspects of the cranial and mandibular cortices, and superior and inferior aspects of the right and left articular pillars and zygapophyseal joints.

- *Effect of mandibular rotation and elevation on C1 and C2 visualization:* The position of the mandible and demonstration of C1 and C2 on a lateral cervical vertebral image are affected by head positioning. The posterior cortices of the mandibular rami are superimposed when the head's midsagittal plane was aligned parallel with the IR. If the posterior cortices of the mandibular rami are not superimposed on a lateral cervical vertebral image, one mandibular ramus is superimposed over the bodies of C1 and/or C2 and the other is situated anteriorly (see Image 15).

- If the chin was elevated adequately to place the acanthiomeatal line parallel with the floor, the mandibular rami are demonstrated anterior to the vertebral column. If the patient's chin was not adequately elevated, the mandibular rami are superimposed over the bodies of C1 and/or C2 (see Image 16).

- *Detecting head and shoulder tilting that causes lateral cervical flexion:* If the patient's head is tilted toward or away from the IR enough to laterally flex the upper cervical column, or if the shoulders are not placed on the same plane but are tilted enough to laterally flex the lower cervical column, the lateral cervical image will demonstrate a superoinferior separation between the right and left articular pillars and zygapophyseal joints of the flexed vertebrae (see Images 15 and 17).

- Head tilting will also result in a superoinferior separation between the cranial cortices and between the mandibular rami. If the head was tilted toward the IR, neither the superior nor the inferior cortices of the cranium nor the mandibular rami are superimposed, and the vertebral foramen of C1 is demonstrated (see Image 17). If the head and upper cervical vertebral column were tilted away from the IR, neither the inferior cortices of the cranium nor the mandibular rami are superimposed, and the posterior arch of C1 remains in profile (see Image 15).

The long axis of the cervical vertebral column is aligned with the long axis of the collimated field.

- Aligning the long axis of the cervical vertebral column with the long axis of the collimated field ensures against flexion or extension of the cervical column and allows for tight collimation. This alignment is obtained by positioning the patient's neck vertically and aligning the midline of the patient's neck with the collimator's longitudinal light line. This alignment places the cervical column in a neutral position.

- *Hyperflexion and hyperextension positioning to evaluate AP mobility of cervical vertebrae:* Hyperflexion and hyperextension lateral cervical vertebral images are obtained to evaluate AP vertebral mobility. For hyperflexion, instruct the patient to tuck the chin into the chest as far as possible (Figure 7-13). For patients who demonstrate extreme degrees of flexion, it may be necessary to place the IR crosswise to include the entire cervical column on the same image. Such an image should meet all the analysis requirements listed for a neutral lateral image, except that the long axis demonstrates forward bending (see Image 18). For hyperextension, instruct the patient to extend the chin up and backward as far as possible (Figure 7-14). Such an image should meet all the analysis requirements listed for a neutral lateral image, except that the long axis demonstrates backward bending (see Image 19).

- If the lateral position is used with the patient in hyperflexion or hyperextension, an arrow pointing in the direction the neck is moving or a flexion or extension marker should be included to indicate the direction of neck movement.

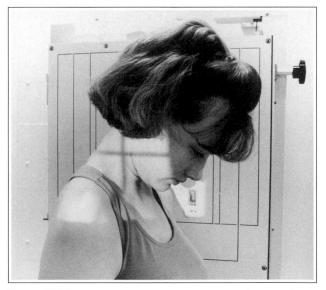

Figure 7-13. Patient positioning for lateral cervical vertebral image with hyperflexion.

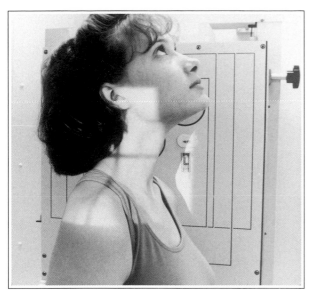

Figure 7-14. Patient positioning for lateral cervical vertebral image with hyperextension.

The fourth cervical vertebra is centered within the collimated field. The sella turcica, clivus, first through seventh cervical vertebrae, and superior half of the first thoracic vertebra and the surrounding soft tissue are included within the field.

- Center a perpendicular central ray to the midcoronal plane at a level halfway between the EAM and the jugular notch in order to center C4 to the collimated field.
- Open the longitudinally and transversely collimated field enough to include the clivus and sella turcica, which is at a level ¾ inch (2 cm) anterosuperior to the EAM. (The clivus, a slanted structure that extends posteriorly off the sella turcica, and the dens are used to determine cervical injury. A line drawn along the clivus should point to the tip of the dens on the normal upper cervical vertebral image.)
- An 8- × 10-inch (18- × 24-cm) IR placed lengthwise should be adequate to include all the required anatomical structures.
- ***Demonstration of C7 and T1 vertebrae:*** The seventh cervical vertebra and first thoracic vertebra are located between the patient's shoulders. This location makes it difficult to demonstrate them because of the great difference in lateral thickness between the neck and the shoulders. The best method to demonstrate C7 is to have the patient hold 5- or 10-lb weights on each arm to depress the shoulders and attempt to move them inferior to C7. Weights are best placed on each arm rather than in each hand, because sometimes the patient's shoulders will elevate when weights are placed in the hands. Without weights, it is often difficult to demonstrate more than six cervical vertebrae (see Image 20). Taking the image on expiration also aids in lowering the shoulders.

- ***Visualization of C7 and T1 in trauma or recumbency:*** For trauma or recumbent patients who do not have upper extremity or shoulder injuries, depress the shoulders by having a qualified assistant, with the consent of a physician, pull down on the patient's arms while the image is taken. To accomplish this, instruct an assistant to wear a protection apron and stand at the end of the imaging table or stretcher, with the patient's feet resting against the assistant's abdomen and the assistant's hands wrapped around the patient's wrists. The assistant should slowly pull on the patient's arms until the shoulders are moved inferiorly as much as possible.
- ***Demonstration C7:*** If even after using weights to depress the patient's shoulders C7 cannot be demonstrated in its entirety, a special image known as the lateral cervicothoracic position (Twining method) should be taken. Refer to p. 400 for specifics.

Lateral Cervical Vertebrae Image Analysis

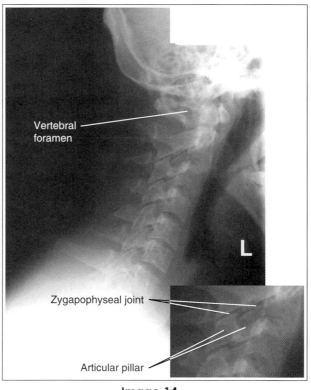

Image 14.

Analysis. The articular pillars and zygapophyseal joints on one side of the patient are situated anterior to those on the other side. The patient was rotated. The inferior cortices of the cranium and mandible are demonstrated without superimposition, and the vertebral foramen of C1 is visualized. The patient's head and upper cervical vertebral column were tilted toward the IR.

Correction. Rotate the patient until the midcoronal plane is aligned perpendicular to the IR, and tilt the head away from the IR until the interpupillary line is perpendicular to the IR.

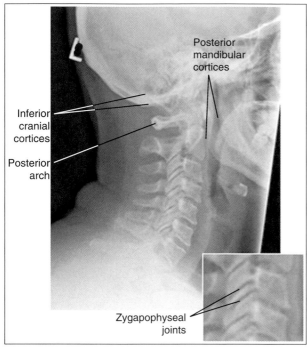

Image 15.

Analysis. The inferior and posterior cortices of the cranium and the mandible are not superimposed; the posterior arch of C1 is demonstrated in profile, and the right and left articular pillars and zygapophyseal joints demonstrate a superoinferior separation. The patient's head was rotated, and the patient's head and upper cervical vertebrae were tilted toward the IR.

Correction. Rotate the head until the midsagittal plane is aligned parallel with the IR, and then tilt the head toward the IR until the interpupillary line is perpendicular to the IR.

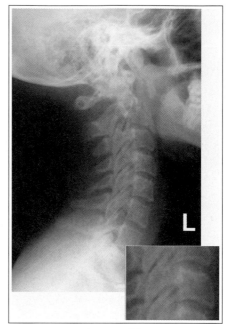

Image 16.

Analysis. The articular pillars and zygapophyseal joints on one side of the patient are situated anterior to those on the other side. The patient was rotated. The cranial and mandibular cortices are accurately aligned, and the mandibular rami are superimposed over the body of C2. The patient's chin was not adequately elevated.

Correction. Rotate the patient until the midcoronal plane is aligned perpendicular to the IR. Elevate the chin until the acanthiomeatal line is aligned parallel with the floor.

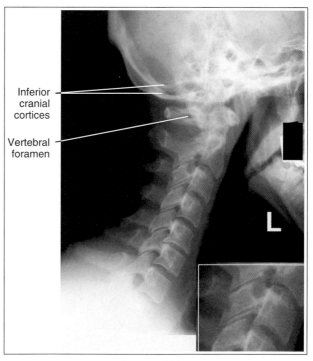

Image 17.

Analysis. The inferior cortices of the cranium and mandible are demonstrated without superimposition, the vertebral foramen of C1 is visualized, and the right and left articular pillars and zygapophyseal joints demonstrate a superoinferior separation. The patient's head and upper cervical vertebrae were tilted toward the IR.

Correction. Tilt the head away from the IR until the interpupillary line is aligned perpendicular to the IR.

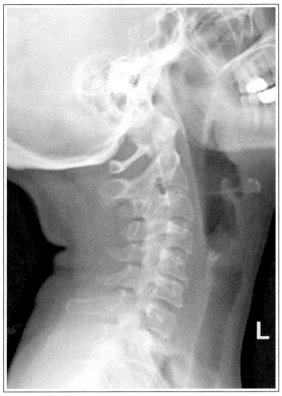

Image 19.

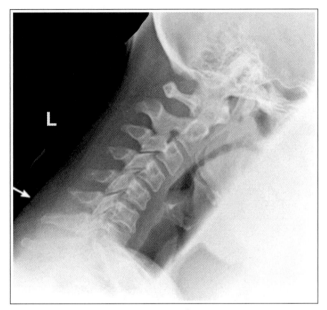

Image 18.

Analysis. The long axis of the cervical vertebral column is not aligned with the long axis of the collimated field. The cervical vertebral column is tilted forward. The patient was in hyperflexion.

Correction. Extend the patient's chin until the eyes are facing forward and the long axis of the neck is aligned with the long axis of the collimated field. If this examination is being performed to evaluate AP mobility, no corrective movement is required.

Analysis. The long axis of the cervical vertebral column is not aligned with the long axis of the collimated field. The cervical vertebral column is tilted backward. The patient was in hyperextension.

Correction. Tuck the patient's chin until the eyes are facing forward and the long axis of the neck is aligned with the long axis of the collimated field. If this examination is being performed to evaluate AP mobility, no corrective movement is required.

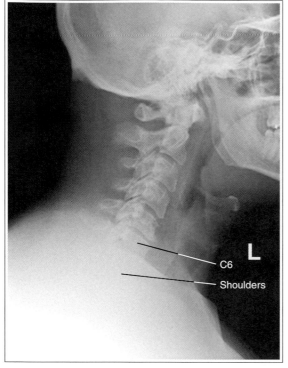

Image 20.

Analysis. The vertebral body of C7 is not demonstrated in its entirety, and the superior body of T1 is not demonstrated. The shoulders were not adequately depressed.

Correction. If possible, have the patient hold 5- to 10-lb weights on each arm to depress the shoulders. If the patient cannot hold weights or if the weights do not sufficiently drop the shoulders, a special image known as the cervicothoracic lateral (Twining method) should be taken to demonstrate this area (see p. 400).

CERVICAL VERTEBRAE: POSTEROANTERIOR OR ANTEROPOSTERIOR AXIAL OBLIQUE PROJECTION (ANTERIOR AND POSTERIOR OBLIQUE POSITIONS)

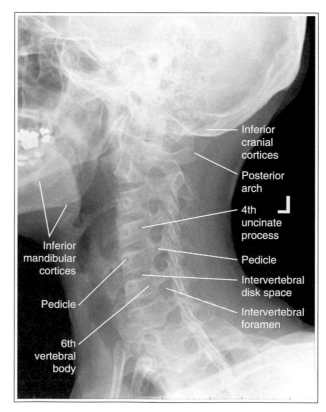

Figure 7-15. Posteroanterior axial oblique cervical vertebral image with cranium in lateral position and with accurate positioning.

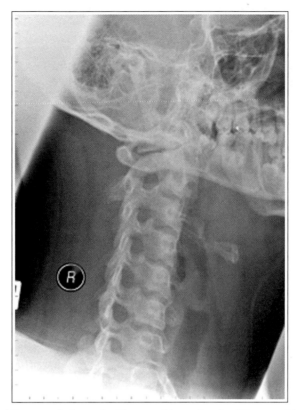

Figure 7-16. Posteroanterior axial oblique cervical vertebral image with cranium in oblique position and with accurate positioning.

Image Analysis

Scatter radiation is controlled.

- *Air-gap technique:* Because this examination uses a long OID, a grid is optional. When the OID is long, scatter radiation that would expose the IR at a short OID is scattered away from the IR. Consequently, much of the scatter radiation is not being directed toward the IR, and a grid is not needed to absorb the scatter. This is also referred to as the *air-gap technique*.

The bony trabecular patterns and cortical outlines of the cervical vertebrae are sharply defined.

- This examination can be taken using anterior ([posteroanterior] PA axial) or posterior (AP axial) oblique positions. The anterior oblique positions place the intervertebral foramina of interest closer to the IR, whereas the posterior oblique positions place the intervertebral foramina of interest farther from the IR. Even when anterior oblique positions are used, some OID remains. Any amount of OID results in magnification and loss of recorded detail. To offset some of this magnification, a 72-inch (183-cm) SID can be used. This decrease in image magnification provides an increase in recorded detail.

The cervical vertebrae have been rotated 45 degrees. The second through seventh intervertebral foramina are open, demonstrating uniformity in size and shape, the pedicles of interest are shown in profile, and the opposite pedicles are aligned with the anterior vertebral bodies. The sternum and sternoclavicular joints, when visible, are demonstrated without vertebral column superimposition.

- To position the intervertebral foramina and pedicles of interest in profile, begin by placing the patient in a recumbent or upright PA/AP axial oblique projection. Rotate the patient from this position until the midcoronal plane is at a 45-degree angle to the imaging table or upright IR. To demonstrate the foramina and pedicles on both sides of the cervical vertebrae, right and left oblique images must be taken. When anterior oblique images (Figure 7-17) are obtained, the foramina and pedicles situated closer to the IR are demonstrated, whereas posterior oblique images (Figure 7-18) demonstrate the foramina and pedicles situated farther from the IR.

- *Effect of incorrect rotation:* If the cervical vertebral rotation is insufficient, the intervertebral foramina are narrowed or obscured, the pedicles are foreshortened, and a portion of the sternum, one sternoclavicular joint, and the vertebral column are superimposed (see Image 21). If the cervical vertebrae are rotated more

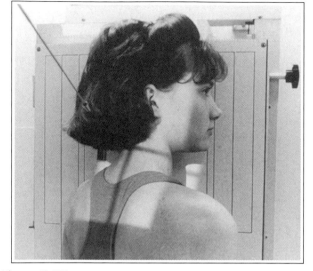

Figure 7-17. Proper patient positioning for posteroanterior axial oblique cervical vertebral image.

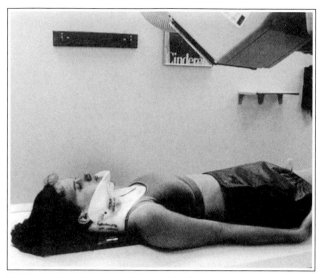

Figure 7-19. Proper patient positioning for anteroposterior axial oblique cervical vertebral image taken to evaluate trauma.

than 45 degrees, one side of the pedicles is partially foreshortened but the other side is aligned with the midline of the vertebral bodies, and the zygapophyseal joints—demonstrated without vertebral body superimposition—are open (see Image 22). Because it is possible for the upper and lower cervical vertebrae to be rotated to different degrees on the same image, one needs to evaluate the entire cervical vertebrae for proper rotation (see Image 23).

- **Positioning for trauma:** When imaging the cervical vertebrae of a trauma patient with suspected subluxation or fracture, obtain the trauma AP axial projection and lateral position and have them evaluated before the patient is moved for the oblique position. The trauma oblique position of the cervical vertebrae is accomplished

by elevating the supine patient's head, neck, and thorax enough to place a lengthwise IR beneath the neck. If the right vertebral foramina and pedicles are of interest, the IR should be shifted to the left enough to align the left mastoid tip with the longitudinal axis of the IR and inferior enough to position the right gonion (C3) with the transverse axis of the IR. Direct the central ray 45 degrees medial to the right side of the patient's neck and 15 degrees cephalically, then center it halfway between the AP surfaces of the neck at the level of the thyroid cartilage (C4) (Figure 7-19). If the left vertebral foramina and pedicles are of interest, shift the IR to the right enough to align the right mastoid tip with the longitudinal axis of the IR and inferior enough to position the left gonion with the transverse axis of the IR. The central ray should be angled and centered as previously described, except that it should be directed to the left side of the patient's neck. A trauma axial oblique cervical image should meet all the analysis requirements listed for a regular AP axial oblique cervical image; the cranium will be in an oblique position (Figure 7-20).

The intervertebral disk spaces are open, the cervical bodies are demonstrated as individual structures and are uniform in shape, and the posterior arch of the atlas is demonstrated without self-superimposition, demonstrating the vertebral foramen. The inferior outline of the outer cranial cortices and the mandibular rami are demonstrated without superimposition.

- The cervical vertebral column demonstrates a lordotic curvature. This curvature, and the shape of the cervical bodies, cause the disk articulating surfaces of the vertebral bodies to slant downward posteriorly to anteriorly.

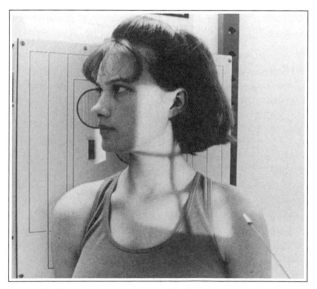

Figure 7-18. Proper patient positioning for anteroposterior axial oblique cervical vertebral image.

- **Importance of central ray angulation:** To obtain open intervertebral disk spaces and undistorted, uniformly shaped vertebral bodies, the central ray must be angled

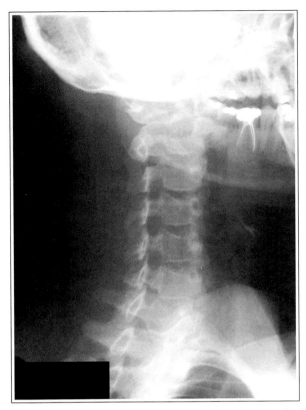

Figure 7-20. Anteroposterior axial oblique cervical vertebral image with accurate positioning taken to evaluate trauma.

in the same direction as the slope of the vertebral bodies. This is accomplished by angling the central ray 15 to 20 degrees caudally for anterior oblique images and 15 to 20 degrees cephalically for posterior oblique images. This angle will also result in demonstration of the atlas's vertebral foramen on oblique images.

- *Effect of inaccurate central ray angulation:* If the central ray is not accurately angled with the intervertebral disk spaces, they are closed and the cervical bodies are not demonstrated as individual structures (see Images 24 and 25). Because this examination can be performed using anterior or posterior oblique positions that require differing central ray angulations, and the typical cervical vertebral series requires the radiographer to change angle directions several times, radiographers should be able to identify an image that was taken with an incorrect angle. Image 24 was taken using a perpendicular central ray, and Image 25 was taken using with the central ray angled in the wrong direction. Note the closed intervertebral disk spaces, distorted cervical bodies, and demonstration of the posterior tubercles within the intervertebral foramina.

- *Positioning for kyphosis:* In patients with severe kyphosis, the lower cervical vertebrae are angled toward the IR because of the greater lordotic curvature of this area. To demonstrate the lower cervical vertebrae with open intervertebral disk spaces and undistorted

cervical bodies, the central ray will need to be angled more than the suggested 15 to 20 degrees for the oblique image. The patient in Image 26 had kyphosis. Note the decrease in intervertebral disk space openness and vertebral body distortion and the demonstration of the zygapophyseal joints through the cervical bodies between the upper and lower cervical regions.

- *Mandibular rami and cranial demonstration:* The distances demonstrated between the inferior cortical outlines of the cranium and the mandibular rami are a result of the angulation placed on the central ray. On anterior oblique cervical images the caudal angle projects the cranial cortex situated farther from the IR approximately $^{1}/_{4}$ inch (0.6 cm) inferiorly and the mandibular ramus situated farther from the IR approximately $^{1}/_{2}$ inch (1.25 cm) inferiorly. The ramus is projected farther inferiorly because it is located at a larger OID than the cranial cortex. On posterior oblique images, the cephalic angle projects the cranial cortex and mandibular rami situated farther from the IR superiorly.

- The distance between these two cortical outlines will be increased or decreased if the patient's head is allowed to tilt toward or away from the IR. Such tilting also causes the upper cervical vertebrae to lean toward or away from the IR. To avoid head and cervical column tilting, position the interpupillary line (imaginary line connecting the outer corners of the eyelids) parallel with the floor.

- *Detecting head tilting:* On anterior oblique images, if the head and upper cervical column are allowed to tilt, the atlas and its posterior arch are distorted. From such an image, one can determine whether the head and upper cervical vertebrae were tilted toward or away from the IR by evaluating the distance demonstrated between the inferior cranial cortices and the inferior mandibular rami. If these distances are increased, the head and upper cervical vertebrae were tilted away from the IR (see Image 27). If these distances are decreased, the head and upper cervical vertebrae were tilted toward the IR.

The cranium is in an oblique or lateral position as defined by the facility.

Oblique cranium: **The upper cervical vertebrae are demonstrated with posterior occipital and mandibular superimposition (see Figure 7-15).**

- The desired position of the patient's head for an AP axial oblique cervical image varies among facilities. If an oblique cranium image is desired, rotate the patient's head 45 degrees with the body. If a lateral cranium image is desired, turn the patient's face away from the side of interest until the head's midsagittal plane is aligned parallel with the IR.

Lateral cranium: **The upper cervical vertebrae are demonstrated without occipital or mandibular superimposition, and the right and left posterior** cortices of the cranium and the mandible are aligned (see Figure 7-16).

- To demonstrate the upper cervical vertebrae without mandibular superimposition and aligned right and left cranial and mandibular cortices on an AP axial oblique cervical image, place the patient's cranium in a lateral position and adjust chin elevation until the acanthiomeatal line is aligned parallel with the floor. If the patient's chin is not properly elevated and/or the patient's head is rotated, the mandibular rami are superimposed over C1 and C2 (see Image 28).

The fourth cervical vertebra is centered within the collimated field. The first through seventh cervical vertebrae, the first thoracic vertebra, and the surrounding soft tissue are included within the field.

- Center a 15- to 20-degree cephalically angled central ray to the patient's midsagittal plane at a level halfway between the EAM and the jugular notch to center C4 to the collimated field.
- Open the longitudinal collimation to the EAM and the jugular notch. Transverse collimation should be to within ½ inch (1.25 cm) of the neck skinline.
- An 8- × 10-inch (18- × 24-cm) IR placed lengthwise should be adequate to include all the required anatomical structures.

Anteroposterior Axial Oblique Cervical Vertebrae Image Analysis

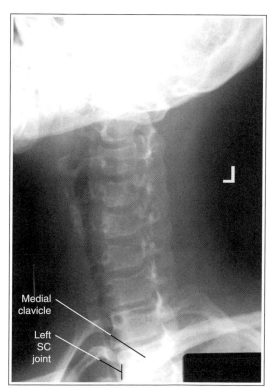

Image 21.

Analysis. This patient was in an LAO position, with the head in an oblique position. The pedicles and intervertebral foramina are obscured, and portions of the left sternoclavicular joint and medial clavicular end are superimposed by the vertebral column. The patient was not rotated the required 45 degrees.

Correction. Increase the patient obliquity until the midcoronal plane is placed at a 45-degree angle with the IR.

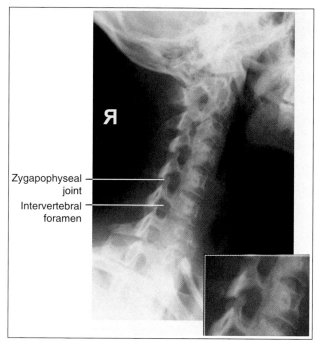

Image 22.

Analysis. This patient was in an RAO position with the patient's head in a lateral position. The intervertebral foramina are demonstrated, the right pedicles are shown although they are not in true profile, the left pedicles are demonstrated in the midline of the vertebral bodies, and the right zygapophyseal joints are demonstrated. The patient was rotated more than 45 degrees.

Correction. Decrease the patient rotation until the midcoronal plane is placed at a 45-degree angle with the IR.

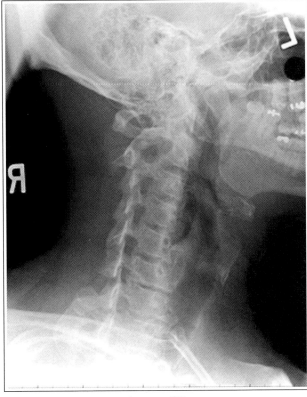

Image 23.

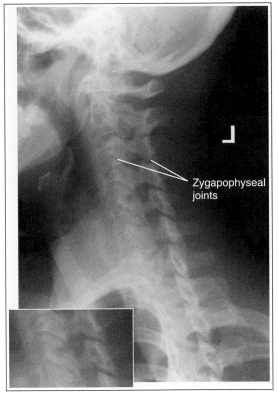

Zygapophyseal joints

Image 24.

Analysis. This patient is in an RAO position with the patient's head in a lateral position. The upper cervical vertebrae demonstrate open and uniformly shaped intervertebral foramina, and the left pedicles are aligned with the anterior vertebral body, indicating that the patient's upper vertebrae were adequately rotated. The lower cervical vertebrae demonstrate the right zygapophyseal joints, narrowed and distorted intervertebral foramina, and the left pedicles aligned closer toward the midline of the vertebral bodies, indicating that the patient's torso was overrotated.

Correction. While maintaining the degree of upper cervical rotation, decrease patient torso rotation until the midcoronal plane is placed at a 45-degree angle with the IR.

Analysis. This patient was in an LAO position, with the head in a lateral position. The intervertebral disk spaces are closed, the cervical bodies are distorted, the posterior tubercles are demonstrated within the intervertebral foramina, the C1 vertebral foramen is not demonstrated, and the inferior mandibular rami and the cranial cortices are demonstrated with superimposition. The central ray was directed perpendicular to the IR.

Correction. Angle the central ray 15 to 20 degrees caudally for anterior oblique images.

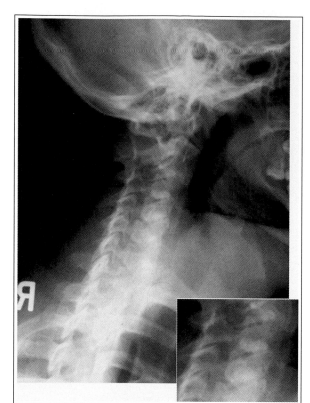

Image 25.

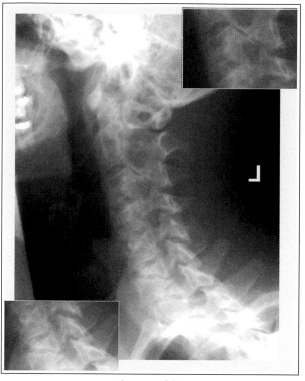

Image 26.

Analysis. This patient was in an RAO position, with the head in a lateral position. The intervertebral disk spaces are closed, the cervical bodies are distorted, the posterior tubercles are demonstrated within the intervertebral foramina, the C1 intervertebral foramen is demonstrated, and the inferior mandibular rami and cranial cortices are shown without superimposition. The central ray was angled 15 to 20 degrees cephalically.

Correction. Angle the central ray 15 to 20 degrees caudally for anterior oblique images.

Analysis. This patient is in an LAO position, with the head in a lateral position. A decrease in intervertebral disk space openness and vertebral body distortion are present, and demonstration of the zygapophyseal joints through the cervical bodies in the lower cervical vertebrae (C5 through C7) is increased. The patient is kyphotic, and the entire cervical spine was not aligned parallel with the IR.

Correction. Align the entire cervical spine parallel with the IR or increase the central ray angulation over the 15 to 20 degrees required for a routine oblique image to better demonstrate the fifth through seventh cervical vertebrae.

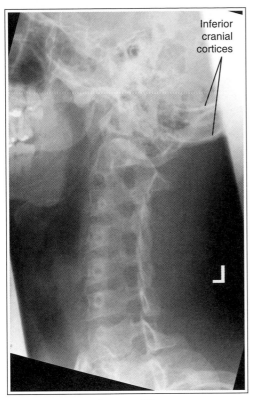

Image 27.

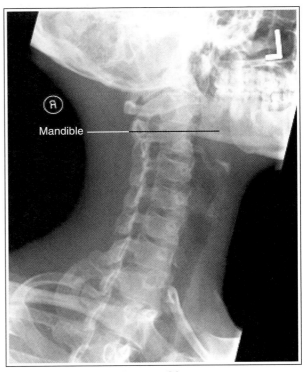

Image 28.

Analysis. This patient was in an LAO position, with the head in a lateral position. The atlas and its posterior arch are obscured. The inferior cranial cortices demonstrate more than ¼ inch (0.6 cm) between them, and the inferior cortices of the mandibular rami demonstrate more than ½ inch (1.25 cm) between them. The first thoracic vertebra is not included in its entirety. The head and the upper cervical vertebrae were tilted away from the IR, and the central ray and IR were positioned too superiorly.

Correction. Tilt the patient's head toward the IR until the interpupillary line is aligned perpendicular to the IR, and move the central ray and IR inferiorly.

Analysis. This patient was in an RAO position, with the head in an oblique position. The mandibular ramus is superimposed over the body of C2.

Correction. To demonstrate C2 without mandibular ramus superimposition, place the patient's head in a lateral position and elevate the patient's chin until the acanthiomeatal line is aligned parallel with the floor.

CERVICOTHORACIC VERTEBRAE

See p. 375 for image analysis criteria for all cervical and thoracic images.

CERVICOTHORACIC VERTEBRAE: LATERAL POSITION (TWINING METHOD)

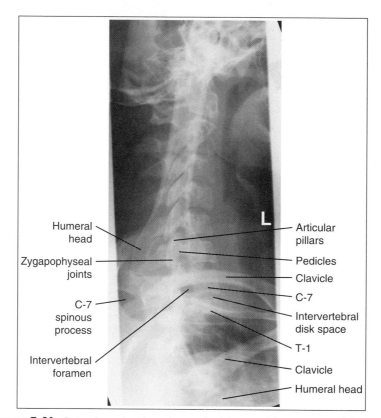

Figure 7-21. Lateral cervicothoracic vertebral image with accurate positioning.

This examination is performed when the routine lateral cervical image does not adequately demonstrate the seventh cervical vertebra or when the routine lateral thoracic image does not demonstrate the first through third thoracic vertebrae.

Image Analysis

Scatter radiation is controlled.

- Use tight collimation, a grid, and a lead sheet placed on the imaging table at the edge of the posteriorly collimated field to reduce the amount of scatter radiation that reaches the IR, providing higher contrast and better visibility of recorded details.

The cervicothoracic vertebrae are demonstrated in a lateral position. The humerus elevated above the patient's head is aligned with the vertebral column, the right and left cervical zygapophyseal joints and **articular pillars are superimposed, and the posterior ribs are superimposed.**

- Position the patient in an upright or a lateral recumbent position. Whether the right or left side of the patient is positioned against the imaging table or upright IR is not significant, although left-side positioning is easier for the technologist. For the recumbent position, flex the patient's knees and hips for support. For the upright position, instruct the patient to evenly distribute weight on both feet. Elevate the arm positioned closer to the IR above the patient's head as high as the patient allows. The forearm and hand may be rested on the head for support in the erect position. Place the other arm against the patient's side, and instruct the patient to depress this shoulder (Figure 7-22) and move it slightly anteriorly.

- This supplementary lateral cervicothoracic method moves the shoulders in opposite directions, overlapping one onto the upper cervical region and the other onto

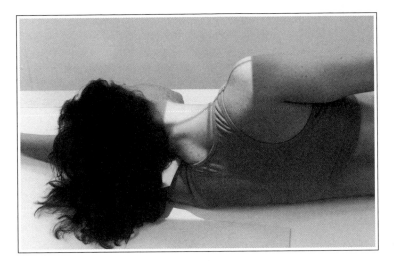

Figure 7-22. Proper patient positioning for recumbent lateral cervicothoracic vertebral image.

the lower thoracic region, allowing visualization of the cervicothoracic area without shoulder superimposition. To demonstrate the fifth through seventh cervical vertebrae and the first through third thoracic vertebrae without shoulder superimposition, the shoulder positioned away from the IR is depressed. Taking the image on expiration will also aid in lowering the shoulder. A 5-degree caudal central ray angulation may be used for a patient who is unable to adequately depress the shoulder positioned farther from the IR. This angle projects the shoulder inferiorly.

- Once the shoulders are positioned, adjust patient head and body rotation to obtain a lateral position. You can avoid cervical rotation by placing the head in a lateral position, and thoracic rotation by resting your extended flat palm against the patient's shoulders and the inferior posterior ribs, then adjusting patient rotation until your hand is positioned perpendicular to the imaging table or upright grid holder.

- *Detecting rotation:* If the patient is rotated, the articular pillars, posterior ribs, zygapophyseal joints, and humeri move away from each other, obscuring the pedicles and distorting the vertebral bodies. When rotation is demonstrated on a lateral cervicothoracic image, determine which side was rotated anteriorly or posteriorly by evaluating the position of the humeral head positioned closer to the IR. If the patient was rotated anteriorly, the humeral head farther from the IR is positioned anteriorly (see Image 29). If the patient was rotated posteriorly, the humeral head closer to the IR is positioned anteriorly, and the humeral head farther from the IR is positioned posteriorly (see Image 30).

- *Positioning for trauma:* When routine cervical images are obtained in a trauma patient with suspected subluxation or fracture and the seventh lateral cervical vertebra is not demonstrated, obtain the lateral cervicothoracic image with the patient's head, neck, and body trunk left as is. Instruct the patient to elevate the arm farther from the x-ray tube and to depress the arm closer to the tube. Then place a grid-cassette against the patient's lateral body surface, centering its transverse axis at a level 1 inch (2.5 cm) superior to the jugular notch (Figure 7-23). Position the central ray horizontal to the posterior neck surface and the center of the grid-cassette. If the shoulder closer to the central ray is not well depressed, a 5-degree caudal angulation is recommended.

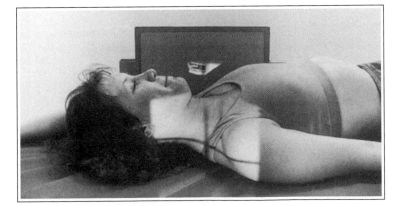

Figure 7-23. Proper patient positioning for lateral cervicothoracic vertebral image taken to evaluate trauma.

The intervertebral disk spaces are open, and the vertebral bodies are demonstrated without distortion.

- To obtain open disk spaces and undistorted vertebral bodies, position the head in a lateral position, with the interpupillary line perpendicular to, and the midsagittal plane parallel with, the upright grid holder or imaging table.
- If the patient is in a recumbent lateral position, it may be necessary to elevate the head on a sponge to place it in a lateral position, preventing cervical column tilting (see Image 31).

The first thoracic vertebra is centered within the collimated field. The fifth through seventh cervical vertebrae and the first through fourth thoracic vertebrae are included within the field.

- Center a perpendicular central ray to the midcoronal plane at a level 1 inch (2.5 cm) superior to the jugular notch or at the level of the vertebra prominens. The seventh cervical vertebra can be identified on a lateral cervicothoracic image by locating the elevated clavicle, which is normally shown traversing the seventh cervical vertebra.
- Open the longitudinal collimated field to the patient's mandibular angle. Transverse collimation should be to within ½ inch (1.25 cm) of the cervical skinline.
- A 10- × 12-inch (24- × 30-cm) IR placed lengthwise should be adequate to include all the required anatomical structures.

Lateral Cervicothoracic Vertebrae Image Analysis

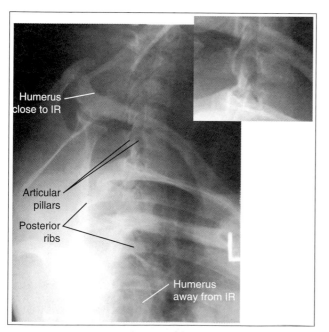

Image 29.

Analysis. The right and left articular pillars, zygapophyseal joints, and posterior ribs are demonstrated without superimposition. The patient's thorax was rotated. The humerus that was raised and situated closer to the IR is demonstrated posterior to the vertebral column. The shoulder that was depressed and positioned farther from the IR was rotated anteriorly.

Correction. Rotate the shoulder positioned farther from the IR posteriorly, until your flat palms placed against the shoulders or the posterior ribs, respectively, are aligned perpendicular to the imaging table and upright grid holder.

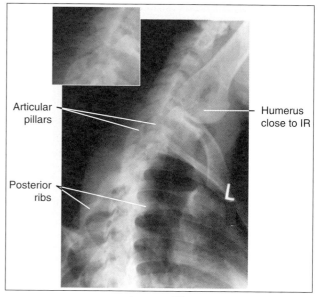

Image 30.

Analysis. The right and left articular pillars, zygapophyseal joints, and posterior ribs are demonstrated without superimposition. The patient's thorax was rotated. The humerus that was raised and situated closer to the IR is demonstrated anterior to the vertebral column. The shoulder that was depressed and positioned farther from the IR was rotated posteriorly.

Correction. Rotate the shoulder positioned farther from the IR anteriorly until your flat palms placed against the shoulders and the posterior ribs, respectively, are aligned perpendicular to the imaging table and upright IR.

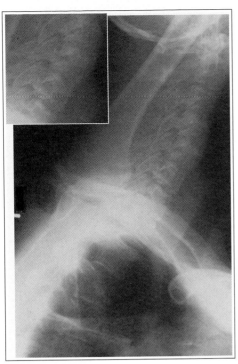

Image 31.

Analysis. The intervertebral disk spaces are closed, and the vertebral bodies are distorted. The patient's cervical vertebral column was not positioned parallel with the IR.

Correction. Position the midsagittal plane of the head and cervical vertebral column parallel with the IR. It may be necessary to prop the head on a sponge to help the patient maintain the position.

THORACIC VERTEBRAE

See p. 375 for image analysis criteria for all cervical and thoracic images.

THORACIC VERTEBRAE: ANTEROPOSTERIOR PROJECTION

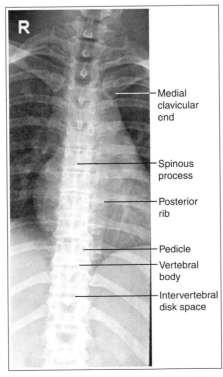

- Medial clavicular end
- Spinous process
- Posterior rib
- Pedicle
- Vertebral body
- Intervertebral disk space

Figure 7-24. Anteroposterior thoracic vertebral image with accurate positioning.

Image Analysis

Contrast and density are adequate to demonstrate the surrounding mediastinum soft tissue and the bony structures of the thoracic vertebrae and connecting posterior ribs. Penetration is sufficient to visualize the bony trabecular patterns and cortical outlines of the vertebral bodies, pedicles, spinous processes, posterior ribs, and transverse processes.

- An optimal 75- to 85-kVp technique sufficiently penetrates the bony and soft-tissue structures of the mediastinum and thoracic vertebrae.
- Use a high-ratio grid and tight collimation to decrease the scatter radiation that reaches the IR, reducing fog, improving the visibility of recorded details, and providing a higher-contrast image.
- When an exposure (mAs) is set that adequately demonstrates the lower thoracic vertebrae (T6 to T12), the upper thoracic vertebrae (T1 to T5) are often overexposed because of the difference in AP body thickness between these two regions. Two methods may be used to achieve uniform density in spite of this difference in thickness. The first method uses a wedge compensating filter, and the second method uses the anode-heel effect.
- *Wedge filter:* The wedge filter absorbs x-ray photons before they reach the patient, thereby decreasing the number of photons exposing the IR where the filter is located. The thicker end of a wedge filter absorbs more photons than the thinner end. When a wedge filter is used, attach it to the x-ray collimator head with the thick end positioned toward the patient's head and the thin end toward the patient's feet. The collimator light projects a shadow of the wedge filter onto the patient's midsagittal plane (Figure 7-25). The number of the upper thoracic vertebrae that should be covered by the filter's shadow depends on the slope of the patient's sternum and upper thorax. Position the thin edge of the

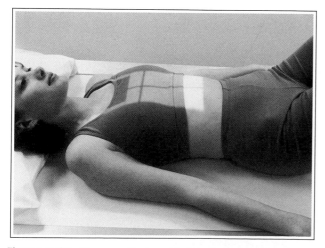

Figure 7-25. Proper patient positioning for anteroposterior thoracic vertebral image with compensating filter.

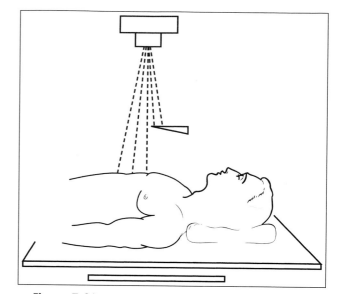

Figure 7-26. Proper placement of compensating filter.

wedge filter's shadow at the inferior sternum and thorax, at the level at which they begin to decline (Figure 7-26). Set exposure factors that adequately expose the lower thorax. If the wedge filter has been accurately positioned, it will absorb the excessive radiation directed toward the upper thorax, thereby resulting in uniform image density throughout the thoracic column. If the wedge filter was inaccurately positioned, a definite density difference will define where the wedge filter was and was not placed. Positioning the filter too inferiorly on the patient results in an underexposed area where the filter was misplaced (see Image 32). Positioning the filter too superiorly results in an overexposed area where the filter should have been placed.

- *Anode-heel effect:* The anode-heel effect works similarly to a filter: it decreases the number of photons reaching the upper thoracic vertebrae and results in decreased density in this area. This method works sufficiently in patients who have very little difference in AP body thickness between their upper and lower thoracic vertebrae but does not provide an adequate density decrease in patients with larger thickness differences. For the latter patients, use the anode-heel effect in combination with a wedge filter. To use the anode-heel effect, position the patient's head and upper thoracic vertebrae at the anode end of the tube and the feet and lower thoracic vertebrae at the cathode end. Then set an exposure (mAs) that adequately demonstrates the middle thoracic vertebrae. Because the anode will absorb some of the photons aimed at the anode end of the IR, the upper thoracic vertebrae will receive less exposure than the lower vertebrae.
- *Expiration versus inspiration image:* Patient respiration determines the amount of contrast and density difference demonstrated between the mediastinum and the vertebral column. These differences are a result of the variation in density (number of atoms per given area) that exists

between the thoracic cavity and the vertebrae. The thoracic cavity is largely composed of air, which contains very few atoms in a given area; the same area of bone, as in the vertebrae, contain many compacted atoms. As radiation goes through the patient's body, fewer photons are absorbed in the thoracic cavity than in the vertebral column, because fewer atoms with which the photons can interact are present in the thoracic cavity. Consequently, more photons will penetrate the thoracic cavity to expose the IR than will penetrate the vertebral column. Taking the exposure on full, suspended expiration can help to decrease the thoracic cavity's image density by reducing the air volume and compressing the tissue in this area (see Figure 7-24). This decreased image density allows better visualization of the posterior ribs and mediastinum region. If the AP thoracic vertebral image is exposed while the patient is in full, suspended inspiration, the thoracic cavity demonstrates increased image density compared with the vertebral column (see Image 33). It should be noted, however, that the contrast created on an AP thoracic vertebral image taken on inspiration can be valuable in detecting thoracic tumors or disease.

The thoracic vertebral column demonstrates an AP projection. The spinous processes are aligned with the midline of the vertebral bodies, the distances from the vertebral column to the medial (sternal) ends of the clavicles are equal, and the distances from the pedicles to the spinous processes are equal on the two sides.

- An AP thoracic vertebral image is obtained by placing the patient supine on the imaging table. Position the shoulders and anterior superior iliac spines (ASISs) at equal distances from the imaging table to prevent rotation, and draw the patient's arms away from the thoracic area to keep them from being tucked beneath the patient (Figure 7-27).

- **Effect of rotation:** The upper and lower thoracic vertebrae can demonstrate rotation independently or simultaneously, depending on which section of the body is rotated. If the patient's shoulders and upper thorax were rotated and the pelvis and lower thorax remained supine, the upper thoracic vertebrae demonstrate rotation. If the patient's pelvis and lower thorax were rotated and the thorax and shoulders remained supine, the lower thoracic vertebrae demonstrate rotation. If the patient's thorax and pelvis were rotated simultaneously, the entire thoracic column demonstrates rotation.

- **Detecting rotation:** Rotation is effectively detected on an AP thoracic image by comparing the distances between pedicles and spinous processes on the same vertebra and the distances between the vertebral column and the medial ends of the clavicles. When no rotation is present, the comparable distances are equal. If one side demonstrates a greater distance, vertebral rotation is present. The side demonstrating a greater distance is the side of the patient positioned closer to the imaging table and the IR (see Image 34).

- **Distinguishing rotation from scoliosis:** In patients with spinal scoliosis the thoracic bodies may appear rotated because of the lateral twisting of the vertebrae. Scoliosis of the vertebral column can be very severe, demonstrating a large amount of lateral deviation, or it can be subtle, demonstrating only a small amount of deviation (Figure 7-28). Severe scoliosis is very

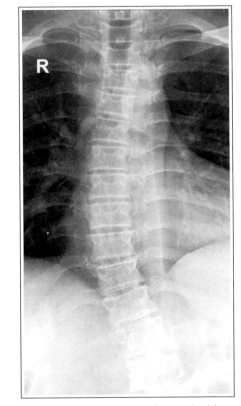

Figure 7-28. Anteroposterior thoracic vertebral image demonstrating spinal scoliosis.

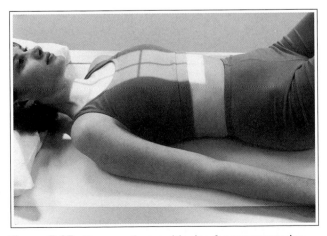

Figure 7-27. Proper patient positioning for anteroposterior thoracic vertebral image without compensating filter.

obvious and is seldom mistaken for patient rotation, whereas subtle scoliotic changes may be easily mistaken for rotation. Although both conditions demonstrate unequal distances between the pedicles and spinous processes, certain clues can be used to distinguish subtle scoliosis from rotation. The long axis of a rotated vertebral column remains straight, whereas the scoliotic vertebral column demonstrates lateral deviation. When the thoracic vertebrae demonstrate rotation, it has been caused by the rotation of the upper or lower torso. Rotation of the middle thoracolumbar vertebrae does not occur unless the upper and lower thoracic vertebrae also demonstrate rotation. On an image from a patient with scoliosis the thoracolumbar vertebrae may demonstrate rotation without corresponding upper or lower vertebral rotation. Familiarity with the difference between a rotated thoracic vertebral column and a scoliotic one prevents unnecessarily repeated procedures in patients with spinal scoliosis.

The intervertebral disk spaces are open, and the vertebral bodies are demonstrated without distortion.

- The thoracic vertebral column demonstrates a kyphotic curvature. Because the thoracic vertebrae have very limited flexion and extension movements, it is difficult to achieve a significant reduction of this curvature. A small reduction can be obtained by placing the patient's head on a thin pillow or sponge and flexing the hips and knees until the lower back rests firmly against the imaging table; both procedures improve the relationship of the upper and lower vertebral disk spaces and bodies with the x-ray beam. The head position reduces the upper vertebral curvature, and the hip and knee position reduces the lower vertebral curvature. If the disk spaces are not aligned parallel with the x-ray beam and the vertebral bodies are not aligned perpendicular to the x-ray beam, it is difficult for the reviewer to evaluate the height of the disk spaces and vertebral bodies (see Image 35).
- *Positioning for kyphosis:* To demonstrate open disk spaces and undistorted vertebral bodies in a patient with excessive spinal kyphosis, it may be necessary to angle the central ray until it is perpendicular to the vertebral area of interest. Because it is painful for such a patient to lie supine on the imaging table, it is best to perform the examination with the patient upright, or in a lateral recumbent position with use of a horizontal beam.

The seventh thoracic vertebra is centered within the collimated field. The seventh cervical vertebra, first through twelfth thoracic vertebrae, first lumbar vertebra, and 2½ inches (6.25 cm) of the posterior ribs and mediastinum on each side of the vertebral column are included within the field.

- Center a perpendicular central ray to the patient's midsagittal plane at a level halfway between the jugular notch and the xiphoid to position the seventh thoracic vertebra in the center of the collimated field.

- Open the longitudinal collimation the full 17-inch (43-cm) IR length for adult patients. Transverse collimation should be to approximately an 8-inch (20-cm) field.
- A 14- × 17-inch (35- × 43-cm) IR placed lengthwise should be adequate to include all the required anatomical structures.

Anteroposterior Thoracic Vertebrae Image Analysis

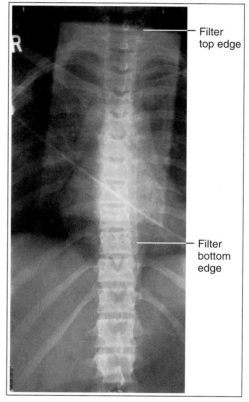

Image 32.

Analysis. The sixth through ninth thoracic vertebrae are underexposed. The wedge compensating filter was positioned too inferiorly.

Correction. Position the shadow of the wedge filter's thin edge at the beginning of the downward slope of the patient's sternum and upper thorax, as demonstrated in Figure 7-25.

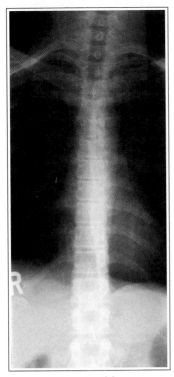

Image 33.

Analysis. The thoracic cavity is overexposed. The image was taken on inspiration.

Correction. Expose the image with the patient in full expiration. If a mediastinal tumor or disease is in question, however, no correction is needed.

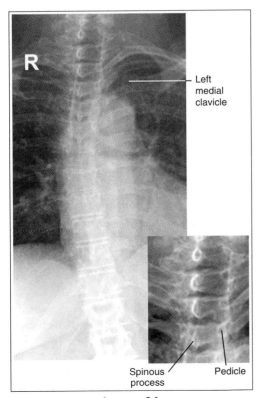

Image 34.

Analysis. The upper cervical vertebrae demonstrate more distance from the left pedicle to the spinous process than from the right pedicle to the spinous process, and the left medial clavicle is demonstrated away from the vertebral column. The patient was rotated toward the left side.

Correction. Rotate the patient toward the right side until the shoulders and ASISs are at equal distances from the imaging table.

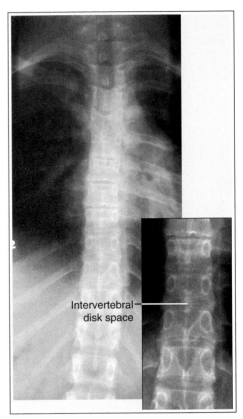

Image 35.

Analysis. The eighth through twelfth intervertebral disk spaces are obscured, and the vertebral bodies distorted. The patient's legs were extended.

Correction. Flex the patient's hips and knees, placing the feet and back firmly against the imaging table.

THORACIC VERTEBRAE: LATERAL POSITION

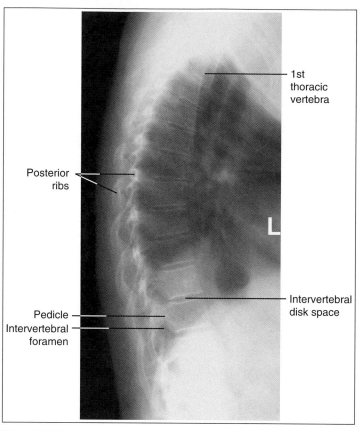

Figure 7-29. Lateral thoracic vertebral image with accurate positioning.

Image Analysis

Scatter radiation is controlled, and thoracic vertebrae are demonstrated through overlying lung and rib structures.

- Use tight collimation, a grid, and a lead sheet placed on the imaging table at the edge of the posteriorly collimated field to reduce the amount of scatter radiation that reaches the IR, providing higher contrast and better visibility of recorded details.
- *Breathing technique:* The thoracic vertebrae have many overlying structures, including the axillary ribs and lungs. Using a long exposure time (3 to 4 seconds) and requiring the patient to breathe shallowly (costal breathing) during the exposure forces a slow and steady, upward and outward movement of the ribs and lungs. This technique is often referred to as *breathing technique.* This movement causes blurring of the ribs and lung markings on the image, providing greater thoracic vertebral demonstration. Deep breathing, which requires movement (elevation) of the sternum and a faster and expanded upward and outward movement of the ribs and lungs,

should be avoided during the breathing technique, because deep breathing results in motion of the thoracic cavity and vertebrae (see Image 36).
- *Note:* If patient motion cannot be avoided when using the extended 3 to 4 seconds for breathing technique, take the image on suspended expiration to reduce the air volume within the thoracic cavity.

The thoracic vertebrae demonstrate a lateral position. The intervertebral foramina are clearly demonstrated, the pedicles are in profile, the posterior surfaces of each vertebral body are superimposed, and no more than ½ inch (1.25 cm) of space is demonstrated between the posterior ribs.

- To obtain a lateral thoracic vertebral image, place the patient on the imaging table in a lateral recumbent position. Whether the patient is lying on the right or left side is not significant, although left-side positioning is easier for the technologist (Figure 7-30). One exception to this guideline is the scoliotic patient, who should be placed on the imaging table so the central ray is directed into the spinal curve. Abduct the patient's arms to a 90-degree angle with the body, to prevent the

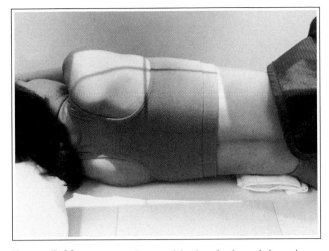

Figure 7-30. Proper patient positioning for lateral thoracic vertebral image.

humeri or their soft tissue from obscuring the thoracic vertebrae. Flex the patient's knees and hips for support, and position a pillow or sponge between the knees. The thickness of the pillow or sponge should be enough to prevent the side of the pelvis situated farther from the IR from rotating anteriorly but not so thick as to cause posterior rotation. To avoid vertebral rotation, align the shoulders, the posterior ribs, and the posterior pelvic wings perpendicular to the imaging table and IR by resting an extended flat palm against each, respectively, then adjusting patient rotation until the hand is positioned perpendicular to the IR.

- *Effect of rotation:* The upper and lower thoracic vertebrae can demonstrate rotation independently or simultaneously, depending on which section of the torso was rotated. If the shoulders and the superoposterior ribs were not placed on top of each other but the posterior pelvic wings and inferoposterior ribs were aligned, the upper thoracic vertebrae demonstrate rotation and the lower thoracic vertebrae demonstrate a true lateral position. If the posterior pelvic wings and inferoposterior ribs were rotated but the shoulders and superoposterior ribs were placed on top of each other, the lower thoracic vertebrae demonstrate rotation and the upper vertebrae demonstrate a lateral position.

- *Detecting rotation:* Rotation can be detected on a lateral thoracic vertebral image by evaluating the superimposition of the right and left posterior surfaces of the vertebral bodies and the amount of posterior rib superimposition. On a nonrotated lateral thoracic image, the posterior surfaces are superimposed and the posterior ribs are nearly superimposed. Because the posterior ribs positioned farther from the IR were placed at a greater OID than the other side, they demonstrate more magnification. This magnification prevents the posterior ribs from being directly superimposed but positions them

approximately ½ inch (1.25 cm) apart. This distance is based on a 40-inch (102-cm) SID. If a longer SID is used, the distance between the posterior ribs is decreased, and if a shorter SID is used, the distance is increased. On rotation, the right and left posterior surfaces of the vertebral bodies are demonstrated one anterior to the other on a lateral image.

- Because the two sides of the thorax and vertebrae are mirror images, it is very difficult to determine from a rotated lateral thoracic image which side of the patient was rotated anteriorly and which posteriorly. If the patient was only slightly rotated, one way of determining which way the patient was rotated is to evaluate the amount of posterior rib superimposition. If the patient's elevated side was rotated posteriorly, the posterior ribs demonstrate more than ½ inch (1.25 cm) of space between them (see Image 37). If the patient's elevated side was rotated anteriorly, the posterior ribs are superimposed on slight rotation (see Image 38) and demonstrate greater separation as rotation of the patient increases.

- *Distinguishing rotation from scoliosis:* On the image of a patient with spinal scoliosis, the lung field may appear rotated owing to the lateral deviation of the vertebral column (see Image 11, Chapter 2, p. 65). On such an image, the posterior ribs demonstrate differing degrees of separation depending on the severity of the scoliosis. View the accompanying AP thoracic image (see Image 2, Chapter 2, p. 59) to confirm this patient condition.

The intervertebral disk spaces are open, and the vertebral bodies are demonstrated without distortion.

- The thoracic vertebral column is capable of lateral flexion. When the patient is placed in a lateral recumbent position, the vertebral column may not be aligned parallel with the imaging table and IR but may sag at the level of the lower thoracic vertebrae, especially in a patient who has wide hips and a narrow waist (Figure 7-31). If the patient's thoracic column is allowed to sag, the

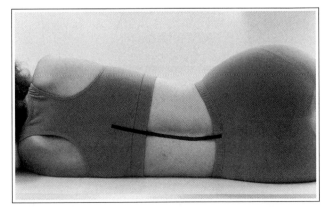

Figure 7-31. Poor alignment of vertebral column with imaging table.

diverging x-ray beams are not aligned parallel with the intervertebral disk spaces and perpendicular with the vertebral bodies. Lateral flexion on a lateral thoracic vertebral image is most evident at the lower thoracic vertebral bodies, where closed disk spaces and distorted vertebral bodies are present (see Image 39). For a patient who has a sagging thoracic column, it may be necessary to tuck an immobilization device between the lateral body surface and the imaging table just superior to the iliac crest, elevating the sagging area. The radiolucent sponge should be thick enough to bring the thoracic vertebral column parallel with the imaging table and IR (see Figure 7-30).

- An alternative method of obtaining open disk spaces and undistorted vertebral bodies in a patient whose thoracic column is sagging is to angle the central ray 10 degrees cephalically for female patients and 15 degrees for male patients. The degree of cephalic angulation used should align the central ray perpendicular to the thoracic vertebral column.

The seventh thoracic vertebra is centered within the collimated field. The seventh cervical vertebra, the first through twelfth thoracic vertebrae, and the first lumbar vertebra are included within the field.

- Center a perpendicular central ray to the inferior scapular angle. With the patient's arm positioned at a 90-degree angle with the body, the inferior scapular angle is placed over the seventh thoracic vertebra.
- Open the longitudinal collimation the full 17-inch (43-cm) IR length for adult patients. Transverse collimation should be to an 8-inch (20-cm) field.
- A 14- × 17-inch (35- × 43-cm) IR placed lengthwise should be adequate to include all the required anatomical structures.
- *Verifying inclusion of all thoracic vertebrae:* When viewing a lateral thoracic image, you can be sure the 12th thoracic vertebra has been included by locating the vertebra that has the last rib attached to it; this is the 12th vertebra. To confirm this finding, follow the posterior vertebral bodies of the lower thoracic and upper lumbar vertebrae, watching for the subtle change in curvature from kyphotic to lordotic. The twelfth thoracic vertebra is located just above it. The first thoracic vertebra can be identified on a lateral thoracic image by counting up from the twelfth thoracic vertebra or by locating the seventh cervical vertebral prominens. The first thoracic vertebra is at the same level as this prominens.
- *Lateral cervicothoracic (Twining method) image:* Because of shoulder thickness and the superimposition of the shoulders over the first through third thoracic vertebrae, it may be necessary to take a supplementary image of this area to demonstrate the thoracic vertebrae. Refer to p. 400 for specifics.

Lateral Thoracic Vertebrae Image Analysis

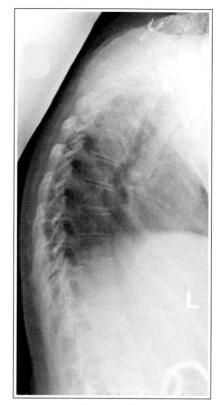

Image 36.

Analysis. The thoracic vertebrae, ribs, and lung markings demonstrate a blurring of the recorded details. The image was exposed using deep breathing technique during the exposure, causing patient motion.

Correction. Instruct the patient to breath shallowly. If the patient is unable to perform costal breathing, take the exposure on suspended expiration.

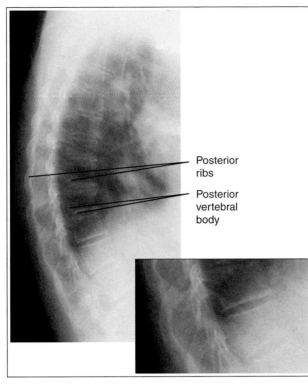

Posterior
ribs

Posterior
vertebral
body

Image 37.

8th posterior
vertebral body

L

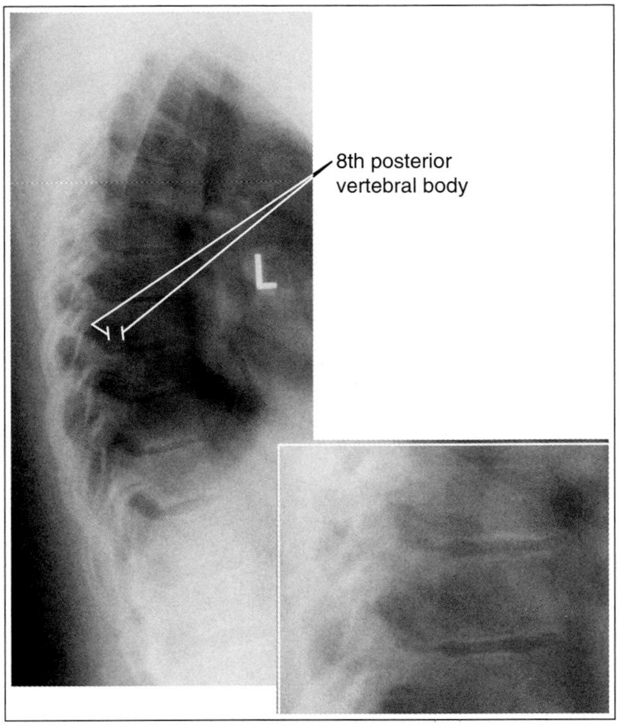

Image 38.

Analysis. The posterior surfaces of the vertebral bodies are demonstrated without superimposition, and more than ½ inch (1.25 cm) of space is demonstrated between the posterior ribs. The elevated side of the thorax was rotated posteriorly.

Correction. Rotate the elevated thorax anteriorly until a flat palm placed against the shoulders, posterior ribs, and posterior pelvic wings is aligned perpendicular to the imaging table. All three areas need to be checked to prevent rotation across the entire spine. The amount of rotation required is half the distance demonstrated between the posterior surfaces of the vertebral bodies.

Analysis. The posterior surfaces of the vertebral bodies are demonstrated without superimposition, and the posterior ribs are superimposed. The elevated side of the thorax was rotated anteriorly.

Correction. Rotate the elevated thorax posteriorly until a flat palm placed against the shoulder, posterior ribs, and posterior pelvic wings is aligned perpendicular to the imaging table. The amount of rotation required is half the distance demonstrated between the posterior surfaces of the vertebral bodies.

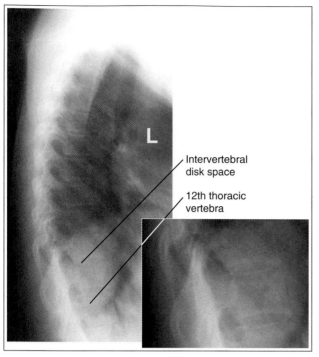

L

Intervertebral
disk space

12th thoracic
vertebra

Image 39.

Analysis. The T8 through T12 intervertebral disk spaces are obscured, and the vertebral bodies distorted. The thoracic vertebral column was not aligned parallel with the imaging table.

Correction. Position a radiolucent sponge between the lateral body surface and imaging table just superior to the iliac crest. The radiolucent sponge should be thick enough to align the thoracic vertebral column parallel with the imaging table. If a sponge cannot be used, the central ray can be angled cephalically until it is perpendicular to the thoracic vertebral column.

CHAPTER 8

Image Analysis of the Lumbar Vertebrae, Sacrum, and Coccyx

The following image analysis criteria are used for all lumbar, sacral, and coccygeal images and should be considered when completing the analysis. Position- and projection-specific criteria relating to these topics are discussed with the other accompanying criteria for that position or projection.

Facility's identification requirements are visible on image as identified in Chapter 1.

A right or left marker, identifying correct side of patient, is present on the image and is not superimposed over anatomy of interest. Specific placement of marker is as described in Chapter 1.

No evidence of preventable artifacts, such as buttons, zippers, and body piercings, is present.

- It is recommended that the patient be instructed to change into a snapless hospital gown before the procedure.

The bony trabecular patterns and cortical outlines of the cervical vertebrae are sharply defined.

- Sharply defined recorded details are obtained when patient motion is controlled, respiration is suspended at exhalation, and a short object–image receptor distance (OID) is maintained. Increased spatial resolution is also obtained when the smallest image receptor (IR) is selected for digital images.

Contrast and density are adequate to demonstrate the soft tissue and bony structures of the lumbar vertebrae, sacrum, and coccyx. Penetration is sufficient to visualize the bony trabecular patterns and cortical outlines of the lumbar vertebrae and the sacral and coccygeal structures.

- An optimal kVp technique, as shown in Table 8-1, sufficiently penetrates lumbar vertebrae and sacral or coccygeal structures and provides the contrast scale necessary to

TABLE 8-1 Technical Data for Imaging Lumbar Vertebrae, Sacrum, and Coccyx				
Position or Projection	**kVp**	**Grid**	**AEC Chamber**	**SID**
AP projection, lumbar vertebrae	75-80	Grid	Center	40-48 inches (100-120 cm)
AP oblique projection, lumbar vertebrae	75-85	Grid	Center	40-48 inches (100-120 cm)
Lateral position, lumbar vertebrae	85-95	Grid	Center	40-48 inches (100-120 cm)
Lateral position, L5-S1 lumbosacral junction	95-100	Grid	Center	40-48 inches (100-120 cm)
AP axial projection, sacrum	75-80	Grid	Center	40-48 inches (100-120 cm)
Lateral position, sacrum	85-95	Grid	Center	40-48 inches (100-120 cm)
AP axial projection, coccyx	75-80	Grid	Center	40-48 inches (100-120 cm)
Lateral position, coccyx	80-85	Grid		40-48 inches (100-120 cm)

AEC, Automatic exposure control; *AP,* anteroposterior; *kVp,* kilovolt peak; *SID,* source–image receptor distance.

visualize the vertebral details. A grid is employed to absorb the scatter radiation produced by the lumbar vertebrae, sacrum, and coccyx, increasing detail visibility. To obtain optimal density, set a manual mAs based on the patient's structure thickness, or choose the appropriate automatic exposure control (AEC) chamber. (See Table 8-1 for specifics.)

The long axis of the imaged structure is aligned with the long axis of the collimated field.

- Aligning the long axis of the imaged structure (mid-sagittal plane) with the long axis of the collimator's longitudinal light line enables tight collimation without clipping needed anatomical structures.

LUMBAR VERTEBRAE: ANTEROPOSTERIOR PROJECTION

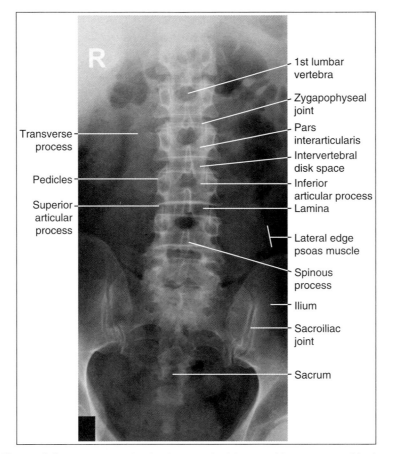

Figure 8-1. Anteroposterior lumbar vertebral image with accurate positioning.

Image Analysis

The psoas muscles are demonstrated.

- **Soft-tissue structures of lumbar vertebrae:** The soft-tissue structures that should be visualized on AP lumbar vertebral images are the psoas muscles. They are located lateral to the lumbar vertebrae, originating at the first lumbar vertebra on each side and extending to the corresponding side's lesser trochanter. They are used in lateral flexion and rotation of the thigh and in flexion of the vertebral column. On an anteroposterior (AP) lumbar image, they are visible on each side of the vertebral bodies as long triangular soft-tissue shadows.

The lumbar vertebrae demonstrate an AP projection. The spinous processes are aligned with the midline of the vertebral bodies, and the distances from the pedicles to the spinous processes and from the sacroiliac joints to the spinous processes are equal on both sides. When demonstrated, the sacrum and coccyx should be centered within the inlet pelvis and aligned with the symphysis pubis.

- An AP lumbar vertebral image is obtained by placing the patient supine on the imaging table. Position the shoulders and anterior superior iliac spines (ASISs) at equal distances from the imaging table to prevent rotation, and draw the arms away from the abdominal area

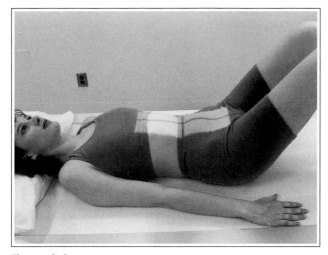

Figure 8-2. Proper patient positioning for anteroposterior lumbar vertebral image.

to prevent them from being tucked beneath the body (Figure 8-2).

- *Effect of rotation:* The upper and lower lumbar vertebrae can demonstrate rotation independently or simultaneously, depending on which section of the body is rotated. If the patient's thorax was rotated and the pelvis remained supine, the upper lumbar vertebrae demonstrate rotation. If the patient's pelvis was rotated and the thorax remained supine, the lower lumbar vertebrae demonstrate rotation. If the patient's thorax and pelvis were rotated simultaneously, the entire lumbar column demonstrates rotation.

- *Detecting rotation:* Rotation is effectively detected on an AP lumbar image by comparing the distances between each pedicle and the spinous processes on the same vertebra and by comparing the distances between each sacroiliac joint and the spinous processes. If no rotation was present, the comparable distances are equal. If one side demonstrates a greater distance, vertebral rotation was present (see Image 1). The side demonstrating the greater distance was the side of the patient positioned closer to the imaging table and IR. Lower lumbar rotation can be easily detected by evaluating the position of the sacrum and coccyx within the pelvic inlet. If no rotation was present, they are centered within the pelvic inlet. On rotation the sacrum and coccyx rotate toward the side of the pelvic inlet positioned farther from the IR.

- *Distinguishing rotation from scoliosis:* In patients with spinal scoliosis, the lumbar bodies may appear rotated owing to the lateral twisting of the vertebrae. Scoliosis of the vertebral column can be very severe, demonstrating a large amount of lateral deviation, or it can be subtle, demonstrating only a small amount of deviation. Severe scoliosis is very obvious and is seldom mistaken for patient rotation (see Image 2), whereas subtle scoliotic changes can be easily mistaken for rotation (see Image 3).

Although both conditions demonstrate unequal distances between the pedicles and spinous processes, certain clues can be used to distinguish subtle scoliosis from rotation. The long axis of a rotated vertebral column remains straight, whereas the scoliotic vertebral column demonstrates lateral deviation. If the lumbar vertebrae demonstrate rotation, it has been caused by the rotation of the upper or lower torso. Rotation of the middle lumbar vertebrae (L3 and L4) does not occur unless the lower thoracic or upper or lower lumbar vertebrae also demonstrate rotation. On a scoliotic image the middle lumbar vertebrae may demonstrate rotation without corresponding upper or lower vertebral rotation. Familiarity with the differences between a rotated lumbar vertebral column and a scoliotic one prevents unnecessary repeated procedures in patients with spinal scoliosis.

The intervertebral disk spaces are open, and the vertebral bodies are demonstrated without distortion.

- When the patient is in a supine position with the legs extended, the lumbar vertebrae have an exaggerated lordotic curvature. Obtaining an AP lumbar image with the patient in this position results in closed intervertebral disk spaces and distorted vertebral bodies, because of the way the x-ray beams are directed at the disk spaces and vertebral bodies (Figure 8-3). To straighten the lumbar vertebral column—thereby aligning the intervertebral disk spaces parallel with and the vertebral bodies perpendicular to the x-ray beam—flex the patient's knees and hips until the lower back rests firmly against the imaging table (Figure 8-4).

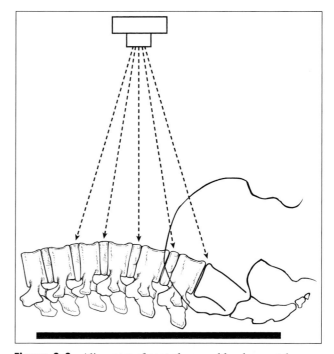

Figure 8-3. Alignment of central ray and lumbar vertebrae when legs are not flexed.

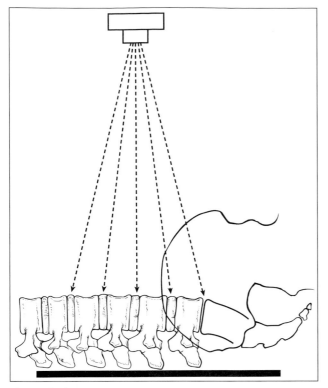

Figure 8-4. Alignment of central ray and lumbar vertebrae when legs are flexed.

- *Effect of lordotic curvature:* On an AP lumbar image, determine how well the central ray paralleled the intervertebral disk spaces by evaluating the openness of the T12 through L3 intervertebral disk spaces and the visibility of the iliac spines without pelvic brim superimposition. If the lordotic curvature was adequately reduced, the disk spaces are open and the iliac spines are only partially demonstrated without pelvic brim superimposition. If the lordotic curvature was not adequately reduced, the intervertebral disk spaces are closed and the iliac spines are demonstrated without pelvic brim superimposition (see Image 4).

If a 14- × 17-inch (35- × 43-cm) IR placed lengthwise was used, **the L4 vertebra and the iliac crest are centered within the collimated field. The twelfth thoracic vertebra, first through fifth lumbar vertebrae, sacroiliac joints, sacrum, coccyx, and psoas muscles are included within the field.**

If an 11- × 14-inch (28- × 35-cm) IR placed lengthwise was used, **the L3 vertebra is centered within the collimated field. The twelfth thoracic vertebra, first through fifth lumbar vertebrae, sacroiliac joints, and psoas muscles are included within the field.**

- Center a perpendicular central ray to the patient's midsagittal plane at the level of the iliac crest for a 14- × 17-inch (35- × 43-cm) IR and at a level 1½ inches (4 cm) superior to the iliac crest for a 11- × 14-inch (28- × 35-cm) IR. Center the IR to the central ray.

- Open the longitudinal collimation the full 17-inch (43-cm) or 14-inch (35-cm) IR length for adult patients. Transverse collimation should be to approximately an 8-inch (20-cm) field.
- *Gonadal shielding:* Gonadal protection shielding should be used on both male and female patients as long as pertinent information is not obscured.

Anteroposterior Lumbar Image Analysis

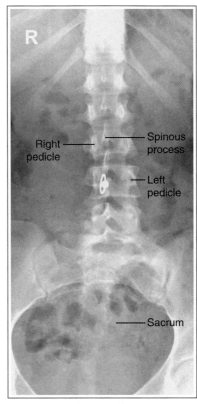

Image 1.

Analysis. The distances from the left pedicles to the spinous processes are less than the distances from the right pedicles to the spinous processes, and the sacrum and coccyx are rotated toward the left lateral inlet pelvis. The patient was rotated onto the right side (right posterior oblique [RPO] position).

Correction. Rotate the patient toward the left side until the shoulders and the ASISs are positioned at equal distances from the IR.

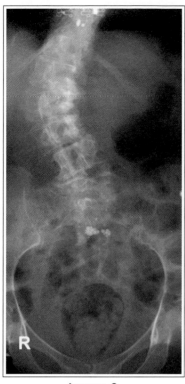

Image 2.

Analysis. The vertebral column demonstrates severe spinal scoliosis.

Correction. No corrective movement is required. An AP lumbar image of a patient with scoliosis appears rotated.

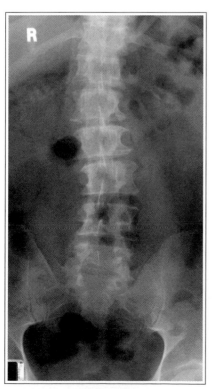

Image 3.

Analysis. The vertebral column deviates laterally at the level of the second through fourth lumbar vertebrae, the sacrum is centered within the pelvic inlet, and the distances from the pedicles to the spinous processes of the eleventh thoracic vertebra and fifth lumbar vertebra are nearly equal. The vertebral column demonstrates subtle spinal scoliosis.

Correction. No corrective movement is required. An AP lumbar image of a patient with scoliosis appears rotated.

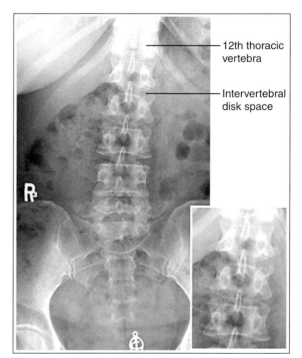

12th thoracic vertebra

Intervertebral disk space

Image 4.

Analysis. The T12 to L3 intervertebral disk spaces are closed, and the lumbar bodies are distorted. The iliac spines are demonstrated without pelvic brim superimposition. The lordotic curvature of the spine was not reduced, as demonstrated in Figure 8-3.

Correction. Flex the hips and knees until the lower back rests firmly against the imaging table, restraightening the lumbar vertebrae as demonstrated in Figure 8-4.

LUMBAR VERTEBRAE: ANTEROPOSTERIOR OBLIQUE PROJECTION (RIGHT POSTERIOR OBLIQUE AND LEFT POSTERIOR OBLIQUE POSITIONS)

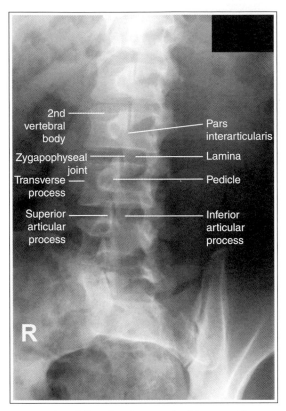

Figure 8-5. Anteroposterior oblique lumbar vertebral image with accurate positioning.

Image Analysis

Zygapophyseal joints are demonstrated with the least amount of magnification.

- This examination can be performed using either a posterior or an anterior oblique position. In the AP (posterior) oblique position (RPO, left posterior oblique [LPO]) (Figure 8-6) the zygapophyseal joints of interest are placed closer to the IR, and in the PA (anterior) oblique position (RAO, LAO) the zygapophyseal joints of interest are positioned farther from the IR, resulting in greater magnification.

The lumbar vertebrae have been adequately rotated. The superior and inferior articular processes are in profile, the zygapophyseal joints are clearly demonstrated, and the pedicles are demonstrated in the midway point between the midpoint of the vertebral bodies and the lateral border of the vertebral bodies. The ears, necks, eyes, feet, and bodies of the "Scottie dogs" are well defined.

- An AP (posterior) oblique lumbar vertebral image is obtained by placing the patient supine on the imaging

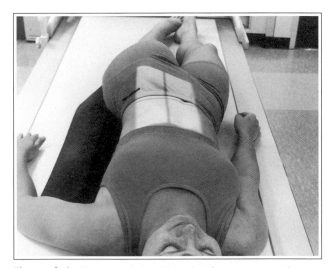

Figure 8-6. Proper patient positioning for anteroposterior (posterior) oblique lumbar vertebral image.

table, then rotating the patient toward the side until the superior and inferior articular processes are positioned in profile. The knee positioned closer to the imaging table may be flexed as needed for support.

- The articular processes are placed in profile by rotating the thorax until the midcoronal plane is at a 45-degree angle with the IR (see Figure 8-6). To demonstrate the right and the left articular processes and zygapophyseal joints of each vertebra, both right and left posterior oblique images must be taken.

- *"Scottie dogs" on oblique lumbar images:* The accuracy of an AP oblique lumbar image is often judged by the demonstration of five "Scottie dogs" that are stacked on top of one another. Figure 8-7 is a close-up of an accurately positioned oblique lumbar vertebra with the "Scottie dog" parts outlined and labeled. It should be noted that the "Scottie dogs" can be identified even on oblique lumbar images with poor positioning. Judge the openness of each zygapophyseal joint to determine whether the lumbar vertebrae have been adequately rotated.

- If a lumbar vertebra was not rotated enough to position the superior and inferior articular processes (ear and front leg of "Scottie dog") in profile, the corresponding zygapophyseal joint is closed, the pedicle (eye of "Scottie dog") is situated closer to the lateral vertebral body border, and more of the lamina (body of "Scottie dog") is demonstrated (see Image 5). If a lumbar vertebra was rotated more than needed to position the superior

and inferior articular processes in profile, the corresponding zygapophyseal joint is closed, the pedicles are demonstrated closer to the vertebral body midline, and less of the lamina is demonstrated (see Image 6).

The third lumbar vertebra is centered within the collimated field. The twelfth thoracic vertebra, first through fifth lumbar vertebrae, first and second sacral segments, and sacroiliac joints are included within the field.

- To place the third lumbar vertebra in the center of the field, center a perpendicular central ray 2 inches (5 cm) medial to the elevated ASIS at a level 1½ inches (4 cm) superior to the iliac crest. Center the IR to the central ray.

- Open the longitudinally collimated field the full 14-inch (35-cm) IR length for adult patients. Transverse collimation should be to an 8-inch (20-cm) field.

- An 11- × 14-inch (28- × 35-cm) IR placed lengthwise should be adequate to include all the required anatomical structures.

- *Gonadal shielding:* Gonadal protection shielding should be used on both male and female patients as long as pertinent information is not obscured. Remember that a shield placed on top of the patient will be greatly magnified.

Anteroposterior Oblique Lumbar Image Analysis

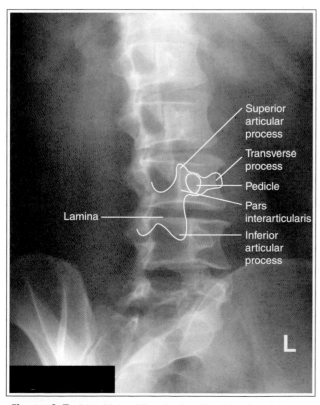

Figure 8-7. Identifying "Scottie dogs" and lumbar anatomy.

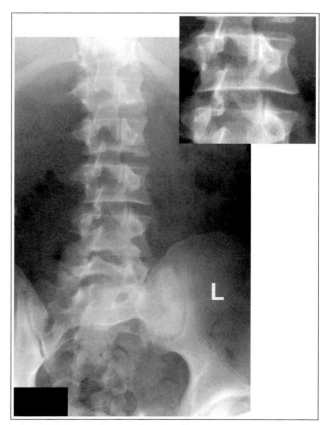

Image 5.

Analysis. The first and second lumbar vertebrae are accurately positioned on this image, indicating that the patient's upper torso was adequately rotated. The third, fourth, and fifth lumbar vertebrae's superior and inferior articular processes are not demonstrated in profile, their corresponding zygapophyseal joint spaces are closed, and their pedicles (eyes of "Scottie dog") are demonstrated closer to the vertebrae's lateral vertebral body borders than to their midlines. The patient's inferior lumbar vertebrae and pelvis were in insufficient obliquity.

Correction. While maintaining the degree of thoracic and upper lumbar vertebral obliquity, increase the lower lumbar vertebral and pelvic rotation.

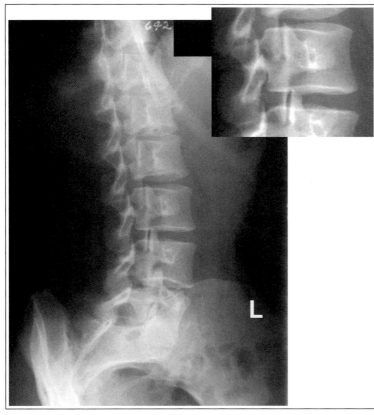

Image 6.

Analysis. The lumbar vertebrae's superior and inferior articular processes are not demonstrated in profile, their corresponding zygapophyseal joint spaces are closed, their laminae are obscured, and the pedicles are aligned with the midline of the vertebral bodies. The patient's upper lumbar vertebrae and thorax were in excessive obliquity.

Correction. Decrease the lumbar vertebral and thoracic rotation to 45 degrees.

LUMBAR VERTEBRAE: LATERAL POSITION

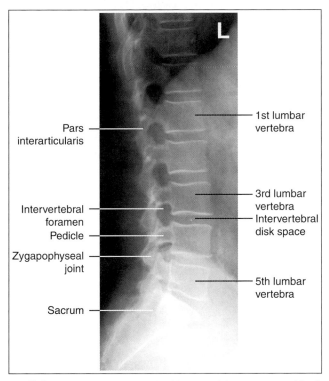

Figure 8-8. Lateral lumbar vertebral image with accurate positioning.

Image Analysis

Scatter radiation is controlled.

- Use tight collimation, a grid, and a lead sheet placed on the imaging table at the edge of the posteriorly collimated field to reduce the amount of scatter radiation that reaches the IR, providing higher contrast and better visibility of recorded details.

The lumbar vertebrae demonstrate a lateral position. The intervertebral foramina are clearly shown, and the spinous processes are in profile. The right and left pedicles and the posterior surfaces of each vertebral body are superimposed.

- To obtain a lateral lumbar image, place the patient on the imaging table in a lateral recumbent position. Whether the patient is lying on the right or left side is insignificant, although left-side positioning is often easier for the technologist. One exception to this guideline is the scoliotic patient, who should be placed on the imaging table so the central ray is directed into the spinal curve (Figure 8-9) to better obtain open intervertebral joint spaces. Determine how the patient's curve is directed by viewing the patient's back and following the curve of the vertebral column and evaluating the AP projection.

Once the patient has been placed on the table, flex the knees and hips for support, and position a pillow or sponge between the knees. The thickness of the pillow or sponge should be sufficient to prevent the side of the pelvis situated farther from the IR from rotating anteriorly, without being so thick as to cause this side to rotate posteriorly (Figure 8-10).

To avoid vertebral rotation, align the shoulders, the posterior ribs, and the posterior pelvic wings perpendicular to the imaging table and IR. This is accomplished by resting your extended flat hand against each structure, individually, then adjusting the patient's rotation until your hand is perpendicular to the IR.

- **Effect of rotation:** The upper and lower lumbar vertebrae can demonstrate rotation independently or simultaneously, depending on which section of the torso is rotated. If the thorax was rotated but the pelvis remained in a lateral position, the upper lumbar vertebrae demonstrate rotation. If the pelvis was rotated but the thorax remained in a lateral position, the lower lumbar vertebrae demonstrate rotation.

- **Detecting rotation:** Rotation can be detected on a lateral lumbar image by evaluating the superimposition of the right and left posterior surfaces of the vertebral bodies. On a nonrotated lateral lumbar image, these posterior surfaces are superimposed, appearing as one. On rotation, these posterior surfaces are not

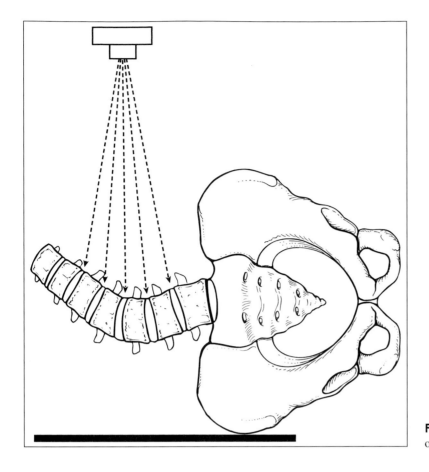

Figure 8-9. Alignment of central ray and scoliotic lumbar vertebral column.

superimposed, but one is demonstrated anterior to the other (see Image 7). Because the two sides of the vertebrae, thorax, and pelvis are mirror images, it is very difficult to determine from a rotated lateral lumbar image which side of the patient was rotated anteriorly and which posteriorly, unless the twelfth posterior ribs are demonstrated. The twelfth posterior rib that demonstrates the greatest magnification and is situated inferiorly is adjacent to the side of the patient positioned farther from the IR.

The intervertebral disk spaces are open, and the vertebral bodies are demonstrated without distortion.

• The lumbar vertebral column is capable of lateral flexion. Therefore when the patient is placed in a lateral recumbent position, the vertebral column may not be aligned parallel with the imaging table and IR but may sag or curve upwardly at the level of the iliac crest (Figure 8-11). If the patient's lumbar column is allowed to sag, the diverging x-ray beams are not aligned parallel with the intervertebral disk spaces and perpendicular

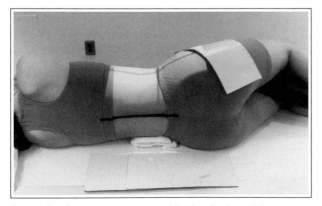

Figure 8-10. Proper patient positioning for lateral lumbar vertebral image.

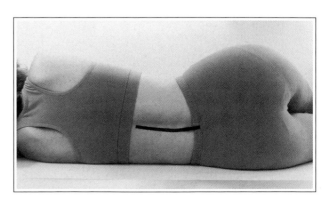

Figure 8-11. Poor alignment of vertebral column and imaging table.

to the vertebral bodies. Lateral lumbar flexion on a lateral vertebral image is most evident at the lower lumbar region, where closed disk spaces and distorted vertebral bodies are present (see Image 8). For a patient who has a sagging lumbar column, it may be necessary to tuck a radiolucent sponge between the lateral body surface and the imaging table just superior to the iliac crest, elevating the sagging area. The sponge should be thick enough to bring the lumbar vertebral column parallel with the imaging table and IR (see Figure 8-10).

- An alternative method of obtaining open disk spaces and undistorted vertebral bodies for a patient whose lumbar column is sagging is to angle the central ray 5 to 8 degrees caudally. This caudal angulation should align the central ray perpendicular to the vertebral column and parallel with the interiliac line (imaginary line connecting the iliac crests).

The lumbar vertebral column is in a neutral position, without anteroposterior flexion or extension. A lordotic curvature is present.

- A neutral position of the lumbar vertebrae is obtained when the long axis of the patient's body is aligned with the long axis of the imaging table. The thoracic and pelvic regions are aligned.
- *Positioning to evaluate AP mobility of lumbar vertebrae:* If the lumbar vertebrae are being imaged in the lateral position to demonstrate AP vertebral mobility, two lateral images should be taken: one with the patient in maximum flexion, and one in maximum extension. For maximum flexion, instruct the patient to flex the shoulders, upper thorax, and knees anteriorly, rolling into a tight ball (Figure 8-12). The resulting image should meet all the requirements listed for a lateral image with accurate positioning, except that the lumbar vertebral column demonstrates a very straight longitudinal axis without lordotic curvature (see Image 9). For maximum extension, instruct the patient to arch the back by extending the shoulders, upper thorax, and legs

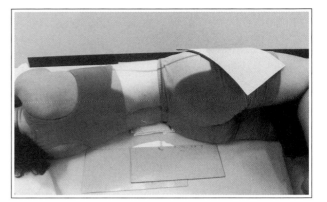

Figure 8-13. Proper patient positioning for lateral (extension) lumbar vertebral image.

as far posteriorly as possible (Figure 8-13). The resulting image should meet all the requirements listed for a lateral image with accurate positioning, except that the lumbar vertebral column demonstrates an increased lordotic curvature (see Image 10).

The long axis of the lumbar vertebral column is aligned with the long axis of the collimated field.

- Aligning the long axis of the lumbar vertebral column with the collimator's longitudinal light line allows tight collimation, which is necessary to reduce the production of scatter radiation.
- The lumbar vertebrae are located in the posterior half of the torso. Their exact posterior location can be determined by palpating the ASIS and posterior iliac wing (at the level of the sacroiliac joint) of the side of the patient situated farther from the IR. The long axis of the lumbar vertebral column is aligned with the coronal plane that is situated halfway between these two structures (Figure 8-14).

If a 14- × 17-inch (35- × 43-cm) IR placed lengthwise was used, **the iliac crest and the fourth lumbar vertebra are centered within the collimated field. The eleventh and twelfth thoracic vertebrae, first through fifth lumbar vertebrae, and sacrum are included within the field.**

If an 11- × 14-inch (28- × 35-cm) IR placed lengthwise was used, **the third lumbar vertebra is centered within the collimated field. The twelfth thoracic vertebra, first through fifth lumbar vertebrae, and L5-S1 intervertebral disk space are included within the field.**

- Center a perpendicular central ray to the coronal plane located halfway between the elevated ASIS and posterior wing, at the level of the iliac crest for a 14- × 17-inch (35- × 43-cm) IR, and at a level 1½ inches (4 cm) superior to the iliac crest for an 11- × 14-inch (28- × 35-cm) IR.
- Open the longitudinal collimation the full 17- or 14-inch (43- or 35-cm) IR length for adult patients. Transverse collimation should be to an 8-inch (20-cm) field.

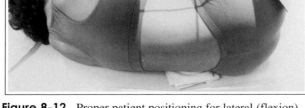

Figure 8-12. Proper patient positioning for lateral (flexion) lumbar vertebral image.

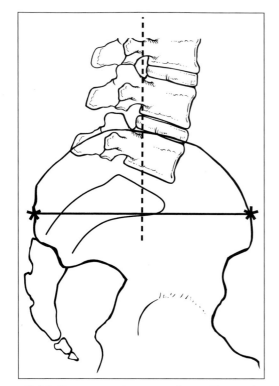

Figure 8-14. Proper central ray centering and long axis placement. Asterisks identify the posterior iliac wing and anterior superior iliac spines.

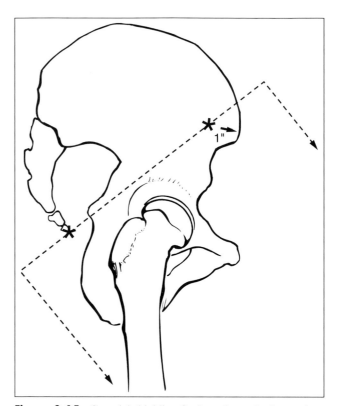

Figure 8-15. Gonadal shielding for lateral vertebral, sacral, and coccygeal images.

- *Supplementary image of the L5-S1 lumbar region:* A coned-down image of the L5-S1 lumbar region is required when a lateral lumbar image is obtained that demonstrates insufficient image density in this area or the L5-S1 joint space is closed. In patients with wide hips, it is often difficult to set exposure factors that adequately demonstrate the upper and lower lumbar regions concurrently. For these patients, set exposure factors that adequately demonstrate the upper lumbar region. Then obtain a tightly collimated lateral image of the L5-S1 lumbar region to demonstrate the lower lumbar area. Follow the procedure and evaluating criteria given in this text for the L5-S1 lumbosacral junction image (see p. 427).

- *Gonadal shielding:* Use gonadal protection shielding on all patients for this procedure. Begin by palpating the patient's coccyx and elevated ASIS. Next, draw an imaginary line connecting the coccyx with a point 1 inch posterior to the ASIS, and position the longitudinal edge of a large flat contact shield or lead half-apron anteriorly against this imaginary line (Figure 8-15). This shielding method can be safely used for patients being imaged for lateral vertebral, sacral, or coccygeal images without fear of obscuring areas of interest (Figure 8-16).

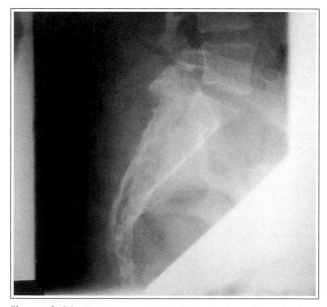

Figure 8-16. Proper gonadal shielding for lateral vertebral, sacral, and coccygeal images.

Lateral Lumbar Vertebrae Image Analysis

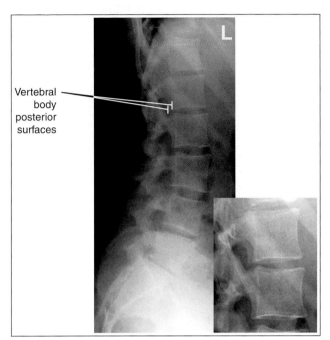

Vertebral body posterior surfaces

Image 7.

Analysis. The posterior surfaces of the first through fourth vertebral bodies and the posterior ribs are demonstrated one anterior to the other. The posterior ribs demonstrating the greater magnification were positioned posteriorly.

Correction. Rotate the side positioned farther from the IR anteriorly until the posterior ribs are superimposed, while maintaining posterior pelvic wing superimposition.

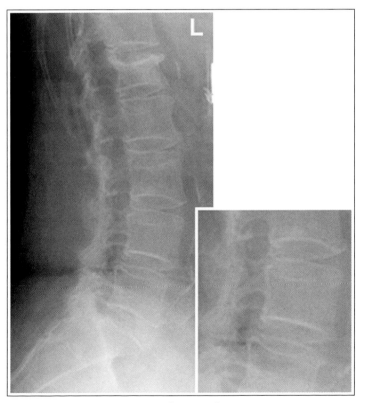

Image 8.

Analysis. The L4-L5 and L5-S1 intervertebral disk spaces are closed, and the third through fifth vertebral bodies are distorted. The lumbar vertebral column was not aligned parallel with the imaging table or IR.

Correction. Position a radiolucent sponge between the patient's lateral body surface and the imaging table just superior to the iliac crest. The sponge should be thick enough only to align the lumbar column parallel with the imaging table and IR.

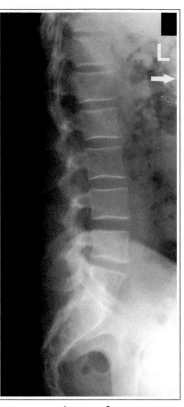

Image 9.

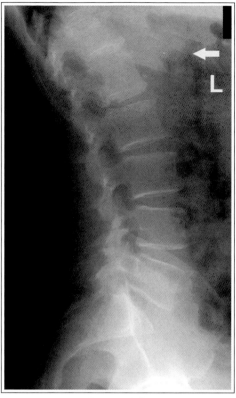

Image 10.

Analysis. The lumbar column demonstrates no lordotic curvature. The patient was in a flexed position, as demonstrated in Figure 8-12.

Correction. If a neutral lateral position is desired, extend the shoulders, upper thorax, and legs posteriorly until the posterior thorax and pelvic wings are aligned with the long axis of the imaging table. If a flexion lumbar image is being performed to evaluate anteroposterior mobility, no corrective movement is required.

Analysis. The lumbar vertebral column demonstrates excess lordotic curvature. The patient was in an extended position, as demonstrated in Figure 8-13.

Correction. If a neutral lateral position is desired, flex the shoulders, upper thorax, and legs anteriorly until the posterior thorax and pelvic wings are aligned with the long axis of the imaging table. If an extended position is desired to evaluate anteroposterior mobility, no corrective movement is required.

L5-S1 LUMBOSACRAL JUNCTION: LATERAL POSITION

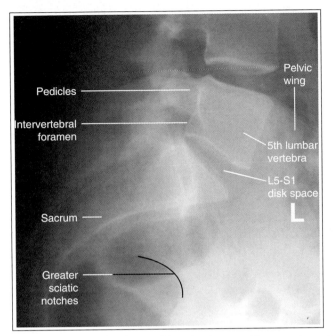

Figure 8-17. Lateral L5-S1 lumbosacral junction image with accurate positioning.

Image Analysis

Scatter radiation is controlled.

- Use tight collimation, a grid, and a lead sheet placed on the imaging table at the edge of the posteriorly collimated field to reduce the amount of scatter radiation that reaches the IR, providing higher contrast and better visibility of recorded details.

The fifth lumbar vertebra and sacrum demonstrate a lateral position. The intervertebral foramina are clearly demonstrated, the right and left pedicles are superimposed and demonstrated in profile, and the greater sciatic notches and pelvic wings are nearly superimposed.

- To obtain a lateral L5-S1 lumbosacral junction image, place the patient on the image table in a lateral recumbent position. Whether the patient is lying on the right or left side is not significant, although the left-side positioning is easier for the technologist. One exception to this guideline is the scoliotic patient, who should be placed on the imaging table so the central ray is directed into the spinal curve to better obtain open intervertebral joint spaces. Determine how the patient's curve is directed by viewing the patient's back and following the curve of the vertebral column and evaluating the AP projection.

   Flex the patient's knees and hips for support, and position a pillow or sponge between the knees. The thickness of the pillow or sponge should be enough to prevent the side of the pelvis situated farther from the

IR from rotating anteriorly, without being so thick as to cause this side to rotate posteriorly (Figure 8-18).

   To avoid vertebral rotation, align the shoulders, posterior ribs, and posterior pelvic wings perpendicular to the imaging table and IR. This is accomplished by resting your extended flat palm against each structure, individually, then adjusting the patient's rotation until your hand is perpendicular to the imaging table.

- *Detecting rotation:* Rotation can be detected on a lateral L5-S1 lumbosacral junction image by evaluating the openness of the intervertebral foramen, and the superimposition of the greater sciatic notches and the femoral heads when seen. On a nonrotated lateral L5-S1 image,

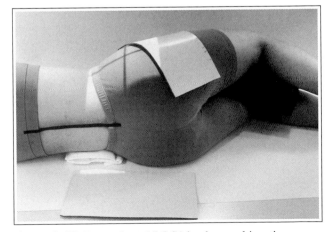

Figure 8-18. Proper lateral L5-S1 lumbosacral junction positioning.

the intervertebral foramen is open, and the greater sciatic notches and the femoral heads are superimposed. On rotation, neither the greater sciatic notches nor the femoral heads are superimposed, but are demonstrated one anterior to the other (see Image 11). Because the two sides of the pelvis are mirror images, it is difficult to determine which side of the patient was rotated anteriorly and which posteriorly on a lateral L5-S1 lumbosacral junction image with poor positioning. When rotation has occurred, it is most common for the side of the patient situated farther from the IR to be rotated anteriorly, owing to the gravitational forward and downward pull on this side's arm and leg, if a sponge is not placed between the patient's knees. If the patient's femoral heads are visible on the image, they may be used to determine rotation. The femoral head that is projected more inferiorly and demonstrates the greatest magnification is the one situated farther from the IR.

The L5-S1 intervertebral disk space is open, the pelvic alae are superimposed, and the sacrum is demonstrated without foreshortening.

- To obtain an open L5-S1 intervertebral disk space, to demonstrate superimposed pelvic alae, and to demonstrate the sacrum without foreshortening, the vertebral column is aligned parallel with the imaging table, the interiliac line is aligned perpendicular to the imaging table, and a perpendicular central ray is used.

- *Detecting lateral lumbar flexion:* The lumbar vertebral column is capable of lateral flexion. If this flexion is not considered during positioning, the diverging x-ray beams will not be aligned parallel with the L5-S1 disk space and perpendicular to the long axis of the sacrum. Lateral lumbar flexion can be detected on an L5-S1 image by evaluating the superimposition of the pelvic alae and the openness of the L5-S1 disk space. A laterally flexed image demonstrates the pelvic alae without superoinferior alignment and a closed L5-S1 disk space (see Image 12).

- *Adjusting for the sagging vertebral column:* The vertebral column of a patient with wide hips and a narrow waist may sag toward the imaging table at the level of the iliac crest (see Figure 8-11). Two methods may be used to achieve accurate positioning in such a patient:
  1. Place a radiolucent sponge between the patient's lateral body surface and the imaging table just superior

to the iliac crest to elevate the vertebral column, aligning it parallel with the imaging table (see Figure 8-18), and use a perpendicular central ray.
  2. Leave the patient positioned as is, and angle the central ray caudally until it parallels the interiliac line (imaginary line connecting the iliac crests).

- *Adjusting for the upwardly curved vertebral column:* The vertebral column of a patient with a large waist may curve upwardly (Figure 8-19). For such a patient, angle the central ray cephalically until it parallels the interiliac line.

The L5-S1 intervertebral disk space is at the center of the collimated field. The fifth lumbar vertebra and the first and second sacral segments are included within the field.

- To place the L5-S1 intervertebral disk space in the center of the field, center a perpendicular central ray to a point 2 inches (5 cm) posterior to the elevated ASIS and 1½ inches (4 cm) inferior to the iliac crest. Center the IR to the central ray.

- Longitudinally collimate 1 inch (2.5 cm) superior to the iliac crest. Transverse collimation should be to an 8-inch (20-cm) field.

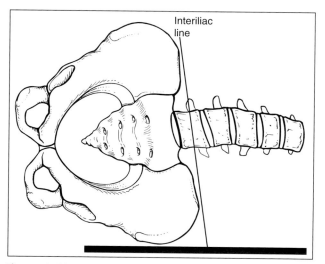

Figure 8-19. Adjusting for upwardly curved vertebral column.

- An 8- × 10-inch (18- × 24-cm) IR placed lengthwise should be adequate to include all the required anatomical structures.
- *Gonadal shielding:* Use gonadal protection shielding on all patients for this procedure. Begin by palpating the patient's coccyx and elevated ASIS. Next, draw an imaginary line connecting the coccyx with a point 1 inch posterior to the ASIS, and position the longitudinal edge of a large flat contact shield or lead half-apron anteriorly against this imaginary line (see Figures 8-15 and 8-16).

Lateral L5-S1 Image Analysis

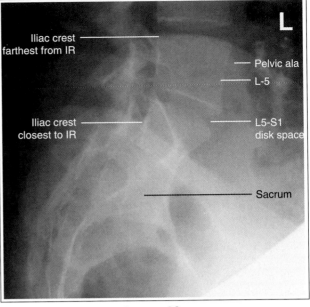

Image 12.

Analysis. The L5-S1 intervertebral disk space is closed, and the pelvic alae are not superimposed. Neither the long axis of the lumbar vertebral column nor the sacrum was aligned parallel with the imaging table, nor were the iliac crests positioned at different transverse levels.

Correction. Position a radiolucent sponge between the patient's lateral body surface and the imaging table just superior to the patient's iliac crest. The sponge should be just thick enough to align the long axis of the vertebral column and sacrum parallel with the imaging table and to place the iliac crests at the same transverse levels.

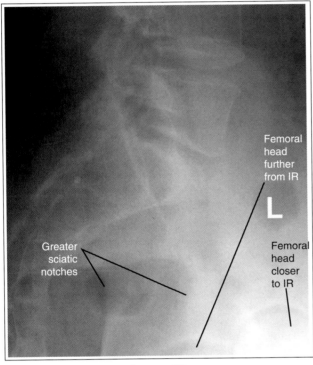

Image 11.

Analysis. The L5-S1 intervertebral foramen is obscured, and the greater sciatic notches and the femoral heads are demonstrated without superimposition. The femoral head positioned closer to the IR was rotated anteriorly.

Correction. Rotate the patient's hip that was positioned farther from the IR toward the opposite hip until the posterior ribs and the posterior pelvic wings are superimposed. From the original position the amount of rotation should be approximately 1 inch (2.5 cm).

SACRUM

See p. 413 for image analysis criteria for all lumbar, sacral, and coccygeal images.

SACRUM: ANTEROPOSTERIOR AXIAL PROJECTION

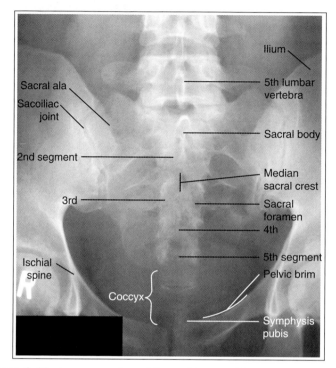

Figure 8-20. Anteroposterior axial sacral image with accurate positioning.

Image Analysis

No evidence suggests that urine, gas, or fecal material is superimposed over the sacrum.

- The patient's urinary bladder should be emptied before the procedure. It is also recommended that the colon be free of gas and fecal material. Elimination of urine, gas, and fecal material from the area superimposed over the sacrum improves its demonstration (Image 13).

The sacrum demonstrates an AP projection. The ischial spines are equally demonstrated and are aligned with the pelvic brim, and the median sacral crest and coccyx are aligned with the symphysis pubis.

- An AP sacrum image is obtained by positioning the patient supine on the imaging table with the legs extended. Position the shoulders and ASISs at equal distances from the imaging table to prevent rotation (Figure 8-21).
- *Detecting rotation:* Rotation is effectively detected on an AP axial sacral image by comparing the amount of iliac spine demonstrated without pelvic brim superimposition and by evaluating the alignment of the median sacral crest and coccyx with the symphysis pubis. If the patient was rotated away from the AP projection, the sacrum shifts toward the side positioned farther from the imaging table and IR, and the pelvic brim and symphysis shift toward the side positioned closer to the imaging table

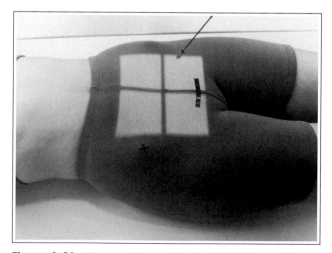

Figure 8-21. Proper patient positioning for anteroposterior axial sacral image.

and IR. If the patient was rotated into an LPO position, the left ischial spine is demonstrated without pelvic brim superimposition, and the median sacral crest and coccyx are not aligned with the symphysis pubis but are rotated toward the patient's right side (see Image 14). If the patient is rotated into an RPO position, the opposite is true; the right ischial spine is demonstrated without pelvic brim superimposition, and the median sacral crest and coccyx are rotated toward the patient's left side (see Image 15).

The first through fifth sacral segments are shown without foreshortening, the sacral foramina demonstrate equal spacing, and the symphysis pubis is not superimposed over any portion of the sacrum.

- When the patient is in a supine position with the legs extended, the lumbar vertebral column demonstrates a lordotic curvature and the sacrum demonstrates a kyphotic curvature (Figure 8-22). To demonstrate the sacrum without foreshortening, a 15-degree cephalad central ray angulation is used. This angle will align the central ray perpendicular to the long axis of the sacrum and parallel with the L5-S1 intervertebral disk space.
- *Effect of misalignment or mispositioning:* If an AP axial sacral image was taken with a perpendicular central ray, the first, second, and third sacral segments are foreshortened (see Image 15). If the image was taken with the patient's legs flexed, the lordotic curvature of the lumbar vertebral column is reduced, and the long axis of the sacrum is positioned closer to parallel with the imaging table and IR. For this positioning a 15-degree cephalad angulation causes elongation of the sacrum and superimposition of the symphysis pubis onto the inferior sacral segments (see Image 16). The same elongation results if the patient's legs remain extended and the central ray is angled more than 15 degrees cephalad.

The third sacral segment is at the center of the collimated field. The fifth lumbar vertebra, first through fifth sacral segments, first coccygeal vertebra, symphysis pubis, and sacroiliac joints are included within the field.

- To place the third sacral segment in the center of the field, center the central ray to the patient's midsagittal plane at a level halfway between an imaginary line connecting the ASISs and the superior symphysis pubis (2 inches superior to the superior symphysis pubis). Center the IR to the central ray, and open the longitudinally collimated field to the symphysis pubis. Transverse collimation should be to approximately an 8-inch (20-cm) field size.
- A 10- × 12-inch (24- × 30-cm) IR placed lengthwise should be adequate to include all the required anatomical structures.
- *Gonadal shielding:* Use gonadal protection shielding on all male patients.

Anteroposterior Sacrum Image Analysis

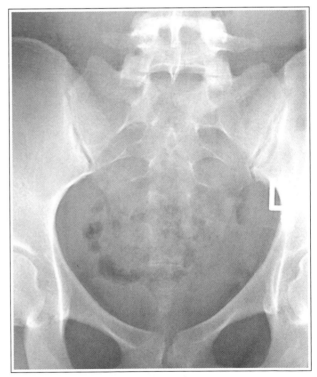

Image 13.

Analysis. Fecal material is superimposed over the sacrum, preventing its visualization.

Correction. Have the patient empty the colon of gas and fecal material before the sacrum is imaged.

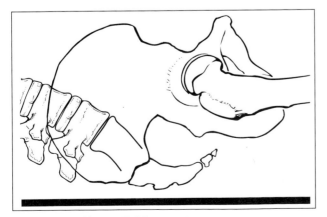

Figure 8-22. Sacral curvature.

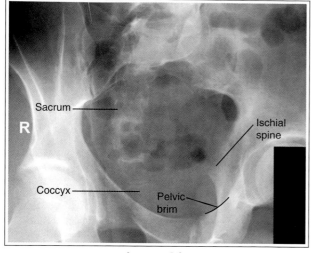

Image 14.

Analysis. The left ischial spine is demonstrated without pelvic brim superimposition, and the median sacral crest and coccyx are rotated toward the right hip. The patient was rotated onto the left side (LPO).

Correction. Rotate the patient toward the right hip until the ASISs are positioned at equal distances from the imaging table.

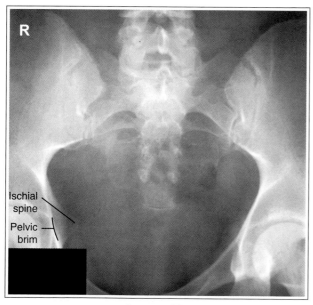

Image 15.

Analysis. The right ischial spine is demonstrated without pelvic brim superimposition, and the first, second, and third sacral segments are foreshortened. The patient was rotated onto the right side (RPO), and the central ray was not angled cephalically enough to align it perpendicular to the long axis of the sacrum.

Correction. Rotate the patient toward the left hip until the ASISs are positioned at equal distances from the imaging table and the patient's legs are fully extended, then angle the central ray 15 degrees cephalad.

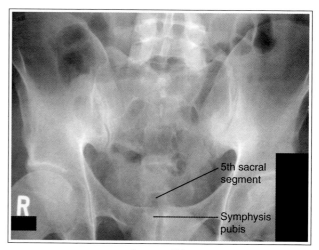

Image 16.

Analysis. The sacrum is elongated, and the symphysis pubis is superimposed over the fifth sacral segment. Either the central ray was angled too cephalically or the patient's legs were not fully extended and a 15-degree central ray angle was used.

Correction. If the patient's legs were extended, decrease the central ray angulation approximately 5 degrees for every 1 inch (2.5 cm) you wish to move the symphysis pubis. This angulation adjustment is based on a 40-inch (102-cm) source–image receptor distance (SID); if a shorter SID is used, the angle adjustment needs to be increased, and if a longer SID is used, the angle adjustment needs to be decreased. For this patient the angulation should be decreased 5 degrees. If the patient's legs were flexed and a 15-degree central ray angle was used, fully extend the patient's legs and use the same angulation.

SACRUM: LATERAL POSITION

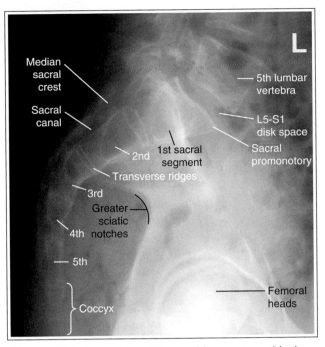

Figure 8-23. Lateral sacral image with accurate positioning.

Image Analysis

Scatter radiation is controlled.

- Use tight collimation, a grid, and a lead sheet placed on the imaging table at the edge of the posteriorly collimated field to reduce the amount of scatter radiation that reaches the IR, providing higher contrast and better visibility of recorded details.

The sacrum demonstrates a lateral position. The median sacral crest is demonstrated in profile, and the greater sciatic notches and the pelvic wings are nearly superimposed.

- To obtain a lateral sacral image, place the patient on the imaging table in a lateral recumbent position. Whether the patient is lying on the right or left side is not significant, although the left-side positioning is easier for the technologist.

   Flex the patient's knees and hips for support, and position a pillow or sponge between the knees. The thickness of the pillow or sponge should be sufficient to prevent the side of the pelvis situated farther from the IR from rotating anteriorly, without being so thick as to cause this side to rotate posteriorly (Figure 8-24).
- To avoid vertebral rotation, align the shoulders, posterior ribs, and posterior pelvic wings perpendicular to the imaging table and IR. This is accomplished by resting your extended flat palm against each structure, individually, then adjusting the patient's rotation until

your hand is positioned perpendicular to the imaging table.

- **Detecting rotation:** Rotation can be detected on a lateral sacral image by evaluating the openness of the intervertebral foramen, and the superimposition of the greater sciatic notches and the femoral heads when seen. On a nonrotated lateral sacral image, the intervertebral foramen is open and the greater sciatic notches and the femoral heads are superimposed. On rotation, neither the greater sciatic notches nor femoral heads are

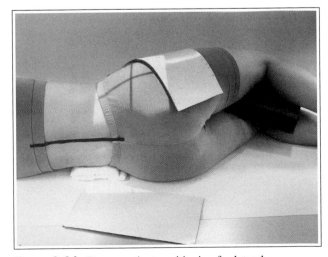

Figure 8-24. Proper patient positioning for lateral sacral image.

superimposed but are demonstrated one anterior to the other (see Image 17). Because the two sides of the pelvis are mirror images, it is difficult to determine which side of the patient was rotated anteriorly and which posteriorly on a lateral sacral image with poor positioning. When rotation has occurred, it is most common for the side of the patient situated farther from the IR to be rotated anteriorly, owing to the gravitational forward and downward pull on this side's arm and leg, if a sponge is not placed between the patient's knees. When visible, the patient's femoral heads may be used to determine rotation. The femoral head that is projected more inferiorly and demonstrates the greater magnification is the one situated farther from the IR.

The L5-S1 intervertebral disk space is open, the greater sciatic notches are superimposed, and the sacrum is demonstrated without foreshortening.

- To obtain an open L5-S1 intervertebral disk space and superimposed greater sciatic notches and to demonstrate the sacrum without foreshortening, the vertebral column is aligned parallel with the imaging table, the interiliac line is aligned perpendicular to the imaging table, and a perpendicular central ray is used.
- *Detecting lateral lumbar flexion:* If the lateral vertebral column is allowed to flex laterally, causing it to sag or curve upwardly, for a lateral sacral image, the image will demonstrate the greater sciatic notches without superoinferior alignment and a closed L5-S1 disk space (see Image 18).
- *Adjusting for the sagging vertebral column:* The vertebral column of a patient with wide hips and a narrow waist may sag toward the imaging table at the level of the iliac crest (see Figure 8-11). Two methods may be used to achieve accurate positioning for such a patient:
  1. Place a radiolucent sponge between the patient's lateral body surface and the imaging table just superior to the iliac crest to elevate the vertebral column, aligning it parallel with the imaging table (see Figure 8-24), and use a perpendicular central ray.
  2. Leave the patient positioned as they are and angle the central ray caudally until it parallels the interiliac line.
- *Adjusting for the upwardly curved vertebral column:* The vertebral column of a patient with a large waist may curve upwardly (see Figure 8-19). For such a patient, angle the central ray cephalically until it parallels the interiliac line.

The third sacral segment is at the center of the collimated field. The fifth lumbar vertebra, first through fifth sacral segments, promontory, and first coccygeal vertebra are included within the field.

- To place the third sacral segment in the center of the field, center a perpendicular central ray to the coronal plane located 3 to 4 inches (7.5 to 10 cm) posterior to the elevated ASIS. Center the IR to the central ray, and

open the longitudinal collimation to include the iliac crest and coccyx. Transverse collimation should be to an 8-inch (20-cm) field.

- A 10- × 12-inch (24- × 30-cm) IR placed lengthwise should be adequate to include all the required anatomical structures.
- *Gonadal shielding:* Use gonadal protection shielding on all patients for this procedure. Begin by palpating the patient's coccyx and elevated ASIS. Next, draw an imaginary line connecting the coccyx with a point 1 inch posterior to the ASIS, and position the longitudinal edge of a large flat contact shield or lead half-apron anteriorly against this imaginary line (see Figures 8-15 and 8-16).

Lateral Sacrum Image Analysis

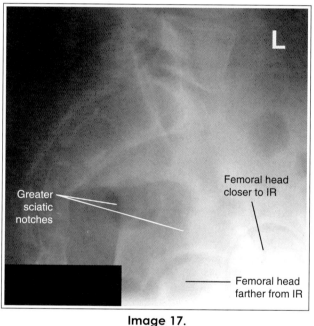

Image 17.

Analysis. The L5-S1 intervertebral foramen is obscured, and the greater sciatic notches and the femoral heads are demonstrated without superimposition. The femoral head positioned closer to the IR was rotated anteriorly.

Correction. Rotate the patient's hip that was positioned farther from the IR toward the opposite hip until the posterior ribs and the posterior pelvic wings are superimposed. From the original position the amount of rotation should be approximately 1 inch (2.5 cm).

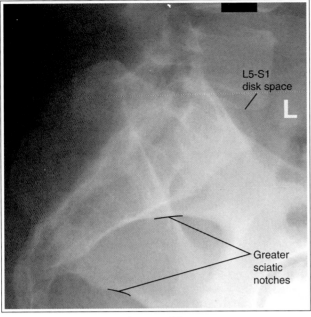

Image 18.

Analysis. The L5-S1 intervertebral disk space is closed, the sacrum is foreshortened, and the greater sciatic notches are demonstrated without superoinferior superimposition. The patient's long axis was not aligned parallel with the imaging table.

Correction. Position the long axis of the lumbar vertebral column and sacrum parallel with the IR. It may be necessary to place a radiolucent sponge between the patient's lateral body surface and the imaging table just superior to the iliac crest. The sponge should be just thick enough to align the lumbar column parallel with the imaging table.

COCCYX

See p. 413 for image analysis criteria for all lumbar, sacral, and coccygeal images.

COCCYX: ANTEROPOSTERIOR AXIAL PROJECTION

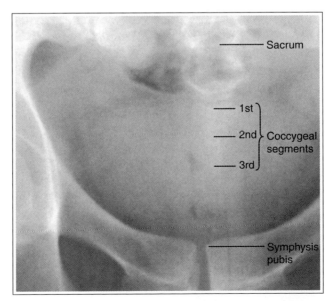

Figure 8-25. Anteroposterior axial coccygeal image with accurate positioning.

Image Analysis

No evidence suggests that urine, gas, or fecal material is superimposed over the sacrum.

• The patient's urinary bladder should be emptied before the procedure. It is also suggested that the colon be free of gas and fecal material. Both procedures will prevent overlap of these materials onto the coccyx, thereby improving its visualization (see Images 19 and 20).

The coccyx demonstrates an AP projection. The coccyx is aligned with the symphysis pubis and is at equal distances from the lateral walls of the inlet pelvis.

• An AP coccyx image is obtained by positioning the patient supine on the imaging table with the legs extended. Position the patient's shoulders and ASISs at equal distances from the imaging table to prevent rotation (Figure 8-26).

• *Detecting rotation:* Rotation is detected on an AP coccyx image by evaluating the alignment of the long axis of the coccyx with the symphysis pubis and by comparing the distances from the coccyx to the lateral walls of the inlet pelvis. If the patient was rotated away from the supine position, the coccyx moves in a direction opposite the direction of the symphysis pubis and is positioned closer to the lateral pelvic wall situated farther from the imaging table and IR. If the patient was rotated into an LPO position, the coccyx is rotated toward the patient's right side (see Image 19). If the patient was rotated into an RPO position, the coccyx is rotated toward the patient's left side.

The first through third coccygeal vertebrae are demonstrated without foreshortening and without symphysis pubis superimposition.

• When the patient is in a supine position with the legs extended, the coccyx curves anteriorly and is located beneath the symphysis pubis. To demonstrate the coccyx without foreshortening and without overlap by the symphysis pubis, a 10-degree caudal central ray angulation is used. This angle aligns the central ray perpendicular to the coccyx and projects the symphysis pubis inferiorly. If the AP projection of the coccyx is taken with a perpendicular central ray, the second and third coccygeal vertebrae are foreshortened and are superimposed by the symphysis pubis (see Image 21).

The coccyx is at the center of the collimated field. The fifth sacral segment, the three coccygeal vertebrae, the symphysis pubis, and the pelvic brim are included within the field.

• To place the coccyx in the center of the field, center the central ray to the patient's midsagittal plane at a level 2 inches (5 cm) superior to the symphysis pubis. Center the IR to the central ray.

• Open the longitudinal collimation to the symphysis pubis. Transverse collimation should be to approximately a 6-inch (15-cm) field size.

• An 8- × 10-inch (18- × 24-cm) IR placed lengthwise should be adequate to include all the required anatomical structures.

• *Gonadal shielding:* Use gonadal protection shielding on all male patients.

Anteroposterior Coccyx Image Analysis

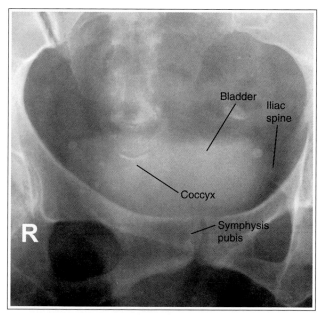

Image 19.

Analysis. The urinary bladder is dense and creating a shadow over the coccyx. The coccyx is not aligned with the symphysis pubis but is situated closer to the right lateral wall of the inlet pelvis. The patient did not empty the urinary bladder and was rotated onto the left side (LPO).

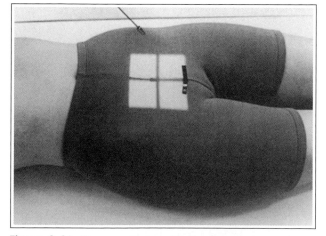

Figure 8-26. Proper patient positioning for anteroposterior axial coccygeal image.

Correction. Have the patient empty the urinary bladder, and rotate the patient toward the right side until the ASISs are positioned at equal distances from the imaging table and IR.

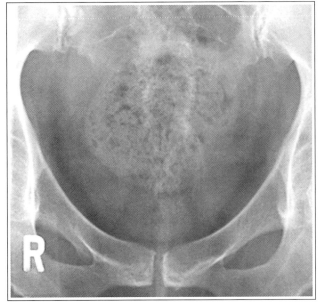

Image 20.

Analysis. Fecal material is superimposed over the coccyx, preventing its visualization.

Correction. Have the patient empty the colon of gas and fecal material before the coccyx is imaged.

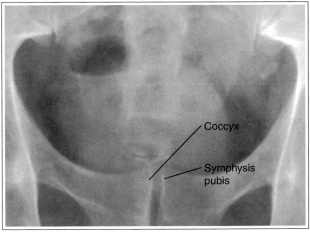

Image 21.

Analysis. The symphysis pubis is superimposed over the coccyx, and the second and third coccygeal vertebrae are foreshortened. The central ray was not angled caudally.

Correction. Angle the central ray approximately 5 degrees for every 1 inch (2.5 cm) you wish to move the symphysis pubis. This angulation adjustment is based on a 40-inch (102-cm) source-image distance (SID); if a shorter SID is used, the angle adjustment needs to be increased, and if a longer SID is used, the angle adjustment needs to be decreased. For this patient, the angulation should be angled 10 degrees caudally.

COCCYX: LATERAL POSITION

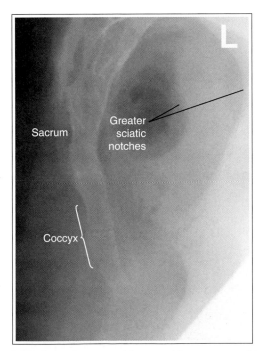

Figure 8-27. Lateral coccygeal image with accurate positioning.

Image Analysis

Scatter radiation is controlled.

- Use tight collimation, a grid, and a lead sheet placed on the imaging table at the edge of the posteriorly collimated field to reduce the amount of scatter radiation that reaches the IR, providing higher contrast and better visibility of recorded details.

The coccyx demonstrates a lateral position. The median sacral crest is demonstrated in profile, and the greater sciatic notches are superimposed.

- To obtain a lateral coccyx image, place the patient on the imaging table in a lateral recumbent position. Whether the patient is lying on the right or left side is not significant, although the left-side positioning is easier for the technologist.

  Flex the patient's knees and hips for support, and position a pillow or sponge between the knees. The thickness of the pillow or sponge should be sufficient to prevent the side of the pelvis situated farther from the IR from rotating anteriorly, without being so thick as to cause this side to rotate posteriorly (Figure 8-28).

- To avoid vertebral rotation, align the shoulders, posterior ribs, and posterior pelvic wings perpendicular to the IR. This is accomplished by resting your extended flat palm against each structure, individually, then adjusting the patient's rotation until your hand is perpendicular to the imaging table and IR.

- *Detecting rotation:* Rotation can be detected on a lateral coccyx image by evaluating the superimposition of the greater sciatic notches. On a nonrotated lateral coccygeal image, the greater sciatic notches are superimposed. On rotation the greater sciatic notches are not superimposed but are demonstrated one anterior to the other, and the coccyx and posteriorly situated ischium are nearly

superimposed on slight rotation and truly superimposed on severe rotation (see Image 22). Because the two sides of the pelvis are mirror images, it is difficult to determine which side of the patient was rotated anteriorly and which posteriorly on a lateral coccygeal image with poor positioning. When rotation has occurred, it is most common for the side of the patient situated farther from the IR to have been rotated anteriorly, if a sponge was not placed between the patient's knees, owing to the gravitational forward and downward pull on this side's arm and leg.

The coccyx is demonstrated without foreshortening.

- To demonstrate the coccyx without foreshortening, the vertebral column is aligned parallel with the imaging table, the interiliac line is aligned perpendicular to the imaging table, and a perpendicular central ray is used.

- *Adjusting for the sagging vertebral column:* The vertebral column of a patient with wide hips and a narrow waist may sag toward the imaging table at the level of the iliac crest (see Figure 8-11). Two methods may be used to achieve accurate positioning in such a patient:
  1. Place a radiolucent sponge between the patient's lateral body surface and the imaging table just superior to the iliac crest to elevate the vertebral column, aligning it parallel with the imaging table (see Figure 8-24), and use a perpendicular central ray.
  2. Leave the patient positioned as is, and angle the central ray caudally until it parallels the interiliac line.

- *Adjusting for the upwardly curved vertebral column:* The vertebral column of a patient with a large waist may curve upwardly (see Figure 8-19). For such a patient, angle the central ray cephalically until it parallels the interiliac line.

The coccyx is at the center of the collimated field. The fifth sacral segment, first through third coccygeal vertebrae, and inferior median sacral crest are included within the field.

- To place the coccyx in the center of the field, center a perpendicular central ray approximately 3½ inches (9 cm) posterior and 2 inches (5 cm) inferior to the elevated ASIS to place the coccyx in the center of the collimated field.

- Because tight collimation is essential to obtain optimal recorded detail visibility, collimate longitudinally and transversely to a 4-inch (10-cm) field. The third coccygeal vertebra is situated slightly more anteriorly than the first coccygeal vertebra. On injury this anterior position may be increased, causing the coccyx to align transversely (see Image 23). When this condition is suspected, transverse collimation should not be too tight.

- An 8- × 10-inch (18- × 24-cm) IR placed lengthwise should be adequate to include all the required anatomical structures.

- *Gonadal shielding:* Use gonadal protection shielding on all patients for this procedure. Begin by palpating the patient's coccyx and elevated ASIS. Next, draw an

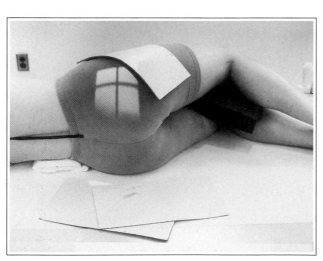

Figure 8-28. Proper patient positioning for lateral coccygeal image.

imaginary line connecting the coccyx with a point 1 inch posterior to the ASIS, and position the longitudinal edge of a large flat contact shield or lead half-apron anteriorly against this imaginary line (see Figure 8-15). This shielding method can be safely used for patients being imaged for lateral vertebral, sacral, or coccygeal images without fear of obscuring areas of interest (see Figure 8-16).

Lateral Coccyx Image Analysis

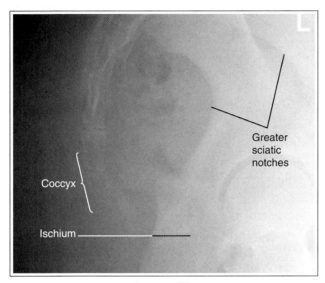

Image 22.

Analysis. The greater sciatic notches are demonstrated one anterior to the other, and the ischium is nearly superimposed over the third coccygeal segment. The pelvis, sacrum, and coccyx were rotated.

Correction. When rotation has occurred, it is most common for the elevated side of the patient to have been rotated anteriorly. Rotate the elevated pelvic wing posteriorly until the posterior pelvic wings are aligned perpendicular to the IR. It may be necessary to position a sponge or pillow between the patient's knees to help maintain this positioning.

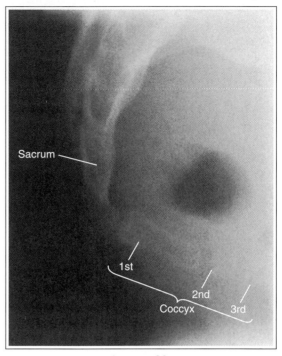

Image 23.

Analysis. The coccyx is aligned transversely, and the third coccygeal vertebra is not included within the collimated field. The transversely collimated field was collimated too tightly.

Correction. Open the transversely collimated field enough to include the third coccygeal vertebra.

Image Analysis of the Sternum and Ribs

STERNUM

The following image analysis criteria are used for all sternum images and should be considered when completing the analysis. Position- and projection-specific criteria relating to these topics are discussed with the other accompanying criteria for that position or projection.

Facility's patient identification requirements are visible on image.

A right or left marker, identifying correct side of patient, is present on the image and is not superimposed over anatomy of interest. Specific placement of marker is as described in Chapter 1.

No evidence of preventable artifacts, such as gown snaps, undergarments, necklaces, and body piercing, is present.

- It is recommended that the patient be instructed to remove all clothing above the waist and change into a snapless hospital gown before the procedure.

The bony trabecular patterns and cortical outlines of the sternum are sharply defined.

- Sharply defined image details are obtained when patient motion and respiration are halted and when a short object–image receptor distance (OID) is maintained. Increased spatial resolution is also obtained when the smallest image receptor (IR) is selected for digital images.

Contrast and density are adequate to demonstrate the surrounding soft tissue and bony structures. Penetration is sufficient to demonstrate the bony trabecular patterns and cortical outlines of the required sternal structures.

- An optimal kilovolt-peak (kVp) technique, as shown in Table 9-1, sufficiently penetrates the sternal structures and provides the contrast scale necessary to demonstrate the recorded details. A grid should be employed to absorb the scatter radiation produced by the thoracic structures,

TABLE 9-1 **Sternal and Rib Technical Data**			
Position or Projection	**kVp**	**Grid**	**SID**
PA oblique projection, sternum	60-70	Grid	30-40 inches (75-100 cm)
Lateral position, sternum	70-75	Grid	72 inches (180 cm)
AP or PA projection, upper ribs	65-70	Grid	40-48 inches (100-120 cm)
AP or PA projection, lower ribs	70-80	Grid	40-48 inches (100-120 cm)
AP or PA oblique, upper ribs	70-75	Grid	40-48 inches (100-120 cm)
AP or PA oblique, lower ribs	70-80	Grid	40-48 inches (100-120 cm)

AP, Anteroposterior; *kVp,* kilovolt peak; *PA,* posteroanterior; *SID,* source–image receptor distance.

increasing detail visibility. To obtain optimal density, set a manual milliampere-seconds (mAs) level based on the patient's thoracic thickness. The appropriate automatic exposure control (AEC) is not recommended for sternum images. (See Table 9-1 for specific recommendations.)

STERNUM: POSTEROANTERIOR OBLIQUE PROJECTION (RIGHT ANTERIOR OBLIQUE POSITION)

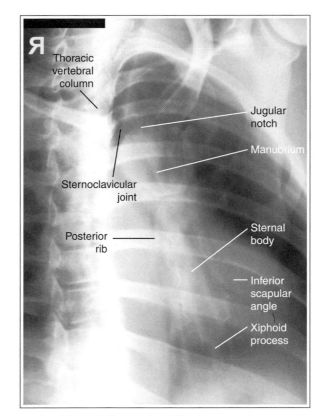

Figure 9-1. Posteroanterior oblique (right anterior oblique) sternum image with accurate positioning.

Image Analysis

The sternum demonstrates homogeneous density.

- *Importance of choosing the right anterior oblique (RAO) position:* The RAO position is used to rotate the sternum from beneath the thoracic vertebrae. It is chosen over the left anterior oblique (LAO) position because the RAO position superimposes the heart shadow over the sternum (see Image 1). Because the air-filled lungs and the heart shadow have different densities, they demonstrate distinctly different degrees of density on an image produced using the same exposure factors. The air-filled lungs demonstrate greater image density than the heart shadow. Positioning the sternum in the heart shadow ensures homogeneous density across the entire sternum. Any portion of the sternum that is positioned outside the heart shadow demonstrates a darker density than the portion positioned within the heart shadow.

The sternum is demonstrated without motion or distortion. The ribs and lung markings are blurred, and the posterior ribs and left scapulae are magnified.

- In the posteroanterior (PA) oblique position, the sternum has many overlying structures—the posterior ribs, lung markings, heart shadow, and left inferior scapula. Specific positioning techniques should be followed to show a sharply defined sternum while magnifying and blurring these overlying structures.
- *Blurring overlying sternal structures:* The source-image receptor distance (SID) recommended for the PA oblique sternum varies among positioning textbooks. It ranges from 30 inches (76 cm) to 40 inches (100 cm). A short (30-inch) SID provides increased magnification and blurring of the posterior ribs and left scapula but also results in a higher patient entrance skin-dosage. Facility protocol dictates the SID.

  Using a long exposure time (3 to 4 seconds) and requiring the patient to breathe shallowly (costal breathing) during the exposure forces upward and outward, and downward and inward movements of the ribs and lungs, thus blurring the posterior ribs and lung markings on the image. Deep breathing requires movement (elevation) of the sternum to provide deep lung expansion and should be avoided during breathing technique because this sternal motion would blur the sternum on the image (see Image 2).

If breathing technique is not employed, the details and cortical outlines of the posterior ribs, left scapula and lung markings are sharply defined, and the increased recorded detail obscures the details of the sternum (see Image 3).

The manubrium, sternoclavicular (SC) joints, sternal body, and xiphoid process are demonstrated within the heart shadow without vertebral superimposition.

- Rotating the patient until the midcoronal plane is angled 15 to 20 degrees to the IR draws the sternum from beneath the thoracic vertebrae (Figure 9-2). This degree of obliquity provides the reviewer a PA oblique projection of the sternum with only a small amount of rotation.

    To sufficiently evaluate an anatomical structure, two images of the area of interest, taken 90 degrees from each other, are obtained. The PA oblique (RAO) and lateral positions are obtained to fulfill this requirement for the sternum. Although these are not exactly 90 degrees from each other, it is necessary to slightly rotate the patient for the PA oblique image to demonstrate the sternum without vertebral superimposition.

- *Determining the required obliquity:* To determine the exact obliquity needed to rotate the sternum away from the thoracic vertebral column on a prone patient, place your fingertips of one hand on the right SC joint and the fingertips of the other hand on the spinous processes of the upper thoracic vertebrae. Rotate the patient until the fingers on the SC joint are positioned just to the left of the fingers on the spinous processes.

- *Evaluating accuracy of obliquity:* When evaluating a PA oblique sternal image, note that patient obliquity

was sufficient when the sternum is located within the heart shadow and the manubrium and right SC joint are shown without vertebral superimposition. If the patient was not adequately rotated, the right SC joint and manubrium are positioned beneath the vertebral column (see Image 4). If patient obliquity was excessive, the sternum is rotated to the left of the heart shadow and the sternum demonstrates excessive transverse foreshortening (see Image 3).

The midsternum is at the center of the collimated field. The jugular notch, SC joints, sternal body, and xiphoid process are included within the field.

- To position the midsternum in the center of the collimated field, align the midsternum to the central ray and midline of the IR (approximately 3 inches to the left of the thoracic spinous processes), then position the top of the IR approximately 1½ inches (3.75 cm) superior to the jugular notch and center a perpendicular central ray to the IR.

- *Determining IR size and collimation:* The size of IR and amount of collimation used for a PA oblique sternum image depends on the age and sex of the patient. The adult male sternum is approximately 7 inches (18 cm) long, but the female sternum is considerably shorter. A 10- × 12-inch (24- × 30-cm) IR should sufficiently accommodate both male and female adult patients. Because chest depth from the thoracic vertebrae to the manubrium is less than from the thoracic vertebrae to the xiphoid process, the manubrium remains closer to the thoracic vertebrae than the xiphoid process when the patient is rotated. The sternum, then, is not aligned with the longitudinal plane but is slightly tilted. Because of this sternal tilt, the transverse collimation should be confined to the thoracic spinous processes and the left inferior angle of the scapula.

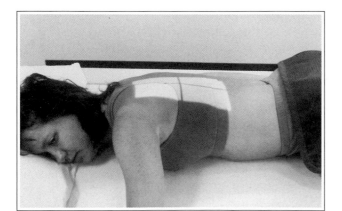

Figure 9-2. Proper patient positioning for posteroanterior oblique (right anterior oblique) sternum image.

Posteroanterior Oblique Sternum Image Analysis

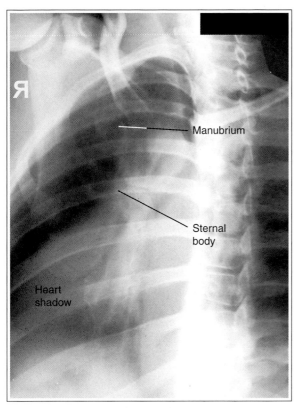

Image 1.

Analysis. The patient was positioned in an LAO position. The thoracic vertebrae are superimposed over the heart shadow, and the sternum is demonstrated to the right of the heart shadow.

Correction. Place the patient in an RAO position.

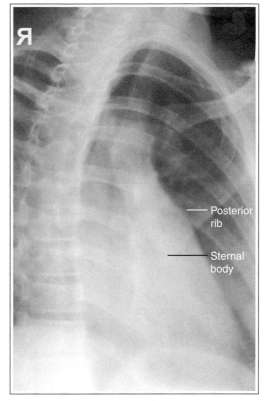

Image 2.

Analysis. The right SC joint is sharply defined, but the sternal body, posterior ribs, and lung markings are blurry. Breathing technique was used for this image, but the patient was breathing deeply instead of shallowly, causing the sternum to move and blur.

Correction. Instruct the patient to breathe shallowly.

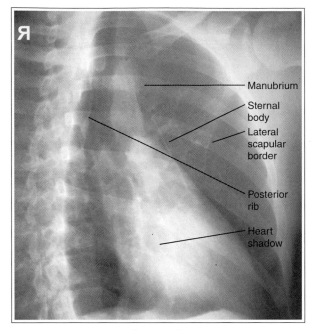

Image 3.

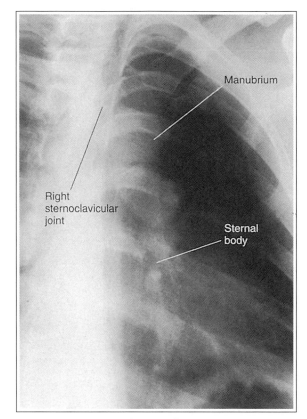

Image 4.

Analysis. The lung markings, posterior ribs, and left scapula are demonstrated without magnification or blurring, making it difficult to distinguish the sternum through these overlying structures. The SID was not shortened, and the patient's breathing was halted for this image. Also, patient obliquity was excessive, as indicated by the position of the sternum to the left of the heart shadow and by the amount of sternum rotation.

Correction. Shorten the SID to 30 inches (76 cm) if it is your facility's protocol, take the exposure while the patient is breathing shallowly, and decrease the degree of patient obliquity.

Analysis. The right SC joint and the right side of the manubrium are superimposed by the thoracic vertebrae. The patient was not rotated enough to move the entire manubrium from beneath the thoracic vertebrae.

Correction. Increase the patient obliquity. Rotate the patient until the palpable right SC joint is positioned to the left of the thoracic vertebrae.

STERNUM: LATERAL POSITION

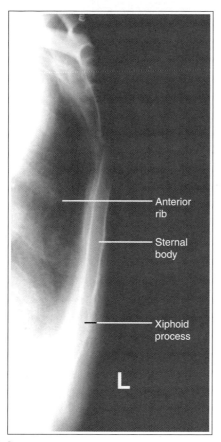

Figure 9-3. Lateral sternum image with accurate positioning.

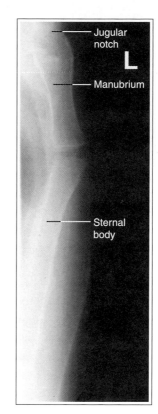

Figure 9-4. Superior lateral sternum image with accurate positioning.

Image Analysis

Contrast, density, and penetration are adequate to show the bony trabecular patterns and cortical outlines of the jugular notch, manubrium, sternal body, and xiphoid process.

- An even density is difficult to obtain over the entire sternum region, because the lower sternum is superimposed by the pectoral (chest) muscles or by the female breast tissue, whereas the upper sternum is free of this superimposition. The amount of density difference between the two halves of the sternum depends on the development of the patient's pectoral muscles and the amount of female breast tissue. Enlargement of either tissue requires an increase in exposure to obtain sufficient density to demonstrate the sternum through them. This increase may overexpose the upper sternum region on the image, requiring an additional image to be taken with a lower exposure so the entire sternum can be demonstrated (Figure 9-4).

- ***Reduce scatter radiation:*** A remarkable amount of scatter radiation is evident on a lateral sternal image anterior to the sternum. One can be certain that if scatter is demonstrated here, it is also overlying the image of the sternum, decreasing the overall image contrast.

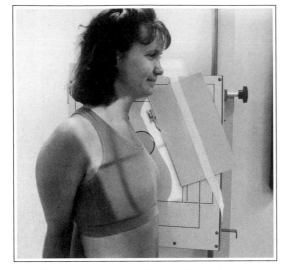

Figure 9-5. Proper patient positioning for lateral sternum image.

To eliminate some of this scatter radiation and produce a higher-contrast image, tightly collimate, use a grid, and place a lead sheet anterior to the sternum close to the patient's skinline (Figure 9-5). For the upright patient the lead sheet may be taped to the upright IR holder.

The sternum and chest demonstrate no rotation; the manubrium, sternal body, and xiphoid process are demonstrated in profile; and the anterior ribs are not superimposed over the sternum.

- To obtain a lateral sternum image, place the patient in an upright position with the right or left lateral aspect of the body against the upright IR holder (see Figure 9-5).
- Avoid chest rotation by aligning the shoulders, the posterior ribs, and the posterior pelvic wings perpendicular to the IR. This alignment, which superimposes each of these posterior body parts on the image, is accomplished by resting your extended flat hand against each structure, individually, and then adjusting the patient's rotation until your hand is perpendicular to the IR. When the thorax is demonstrated without rotation, the sternum is in profile and the anterior ribs are superimposed over each other instead of over or under the sternum.
- *Lateral sternal image in supine position:* If the patient is unable to be positioned upright, a lateral sternum image can be accomplished with the patient supine. In this position, rest the patient's arms against the sides, position a grid-cassette vertically against the patient's arm, and use a horizontal beam. All other positioning and analysis requirements are the same as for an upright image.
- *Detecting rotation and determining how to reposition the rotated patient:* Rotation is effectively detected on a lateral sternum image by evaluating the degree of anterior rib and sternal superimposition. If a lateral sternum image demonstrates rotation, the right and left

anterior ribs are not superimposed; one side is positioned anterior to the sternum, and the other side is positioned posterior to the sternum.

Determine how to reposition after obtaining a rotated image by using the heart shadow to identify the right and left anterior ribs. Because the heart shadow is located in the left chest cavity and extends anteroinferiorly, outlining the superior border of the heart shadow enables recognition of the left side of the chest. If the left lung and ribs were positioned anterior to the sternum, as demonstrated in Figure 9-6, the outline of the superior heart shadow continues beyond the sternum and into the anteriorly located lung (see Image 5). If the right lung and ribs were positioned anterior to the sternum, as demonstrated in Figure 9-7, the superior heart shadow does not continue into the anteriorly situated lung, but ends at the sternum (see Image 6). Once the right and left sides of the chest have been identified, reposition the patient by rotating the thorax. If the left lung and ribs were anteriorly positioned, rotate the left thorax posteriorly. If the right lung and ribs were anteriorly positioned, rotate the right thorax posteriorly.

- *Respiration:* Elevation of the sternum, resulting from deep suspended inspiration, aids in better sternal demonstration by drawing the sternum away from the anterior ribs.

No superimposition of humeral soft tissue over the sternum is present.

- Extending the patient's arms behind the back with the hands clasped positions the humeral soft tissue away from the sternum.

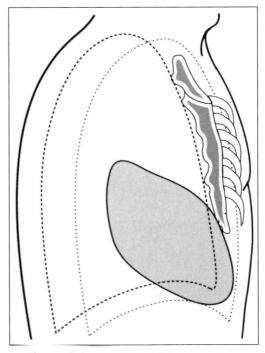

Figure 9-6. Rotation—left lung anterior.

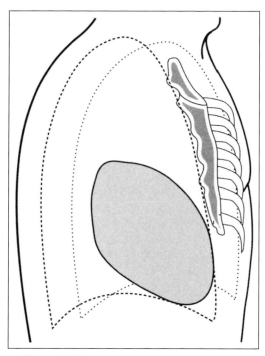

Figure 9-7. Rotation—right lung anterior.

The midsternum is at the center of the collimated field. The jugular notch, sternal body, and xiphoid process are included within the field.

- To position the midsternum in the center of the collimated field, place the top edge of the IR 1½ inches (4 cm) above the jugular notch, then align the image receptor's long axis and a perpendicular central ray to the midsternum. Use the sternal skin surface when determining the location of the midsternum. Do not be thrown off by the vastness of the patient's pectoral muscles or breast tissue; these structures are situated anterior to the sternum and its skin surface.
- A 72-inch (180-cm) SID is used to minimize the sternal magnification that would result because of the long sternum-to-IR distance.

Lateral Sternum Image Analysis

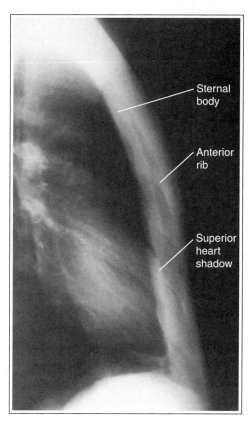

Sternal body

Anterior rib

Superior heart shadow

Image 5.

Analysis. The anterior ribs are not superimposed, and the sternum is not in profile, indicating that the chest was rotated. The superior heart shadow extends anterior to the sternum and into the anteriorly situated lung, verifying it as the left lung. The patient was positioned with the left thorax rotated anteriorly and the right thorax rotated posteriorly.

Correction. Position the right thorax slightly anteriorly.

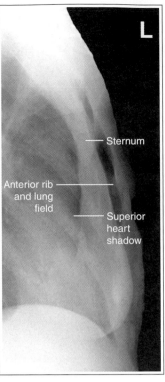

Sternum

Anterior rib and lung field

Superior heart shadow

Image 6.

Analysis. The anterior ribs are not superimposed, and the sternum is not in profile, indicating that the chest was rotated. The superior heart shadow does not extend beyond the sternum, verifying that the right lung is situated anterior to the sternum, and the left lung is situated posterior. The patient was positioned with the right thorax rotated anteriorly and the left thorax rotated posteriorly.

Correction. Position the left thorax posteriorly.

RIBS

The following image analysis criteria are used for all rib images and should be considered when completing the analysis. Position- and projection-specific criteria relating to these topics are discussed with the other accompanying criteria for that position or projection.

Facility's patient identification requirements are visible on image.

A right or left marker, identifying correct side of patient, is present on the image and is not super-imposed over anatomy of interest. Specific placement of marker is as described in Chapter 1. A rib marker is present when requested by facility.

- Many facilities require that the technologist tape a rib marker (lead "BB") on the patient's skin near the area where the ribs are tender. This aids the reviewer in pinpointing the exact location of potential injury.

No evidence of preventable artifacts, such as under-garments, necklaces, belts, buttons, gown snaps, and body piercings, is present.

- It is recommended the patient remove all clothing above the waist and change into a snapless hospital gown before the procedure.

The bony trabecular patterns and cortical outlines of the ribs are sharply defined.

- Sharply defined image details are obtained when patient motion is controlled, when respiration is suspended on full inhalation for above-diaphragm and full exhalation

for below-diaphragm ribs, and when a short OID is maintained.

Contrast, density, and penetration are adequate to demonstrate the surrounding chest and intra-abdominal soft tissue, the cortical outlines of the anterior, posterior, and axillary ribs, and the vertebral column.

- A lower kVp, as demonstrated in Table 9-1, would best define the upper ribs that surround the lateral portion of the lung field without overpenetrating the air-filled lungs. When the lower ribs are of interest, a slightly higher kVp is needed to penetrate the denser abdominal structures and demonstrate the ribs while still maintaining a relatively high image contrast. A grid should be employed to absorb the scatter radiation produced by the thorax and abdomen, increasing detail visibility. To obtain optimal density, set a manual mAs level based on the patient's thoracic or abdominal thickness.
- *Soft-tissue structures of interest:* The demonstration of the soft-tissue structures that surround the ribs is also very important. When an upper rib fracture is suspected, the surrounding upper thorax, axillary, and neck soft tissues and vascular lung markings are carefully studied for signs (hematoma, a presence of air, etc.) that indicate associated lung pathology (pneumothorax, interstitial emphysema, etc.) or rupture of the trachea, bronchus, or aorta. When a lower rib fracture is suspected, the upper abdominal tissue is examined for signs of associated injury to the kidney, liver, spleen, or diaphragm.

RIBS: ANTEROPOSTERIOR OR POSTEROANTERIOR PROJECTION (ABOVE OR BELOW DIAPHRAGM)

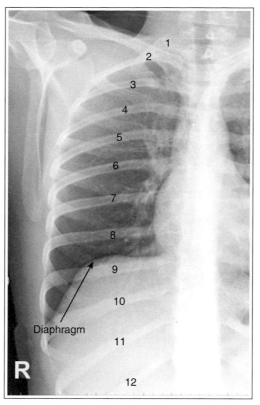

Figure 9-8. Anteroposterior above-diaphragm rib image with accurate positioning.

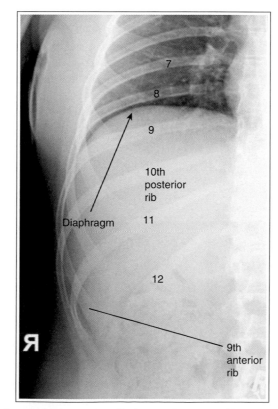

Figure 9-9. Posteroanterior below-diaphragm rib image with accurate positioning.

Alternative IR size and centering method when both sides of the ribs are on the same image: It should be noted that some positioning textbooks suggest that PA or AP above- and below-diaphragm rib images be taken to include both sides of the ribs on the same image. For this positioning, the IR is positioned crosswise and centering is to the midsagittal plane instead of halfway between the midsagittal plane and lateral rib surface.

Image Analysis

Rib magnification is kept to a minimum.

- *AP versus PA projection:* When the patient complains of anterior rib pain, obtain the image in a PA projection, to place the anterior ribs closer to the IR. When the posterior ribs are the affected ribs, take the image in an AP projection, to place the posterior ribs closer to the IR.

  Compare the difference in posterior rib detail sharpness in Figures 9-8 and 9-9. Figure 9-8 was obtained in an AP projection, and Figure 9-9 in a PA projection. Note how the posterior ribs in Figure 9-9 are magnified, demonstrating less detail sharpness than the posterior ribs in Figure 9-8, which were positioned closer to the IR for the image.

The thorax demonstrates no rotation. The thoracic vertebrae–rib head articulations are demonstrated, the sternum and vertebral column are superimposed, and the distances from the vertebral column to the sternal ends of the clavicles, when demonstrated, are equal.

- Thoracic and rib rotation are avoided on the AP projection by flexing the patient's knees and placing the feet flat against the table. The shoulders should also be positioned at equal distances from the imaging table. (Figure 9-10)

  For the kyphotic patient, it may be necessary to place a sponge under each shoulder or obtain the image with

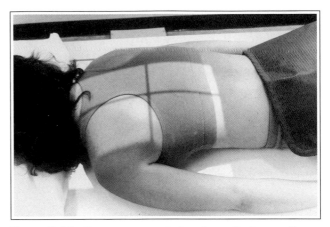

Figure 9-11. Proper posteroanterior, above-diaphragm rib positioning.

the patient in an upright position to avoid rotation of the upper thorax. Preventing rotation in the PA projection is slightly more difficult. It is best accomplished by placing the patient's chin on a radiolucent sponge so he or she can look straight ahead and still be able to breathe, as well as by positioning shoulders and anterosuperior iliac spines (ASISs) at equal distances from the table (Figure 9-11).

For the patient who has excessive abdominal tissue and has a tendency to roll to one side in the PA projection, it may be necessary to place a radiolucent sponge under the side of the lower abdomen toward which the patient is leaning or to obtain the image with the patient in an upright position to avoid thoracic rotation.

- *Detecting rotation:* Rotation is effectively detected on an AP or PA rib image by evaluating the sternum and vertebral column superimposition and by comparing the distances between the vertebral column and the sternal ends of the clavicles. When an image of the ribs demonstrates rotation and the patient was in an AP projection, the side of the patient positioned closer to the IR demonstrates the sternum and the SC joint without vertebral column superimposition (see Image 7). The opposite is true for a PA projection: the side of the chest positioned farther from the IR demonstrates the sternum and the SC joint without vertebral column superimposition (see Image 8).
- *Rotation versus scoliosis:* In images of patients with spinal scoliosis, the ribs and vertebral column will appear rotated because of the lateral deviation of the vertebrae (Image 9). Become familiar with this condition to prevent unnecessarily repeated procedures on these patients.

ANTEROPOSTERIOR AND POSTEROANTERIOR PROJECTIONS OF RIBS ABOVE DIAPHRAGM
The scapulae are located outside the lung field, and the chin does not obscure the superior ribs.

- For the AP projection, position the scapulae outside the lung field by placing the back of the patient's hands on

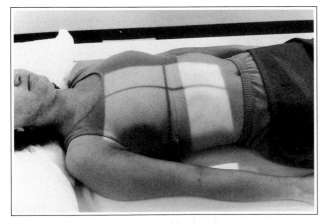

Figure 9-10. Proper patient positioning for anteroposterior below-diaphragm rib image.

the hips or under the patient's head and rotating the elbows and shoulders anteriorly.

- For the PA projection, position the scapulae outside the lung field by abducting and internally rotating the patient's arms, forcing the shoulders to rotate anteriorly.
- To avoid rotation, it is best to position the two arms in the same manner even when only one side of the thorax is being imaged. If the scapula is not drawn away from the lung field, it is demonstrated in the upper ribs (see Image 10).
- Elevate the chin to position it superior to the upper ribs.

Nine posterior ribs are demonstrated above the diaphragm, indicating full lung aeration.

- The number of ribs demonstrated above the diaphragm is determined by the depth of patient inspiration. In full inspiration, when the patient is recumbent, approximately nine posterior ribs are demonstrated above the diaphragm. When the patient is in an upright position, 10 or 11 posterior ribs will be demonstrated. If the patient does not fully inhale, the inferior ribs are demonstrated below the diaphragm. Any ribs situated below the diaphragm are not well demonstrated, because an increase in exposure would be needed to penetrate the abdominal tissue they surround. To maximize the number of ribs located above the diaphragm, the exposure should be taken with the patient in full inspiration.

The seventh posterior rib is at the center of the collimated field. The affected side's first through ninth ribs and the vertebral column are included within the field.

- In the AP projection, to place the seventh posterior rib at the center of the image, center a perpendicular central ray halfway between the midsagittal plane and the affected lateral rib surface at a level halfway between the jugular notch and the xiphoid process.
- In the PA projection, center a perpendicular central ray halfway between the midsagittal plane and the affected lateral rib surface at the level of the inferior scapular angle. Palpate the scapular angle with the arm next to the patient's body. After accurate centering has been accomplished, abduct the arm to position it out of the collimated field. Abducting the arm shifts the inferior scapular angle laterally and inferiorly, so centering should be accomplished before arm abduction.
- Once the central ray is centered, collimate transversely to the thoracic vertebral column and the patient's lateral skinline. Because above-diaphragm ribs are imaged on inspiration, causing the thorax to expand transversely, perform the transverse collimation with the patient in deep inspiration. Open the longitudinal collimation the full 17-inch (43-cm) IR length.
- A 14- × 17-inch (35- × 43-cm) IR placed lengthwise should be adequate to include all the required anatomical structures.

ANTEROPOSTERIOR AND POSTEROANTERIOR PROJECTIONS OF RIBS BELOW DIAPHRAGM
The eighth through twelfth posterior ribs are demonstrated below the diaphragm.

- The number of ribs demonstrated below the diaphragm is determined by the depth of patient inspiration. In full inspiration, up to 10 posterior ribs may be demonstrated above the diaphragm (see Image 11). To maximize demonstration of the lower ribs the exposure should be obtained on expiration. In expiration, only seven or eight posterior ribs are clearly visible above the diaphragm, and four or five ribs are demonstrated below the diaphragm. When below-diaphragm ribs are imaged, it is necessary to use a higher kVp and exposure than needed for the above-diaphragm ribs, to penetrate the denser abdominal tissue. Any ribs situated above the diaphragm for this image may be too dark to evaluate.

The tenth posterior rib is at the center of the collimated field. A portion of the thoracic and lumbar vertebral column and the eighth through twelfth ribs of affected side of the patient are included within the field.

- To center the tenth posterior rib in the center of the field and include the eighth through twelfth ribs on the AP and PA below-diaphragm rib projections, place the lower edge of the IR at the level of the iliac crest and center the image receptor's long axis halfway between the midsagittal plane and the affected lateral rib surface. Center a perpendicular central ray to the IR.
- For a hypersthenic patient with a short, wide thorax, the centering needs to be positioned slightly higher. Place the lower border of the IR approximately 2 inches (5 cm) above the iliac crest.
- Transversely collimate to the vertebral column and the patient's lateral skinline. Open the longitudinal collimation the full 17-inch (43-cm) field size.
- A 14- × 17-inch (35- × 43-cm) IR placed lengthwise should be adequate to include all the anatomical structures.

Anteroposterior or Posteroanterior Rib Image Analysis

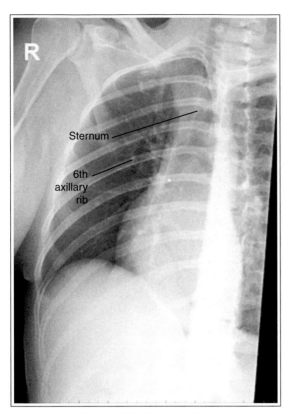

Image 7. AP projection.

Analysis. The sternum is demonstrated to the right of the patient's vertebral column. The patient was rotated. In an AP projection, the sternum is rotated toward the side that was positioned closer to the IR. For this image, the patient was rotated toward the right side.

Correction. Position the patient in an AP projection by flexing his or her knees and placing his or her shoulders at equal distances from the imaging table.

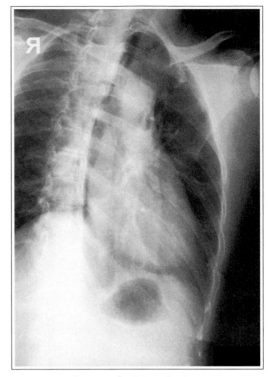

Image 8. PA projection.

Analysis. The sternum and the SC joints are demonstrated to the left of the patient's vertebral column. The patient was rotated. In a PA projection the sternum and SC joints are rotated toward the side that was positioned farther from the IR. For this image the patient was rolled toward the right side, away from the left side.

Correction. Position the patient in a PA projection by having the patient look straight ahead with the chin elevated on a sponge. The shoulders and the ASISs should be positioned at equal distances from the imaging table.

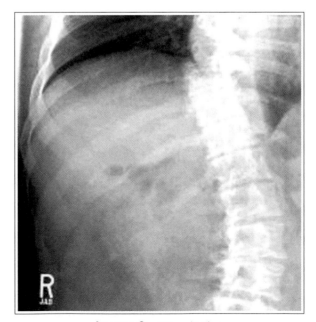

Image 9. AP projection.

Analysis. The distances from the vertebral column to the lateral rib edges down the length of the thoracic region vary, indicating that the patient has spinal scoliosis.

Correction. No corrective movement is required.

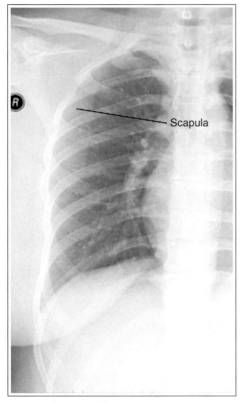

Image 10. AP projection.

Analysis. The left scapula is superimposed over the upper lateral rib field. The left elbow and shoulder were not rotated anteriorly.

Correction. If the patient's condition allows, place the back of the patient's hands on the hips, and rotate the elbows and shoulders anteriorly.

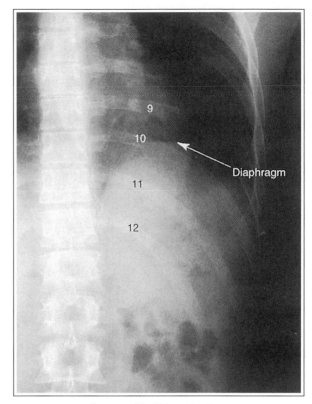

Image 11. PA projection.

Analysis. For this below-diaphragm rib image, only three posterior ribs are demonstrated below the diaphragm. The image was exposed after the patient had taken a deep breath.

Correction. To demonstrate more posterior ribs below the diaphragm, the image should be exposed after the patient exhales.

RIBS: ANTEROPOSTERIOR OBLIQUE PROJECTION (POSTERIOR OBLIQUE POSITION, ABOVE OR BELOW DIAPHRAGM)

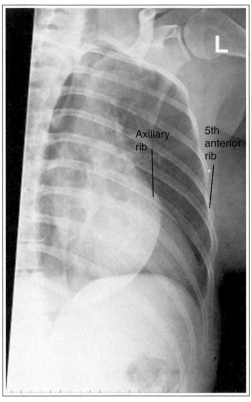

Figure 9-12. Anteroposterior (posterior) oblique, above-diaphragm rib image with accurate positioning.

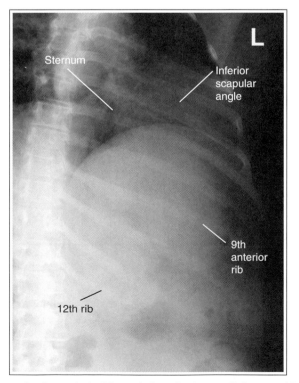

Figure 9-13. Anteroposterior (posterior) oblique, below-diaphragm rib image with accurate positioning.

The posterior oblique position should be the position performed routinely, because it positions the axillary (lateral) ribs closer to the IR.

Image Analysis

Rib magnification is kept to a minimum.

- *Posterior versus anterior oblique:* To provide maximum axillary rib detail, posterior oblique positions (right posterior oblique [RPO], left posterior oblique [LPO]) should be routinely performed. In the RPO and LPO positions the axillary ribs are placed closer to the IR than in the RAO and LAO positions, resulting in less rib magnification and greater recorded detail. Image 12 demonstrates below-diaphragm ribs exposed with the patient in an anterior oblique position. Compare this image with the posterior oblique rib image in Figure 9-12. Note the greater magnification and loss of detail of the ribs and the increased visualization (Image 12).

The thorax has been rotated 45 degrees. The inferior sternal body is located halfway between the lateral rib surface and the vertebral column, and the axillary ribs are free of superimposition. The axillary ribs are demonstrated without superimposition and are located in the center of the collimated field, and the anterior ribs are located at the lateral edge.

- Rotating the patient until the midcoronal plane is angled 45 degrees with the IR provides the reviewer with an additional perspective of the axillary ribs, without the self-superimposition demonstrated on the AP or PA projection.

  To open up the curvature of the axillary ribs, rotate the patient toward the affected side for a posterior oblique position and away from the affected side for an anterior oblique position (Figures 9-14 and 9-15). If the patient is

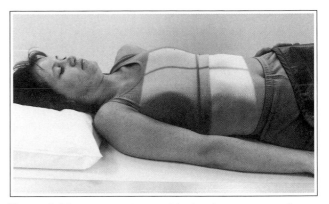

Figure 9-15. Proper patient positioning for anteroposterior (posterior) oblique, below-diaphragm rib image.

rotated in the opposite direction, the axillary ribs demonstrate greater self-superimposition (see Image 13).

- *Determining accuracy of rotation:* Because the sternum rotates toward the affected axillary ribs on thoracic rotation, the position of the sternum can be used to identify accuracy of patient rotation. If the inferior sternum is positioned halfway between the vertebral column and the anterior ribs, the patient was rotated 45 degrees and the axillary ribs are "opened." When the desired 45-degree obliquity has not been obtained, view the position of the inferior sternum to determine how to reposition the patient. If the sternal body is demonstrated next to the vertebral column, the patient was insufficiently rotated (see Image 14). If the inferior sternal body is demonstrated laterally, the patient was rotated more than 45 degrees.

POSTERIOR OBLIQUE IMAGES OF RIBS ABOVE THE DIAPHRAGM

Ten axillary ribs are demonstrated above the diaphragm, indicating full lung aeration.

- The number of ribs demonstrated above the diaphragm is determined by the depth of patient inspiration. In full inspiration, when the patient is recumbent, 10 axillary ribs are usually demonstrated above the diaphragm. When the patient is in an upright position, 10 or 11 axillary ribs are demonstrated. If the patient does not fully inhale, the inferior axillary ribs are positioned below the diaphragm. Any ribs situated below the diaphragm are not well demonstrated, because an increase in exposure would be needed to penetrate the abdominal tissue they surround. To maximize the number of ribs located above the diaphragm, take the exposure with the patient in full inspiration.

The seventh axillary rib is at the center of the collimated field. The first through tenth axillary ribs of the affected side and the thoracic vertebral column are included within the field.

- For posterior oblique axillary rib images (RPO or LPO), the seventh posterior rib is placed at the center of

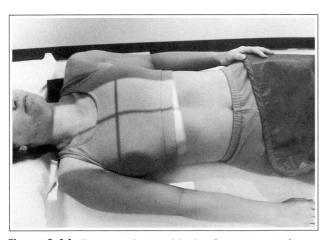

Figure 9-14. Proper patient positioning for anteroposterior (posterior) oblique, above-diaphragm rib image.

the image by centering a perpendicular central ray halfway between the midsagittal plane and the affected lateral rib surface at a level halfway between the jugular notch and the xiphoid process.

- Once the central ray is centered, collimate transversely to the thoracic vertebral column and the patient's lateral skinline. Because above-diaphragm ribs are imaged on inspiration, causing the thorax to expand transversely, perform the transverse collimation with the patient in deep inspiration. Open the longitudinal collimation the full 17-inch (43-cm) IR length.
- A 14- × 17-inch (35- × 43-cm) IR placed lengthwise should be adequate to include all the required anatomical structures.

POSTERIOR OBLIQUE IMAGES OF RIBS BELOW THE DIAPHRAGM

The ninth through twelfth axillary ribs are demonstrated below the diaphragm

- The number of ribs located below the diaphragm is determined by the depth of patient inspiration. In full suspended inspiration, up to 10 axillary ribs may be demonstrated above the diaphragm. In expiration only seven or eight axillary ribs are clearly visible above the diaphragm, and four or five ribs are demonstrated below the diaphragm. When below-diaphragm ribs are imaged, it is necessary to use a higher kVp and exposure than needed for the above-diaphragm ribs, to penetrate the denser abdominal tissue. Any ribs situated above the diaphragm for this image may be too dark to evaluate. To maximize the number of ribs located below the diaphragm, take the exposure on full suspended expiration.

The tenth axillary rib is at the center of the collimated field. A portion of the thoracic and lumbar vertebral column and the eighth through twelfth axillary ribs of the affected side of the patient are included within the field.

- To place the tenth axillary rib in the center of the collimated field for posterior oblique (RPO, LPO) axillary rib images, place the lower edge of the IR at the level of the iliac crest and center the image receptor's long axis halfway between the midsagittal plane and the affected lateral rib surface. Center a perpendicular central ray to the IR.

  For a hypersthenic patient with a short, wide thorax, the centering needs to be positioned slightly higher. Place the lower border of the IR approximately 2 inches (5 cm) above the iliac crest.
- Transversely collimate to the vertebral column and the patient's lateral skinline. Open the longitudinal collimation the full 17-inch (43-cm) field size.
- A 14- × 17-inch (35- × 43-cm) IR placed lengthwise should be adequate to include all the anatomical structures.

Anteroposterior Oblique Rib Image Analysis

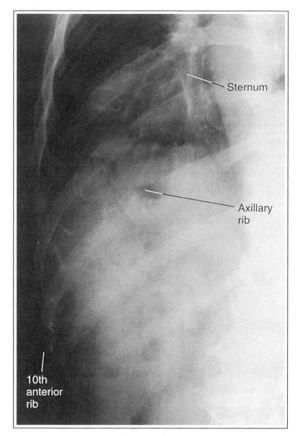

Image 12.

Analysis. This is an anterior oblique image of the lower ribs. The sternum demonstrates sharply defined cortical outlines, but the axillary ribs are magnified and demonstrate little definition.

Correction. The axillary ribs would demonstrate greater definition if a posterior oblique image had been taken instead. Replace an RAO position with an LPO position to demonstrate the left axillary ribs. Replace an LAO position with an RPO position to demonstrate the right axillary ribs.

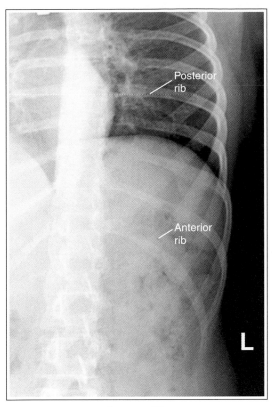

Image 13.

Image 14.

Analysis. The axillary ribs demonstrate greater self-superimposition, and the sternum is rotated away from the affected ribs. The patient was rotated in the wrong direction.

Correction. For posterior oblique positions, rotate the patient toward the affected side. For anterior oblique positions, rotate the patient away from the affected side.

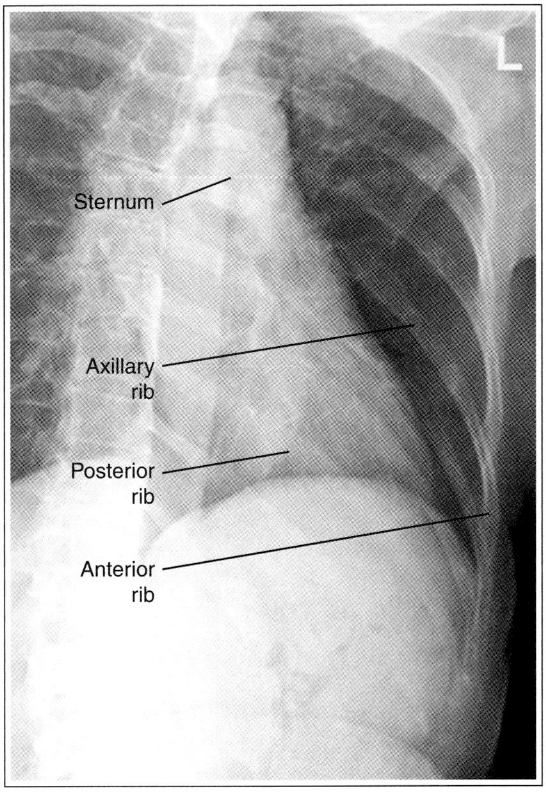

Analysis. The sternal body is not positioned halfway between the vertebral column and the affected lateral rib surface. The sternum is situated next to the vertebral column. The patient was rotated less than 45 degrees.

Correction. Increase the degree of patient obliquity until the midcoronal plane is angled 45 degrees with the IR.

Image Analysis of the Cranium

CRANIUM, FACIAL BONES, SINUSES, MANDIBLE, AND PETROMASTOID PORTION

The following image analysis criteria are used for all cranium, facial bone, sinus, and petromastoid portion images and should be considered when the analysis is performed. Position- or projection-specific criteria relating to these topics are discussed with the other accompanying criteria for that position or projection.

Facility's patient identification requirements are visible on image.

A right or left marker, identifying correct side of patient, is present on the image and is not super-imposed over anatomy of interest. Specific placement of marker is as described in Chapter 1.

No evidence of preventable artifacts, such as hairpins, hair ornaments, removable dental structures, earrings, and hearing aids, is present.

The bony trabecular patterns and cortical outlines of the cranium, facial bones, and mandible, as well as the sinuses and mastoid cells, are sharply defined.

- Sharply defined recorded details are obtained when patient motion is controlled, using a small focal spot, and a short object–image receptor distance (OID) is maintained. Increased spatial resolution is also obtained when the smallest image receptor (IR) is selected for digital images.

Contrast and density are adequate to demonstrate the air-filled cavities, sinuses, and mastoids when present and the bony structures of the cranium, facial bones, and mandible when present. Penetration is sufficient to visualize the bony trabecular patterns and cortical outlines.

- An optimal kilovolt-peak (kVp) technique, as shown in Table 10-1, sufficiently penetrates the structures as indicated and provides a contrast scale necessary to visualize the needed details. Use a grid to absorb the scatter radiation, providing a higher-contrast image. To obtain optimal density, set a manual milliampere-seconds (mAs) level based on the patient's part thickness, or choose the appropriate automatic exposure control (AEC) chamber when recommended. (See Table 10-1 for specifics.)

TABLE 10-1 Cranium, Facial Bones, Sinuses, Mandible, and Petromastoid Portion Technical Data

Position or Projection	Structure	kVp	Grid	AEC Chamber(s)	SID
AP or PA projection	Cranium	70-80	Grid	Center	40-48 inches (100-120 cm)
	Mandible	70-80	Grid		
PA axial (Caldwell) projection	Cranium	70-80	Grid	Center	40-48 inches (100-120 cm)
	Facial bones	70-80	Grid	Center	
	Sinuses	70-80	Grid	Center	
AP axial (Towne) projection	Cranium	70-80	Grid	Center	40-48 inches (100-120 cm)
	Mandible	70-80	Grid		
	Petromastoid portion	70-80	Grid	Center	
Lateral position	Cranium	70-80	Grid	Center	40-48 inches (100-120 cm)
	Facial bones	70-80	Grid	Center	
	Sinuses	50-60	Grid		
	Nasal bones	70-80	Grid		
Submentovertex (Schueller) projection	Cranium	70-80	Grid	Center	40-48 inches (100-120 cm)
	Mandible	70-80	Grid	Center	
	Sinuses	70-80	Grid	Center	
	Zygomatic arches	60-70	Nongrid		
Parietoacanthial (Waters) projection	Facial bones	70-80	Grid	Center	40-48 inches (100-120 cm)
	Sinuses	70-80	Grid	Center	
Parietoorbital oblique (Rhese) projection	Optic canal and foramen	70-80	Grid		40-48 inches (100-120 cm)
Tangential (superoinferior) projection	Nasal bones	50-60			40-48 inches (100-120 cm)
Axiolateral oblique (modified Law) projection	Petromastoid portion	70-80	Grid		40-48 inches (100-120 cm)
Axiolateral oblique (Stenvers) projection	Petromastoid portion	70-80	Grid	Center	40-48 inches (100-120 cm)

AEC, Automatic exposure control; *AP,* anteroposterior; *kVp,* kilovolt peak; *SID,* source–image receptor distance; *PA,* posteroanterior.

CRANIUM AND MANDIBLE: POSTEROANTERIOR OR ANTEROPOSTERIOR PROJECTION

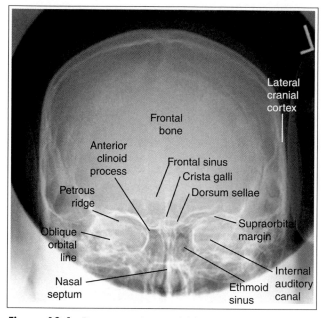

Figure 10-1. Posteroanterior cranial image with accurate positioning.

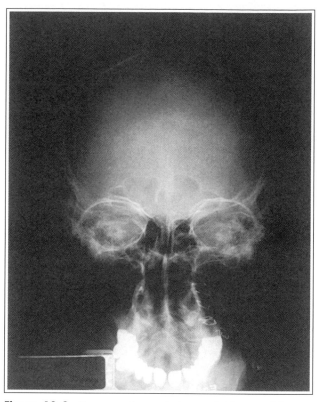

Figure 10-2. Trauma anteroposterior cranial image with accurate positioning.

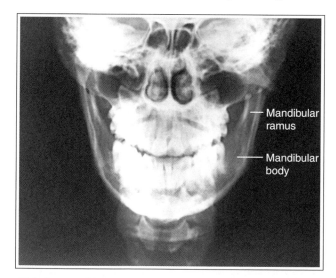

Figure 10-3. Posteroanterior mandible image with accurate positioning. (*From Ballinger PW, Frank ED: Merrill's atlas of radiographic positions and radiologic procedures, vol 2, ed 10, St Louis, 2005, Elsevier, p 382*).

Image Analysis

The cranium and mandible demonstrate a posteroanterior (PA) projection. The distances from the lateral margin of orbits to the lateral cranial cortex; from the crista galli to the lateral cranial cortices; and

from the mandibular rami to the lateral cervical vertebrae on both sides are equal.

- A PA projection of the cranium is obtained by positioning the patient in an upright or recumbent prone position with the nose and forehead resting against the upright IR holder or imaging table (Figure 10-4). Positioning the

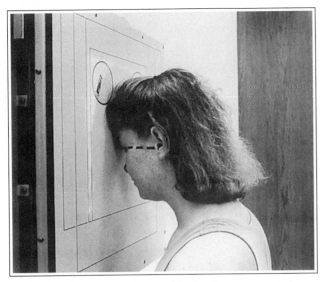

Figure 10-4. Proper patient positioning for posteroanterior cranial image.

midsagittal plane perpendicular to the IR prevents skull rotation. The best method of accomplishing this goal is to place an extended flat palm next to each lateral parietal bone. Then adjust the head rotation until your hands are perpendicular to the IR and parallel with each other.

- *Detecting head rotation:* Head rotation is present on a PA projection if the distance from the lateral margins of orbit to the lateral cranial cortices on one side is greater than on the other side, the distance from the crista galli to the lateral cranial margin on one side is greater than on the other side, and the distance from the mandibular rami on one side is greater than on the other side (see Image 1). The patient's face was rotated away from the side demonstrating the greater distance.

- *Trauma anteroposterior (AP) projection of cranium:* For the trauma AP projection of the cranium the patient is placed supine on the imaging table. If injury to cervical vertebrae is suspected, do not adjust the patient's head rotation. Take the image with the head positioned as is. If a cervical vertebral injury is not in question, adjust the patient's head until the midsagittal plane is perpendicular to the IR, to prevent rotation.

- An AP skull image should meet all the requirements listed for the PA cranial image, although some features of the cranium appear different. The AP projection demonstrates increased orbital magnification and less distance from the oblique orbital line to the lateral cranial cortices than the PA projection. These differences result from greater magnification of the anatomy situated farther from the IR. In the AP projection the orbits are positioned farther from the IR than the lateral parietal bones, whereas in the PA projection the lateral parietal bones are farther from the IR.

The anterior clinoids and dorsum sellae are demonstrated superior to the ethmoid sinuses. The petrous ridges are superimposed over the supraorbital margins, and the internal acoustic meatus are demonstrated horizontally through the center of the orbits.

- To position the anterior clinoids and dorsum sellae superior to the ethmoid sinuses, lower or tuck the patient's chin toward the chest until the orbitomeatal line (OML) (imaginary line connecting the outer eye canthus and the external acoustic opening) is perpendicular to the IR. This positioning moves the frontal bone inferiorly, until it is parallel with the IR, and the orbits inferiorly, until the supraorbital margins are situated beneath the petrous ridges, and places the petrous pyramids and internal acoustic meatus within the orbits.

- *Adjusting central ray for poor OML alignment:* If the patient is unable to tuck the chin adequately to position the OML perpendicular to the IR, the central ray angle may be adjusted to compensate. Instruct the patient to tuck the chin to place the OML as close as possible to perpendicular to the IR. Then angle the central ray parallel with the patient's OML (easily accomplished by aligning the collimator's transverse light line with the patient's OML).

- *Detecting poor OML alignment:* Poor OML alignment can be detected on a PA cranial or mandibular image by evaluating the relationship of the petrous ridges and supraorbital margin. If the patient's chin was not adequately tucked to bring the OML perpendicular to the IR, the petrous ridges are demonstrated inferior to the supraorbital margins, the internal acoustic meatus are obscured by the infraorbital margins, and the dorsum sellae and anterior clinoids are demonstrated within the ethmoid sinuses (see Image 2). If the patient's chin was tucked more than needed to bring the OML perpendicular to the IR, the petrous ridges are demonstrated superior to the supraorbital margins, the internal acoustic meatus are distorted, and the dorsum sellae and anterior clinoids are visualized more clearly superior to the ethmoid sinuses (see Images 3 and 4). When adjusting for poor OML alignment, adjust the patient's head the full distance demonstrated between the petrous ridges and supraorbital margins.

- *Trauma AP projection:* For a trauma AP projection of the cranium or mandible when a cervical vertebrae injury is not in question, adjust the patient's head as described for the PA projection. If a cervical vertebrae injury is suspected, do not adjust the patient's head position, or greater cervical injury may result. Instead, angle the central ray through the OML, as demonstrated in Figure 10-5. The angulation required varies according to the chin elevation provided by the cervical collar but is most often between 10 and 15 degrees caudad.

- *Correcting the central ray angulation for a trauma AP projection:* For the trauma AP projection, the central ray angulation determines the relationship of the petrous ridges and the supraorbital margins. For a trauma AP skull image that demonstrates poor supraorbital margin and petrous ridge superimposition, adjust the angulation in

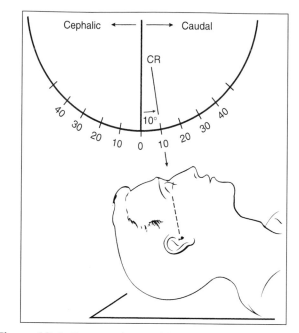

Figure 10-5. Proper patient positioning for anteroposterior cranial image. *CR*, central ray. *(Reproduced with permission from Martensen K: Trauma Skulls [In-Service Reviews in Radiologic Technology, vol 15, no 5], Birmingham, Ala, 1991, Educational Reviews.)*

the direction in which the orbits are to move. If the petrous ridges are demonstrated inferior to the supraorbital margins, the central ray was angled too cephalically and should be decreased (adjusted caudally) (see Images 5 and 6). If the petrous ridges are demonstrated superior to the supraorbital margins, the central ray was not angled cephalically enough and should be increased (see Image 7).

Mandible: **The bottom and top teeth are next to each other.**

- The bottom and top teeth are positioned next to each other when the patient's jaw is closed, with teeth and lips placed together. This places the mandible in a PA instead of a PA axial projection.
- *Patients who are unable to close jaw:* For patients who are unable to close the jaw for the PA projection, the mandible will be tilted (Image 6). For a PA projection of the mandible, the central ray should be angled cephalically until it is aligned with the palpable posterior mandibular rami.

The crista galli and nasal septum are aligned with the long axis of the IR, and the supraorbital margins and the temporomandibular joints (TMJs) are demonstrated on the same horizontal plane.

- Aligning the head's midsagittal plane with the long axis of the IR ensures that the cranium and mandible are demonstrated without tilting. Head tilting does not change any anatomical relationships for this position, although

severe tilting prevents tight collimation and makes viewing the image slightly more awkward.

Cranium: **The dorsum sellae is centered within the collimated field. The outer cranial cortex and the maxillary sinuses are included within the field.**

- Center a perpendicular central ray to the glabella (area located on the midsagittal plane at the level of the eyebrows) to place the dorsum sellae in the center of the collimated field and include the top of the cranium. Center the IR to the central ray.
- Open the longitudinal and transverse collimation to within $\frac{1}{2}$ inch (1.25 cm) of the head skinline, or use a circle diaphragm.
- A 10- × 12-inch (24- × 30-cm) IR placed lengthwise should be adequate to include all the required anatomical structures.

Mandible: **A point midway between the mandibular rami is centered within the collimated field. The entire mandible is included within the field.**

- Center a perpendicular central ray to exit the acanthion (junction of nose and upper lip). Center the IR to the central ray.
- Open the longitudinal collimation to include the patient's orbits and chin, and transversely collimate to within $\frac{1}{2}$ inch (1.25 cm) of the lateral skinline or use a circle diaphragm.
- An 8- × 10-inch (18- × 24-cm) IR placed lengthwise should be adequate to include all the required anatomical structures.

Posteroanterior or Anteroposterior Cranium and Mandible Image Analysis

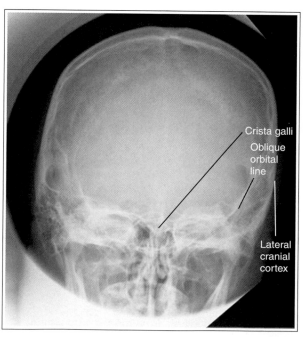

Image 1. PA projection skull.

Analysis. The distances from the lateral orbital margins to the lateral cranial cortices and from the crista galli to the lateral cranial cortex on the right side are greater than the same distances on the left side. The patient's face was rotated toward the left side.

Correction. Rotate the patient's face toward the right side until the midsagittal plane is aligned perpendicular to the IR.

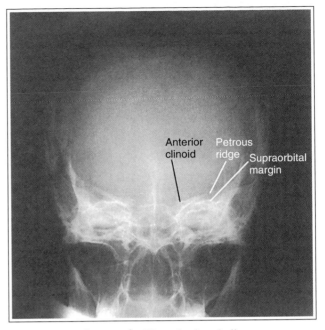

Image 3. PA projection skull.

Analysis. The petrous ridges are demonstrated superior to the supraorbital margins, and the internal acoustic meatus are obscured. The patient's chin was tucked more than needed to position the OML perpendicular to the IR.

Correction. Extend the chin, moving it away from the thorax until the OML is aligned perpendicular to the IR or move it half the distance demonstrated between the petrous ridges and supraorbital margins.

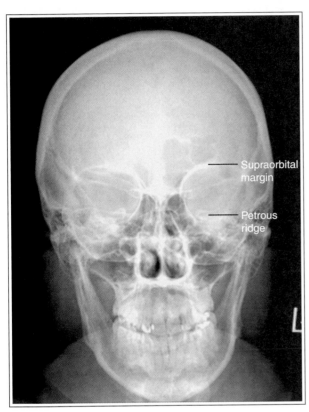

Image 2. PA projection skull.

Analysis. The petrous ridges are demonstrated inferior to the supraorbital margins, and the dorsum sellae and anterior clinoids are demonstrated within the ethmoid sinuses. The patient's chin was not tucked enough to position the OML perpendicular to the IR.

Correction. Tuck the chin until the OML is aligned perpendicular to the IR or move it half the distance demonstrated between the petrous ridges and supraorbital margins.

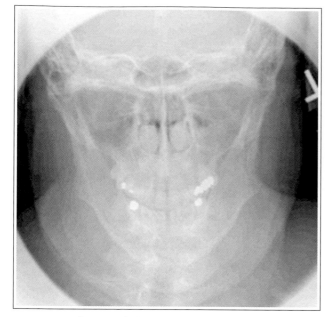

Image 4. PA projection mandible.

Analysis. The petrous ridges are demonstrated superior to the supraorbital margins, and the internal acoustic meatus are obscured. The patient's chin was tucked more than needed to position the OML perpendicular to the IR.

Correction. Extend the chin, moving it away from the thorax until the OML is aligned perpendicular to the IR or move it half the distance demonstrated between the petrous ridges and supraorbital margins.

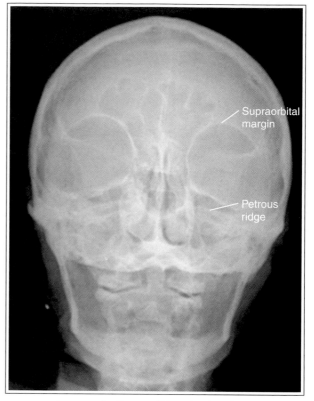

Image 5. Trauma AP projection skull.

Analysis. The petrous ridges are demonstrated inferior to the supraorbital margins, and the dorsum sellae and anterior clinoids are demonstrated within the ethmoid sinuses. The chin was not tucked enough to position the OML perpendicular to the IR, or the central ray was angled too cephalically.

Correction. The supraorbital margins need be moved toward the petrous ridges. To accomplish this, tuck the chin until the OML is aligned perpendicular to the IR or adjust the central ray angulation caudally. The amount of adjustment needed is approximately 5 degrees for every $\frac{1}{4}$ inch (0.6 cm) of distance demonstrated between the petrous ridges and the supraorbital margins.

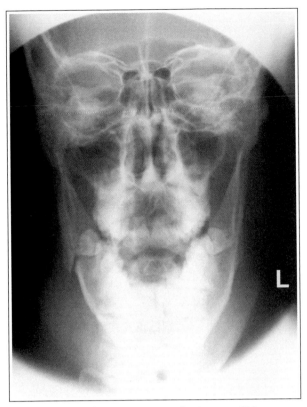

Image 6. Trauma AP projection mandible.

Analysis. The petrous ridges are demonstrated inferior to the supraorbital margins, the dorsum sellae and anterior clinoids are demonstrated within the ethmoid sinuses, and the mandible is elongated. The patient's chin was not tucked enough to position the OML perpendicular to the IR, or the central ray was not aligned parallel with the OML. The patient's jaw was not closed owing to a fracture.

Correction. If the patient is able, tuck the chin until the OML is perpendicular to the IR and close the patient's mouth. If the patient is unable to move, adjust the central ray angulation caudally until it is aligned parallel with the OML to best demonstrate the TMJ area. To best demonstrate the mandible when the jaw is open in an AP projection, angle the central ray cephalically until it is aligned with the posterior mandibular rami.

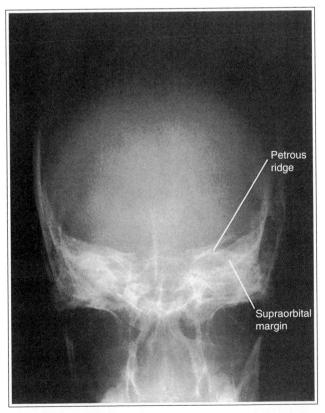

Petrous
ridge

Supraorbital
margin

Image 7. AP projection skull.

Analysis. The petrous ridges are demonstrated superior to the supraorbital margins. The chin was tucked more than needed to position the OML perpendicular to the IR, or the central ray was not angled cephalically enough to align it parallel with the OML.

Correction. The supraorbital margins need be moved toward the petrous ridges. To accomplish this, elevate the chin until the OML is aligned perpendicular to the IR, or adjust the central ray angulation cephalically until it is parallel with the OML.

CRANIUM, FACIAL BONES, AND SINUSES: POSTEROANTERIOR AXIAL PROJECTION (CALDWELL METHOD)

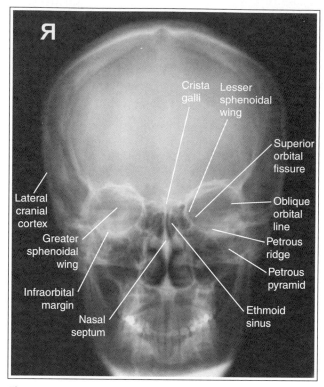

Figure 10-6. Posteroanterior axial (Caldwell) cranial image with accurate positioning.

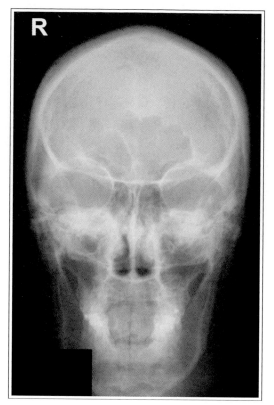

Figure 10-7. Anteroposterior axial (Caldwell) cranial image with accurate positioning.

Image Analysis

The cranium is demonstrated without rotation. The distances from the lateral orbital margins to the lateral cranial cortices on both sides and from the crista galli to the lateral cranial cortices on both sides are equal.

- A PA axial (Caldwell) projection of the cranium is obtained by positioning the patient in an upright or recumbent prone position with the nose and forehead resting against the upright IR holder or imaging table (Figure 10-8). Position the midsagittal plane perpendicular to the IR to prevent rotation.

- *Detecting rotation:* Head rotation is present on an AP axial (Caldwell) projection if the distance from the lateral orbital margin to the lateral cranial cortex on one side is greater than that on the other side and if the distance from the crista galli to the lateral cranial cortex is greater on one side than on the other side (Image 8). The patient's face was rotated away from the side demonstrating the greater distance.

- *Positioning for trauma AP axial (Caldwell) projection:* For the trauma AP axial (Caldwell) projection of the cranium, the patient is placed supine on the imaging table. If a cervical vertebral injury is suspected, do not adjust the patient's head rotation. Take the image with the head positioned as is. If a cervical vertebral injury is not in

question, adjust the patient's head until the midsagittal plane is perpendicular to the IR to prevent rotation.

- An AP axial (Caldwell) image should meet all the requirements listed for a PA (Caldwell) image, although some features of the cranium appear different. The AP projection demonstrates greater orbital magnification and less distance from the oblique orbital lines

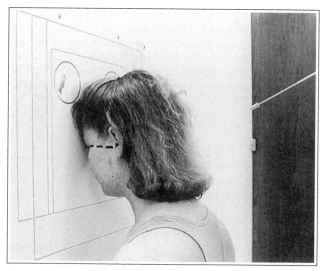

Figure 10-8. Proper patient positioning for posteroanterior axial (Caldwell) cranial image.

to the lateral cranial cortices than the PA projection. (Compare Figures 10-6 and 10-7.)

The petrous ridges are demonstrated horizontally through the lower third of the orbits, the petrous pyramids are superimposed over the infraorbital margins, and the superior orbital fissures are demonstrated within the orbits.

- Accurate petrous ridge and pyramid placement within the lowest third of the orbits is accomplished when the patient's chin is lowered or tucked toward the chest until the OML is aligned perpendicular to the IR. This positioning moves the frontal bone inferiorly until it is parallel with the IR and the orbits inferiorly until the supraorbital margins are situated beneath the petrous ridges, and places the pyramids and internal acoustic meatus within the orbits just as they are positioned for a PA skull projection.

- For the PA axial (Caldwell) projection, a 15-degree caudal central ray angulation is then used to align the central ray perpendicular to the frontal and ethmoid sinuses, orbital margins, superior orbital fissures, nasal septum, and anterior nasal spine. This angulation also projects the petrous ridges and pyramids inferiorly, onto the lowest third of the orbits.

- *Adjusting the central ray for poor OML alignment:* For a patient who is unable to tuck the chin adequately to position the OML perpendicular to the IR, the central ray angulation may be adjusted to compensate. Instruct the patient to tuck the chin to position the OML as close as possible to perpendicular to the IR. Angle the central ray parallel with the patient's OML (this is easily accomplished by aligning the collimator's transverse light line with the patient's OML). Then adjust the central ray 15 degrees caudally from the angle that resulted when the central ray was parallel with the OML.

- *Detecting poor OML–central ray alignment:* Poor OML–central ray alignment can be detected on the image by evaluating the relationship of the petrous ridges and the orbits. If the patient's chin was not adequately tucked to bring the OML perpendicular to the IR, or if the OML was adequately positioned but the central ray was angled more than 15 degrees caudally, the petrous ridges are demonstrated inferior to the infraorbital margins (see Image 9). If the patient's chin was tucked more than needed to bring the OML perpendicular to the IR, or if the OML was adequately positioned but the central ray was angled less than 15 degrees caudally, the petrous ridges and pyramids are demonstrated in the upper half of the orbits (see Image 10).

- *Central ray angulation for a trauma AP axial (Caldwell) projection:* For a trauma AP axial (Caldwell) projection of the cranium if no possibility of a cervical vertebrae injury exists, adjust the patient's head as described for the PA axial (Caldwell) projection. If a cervical vertebrae injury is suspected, do not adjust the patient's head position, or increased cervical injury may result.

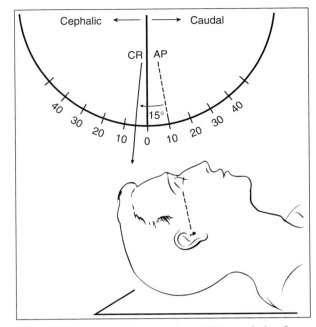

Figure 10-9. Determining central ray *(CR)* angulation for trauma anteroposterior axial (Caldwell) cranial image. *AP,* anteroposterior projection. *(Reproduced with permission from Martensen K:* Trauma Skulls *[In-Service Reviews in Radiologic Technology, vol 15, no 5], Birmingham, Ala, 1991, Educational Reviews.)*

Instead, begin by angling the central ray parallel with the OML, as demonstrated in Figure 10-9. The angulation required to do this varies according to the chin elevation provided by the cervical collar, but is most often between 10 and 15 degrees caudad. From this angulation, adjust the central ray 15 degrees cephalad (a cephalic angulation is used instead of a caudal angle because the patient is now in an AP projection) to align the angle 15 degrees from the OML, as demonstrated in Figure 10-9. For example, if a 10-degree caudal angle was needed to position the central ray parallel with the OML, a 5-degree cephalic angulation would be required for the AP axial (Caldwell) projection—15 degrees cephalad from the OML.

- *Correcting the central ray angulation for a trauma AP axial (Caldwell) projection:* For the trauma AP axial (Caldwell) projection, the central ray angulation determines the relationship of the petrous ridges and the orbits. For an AP axial (Caldwell) cranial image that demonstrates a poor petrous ridge and orbital relationship, adjust the central ray angulation in the direction in which you want the orbits to move. If the petrous ridges are demonstrated inferior to the infraorbital margins, the central ray was angled too cephalically and should be decreased. (The petrous ridge and orbital relationship obtained would be similar to that shown in Image 9.) If the petrous ridges are demonstrated in the superior half of the orbits, the central ray was not angled cephalically enough and should be increased. (The petrous ridge and orbital relationship obtained would be similar to that shown in Image 10.)

The crista galli and nasal septum are aligned with the long axis of the IR, and the supraorbital margins are demonstrated on the same horizontal plane.

- Aligning the head's midsagittal plane with the long axis of the IR ensures that the patient's cranium is demonstrated without tilting. Slight tilting does not change any anatomical relationships for this position, although it does prevent tight collimation and makes viewing the image slightly more awkward.

Cranium: **The ethmoid sinuses are centered within the collimated field. The outer cranial cortex and the ethmoid sinuses are included within the field.**

- Centering a 15-degree caudally angled central ray to exit at the nasion (depression at the bridge of the nose) places the ethmoid sinuses in the center of the collimated field. A slightly higher centering may be needed if the entire cranial cortex is required on the image. Center the IR to the central ray.
- Open the longitudinal and transverse collimation to within ½ inch (1.25 cm) of the head skinline, or use a circle diaphragm, for an image of the cranium.
- An 8- × 10-inch (18- × 24-cm) IR placed lengthwise is sufficient when facial bones and sinuses are imaged.

Facial bones and sinuses: **The ethmoid sinuses are centered within the collimated field. The frontal and ethmoid sinuses and the lateral cranial cortices are included within the field.**

- Centering a 15-degree caudally angled central ray to exit at the nasion, places the ethmoid sinuses in the center of the collimated field. A slightly higher centering may be needed if the entire cranial cortex is required on the image. Center the IR to the central ray.
- Open the longitudinal and transverse collimation to within 1 inch (2.5 cm) of the sinus cavities, or use a circle diaphragm, for an image of the facial bones or sinuses.
- A 10- × 12-inch (24- × 30-cm) IR placed lengthwise should be adequate to include all required anatomical structures when the cranium is imaged.

Posteroanterior Axial Cranium, Facial Bone, and Sinus Image Analysis

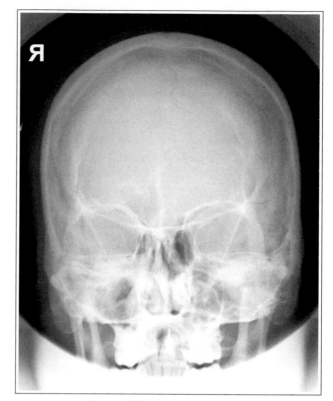

Image 8. PA axial projection.

Analysis. The distances from the lateral orbital margins to the lateral cranial cortices and from the crista galli to the lateral cranial cortex are greater on the left side than on the right side. The patient's face was rotated toward the right side. The petrous ridges are demonstrated inferior to the infraorbital margins. The patient's chin was not tucked enough to position the OML perpendicular to the IR.

Correction. Rotate the patient's face toward the left side, and tuck the chin to bring the OML perpendicular to the IR.

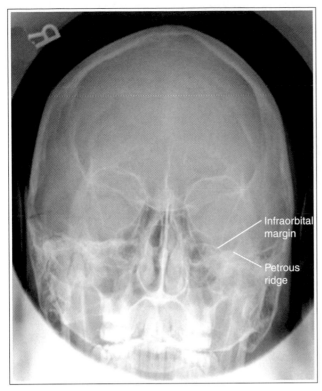

Image 9. Trauma AP axial projection.

Analysis. The petrous ridges are demonstrated inferior to the infraorbital margins. The patient's chin was not tucked enough to position the OML perpendicular to the IR, or the central ray was angled too cephalically.

Correction. The infraorbital margins need to be moved toward the petrous ridges. To accomplish this, tuck the chin until the OML is aligned perpendicular to the IR, or adjust the central ray angulation caudally. The amount of adjustment needed is approximately 5 degrees for every ¼ inch (0.6 cm) of distance demonstrated between where the petrous ridges are and where they should be on a PA axial (Caldwell) projection image with accurate positioning.

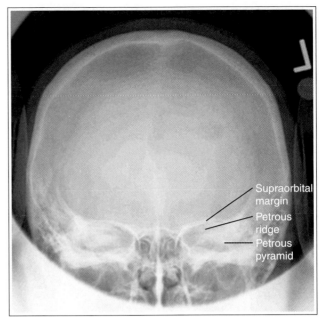

Image 10. Trauma AP axial projection.

Analysis. The petrous ridges and pyramids are demonstrated in the superior half of the orbits. The patient's chin was tucked more than needed to position the OML perpendicular to the IR, or the central ray was angled more caudally.

Correction. Elevate the chin until the OML is perpendicular to the IR, or adjust the central ray angulation cephalically.

CRANIUM, MANDIBLE, AND PETROMASTOID PORTION: ANTEROPOSTERIOR AXIAL PROJECTION (TOWNE METHOD)

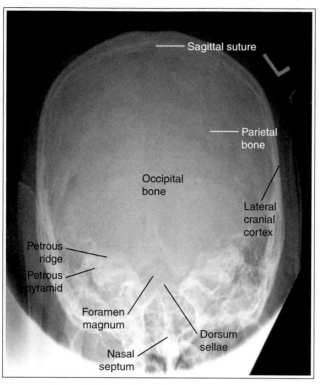

Figure 10-10. Anteroposterior axial (Towne) cranial and mastoid image with accurate positioning.

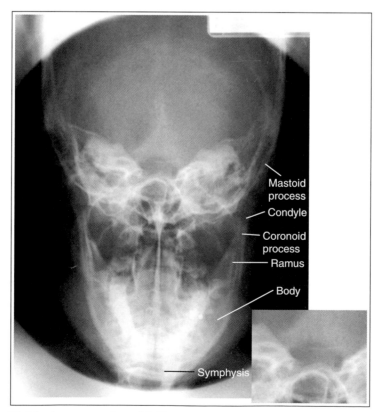

Figure 10-11. Anteroposterior axial (Towne) mandible image with accurate positioning.

Image Analysis

The cranium is demonstrated without rotation. The distances from the posterior clinoid process to the lateral borders of the foramen magnum on both sides and the mandibular necks to the lateral cervical vertebrae on both sides are equal, the petrous ridges are symmetrical, and the dorsum sellae is centered within the foramen magnum.

- An AP axial (Towne) projection of the cranium, petro-mastoid portion, or mandible is obtained by positioning the patient in an upright AP projection or supine position with the posterior head resting against the upright IR holder or imaging table (Figure 10-12). Position the midsagittal plane perpendicular to the IR to prevent cranial rotation. The best method of accomplishing this goal is to place an extended flat palm next to each lateral parietal bone and then to adjust patient head rotation until your hands are perpendicular to the IR and parallel with each other.

- *Detecting head rotation:* Head rotation was present on an AP axial (Towne) image if the distance from the posterior clinoid process and dorsum sellae to the lateral border of the foramen magnum is greater on one side and the distance from the mandibular neck to the cervical vertebrae is greater on one side than on the other side. The patient's face was rotated toward the side demonstrating the least distance from the posterior clinoid process and dorsum sellae to the lateral foramen magnum (Image 11) and from the mandibular neck to the cervical vertebrae.

- *Positioning for trauma:* For a trauma AP axial (Towne) projection of the cranium and mandible, the patient is positioned supine on the imaging table. If a cervical

vertebral injury is suspected, do not adjust the patient's head rotation. Take the image with the head positioned as is. If no possibility of a cervical vertebral injury exists, adjust the patient's head until the midsagittal plane is positioned perpendicular to the IR, to prevent rotation.

Cranium and petromastoid portion: **The dorsum sellae and posterior clinoids are demonstrated within the foramen magnum without foreshortening or superimposition of the atlas's posterior arch.**

Mandible: **The dorsum sellae and posterior clinoids are at the level of the superior foramen magnum. The mandibular condyles and fossae are clearly demonstrated, with minimal mastoid superimposition.**

- A combination of patient positioning and central ray angulation accurately demonstrates the dorsum sellae and posterior clinoids within the foramen magnum. To accomplish proper patient positioning, tuck the chin until the OML is aligned perpendicular to the IR. This positioning aligns an imaginary line connecting the dorsum sellae and foramen magnum at a 30-degree angle with the IR and the OML.

- *Cranium and petromastoid portion:* The central ray needs to be aligned parallel with the OML to project the dorsum sellae into the foramen magnum. This explains the need for a 30-degree caudal angulation for the AP axial (Towne) projection of the cranium and mastoid.

- *Mandible:* To position the dorsum sellae at the level of the superior foramen magnum and align the central ray with the TMJs, a 35- to 40-degree caudal angulation is used for the AP axial projection of the mandible.

- *Poor OML alignment:* If a patient tucked the chin more than needed to position the OML perpendicular to the IR, the dorsum sellae will be demonstrated superior to the foramen magnum (Images 12 and 13). If the patient tucked the chin less than needed to align the OML perpendicular to the IR, the dorsum sellae will be foreshortened and will be superimposed over the atlas's posterior arch (Image 14).

- *Adjusting for poor OML alignment and determining central ray angulation for trauma patients:* In a patient who is unable to tuck the chin adequately to position the OML perpendicular to the IR because of cervical trauma or stiffness, the central ray angulation may be adjusted to compensate. If the patient is able to place the infraorbitomeatal line (IOML) perpendicular to the IR, use a 37-degree caudal angle. If the patient is unable to tuck until the IOML or OML is perpendicular, instruct the patient to tuck the chin to position the OML as close as possible to perpendicular to the IR. Angle the central ray parallel with the OML (easily accomplished by aligning the collimator's transverse light line with the patient's OML), then adjust the central ray 30 degrees caudally from the angle obtained when the central ray was parallel with the OML to obtain an AP axial cranium and mastoid image (Figure 10-13), and 35 to 40 degrees

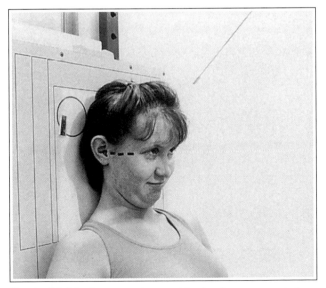

Figure 10-12. Proper patient positioning for anteroposterior axial (Towne) cranial image.

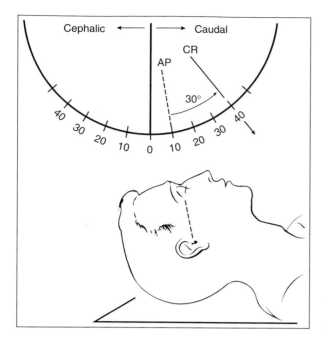

Figure 10-13. Determine central ray *(CR)* angulation for anteroposterior axial cranial image in a trauma patient. *AP,* Anteroposterior projection. *(Reproduced with permission from Martensen K:* Trauma Skulls. *[In-Service Reviews in Radiologic Technology, vol 15, no 5.] Birmingham, AL: Educational Reviews, 1991.)*

caudally from the angle obtained to obtain an AP axial mandible image. The angle used for this projection should not exceed 45 degrees, or excessive distortion will result.

The sagittal suture and nasal septum are aligned with the long axis of the collimated field.

- Aligning the head's midsagittal plane with the long axis of the collimator's longitudinal light line ensures that the patient's cranium is demonstrated without tilting. Head tilting changes the alignment of the central ray, dorsum sellae, and foramen magnum by positioning the dorsum sellae laterally to the central ray and foramen magnum.

Cranium and petromastoid portion: **The inferior occipital bone is centered within the collimated field. The outer cranial cortex, petrous ridges, dorsum sellae, and foramen magnum are included within the field.**

- Center the central ray to the midsagittal plane at a level 2½ inches (6 cm) above the glabella. Center the IR to the central ray.
- Open the longitudinally and transversely collimated field to within ½ inch (1.25 cm) of the head skinline, or use a circle diaphragm.
- A 10- × 12-inch (24- × 30-cm) IR placed lengthwise should be adequate to include all the required anatomical structures.

Mandible: **A point midway between the mandibular rami is centered within the collimated field. The entire mandible and temporomandibular fossae are included within the field.**

- Center the central ray to the midsagittal plane at the level of the glabella. Center the IR to the central ray.
- Open the longitudinally and transversely collimated field to within ½ inch (1.25 cm) of the head skinline, or use a circle diaphragm.
- An 8- × 10-inch (18- × 24-cm) IR placed lengthwise should be adequate to include all the required anatomical structures.

Anteroposterior Axial Cranium, Mandible, and Petromastoid Portion Image Analysis

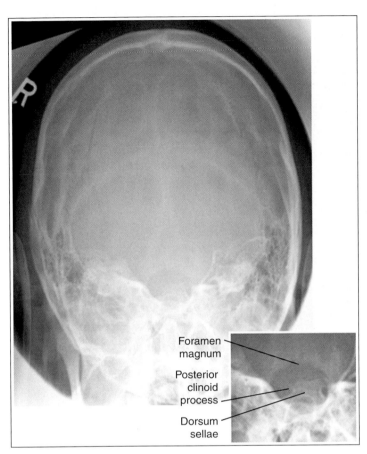

Foramen magnum

Posterior clinoid process

Dorsum sellae

Image 11.

Analysis. The distance from the posterior clinoid process to the lateral foramen magnum is less on the patient's left side than on the right side. The patient's face was rotated toward the left side.

Correction. Rotate the patient's face toward the right side until the midsagittal plane is perpendicular to the IR.

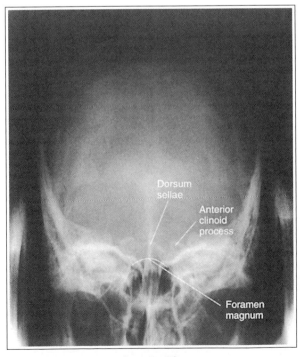

Dorsum sellae

Anterior clinoid process

Foramen magnum

Image 12.

Analysis. The dorsum sellae and anterior clinoids are demonstrated superior to the foramen magnum. Either the patient's chin was not tucked enough or the central ray was not angled caudally enough to form a 30-degree angle with the OML.

Correction. Tuck the patient's chin until the OML is perpendicular to the IR. The amount of movement needed is the full distance demonstrated between where the foramen magnum is located and where it should be located on an AP axial (Towne) projection with accurate positioning. If the patient is unable to tuck the chin any further, leave the patient's chin positioned as is, and angle the central ray caudally approximately 5 degrees for every ¼ inch (0.6 cm) of distance demonstrated between where the foramen magnum is located on this image and where it should be on an AP axial (Towne) projection with accurate positioning.

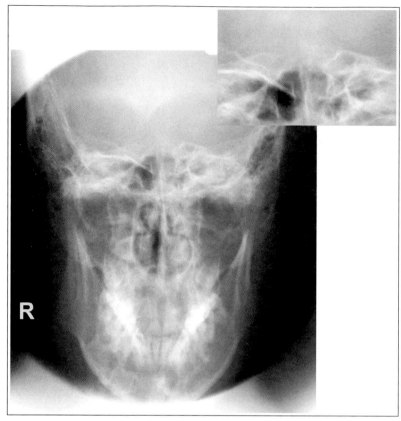

Image 13.

Analysis. The dorsum sellae and anterior clinoids are demonstrated superior to the foramen magnum. Either the patient's chin was not tucked enough or the central ray was not angled cephalically enough to form a 30-degree angle with the OML.

Correction. Tuck the patient's chin until the OML is perpendicular to the IR. The amount of movement needed is the full distance demonstrated between where the foramen magnum is located and where it should be located on an AP axial (Towne) projection with accurate positioning. If the patient is unable to tuck the chin any further, leave the patient's chin positioned as is and adjust the central ray angulation caudally.

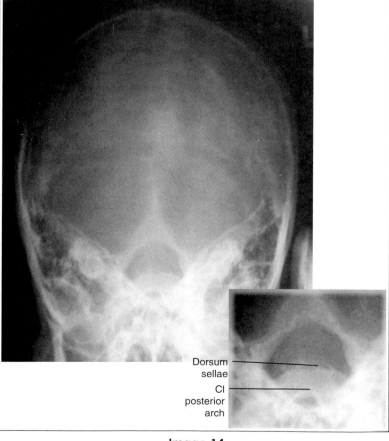

Dorsum sellae
CI posterior arch

Image 14.

Analysis. The dorsum sellae is foreshortened and is superimposed over the atlas's posterior arch. Either the patient's chin was tucked more than needed to bring the OML perpendicular to the IR or the central ray was angled more caudally than needed to form a 30-degree angle with the OML.

Correction. Elevate the patient's chin until the OML is perpendicular to the IR. The amount of movement needed is the full distance needed to position the posterior arch inferior to the dorsum sellae. If the patient is unable to tuck the chin any further, angle the central ray cephalically approximately 5 degrees for every $1/4$ inch (0.6 cm) of the posterior arch that is demonstrated.

CRANIUM, FACIAL BONES, NASAL BONES, AND SINUSES: LATERAL POSITION

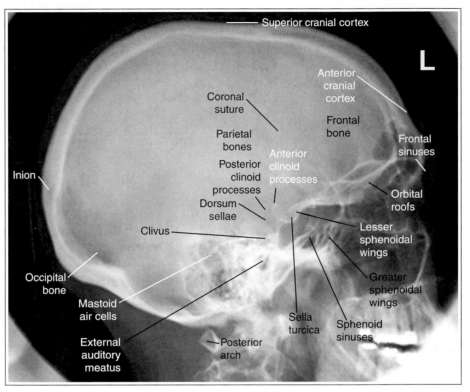

Figure 10-14. Lateral cranial image with accurate positioning.

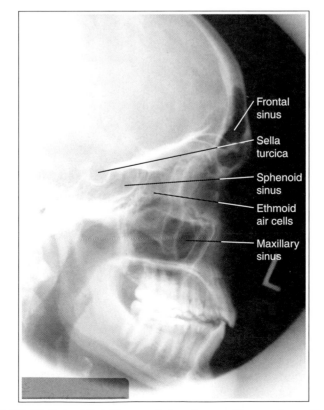

Figure 10-15. Lateral facial bone and sinus image with accurate positioning.

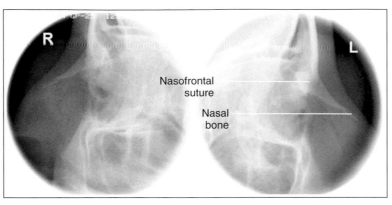

Figure 10-16. Lateral nasal bone image with accurate positioning.

Image Analysis

The cranium, facial bones, sinuses, and nasal bones are in a lateral position. When visualized the sella turcica is demonstrated in profile, and the orbital roofs, mandibular rami, greater wings of the sphenoid, external acoustic canals, zygomatic bones, and cranial cortices are superimposed.

- Achieve a lateral position of the cranium, facial bones, sinuses, and nasal bones by placing the patient in an upright PA projection or recumbent prone position with the affected side of the head against the upright IR holder or imaging table.

- To demonstrate air-fluid levels within the sinus cavities, this projection should be taken in an upright position. In this position the thick, gelatin-like sinus fluid settles to the lowest position, creating an air-fluid line that shows the reviewer the amount of fluid present.

- Rotate the patient's head and body as needed to place the head in a lateral position, with the head's midsagittal plane parallel with the IR and the interpupillary line (IPL—an imaginary line connecting the outer corners of the eyelids) perpendicular to the IR (Figure 10-17). It may be necessary to position a sponge beneath the patient's chin or head to help maintain precise positioning.

- *Positioning for trauma:* A trauma lateral cranial image is accomplished by placing a crosswise IR vertically against the patient's lateral cranium and directing a horizontal beam to a point 2 inches (5 cm) superior to the external acoustic meatus (EAM). For a patient whose head position can be manipulated, elevate the occiput on a radiolucent sponge and adjust the head until the midsagittal plane is parallel with the IR. If a cervical vertebral injury is suspected, do not adjust the patient's head; take the image with the head positioned as is, and position the IR 1 inch (2.5 cm) below the occipital bone.

- *Detecting rotation:* Accurate positioning of the head's midsagittal plane is essential to prevent rotation and tilting of the cranium, facial bones, sinuses, and nasal bones. If the patient's head was not adequately turned to position the midsagittal plane parallel with the IR,

rotation results. Rotation causes distortion of the sella turcica and situates one of the mandibular rami, greater wings of the sphenoid, external acoustic canals, zygomatic bones, and anterior cranial cortices anterior to the other on a lateral image (see Image 15). Because the two sides of the cranium are mirror images, it is very difficult to determine which way the face was rotated when studying lateral images with poor positioning. Paying close attention to initial positioning may give you an idea as to which way the patient has a tendency to lean. Routinely patients tend to rotate their faces and lean the tops of their heads toward the IR.

- *Distinguishing tilting from rotation:* If the patient's head was tilted toward or away from the IR, preventing the midsagittal plane from aligning parallel with the IR or the IPL from aligning perpendicular to the IR, tilting of the cranium, facial bones, sinuses, and nasal bones results. Tilting can be distinguished from rotation on lateral images by studying the superimposition of the orbital roofs, the greater wings of the sphenoid, the external

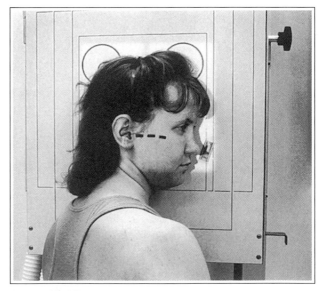

Figure 10-17. Proper patient positioning for lateral cranial image.

acoustic canals, the zygomatic bones, and the inferior cranial cortices. If the patient's head was tilted, one of each corresponding structure is demonstrated superior to the other. The direction of the head tilt, toward or away from the IR, can be determined by evaluating the degree of atlas (C1) vertebral foramen visualization. If the top of the head is tilted toward the IR, the foramen will not be visualized, and if the tip of the head is tilted away from the IR, the foramen will be seen (see Image 16).

Cranium: **The posteroinferior occipital bone and posterior arch of the atlas are free of superimposition.**

- Adjusting the chin to bring the IOML perpendicular to the front edge of the IR positions the posteroinferior cranium superior to the posterior arch of the atlas, preventing their superimposition.

Cranium: **An area 2 inches (5 cm) superior to the EAM is centered within the collimated field. The outer cranial cortex is included within the field.**

- Centering a perpendicular central ray to a point 2 inches (5 cm) superior to the EAM positions the cranium in the center of the collimated field.
- Open the longitudinally and transversely collimated field to within ½ inch (1.25 cm) of the patient's head skinline, or use a circle diaphragm.
- A 10- × 12-inch (24- × 30-cm) IR placed crosswise should be adequate to include all the required anatomical structures.

Facial bones and sinuses: **The zygoma and greater wings of the sphenoid are centered within the collimated field. Included within the field are the frontal, ethmoid, sphenoid, and maxillary sinuses, greater wings of the sphenoid, orbital roofs, sella turcica, zygoma, and mandible.**

- Centering a perpendicular central ray to the zygoma (midway between the outer canthus and EAM) positions the zygoma and greater wings of the sphenoid in the center of the collimated field. Center the IR to the central ray.
- Open the longitudinally and transversely collimated field to include the mandible and frontal sinuses and transversely collimate to within ½ inch (1.25 cm) of the anterior skinline or use a circle diaphragm.
- An 8- × 10-inch (18- × 24-cm) IR placed lengthwise should be adequate to include all the required anatomical structures.

Nasal bones: **The nasal bones are centered within the collimated field. Included within the field are the nasal bones, with surrounding soft tissue, anterior nasal**

spine of maxilla, **and the most anterior aspects of the cranial cortices, orbital roofs, and zygomatic bones.**

- Center a perpendicular central ray ½ inch (1.25 cm) inferior to the nasion to center the nasal bones to the center of the collimated field. Center the IR to the central ray.
- Open the longitudinal field to include the frontal sinuses and transversely collimated field to within ½ inch (1.25 cm) of the nose skinline or use a small circle diaphragm.
- An 8- × 10-inch (18- × 24-cm) detailed screen-film or computed radiography IR placed lengthwise should be adequate to include all the required anatomical structures. A small focal spot will increase detail sharpness. Both right and left lateral images of the nasal bones are routinely requested.

Lateral Cranium, Facial Bone, Sinus, and Nasal Bone Image Analysis

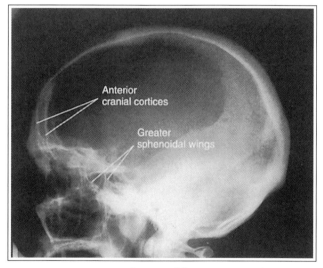

Image 15.

Analysis. The greater wings of the sphenoid and the anterior cranial cortices are demonstrated without superimposition. One of each corresponding structure is demonstrated anterior to the other. The patient's head was rotated.

Correction. Position the cranium's midsagittal plane parallel with the IR.

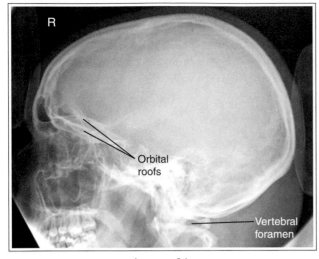

Image 16.

Analysis. The orbital roofs, the EAM, and the inferior cranial cortices are demonstrated without superimposition. One of each corresponding structure is demonstrated superior to the other and the atlas vertebral foramen is visualized. The patient's head was tilted away from the IR.

Correction. Tilt the top of the head toward the IR until the cranium's midsagittal plane is parallel with the IR and the IPL is perpendicular to the IR.

CRANIUM, MANDIBLE, AND SINUSES: SUBMENTOVERTEX PROJECTION (SCHUELLER METHOD)

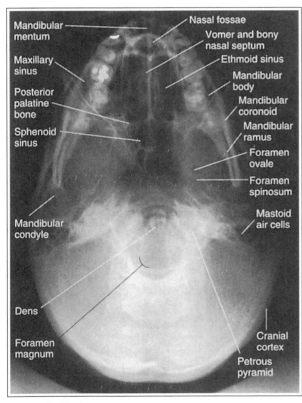

Figure 10-18. Submentovertex (Schueller) cranial image with accurate positioning.

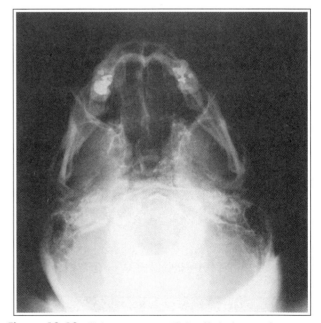

Figure 10-19. Submentovertex (Schueller) sinus and mandible image with accurate positioning.

Image Analysis

The mandibular mentum and nasal fossae are demonstrated just anterior to the ethmoid sinuses.

- The SMV projection (Schueller position) is accomplished by placing the patient in an upright AP projection with the cranial vertex resting against the upright IR holder or imaging table. Continue to elevate the chin and hyperextend the patient's neck until the IOML is parallel to the upright IR holder or imaging table (Figure 10-20). For a patient with a retracted jaw, it may be necessary to raise the chin and extend the patient's neck beyond the IOML to position the mandibular mentum anterior to the frontal bone.
- If the patient is unable to align the IOML parallel with the imaging table, extend the patient's neck as far as possible, and angle the central ray cephalad until it is aligned perpendicular to the IOML.
- ***Effect of mispositioning IOML:*** Mispositioning of the mandibular mentum and ethmoid sinuses on an SMV (Schueller) position obscures the nasal fossae, ethmoid sinuses, and foramen ovale and spinosum. If the patient's neck was overextended, the mandibular mentum is demonstrated too far anterior to the ethmoid sinuses (see Image 17). If the patient's neck was underextended, the mandibular mentum is demonstrated posterior to the ethmoid sinuses (see Image 18).

The distances from the mandibular ramus and body to the lateral cranial cortex on both sides are equal.

- Positioning the cranium's midsagittal plane perpendicular to the IR prevents cranial tilting.
- ***Detecting head tilting:*** Cranial tilting can be identified on an SMV projection of the head by comparing the distances from the mandibular ramus and body with the distance to the corresponding lateral cranial cortex

on either side. If the head was not tilted, the distances are equal. If the head was tilted the distance is greater on the side toward which the cranial vertex was tilted (see Image 19).

The vomer, bony nasal septum, and dens are aligned with the long axis of the collimated field.

- Turning the patient's face until the midsagittal plane is aligned with the long axis of the collimator's longitudinal light line ensures that the patient's head is not rotated. Rotation does not change any anatomical relationships for this position, although it does prevent tight collimation and makes viewing of the image slightly more awkward.

Cranium: **The dens is centered within the collimated field. The mandible and the outer cranial cortices are included within the field.**

- Centering a perpendicular central ray to the midsagittal plane (midway between the mandibular angles), ¾ inch (2 cm) anterior to the level of the EAM places the dens in the center of the collimated field. Center the IR to the central ray.
- Open the longitudinally and transversely collimated field to within ½ inch (1.25 cm) of the patient's lateral head skinline and mandibular mentum, or use a circle diaphragm.
- A 10- × 12-inch (24- × 30-cm) IR placed lengthwise should be adequate to include all the required anatomical structures.

Sinuses and mandible: **The sphenoid sinuses are centered within the collimated field. The mandible, lateral cranial cortices, and mastoid air cells are included within the field.**

- Centering a perpendicular central ray to the midsagittal plane at a level 1½ to 2 inches (4 to 5 cm) inferior to the mandibular symphysis places the ethmoid sinuses in the center of the collimated field.
- Open the longitudinally and transversely collimated field to within ½ inch (1.25 cm) of the patient's lateral head skinline and mandibular symphysis, or use a circle diaphragm.
- An 8- × 10-inch (18- × 24-cm) IR placed lengthwise should be adequate to include all the required anatomical structures.

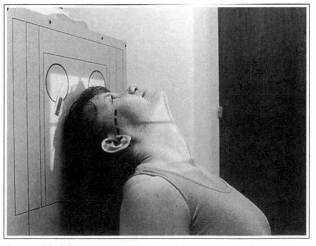

Figure 10-20. Proper patient positioning for submentovertex (Schueller) cranial image.

Submentovertex Cranium, Sinus, and Mandible Image Analysis

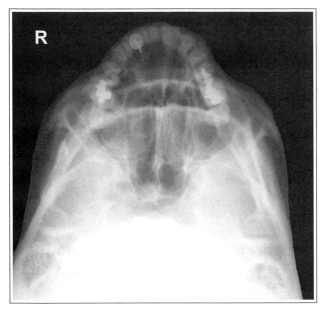

Image 17.

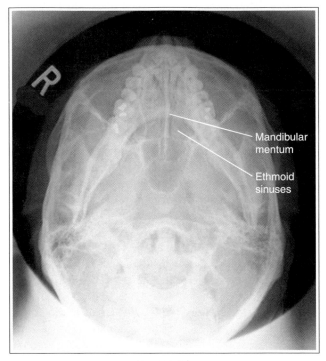

Image 18.

Analysis. The mandibular mentum is demonstrated too far anterior to the ethmoid sinuses. The patient's neck was overextended, preventing the IOML from being positioned parallel with the IR. If the central ray was angled to accomplish this image, it was angled too cephalically.

Correction. Depress the patient's chin until the IOML is aligned parallel with the IR. The amount of movement needed is half the distance demonstrated between the mandibular mentum and the ethmoid sinuses. If the central ray was angled, adjust the angulation 5 degrees caudally for every $\frac{1}{4}$ inch (0.6 cm) of distance demonstrated between the mandibular mentum and anterior ethmoid sinuses.

Analysis. The mandibular mentum is demonstrated posterior to the ethmoid sinuses. The patient's neck was underextended, preventing the IOML from being positioned parallel with the IR.

Correction. Elevate the patient's chin until the IOML is aligned parallel with the IR. The amount of movement needed is half the distance demonstrated between the mandibular mentum and the ethmoid sinuses. If the patient is unable to elevate the chin or hyperextend the neck any further, leave the position as is and angle the central ray cephalad either until it is perpendicular to the IOML or 5 degrees cephalad for every $\frac{1}{4}$ inch (0.6 cm) of distance demonstrated between the mandibular mentum and the anterior ethmoid sinuses.

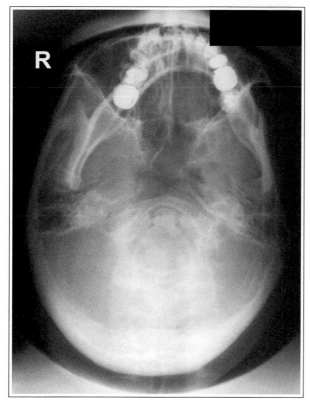

Image 19.

Analysis. The distance from the right mandibular ramus and body to its corresponding lateral cranial cortex is greater than the distance from the left mandibular ramus and body to its corresponding lateral cranial cortex. The patient's cranial vertex was tilted toward the right side.

Correction. Tilt the patient's cranial vertex toward the left side until the cranium's midsagittal plane is perpendicular to the IR.

FACIAL BONES AND SINUSES: PARIETOACANTHIAL AND ACANTHIOPARIETAL PROJECTION (WATERS AND OPEN-MOUTH METHODS)

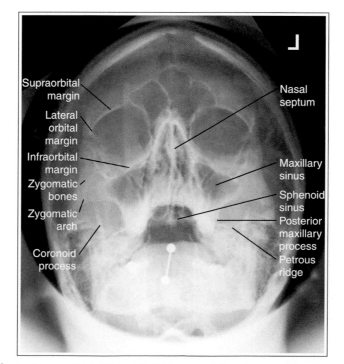

Figure 10-21. Parietoacanthial (Waters) facial bone and sinus image with accurate positioning.

Image Analysis

The cranium is demonstrated without rotation. The distances from the lateral orbital margin to the lateral cranial cortex and the distance from the bony nasal septum to the lateral cranial cortex on both sides are equal.

- The parietoacanthial (Waters) projection of the cranium is obtained by positioning the patient in an upright or recumbent prone position with the neck extended and the chin resting against the upright IR holder or imaging table (Figure 10-22).

- To demonstrate air-fluid levels within the maxillary sinus cavities, this projection should be taken with the patient in an upright position. The thick, gelatin-like sinus fluid then settles to the lowest level in the sinus cavity, creating an air-fluid line that shows the reviewer the amount of fluid present.

- To prevent cranial rotation, position an extended flat palm next to each lateral parietal bone. Then adjust the head rotation until your hands are perpendicular to the IR and parallel with each other.

- *Detecting head rotation:* Head rotation is present on a parietoacanthial (Waters) projection if the distance from the lateral orbital margin to the lateral cranial cortex on one side is greater than on the other side and if the distance from the bony nasal septum to the lateral cranial cortex on one side is greater than on the other side (see Image 20). The patient's face was rotated away from the side demonstrating the greater distance.

- *Positioning for trauma acanthioparietal (Waters) projection:* For the trauma acanthioparietal (Waters) projection of the cranium, the patient is supine on the imaging table. If a cervical vertebral injury is suspected, do not adjust the patient's head rotation, but take the image with the head positioned as is. If a cervical vertebral injury is not in question, adjust the patient's head to prevent rotation. An acanthioparietal projection image should meet all the requirements listed for a parietoacanthial projection image, although some features of the cranium appear different. The acanthioparietal projection demonstrates greater orbital magnification and less distance from the lateral orbital margin to the lateral cranial cortices than does the parietoacanthial projection (compare Figure 10-21 and Image 23). These differences result from greater magnification of the anatomy situated farther from the IR. With the acanthioparietal projection the orbits are situated farther from the IR than the parietal bones, whereas in the parietoacanthial projection, the parietal bones are positioned farther from the IR.

The petrous ridges are demonstrated inferior to the maxillary sinuses and extend laterally from the posterior maxillary alveolar process.

- To accurately position the petrous ridges inferior to the maxillary sinuses, elevate the patient's chin until the OML is at a 37-degree angle with IR. Chin elevation moves the maxillary sinuses superior to the petrous ridges. This is best accomplished by positioning the mentomeatal line (MML—imaginary line connecting the chin with the external ear opening) perpendicular to the IR. If an open-mouth Waters position is required, do not have patient drop jaw until *after* the MML has been positioned perpendicular to the IR (Figure 10-23).

- *Adjusting the central ray for poor MML alignment:* For a patient who is unable to elevate the chin adequately to position the MML perpendicular to the IR, the central ray may be adjusted to compensate. Instruct the patient to elevate the chin to position the MML as close as possible to perpendicular to the IR. Then angle the central ray until it is parallel with the MML. This method should not be

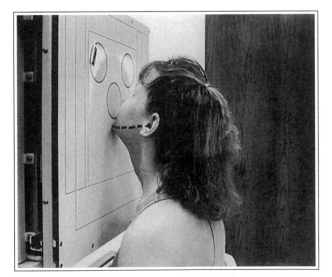

Figure 10-22. Proper patient positioning for parietoacanthial (Waters) facial bone and sinus image.

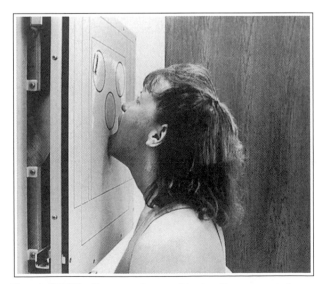

Figure 10-23. Proper patient positioning for open-mouth parietoacanthial (Waters) sinus image.

used if the maxillary sinuses are being evaluated for air-fluid levels. *Unless the central ray remains horizontal, the air-fluid level is obscured or appears higher.*

- **Detecting poor MML positioning:** Poor MML positioning can be detected by evaluating the position of the petrous ridges and posterior maxillary alveolar process. If the patient's chin was not adequately elevated to bring the MML perpendicular to the IR, the petrous ridges are demonstrated superior to the posterior maxillary alveolar process superimposing the maxillary sinuses (see Images 20 and 21). If the patient's chin was elevated more than needed to position the MML perpendicular to the IR, the petrous ridges are demonstrated inferior to the maxillary sinuses and posterior maxillary alveolar process, and the maxillary sinuses are superimposed over the posterior molars and alveolar process (see Image 22).

- **Central ray angulation for acanthioparietal projection:** For the acanthioparietal projection of the cranium, if a cervical vertebrae injury is not suspected, adjust the patient's head as described for the parietoacanthial projection. If a cervical vertebrae injury is suspected, do not adjust the patient's head position or increased cervical injury might result. Instead, angle the central ray cephalically until it is aligned parallel with the MML. If the MML is difficult to use or if the patient's mouth is open, the central ray may also be adjusted 37 degrees cephalically from the OML to obtain identical anatomical relationships (Figure 10-24).

- **Correcting the central ray angulation for a trauma acanthioparietal projection:** For the trauma acanthioparietal projection, the central ray angulation determines the relationship of the petrous ridges to the maxillary sinuses and posterior maxillary alveolar process. For an acanthioparietal image that demonstrates poor petrous ridge positioning, adjust the central ray angulation in the direction in which you want the maxillary sinuses and posterior maxillary alveolar process to move. Because they are situated farther from the IR than the maxillary sinuses, their position is most affected by an angulation change. If the petrous ridges are demonstrated within the maxillary sinuses and superior to the posterior maxillary alveolar process, the central ray was angled too caudally (see Image 23). If the petrous ridges are demonstrated inferior to the maxillary sinuses and posterior maxillary alveolar process, and the posterior molars and maxillary alveolar process are superimposed over the maxillary sinuses, the central ray was angled too cephalically. (The petrous ridge and posterior maxillary alveolar relationship would be similar to that shown in Image 22.)

- **Modified Waters method:** A modified Waters method is used to position the orbital floors perpendicular to the IR and parallel to the central ray for increased demonstration of the orbital floors—a modified Waters method. This examination is commonly obtained to rule out fractures of the orbits and demonstrate foreign bodies in the eyes. The modified Waters method is accomplished by positioning the patient as described for the Waters method, with one exception: The patient's chin is elevated only until the OML is at a 55-degree angle with the IR. In this position the petrous ridges will be demonstrated within the maxillary sinuses rather than inferior to them (Figure 10-25).

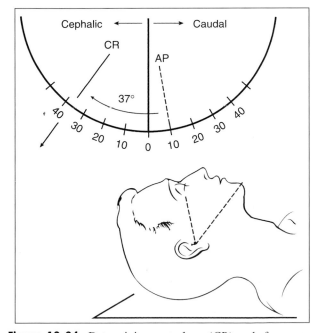

Figure 10-24. Determining central ray *(CR)* angle for acanthioparietal (Waters) facial bone and sinus image in a trauma patient. *AP,* Anteroposterior projection.

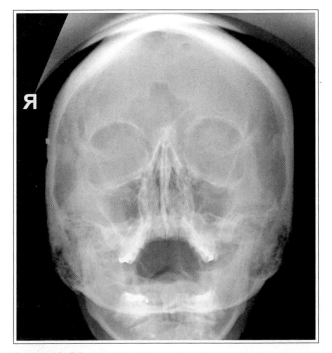

Figure 10-25. Modified Waters facial bone and sinus image with accurate positioning.

The bony nasal septum is aligned with the long axis of the collimated field, and the infraorbital margins are demonstrated on the same horizontal plane.

- Aligning the cranium's midsagittal plane with the collimator's longitudinal light line controls tilting of the patient's head. Tilting does not change any anatomical relationships for this projection, but it does prevent tight collimation and makes viewing the image slightly more awkward.

The anterior nasal spine is at the center of the collimated field. The frontal and maxillary (and sphenoid on the open-mouth position) sinuses and the lateral cranial cortices are included within the field.

- Centering a perpendicular central ray to the acanthion (area located at the midsagittal plane where the nose and upper lip meet) places the anterior nasal spine in the center of the collimated field. Center the IR to the central ray.
- Open the longitudinally and transversely collimated fields to within 1 inch (2.5 cm) of palpable orbits and zygomatic arches, or use a circle diaphragm.
- An 8- × 10-inch (18- × 24-cm) IR placed lengthwise should be adequate to include all required anatomical structures.

Parietoacanthial and Acanthioparietal Facial Bone and Sinus Image Analysis

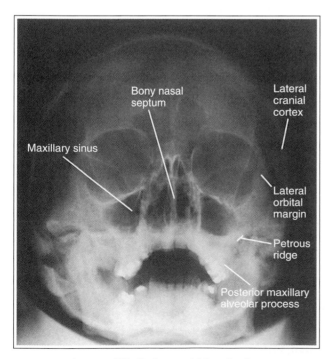

Image 20. Parietocanthial projection.

Analysis. The distances from the lateral orbital margin to the lateral cranial cortex and from the bony nasal septum to the lateral cranial cortex on the right side of the patient are greater than the same distances on the left side. The petrous ridges are demonstrated within the maxillary sinuses and superior to the posterior maxillary alveolar process. The patient's face was rotated toward the left side, and the chin was not elevated enough to position the MML perpendicular to the IR.

Correction. Rotate the patient's face toward the right side until the midsagittal plane is perpendicular with the IR. Elevate the patient's chin until the MML is perpendicular to the IR. The amount of movement needed is the full distance demonstrated between the petrous ridges and the posterior maxillary alveolar process. If the patient is unable to elevate the chin any further, leave the chin positioned as is and angle the central ray caudally approximately 5 degrees for every 1/4 inch (0.6 cm) of distance demonstrated between the petrous ridges and the posterior maxillary alveolar process.

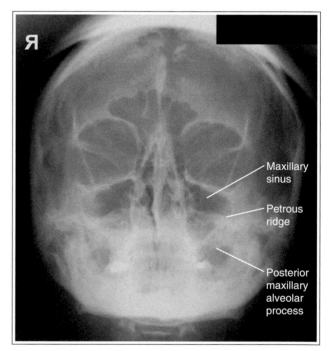

Image 21. Parietocanthial projection.

Analysis. The petrous ridges are demonstrated within the maxillary sinuses and superior to the posterior maxillary alveolar process. The patient's chin was not elevated enough to position the MML perpendicular to the IR. If this petrous ridge and posterior maxillary alveolar process relationship was obtained on a trauma acanthioparietal projection image, the central ray was angled too caudally.

Correction. Elevate the patient's chin until the MML is perpendicular to the IR. The amount of movement needed is the full distance between the petrous ridges and the posterior maxillary alveolar process. If the patient is unable to further elevate the chin, leave the patient's chin positioned as is and angle the central ray caudally approximately 5 degrees for every ¼ inch (0.6 cm) of distance demonstrated between the petrous ridges and the posterior maxillary alveolar process. This should align the central ray parallel with the MML when the patient's mouth is closed.

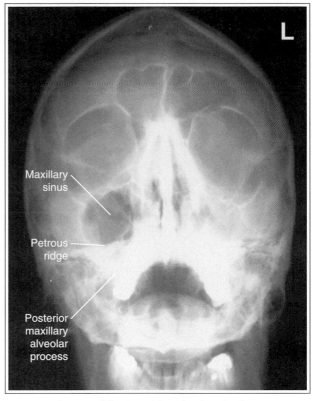

Image 23. Acanthioparietal projection.

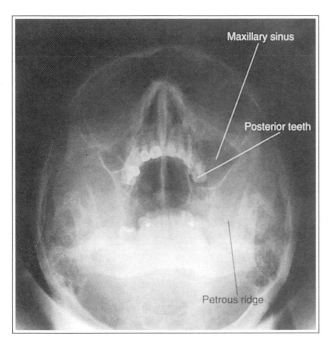

Image 22. Parietoacanthial projection.

Analysis. The petrous ridges are inferior to the maxillary sinuses and the posterior maxillary alveolar process. The patient's chin was elevated more than needed to align the MML perpendicular to the IR.

Correction. Depress the patient's chin until the MML is perpendicular to the IR. The amount of movement needed is the full distance demonstrated between the petrous ridges and the posterior maxillary alveolar process.

Analysis. The petrous ridges are demonstrated within the maxillary sinuses and superior to the posterior maxillary alveolar process. Either the patient's chin was not elevated enough to position the MML perpendicular to the IR, or the central ray was angled too caudally.

Correction. Elevate the patient's chin until the MML is perpendicular to the IR. The amount of movement needed is the full distance demonstrated between the petrous ridges and the posterior maxillary alveolar process. If the patient is unable to elevate the chin any further, leave the patient's chin positioned as is and angle the central ray cephalically approximately 5 degrees for every ¼ inch (0.6 cm) of distance demonstrated between the petrous ridges and the posterior maxillary alveolar process.

OPTIC CANAL AND FORAMEN: PARIETOORBITAL OBLIQUE PROJECTION (RHESE METHOD)

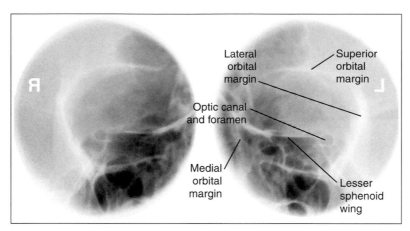

Figure 10-26. Bilateral parietoorbital (Rhese) image with accurate positioning.

Image Analysis

The optic canal is demonstrated on end, and the optic foramen is open and demonstrated in the lower half of the orbit, adjacent to the lateral orbital margin.

- To obtain a parietoorbital oblique image of the optic canal and foramen, position the patient in an upright seated or prone position. Begin with the patient's head in a PA projection. Tuck the patient's chin until the acanthiomeatal line (AML—imaginary line connecting the acanthion and EAM) is perpendicular to the IR and the IPL is level (parallel with the floor if the patient is seated). From this position, rotate the head toward the affected orbit (orbit positioned closer to IR) until the midsagittal plane is at a 53-degree angle with the IR (Figure 10-27). Accurate AML positioning places the optic foramen in the lower half of the orbit, head

rotation places it adjacent to the lateral orbital margin, and accuracy in both situations is required to achieve an open optic canal and foramen.

- ***Inaccurate AML alignment and head rotation:*** A closed optic canal and foramen will result from poor AML positioning and poor head rotation. Which positioning error has caused poor optic canal and foramen alignment can be identified by evaluating the optic foramen placement within the orbit. If the patient's chin is not tucked enough to position the AML perpendicular to the IR, the optic foramen will be superimposed over the inferior orbital margin; and if the chin is tucked more than needed, the optic foramen will be situated in the superior half of the orbit. If the patient's head is rotated less than 53 degrees, the optic foramen will be situated closer to the center of the orbit; and if the patient's head is rotated more than 53 degrees, the optic foramen will be superimposed over the lateral orbital margin.

The optic canal and foramen are centered within the collimated field. Included within the field are the optic canal and foramen, lesser wing of sphenoid, and orbital margins.

- Centering a perpendicular central ray to the orbit closer to or adjacent to the IR will position the optic canal and foramen in the center of the collimated field. Center the IR to the central ray.
- Open the longitudinally and transversely collimated fields to within 1 inch (2.5 cm) of the downside orbital margins, or use a small circle diaphragm.
- An 8- × 10-inch (18- × 24-cm) IR placed lengthwise should be adequate to include all the required anatomical structures. Both right and left parietoorbital oblique images are routinely requested for comparison purposes.

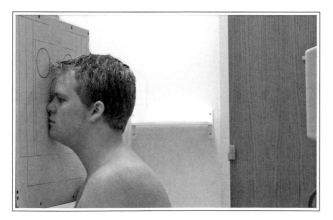

Figure 10-27. Proper patient positioning for parietoorbital (Rhese) image.

NASAL BONES: TANGENTIAL PROJECTION (SUPEROINFERIOR PROJECTION)

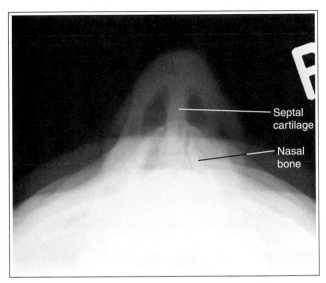

Figure 10-28. Tangential (superoinferior) nasal bone image with accurate positioning.

Image Analysis

Equal soft tissue is demonstrated from the nasal bones to the lateral soft tissue on both sides.

- The tangential projection of the nasal bones is obtained by positioning the patient seated in a chair at the end of the imaging table or in a prone position on the imaging table. The chin is extended and is placed on an IR that is resting on a 45-degree angled sponge. Chin elevation and depression is adjusted until the glabelloalveolar line (GAL) is perpendicular to the IR (Figure 10-29). To obtain equal amounts of soft tissue on both sides of

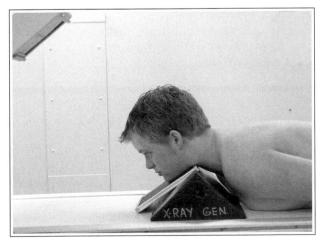

Figure 10-29. Proper patient positioning for tangential (superoinferior) nasal bone image.

the nasal bones, tilt the head as needed to align the cranial midsagittal plane perpendicular to the IR.

- If the cranial midsagittal plane is not aligned perpendicular to the IR, more soft-tissue width will be demonstrated from the nasal bone to the lateral soft tissue on the side toward which the patient's chin is rotated and less on the side toward which the patient's cranium is rotated.

The petrous ridges are demonstrated inferior to the maxillary sinuses and extend laterally from the posterior maxillary alveolar process.

- When the GAL is aligned perpendicular to the IR, the posterior nasal bones are demonstrated without glabella and alveolar ridge superimposition. If the GAL is not aligned perpendicular to the IR, the posterior nasal bones will be obscured. If the patient is unable to elevate the chin enough to position the GAL perpendicular to the IR, the central ray may be angled toward the patient until it is aligned parallel with the GAL.

The nasal bones are at the center of the collimated field. The nasal bones and the surrounding nasal soft tissue are included within the field.

- Centering a perpendicular central ray to the nasion positions the nasal bones in the center of the collimated field.
- An 8- × 10-inch (18- × 24-cm) detailed screen-film or computed radiography IR placed lengthwise should be adequate to include all the required anatomical structures. A small focal spot will increase detail sharpness.
- Open the longitudinally and transversely collimated fields to within ½ inch (1.25 cm) of the nasal skinline, or use a circle diaphragm.

PETROMASTOID PORTION: AXIOLATERAL OBLIQUE PROJECTION (MODIFIED LAW METHOD)

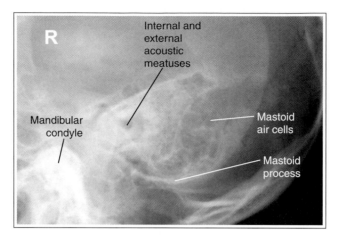

Figure 10-30. Axiolateral oblique (modified Law) petromastoid image with accurate positioning.

Image Analysis

The TMJ, the mastoid process, and air cells positioned farther from the IR are demonstrated anterior to the TMJ, the mastoid process, and air cells positioned closer to the IR.

- To obtain an axiolateral oblique image of the petromastoid portion, position the patient in an upright PA projection or recumbent prone position, with the affected side of the head against the upright IR holder or imaging table in a lateral position. Adjust the chin to bring the IOML perpendicular to the front edge of the IR, and rotate the patient's face toward the IR until the cranium's midsagittal plane and IR form a 15-degree angle (Figure 10-31). Adequate head rotation positions the TMJ, and the mastoid process and air cells placed farther from the IR anterior to those situated closer to the IR. Failure to adequately rotate the face toward the

IR will result in anteroposterior superimposition of the right and left mastoid processes and air cells.

The TMJ, the mastoid process, and air cells positioned farther from the IR are demonstrated inferior to the TMJ, the mastoid process, and air cells positioned closer to the IR.

- The mastoid process and air cells situated farther from the IR are projected inferiorly the needed amount when the patient's IPL is level and a 15-degree caudad central ray angle is used. Failure to adequately position the IPL and angle the central ray will result in inferosuperior superimposition of the right and left mastoid processes and air cells.

The ear auricles are demonstrated anterior to the mastoid processes.

- The auricle of each ear should be taped forward with adhesive tape before positioning to prevent them from being superimposed over the mastoid air cells.

The mastoid process situated closer to the IR is centered within the collimated field. Included within the field are the mastoid cells, lateral portion of the petrous pyramid, and internal and external acoustic meatus.

- Centering the angled central ray 2 inches (5 cm) posterior and 2 inches (5 cm) superior to the upper EAM places the mastoid process of the side situated closer to the IR in the center of the collimated field. Center the IR to the central ray.
- Open the longitudinally and transversely collimated fields to within 1 inch (2.5 cm) of the downside mastoid process, or use a small circle diaphragm.
- An 8- × 10-inch (18- × 24-cm) IR placed lengthwise should be adequate to include all the required anatomical structures. Both right and left axiolateral petromastoid images are routinely requested for comparison purposes.

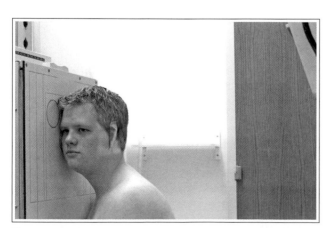

Figure 10-31. Proper patient positioning for axiolateral oblique (modified Law) petromastoid portion image.

PETROMASTOID PORTION: AXIOLATERAL OBLIQUE PROJECTION (STENVERS METHOD, POSTERIOR PROFILE)

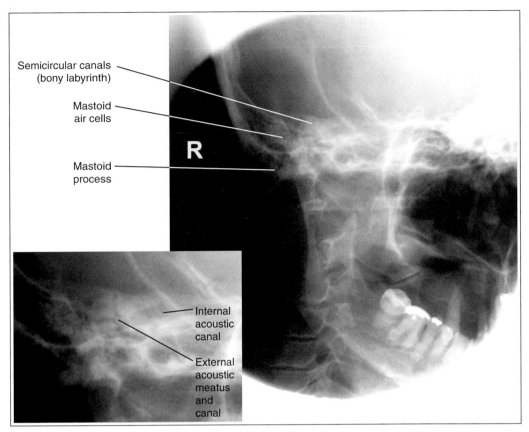

Semicircular canals
(bony labyrinth)

Mastoid
air cells

Mastoid
process

R

Internal
acoustic
canal

External
acoustic
meatus
and
canal

Figure 10-32. Axiolateral oblique (Stenvers) image with accurate positioning.

Image Analysis

The petrous pyramid and mastoid process of interest are in profile, the semicircular canals (bony labyrinth) are in profile and is at the same longitudinal level as the posterior margin of the mandibular rami, the internal acoustic canal (IAC) is demonstrated without foreshortening, and the cervical vertebral column is superimposed over the mandibular rami.

- To obtain an axiolateral oblique image of the petromastoid portion, position the patient in an upright seated or prone position. Begin with the patient's head in a PA projection. Tuck the patient's chin until the IOML is perpendicular to the IR and the IPL is level (parallel with the floor if the patient is seated). From this position, rotate the head toward the affected mastoid (mastoid positioned closest to IR) until the midsagittal plane is at a 40- to 54-degree angle with the IR (Figure 10-33). Accurate head rotation positions the petrous pyramid and semicircular canals of interest in profile, demonstrating the IAC without foreshortening, and superimposing the vertebral column over the mandibular rami.

Skull shape and the degree of head rotation: The shape of the skull determines the degree of rotation needed to accomplish accurate positioning. The average skull shape (mesocephalic) demonstrates the petrous pyramids at a 45-degree angle with the midsagittal plane, so the head should be rotated 45 degrees for this patient type. For the

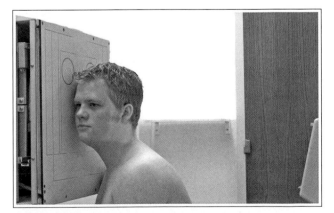

Figure 10-33. Proper patient positioning for axiolateral oblique (Stenvers) petromastoid portion image.

patient who demonstrates a short, broad skull type (brachycephalic), closer to 54 degrees of rotation will be required because the petrous pyramids arc at a 54-degree angle with the midsagittal plane. The patient with a long, narrow skull type (dolichocephalic) will require closer to 40 degrees of rotation because the petrous pyramids are at a 40-degree angle with the midsagittal plane.

Inaccurate head rotation: If the patient's head is rotated less than the required amount, the IAC is foreshortened, the semicircular canals are not in profile and is demonstrated anterior to the posterior margin of the mandibular rami, and the cervical vertebral column is not superimposed over the entire mandibular rami (Image 24). If the patient's head is rotated more than the required amount, the IAC is foreshortened, the semicircular canals are not in profile and is demonstrated posterior to the posterior margin of the mandibular rami, and the cervical column is not superimposed over the entire mandibular rami (Image 25).

Axiolateral oblique projection (Arcelin method, anterior profile): The Arcelin method is a reversed Stenvers method and is used for patients who must remain supine. To obtain this position, rotate the patient's head 45 degrees away from the side of interest (side positioned farther from the IR is the side of interest), and adjust the chin until the IOML is perpendicular to the imaging table. Angle the central ray 10 degrees caudally, and center it 1 inch (2.5 cm) anterior and ¾ inch (2 cm) superior to the elevated EAM.

The supraorbital margin and the petrous ridge of interest are on the same transverse plane.

To position the supraorbital margin and petrous ridge on the same transverse plane, position the IOML perpendicular to the IR and level the IPL before the head is rotated. This positioning, with the required 12-degree cephalic central ray angulation, aligns the central ray perpendicular to the petrous pyramid and semicircular canals, demonstrating them in profile and without foreshortening.

Inaccurate IOML alignment: Inadequate alignment of the petrous pyramid and central ray will result in the IAC and bony labyrinth being obscured on the resulting image. If the patient's chin is not tucked enough to position the IOML perpendicular to the IR, the supraorbital margin is demonstrated superior to the petrous ridge (Image 26). This same image is obtained if the image is taken without the 12-degree cephalic central ray angulation. If the patient's chin is tucked more than needed to position the IOML perpendicular to the IR, the supraorbital margin is inferior to the petrous ridge (Image 27).

The IAC and semicircular canals are centered within the collimated field. Included within the field are the mastoid air cells, petrous pyramid and ridge, semicircular canals, tympanic cavity, and IAC.

- Centering a 12-degree cephalically angled central ray 3 to 4 inches (7 to 10 cm) posterior and ½ inch (1.25 cm) inferior to the upside EAM will position the IAC and

semicircular canals in the center of the collimated field. Center the IR to the central ray.

- To best be able to analyze axiolateral oblique images of the mastoids, the supraorbital margin and mandibular rami must be included. To demonstrate these structures, open the longitudinal collimation field to the mandibular angle and open the transverse collimation field to include the mastoid process of interest or use a circle diaphragm.
- An 8- × 10-inch (18- × 24-cm) IR placed lengthwise should be adequate to include all the required anatomical structures. Both right and left axiolateral oblique images are routinely requested for comparison purposes.

Axiolateral Oblique (Stenvers) Mastoid Image Analysis

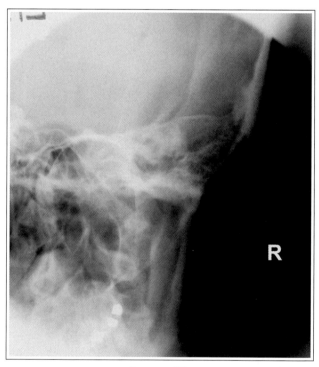

Image 24.

Analysis. The IAC is foreshortened, the semicircular canals are not in profile and is shown anterior to the posterior margin of the mandibular rami, and the cervical vertebral column is not superimposed over the entire mandibular rami. The patient's head was rotated less than the required amount to place the petrous pyramid parallel with the IR.

Correction. Increase the degree of head rotation.

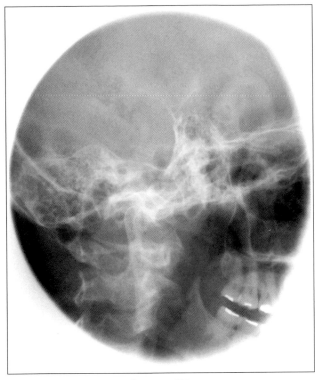

Image 25.

Analysis. The IAC is foreshortened, the semicircular canals are not in profile and is shown posterior to the posterior margin of the mandibular rami, and the cervical column is not superimposed over the entire mandibular rami. The patient's head was rotated more than the required amount to place the petrous pyramid parallel with the IR.

Correction. Decrease the degree of patient head rotation.

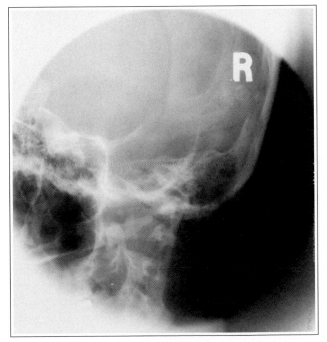

Image 26.

Analysis. The IAC and semicircular canals are obscured, and the supraorbital margin is demonstrated superior to the petrous ridge. The patient's chin was not tucked enough to position the IOML perpendicular to the IR, or the image was obtained without the required 12-degree cephalic central ray angulation.

Correction. Tuck the patient's chin toward the chest until the IOML is aligned perpendicular to the IR. If the central ray was not angled, use the same positioning and add the angle as required.

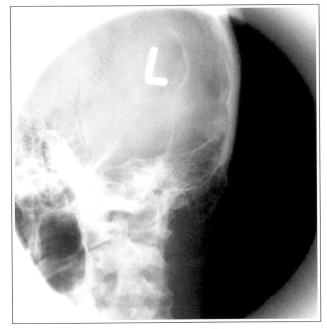

Image 27.

Analysis. The IAC and semicircular canals are obscured, and the supraorbital margin is demonstrated inferior to the petrous ridge. The patient's chin was tucked more than needed to position the IOML perpendicular to the IR (entire line is on the same transverse plane).

Correction. Elevate the patient's chin away from the chest until the IOML is aligned perpendicular to the IR (entire line on the same transverse plane).

Image Analysis of the Digestive System

The following image analysis criteria are used for all digestive system images and should be considered when completing the analysis. Position- or projection-specific criteria relating to these topics are discussed with the other accompanying criteria for that position or projection.

Facility's identification requirements are visible on image as identified in Chapter 1.

A right or left marker, identifying correct side of patient, is present on image and is not superimposed over anatomy of interest. Specific placement of marker is as described in Chapter 1.

Radiation practices, as defined in Chapter 1, have been followed.

No evidence of preventable artifacts, such as buttons, zippers, undergarments, and body piercings, is present, and the digestive structures of interest are free of residual debris and fluid.

- The patient should be instructed to remove outer clothing and any underclothes containing artifacts, then to change into a snapless hospital gown before the procedure.
- *Pendulous breasts:* Pendulous breasts may overlap the colic flexures unless they are shifted superiorly and laterally. Such movement also prevents excessive radiation exposure to the breasts.

PREPARATION PROCEDURES

- *Esophagram preparation:* No preparation procedures are required when the esophagus is imaged, but if an esophagus and stomach examination is being performed, the stomach and duodenum preparation is to be followed.

- *Stomach and duodenum preparation:* Adequate preparation of the upper gastrointestinal (GI) system eliminates residual stomach debris, which may obscure abnormalities, and prevents excessive fluid from accumulating in the stomach, which could dilute the barium suspension enough to interfere with optimal mucosal coating (see Image 5). The preparation procedure for the upper GI system includes NPO (nothing orally) after midnight or at least 8 hours before the examination, and avoidance of gum and tobacco products before the procedure.

- *Small intestine preparation:* Optimal preparation of the small intestine for a small bowel study is obtained through a patient preparation procedure that includes a low-residue diet for 1 to 2 days before the examination, NPO after midnight and until the examination, and avoidance of gum and tobacco products before the examination (these are thought to increase salivation and gastric secretions).

- *Large intestine preparation:* Adequate cleansing of the large intestine for a barium enema is obtained through a patient preparation procedure including a low-residue diet for 2 to 3 days before the examination, followed by a clear liquid diet 1 day before the examination, laxatives the afternoon before the examination, and a suppository or cleansing enema the morning of the examination. Remaining fecal material may obscure the mucosal surfaces and, when barium coated, may mimic polyps and small tumors; remaining residual fluid causes dilution of the barium suspension, resulting in poor mucosal coating and coating artifacts (see Image 11).

On arrival in the fluoroscopic department the patient should be questioned to determine whether proper preparation instructions were given and followed. Adequate preparation can be assumed if the patient's last bowel movement lacked solid fecal material.

The GI structures and cortical outlines of the bony structures are sharply defined.

- Sharply defined recorded details are obtained when patient motion is controlled, respiration is halted, a short exposure time is used, and a short object–image receptor distance (OID) is maintained.

  For most digestive system images the patient is positioned with the anterior surface placed closer to the IR, since this will place the organs at the shortest OID for most patients. The halting of respiration is especially important when the patient is positioned with the anterior surface down, because breathing may cause the entire torso to move.

  Short exposure times are needed when imaging the digestive system, to control the image blur that may result from peristaltic activity within the system. Peristalsis is the contraction and relaxation movement of the smooth muscles in the walls of the digestive system that mixes food and secretions and moves the materials through the system. Peristaltic activity of the stomach and large

or small intestine can be identified on an image by sharp bony cortices and blurry gastric and intestinal gases or barium (see Image 9).

Contrast, density, and penetration are adequate to demonstrate the barium-coated mucosal surface patterns and intestinal contours while providing uniform grayness within the air-filled stomach or intestine.

- An optimal kilovolt-peak (kVp) technique, as shown in Table 11-1, sufficiently penetrates the barium-coated mucosal surface and provides the contrast needed to distinguish the mucosal patterns. Use a grid to reduce the scatter radiation that reaches the IR, thereby reducing fog, increasing the visibility of the recorded details, and providing a higher-contrast image. To obtain optimal density, set a manual milliampere-seconds (mAs) level based on the patient's abdominal thickness or choose the appropriate automatic exposure control (AEC) (see Table 11-1 for details). For double-contrast examinations, using the AEC may be contraindicated because choosing

TABLE 11-1 Digestive System Technical Data

Position/Projection	kVp	Grid	AEC Chamber(s)	SID
UPPER GASTROINTESTINAL SYSTEM				
PA Oblique (RAO) projection, esophagus	SC = 100-110	Grid	Center	40-48 inches (100-120 cm)
Lateral projection, esophagus	SC = 100-110	Grid	Center	40-48 inches (100-120 cm)
AP or PA projection, esophagus	SC = 100-110	Grid	Center	40-48 inches (100-120 cm)
PA oblique (RAO) projection, stomach	SC = 100-110 DC = 80-90	Grid	Center	40-48 inches (100-120 cm)
PA projection, stomach	SC = 100-110 DC = 80-90	Grid	Center	40-48 inches (100-120 cm)
Right lateral position, stomach	SC = 100-110 DC = 80-90	Grid	Center	40-48 inches (100-120 cm)
AP oblique (LPO) projection, stomach	SC = 100-110 DC = 80-90	Grid	Center	40-48 inches (100-120 cm)
AP projection, stomach	SC = 100-110 DC = 80-90	Grid	Center	40-48 inches (100-120 cm)
SMALL INTESTINE				
PA or AP projection	SC = 100-125	Grid	All three	40-48 inches (100-120 cm)
LARGE INTESTINE				
PA or AP projection	SC = 100-125 DC = 80-90	Grid	All three	40-48 inches (100-120 cm)
Lateral (rectum) position	SC = 100-125 DC = 80-90	Grid	Center	40-48 inches (100-120 cm)
AP or PA (lateral) decubitus projection	DC = 80-90	Grid	All three	40-48 inches (100-120 cm)
PA oblique (RAO) projection	SC = 100-125 DC = 80-90	Grid	All three	40-48 inches (100-120 cm)
PA oblique (LAO) projection	SC = 100-125 DC = 80-90	Grid	All three	40-48 inches (100-120 cm)
PA or AP axial projection	SC = 100-125 DC = 80-90	Grid	All three	40-48 inches (100-120 cm)

AEC, Automatic exposure control; *AP*, anteroposterior; *DC*, double contrast; *kVp*, kilovolt-peak; *LPO*, left posterior oblique; *PA*, posteroanterior; *RAO*, right anterior oblique; *SC*, single contrast; *SID*, source–image receptor distance.

the cell beneath the barium pool may result in overexposure of the area containing the air contrast (see Image 6).

The long axis of the lumbar vertebral column is aligned with the long axis of the collimated field.

- Aligning the midsagittal plane with the long axis of the collimated field will allow for tight collimation.

The required upper and lower intestinal structures are included on the image. Adjustments in patient positioning, central ray centering, and IR size and direction are made to accommodate the patient's habitus.

- *Body habitus:* The body habitus determines the size, shape, and position of the stomach and the abdominal cavity placement of the large intestine. Being familiar with these differences will help the technologist to adjust the central ray centering and IR placement for optimal demonstration of the required digestive structures.

  Hypersthenic: The hypersthenic patient's abdomen is broad and deep from anterior to posterior; the stomach is positioned high in the abdomen and lies transversely at the level of the T9 to T12, with the duodenal bulb at the level of T11 to T12. The colic flexures and transverse colon tend to be positioned high in the abdomen (Figure 11-1). Using the sthenic patient as the reference point, this habitus will require a more superior and medial central ray centering and image receptor (IR) placement for anteroposterior (AP) and posteroanterior (PA) projections, a more superior and anterior central ray centering and IR placement for the lateral position

of the stomach, and two crosswise IRs to include the entire large intestine for barium enema images.

  Asthenic: The asthenic patient's abdomen is narrow and the stomach is positioned low in the abdomen and runs vertically along the left side of the vertebral column, typically extending from T11 to L5, with the duodenal bulb at the level of L3 to L4. The small and large intestinal structures tend to be positioned low in the abdomen (Figure 11-2). Using the sthenic patient as the reference point, this habitus will require lower and more lateral centering of the central ray for stomach images.

  Sthenic: The sthenic habitus is the most common. The abdomen is less broad than the hypersthenic habitus, yet not as narrow as the asthenic. The stomach also rests at a position between the hypersthenic and asthenic habitus and typically extends from T10 to L2, with the duodenal bulb at the level of L1 to L2. The small and large intestinal structures tend to be centered within the abdomen (Figure 11-3).

The image was taken on full suspended expiration. The diaphragm dome is located superior to the ninth posterior ribs.

- From full inspiration to expiration the diaphragm position moves from an inferior to a superior position. This movement also changes the pressure placed on the abdominal structures. On full expiration the right side of the diaphragm dome is at the same transverse level as the eighth thoracic vertebrae, whereas on inspiration it may be found at the same transverse level as the ninth

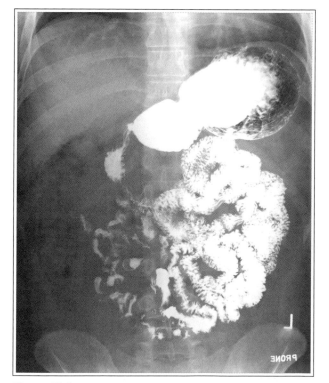

Figure 11-1. *Posteroanterior projection of hypersthenic patient.*

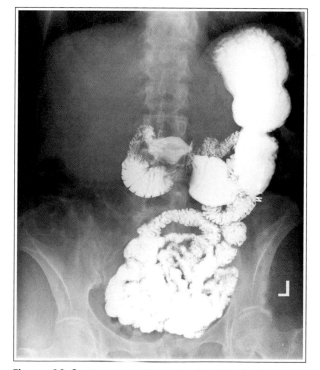

Figure 11-2. *Posteroanterior projection of asthenic patient.*

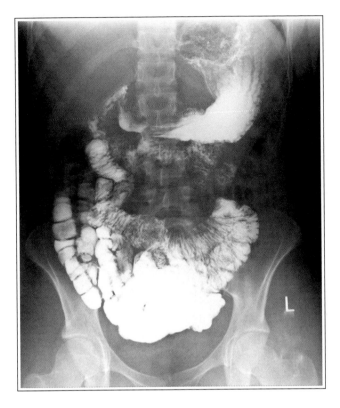

Figure 11-3. Posteroanterior projection of sthenic patient.

or tenth posterior rib. Exposing upper GI images and images of the small and large intestines on full expiration allows increased abdominal space for the structures to be demonstrated without segment overlapping and foreshortening (see Image 7).

ESOPHAGRAM

Upper Gastrointestinal System: the Esophagram

The esophagus is filled with barium, demonstrating its contour.

- *Contrast:* The goal of the esophagram is to demonstrate the workings and appearance of the pharynx and esophagus. This is accomplished through the fluoroscopic procedure and overhead images that are obtained in an esophagram. Barium is used to demonstrate the pharynx and esophagus during this examination. A 30% to 50% weight or volume barium suspension is ingested continuously during the exposure, or two to three spoonfuls with toothpaste consistency; thick barium is ingested before exposing the esophagus, filling it with barium. The patient may also be asked to swallow cotton balls soaked in thin barium, barium-filled gelatin capsules, barium tablets, or marshmallows when a radiolucent foreign body or stricture is suspected. Adequate filling of the esophagus has occurred when the entire column is filled with barium. Only aspects of the esophagus that are filled with barium will be adequately demonstrated (see Images 1 and 3).

For the overhead images a glass of barium is placed on the imaging table in the patient's hand and the straw in the mouth so the patient can ingest barium during the exposure, or the patient is asked to swallow two spoonfuls of thick barium and then given a third that is swallowed directly before the exposure.

ESOPHAGRAM: POSTEROANTERIOR OBLIQUE PROJECTION (RIGHT ANTERIOR OBLIQUE POSITION)

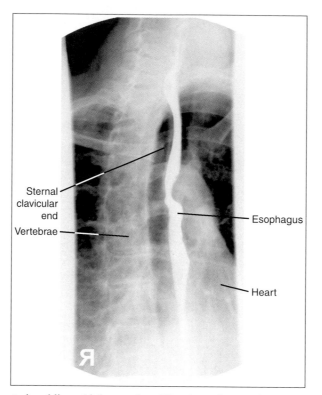

Figure 11-4. Posteroanterior oblique (right anterior oblique) esophagram image with accurate positioning.

Image Analysis

The barium-filled esophagus is demonstrated between the vertebrae and heart shadow, and approximately ½ inch (1.25 cm) of the right sternal (medial) clavicular end is demonstrated to the left of the vertebrae.

- A PA oblique (right anterior oblique [RAO]) esophagram image is obtained by placing the patient prone on the imaging table, then rotating the torso toward the right side until the midcoronal plane is at a 35- to 40-degree angle with the imaging table (Figure 11-5). The patient's left elbow and knee may be flexed and used to support the body rotation.
- *Inaccurate patient rotation:* If less than the desired 35 to 40 degrees of obliquity is obtained on an esophagram image, the vertebrae will be superimposed over the esophagus and the right sternal clavicular end (see Image 2). If the patient is rotated more than 40 degrees, more than ½ inch (1.25 cm) of the right sternal clavicular end will be demonstrated to the left of the vertebrae.

The midesophagus, at the level of T5 to T6, is at the center of the collimated field. The entire esophagus is included within the field.

- To place the midesophagus in the center of the field, center a perpendicular central ray approximately 3 inches (7.5 cm) to the left of the spinous processes and 2 to 3 inches (5 to 7.5 cm) inferior to the jugular notch. Center the IR to the central ray.
- Open the longitudinally collimated field the full 17-inch (43-cm) IR length. Transverse collimation should be to a 6-inch (15-cm) field size.
- A 14- × 17-inch (35- × 43-cm) IR placed lengthwise should be adequate to include all the required anatomical structures.

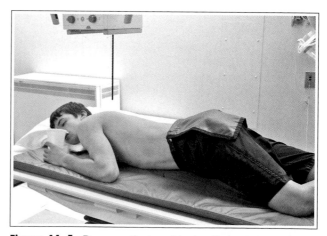

Figure 11-5. Proper patient positioning for posteroanterior oblique esophagram image.

Posteroanterior Oblique (Right Anterior Oblique) Esophagram Image Analysis

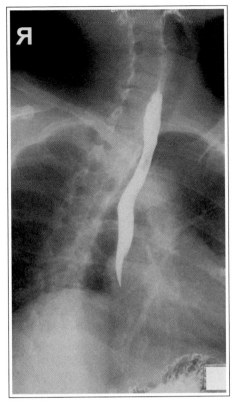

Image 1.

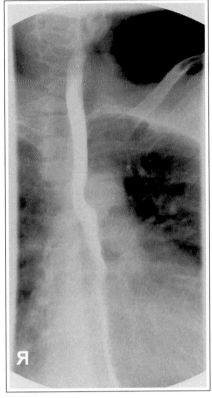

Image 2.

Analysis. The superior and inferior ends of the esophagus are not filled with barium.

Correction. The patient should drink barium continuously during the exposure or should swallow two spoonfuls of thick barium and then be given a third that is swallowed directly before the exposure.

Analysis. The vertebrae are superimposed over the right sternal clavicular end and a portion of the esophagus. The patient was rotated less than the required 35 to 40 degrees.

Correction. Increase the degree of patient obliquity until the midcoronal plane is at a 35- to 40-degree angle with the imaging table.

ESOPHAGRAM: LATERAL POSITION

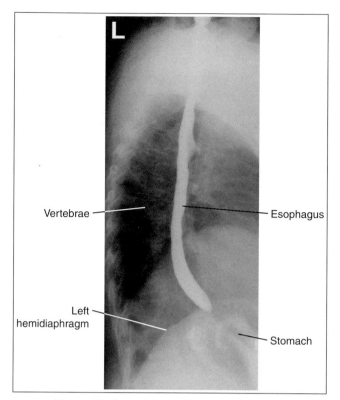

Figure 11-6. Left lateral esophagram image.

Image Analysis

A lateral barium-filled esophagus image is demonstrated. The esophagus is positioned anterior to the thoracic vertebrae, the posterior surfaces of each vertebral body are superimposed, and no more than $\frac{1}{2}$ inch (1.25 cm) of space is demonstrated between the posterior ribs.

- To obtain a lateral esophogram image, place the patient on the imaging table in a lateral recumbent position. Whether the patient is lying on the right or left side is not significant, although left-side positioning is easier for the technologist (Figure 11-7). Flex the patient's knees

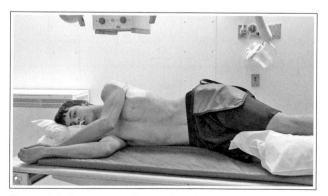

Figure 11-7. Proper patient positioning for lateral esophagram image with arms at 90 degrees.

and hips for support, and position a pillow or sponge between the knees. The pillow or sponge should be enough to prevent the side of the pelvis situated farther from the IR from rotating anteriorly but not so thick as to cause posterior rotation. To avoid vertebral rotation, align the shoulders, the posterior ribs, and the posterior pelvis perpendicular to the imaging table and IR by resting an extended flat palm against each, respectively, then adjusting patient rotation until the hand is positioned perpendicular to the IR.

- **Detecting thorax rotation:** Rotation can be detected on a lateral esophagram image by evaluating superimposition of the right and left posterior surfaces of the vertebral bodies and superimposition of the posterior ribs. Because the two sides of the thorax and vertebrae are mirror images, it is very difficult to determine from a rotated lateral esophagram image which side of the patient was rotated anteriorly and which posteriorly. If the patient was only slightly rotated, one way of determining which way the patient was rotated is to evaluate the amount of posterior rib superimposition. If the patient's elevated side was rotated posteriorly, the posterior ribs demonstrate more than $\frac{1}{2}$ inch (1.25 cm) of space between them (see p. 411, Image 37). If the patient's elevated side was rotated anteriorly, the posterior ribs are superimposed on slight rotation (see p. 411, Image 38) and demonstrate greater separation as rotation of the patient increases.

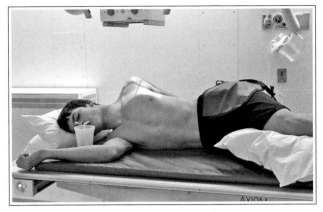

Figure 11-8. Proper patient positioning for lateral esophagram image with shoulders rotated.

No superimposition of shoulders or humeri over the esophagus is present.

- *Humeral and shoulder positioning*: Placing the humeri anteriorly at a 90-degree angle with the torso or separating the shoulders by positioning the arm and shoulder closer to the imaging table slightly forward and the arm and shoulder farther away from the imaging table back, while maintaining a lateral thorax (Figure 11-8), prevents the shoulders and humeri from being superimposed over the esophagus.

The midesophagus, at the level of T5 to T6, is at the center of the collimated field. The entire esophagus is included within the field.

- Center a perpendicular central ray to the midcoronal plane at a level 2 to 3 inches (5 to 7.5 cm) inferior to the jugular notch, to center the midesophagus at the center of the collimated field. Center the IR to the central ray.
- Open the longitudinally collimated field the full 17-inch (43-cm) IR length. Transverse collimation should be to a 6-inch (15-cm) field size.
- A 14- × 17-inch (35- × 43-cm) IR placed lengthwise should be adequate to include all the required anatomical structures.

Lateral Esophagram Image Analysis

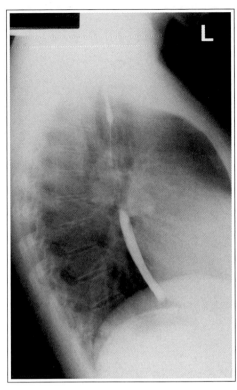

Image 3.

Analysis. The superior and middle ends of the esophagus are not filled with barium.

Correction. The patient should drink barium continuously during the exposure or should swallow two spoonfuls of thick barium and then be given a third that is swallowed directly before the exposure.

ESOPHAGRAM: POSTEROANTERIOR PROJECTION

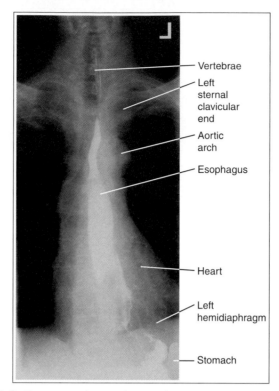

Figure 11-9. Posteroanterior esophagram image with accurate positioning.

A PA projection is demonstrated. The distances from the vertebral column to the sternal (medial) ends of the clavicles are equal, and the vertebrae are superimposed over the esophagus.

- To obtain a PA esophagus image, place the patient prone on the imaging table. Position the shoulders and anterior superior iliac spines (ASISs) at equal distances from the imaging table to prevent rotation, and draw the patient's arms away from the abdominal area to prevent them from being superimposed over the abdominal region (Figure 11-10). Special attention should be given to female patients who have had one breast removed. *The side of the patient on which the breast was removed may need to be placed at a greater OID than the opposite side to prevent rotation.*

- **Detecting rotation:** Rotation is readily detected on a PA esophagus image by evaluating the position of the esophagus with respect to the vertebrae and the distances from the vertebral column to the sternal clavicular ends. On a nonrotated esophagus image, the vertebrae and esophagus are superimposed and the distances from the vertebrae to the sternal clavicular ends are equal on both sides. On a rotated PA projection, the side of the vertebrae toward which the esophagus is rotated and the sternal clavicular end that demonstrates less vertebral column superimposition represents the side of the chest positioned farther from the IR (see Image 4).

The midesophagus at the level of T5 to T6 is at the center of the collimated field. The entire esophagus is included within the field.

- Center a perpendicular central ray to the midsagittal plane at a level 2 to 3 inches (5 to 7.5 cm) inferior to the

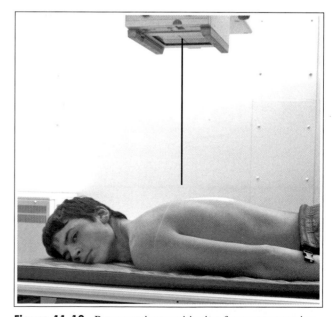

Figure 11-10. Proper patient positioning for posteroanterior esophagram image.

jugular notch for the AP projection and at the level of T5 to T6 (2 to 3 inches superior to the inferior scapular angle) for the PA projection to center the midesophagus at the center of the collimated field. Center the IR to the central ray.

- Open the longitudinally collimated field the full 14-inch (35-cm) IR length. Transverse collimation should be to a 6-inch (15-cm) field size.
- A 14- × 17-inch (35- × 43-cm) IR placed lengthwise should be adequate to include all the required anatomical structures.

Posteroanterior Esophagram Image Analysis

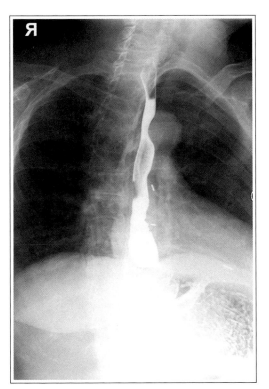

Image 4.

Analysis. The esophagus is to the left of the vertebrae, and the left sternal clavicular end is demonstrated without vertebral column superimposition. The patient was rotated toward the right side.

Correction. Position the left shoulder closer to the IR until the shoulders are at equal distances from the IR.

STOMACH AND DUODENUM

Single contrast: **The stomach and duodenum is barium filled, demonstrating the contour of the stomach and lumen.**

- The single-contrast stomach and duodenum image demonstrates barium-filled organs with normally present gas. The primary goal of a single-contrast upper GI study is to demonstrate abnormalities of the stomach and lumen contour. A 30% to 50% weight or volume barium suspension is typically used for this study.

Double contrast: **The stomach and duodenum demonstrate adequate distention and mucosal covering. The rugae (longitudinal gastric folds) are smoothed out, the gastric surface pattern is demonstrated, and a thin, uniform barium line is visible along the contour of the stomach.**

- The goal of a double-contrast study is to visualize abnormalities in the mucosal details, and contour and lumen of the stomach and duodenum.

TABLE 11-2 Double-Contrast Filling of Upper Gastrointestinal System		
Stomach	**Barium-Filled Structures**	**Air-Filled Structures**
Right anterior oblique position	Pylorus, duodenum	Fundus
Posteroanterior projection	Pylorus, duodenum	Fundus
Right lateral position	Pylorus, duodenum, body	Fundus
Left posterior oblique position	Fundus	Pylorus, duodenum
Anteroposterior projection	Fundus	Pylorus, duodenum, body

The negative (radiolucent) contrast is most commonly obtained by having the patient swallow effervescent granules, powder, or tablets that rapidly release 300 to 400 ml of carbon dioxide on contact with the fluid in the stomach. The carbon dioxide provides the gastric distention and smoothing of the rugae.

The positive (radiopaque) contrast is obtained by having the patient drink a high-density, up to 250% weight or volume, barium suspension. The barium provides the thin coating that covers the mucosal surface. To obtain adequate mucosal coating of the area, the barium is washed over the gastric surface by having the patient turn 360 degrees and then positioning the patient so the barium pool will be placed away from the area of interest. Because the barium will slowly flow toward the lowest level after coating, to maintain an optimal mucosal covering the patient should be rotated between images or the sequence of images should be taken to optimize coating of the area of interest. Table 11-2 indicates where the barium will pool and what aspect of the upper GI tract is best demonstrated in the most commonly obtained stomach and duodenum images.

Failure to obtain good mucosal coating may result in missed or simulated lesions. The quality of the mucosal coating depends on the properties of the barium suspension, the volume of barium and gas, the frequency of washing, and the amount of fluid or secretions and viscosity of mucus in the stomach. Although proper double-contrast filling is primarily the fluoroscopist's responsibility, the technologist's scope of practice does play a part in some of the causes of poor coating, such as using the wrong type of barium, improperly preparing the barium suspension, or performing poor lower intestine preparation. A thorough mixing of the barium suspension is required before the patient ingests the material.

STOMACH AND DUODENUM: POSTEROANTERIOR OBLIQUE PROJECTION (RIGHT ANTERIOR OBLIQUE POSITION)

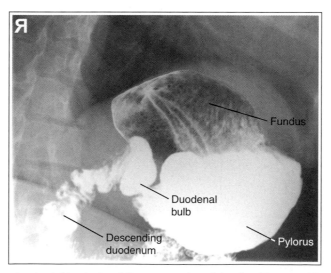

Figure 11-11. Hypersthenic right anterior oblique stomach and duodenal image with accurate positioning.

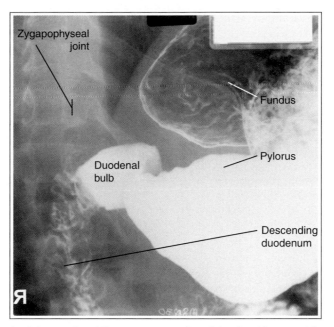

Figure 11-12. Sthenic right anterior oblique spot stomach and duodenal image with accurate positioning.

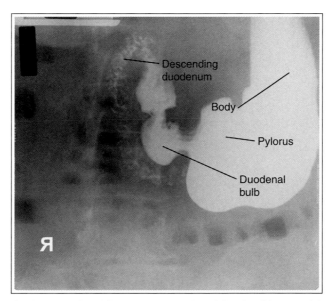

Figure 11-13. Asthenic right anterior oblique spot stomach and duodenal image with accurate positioning.

Image Analysis

Contrast distribution: Air contrast is demonstrated in the fundus, and barium is visible in the pylorus, duodenal bulb, and descending duodenum.

An optimal RAO stomach image has been obtained when the lumbar vertebrae demonstrate an oblique position, with the degree of obliquity adequate for the body habitus, and when the correct aspect of the stomach, as defined by the body habitus, is in profile.

Hypersthenic habitus: The patient has been rotated 70 degrees, as identified by the demonstration of the left lumbar zygapophyseal joints in the posterior third of the vertebral bodies. The duodenal bulb and descending duodenum are in profile, and the long axis of the stomach demonstrates foreshortening with a closed lesser curvature (Figure 11-11).

Sthenic habitus: The patient has been rotated approximately 45 degrees, as identified by the demonstration of the left lumbar zygapophyseal joints at the midline of the vertebral bodies. The duodenal bulb and descending duodenum arc in profile, and the long axis of the stomach is partially foreshortened with a partially closed lesser curvature (Figure 11-12).

Asthenic habitus: The patient has been rotated approximately 40 degrees, as identified by the demonstration of the left lumbar zygapophyseal joints in the anterior third of the vertebral bodies. The duodenal bulb and descending duodenum are in profile, the long axis of the stomach is demonstrated without foreshortening, and the lesser curvature is open (Figure 11-13).

- A PA oblique (RAO) stomach image is obtained by placing the patient prone on the imaging table, and then rotating the torso toward the right side until the midcoronal plane is at a 40- to 70-degree angle with the imaging table (Figure 11-14). The patient's left elbow and knee may be flexed and used to support the body rotation. In general, hypersthenic habitus patients require approximately 70 degrees of obliquity, and the asthenic habitus approximately 40 degrees. The difference in the degree of obliquity for the body habitus is a result of the difference in the amount of superimposition of the pylorus and duodenal bulb that exists among patients with different habitus.

The pylorus is centered within the collimated field. The stomach and duodenal loop are included within the field.

- To place the pylorus in the center of the field, center a perpendicular central ray halfway between the vertebrae

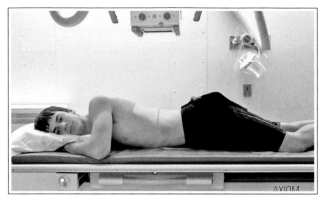

Figure 11-14. Proper patient positioning for posteroanterior oblique (right anterior oblique) stomach and duodenal image.

and lateral rib border of the elevated side at a level 1 to 2 inches (2.5 to 5 cm) superior to the inferior rib margin for the sthenic habitus. Center the central ray at a level 2 inches (5 cm) superior to the sthenic patient centering for the hypersthenic habitus, and at a level 2 inches inferior for the asthenic habitus. Center the IR to the central ray.

- Open the longitudinally collimated field the full 14-inch (35-cm) IR length. Transverse collimation should be to the vertebrae and lateral rib border.
- An 11- × 14-inch (28- × 35-cm) IR placed lengthwise should be adequate to include all the required anatomical structures.

STOMACH AND DUODENUM: POSTEROANTERIOR PROJECTION

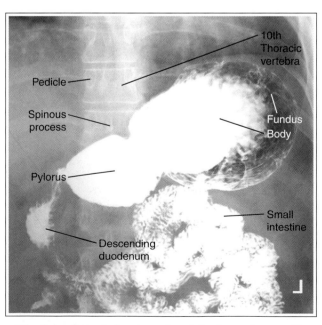

Figure 11-15. Hypersthenic posteroanterior stomach and duodenum image with accurate positioning.

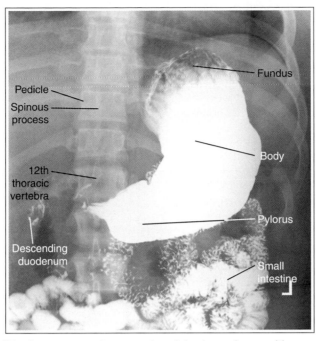

Figure 11-16. Sthenic posteroanterior stomach and duodenum image with accurate positioning.

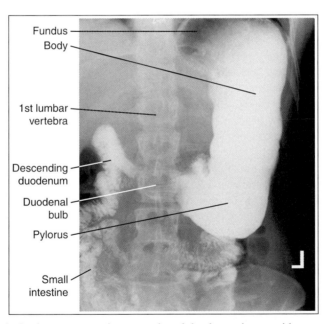

Figure 11-17. Asthenic posteroanterior stomach and duodenum image with accurate positioning.

Image Analysis

Contrast distribution: Air contrast is demonstrated in the fundus, and barium is visible in the body and pylorus.

An optimal PA stomach and duodenum image has been obtained when the spinous processes are aligned with the midline of the vertebral bodies, the distances from the pedicles to the spinous processes are the same on both sides, and the correct aspect of the stomach, as defined by the body habitus, is in profile.

Hypersthenic habitus: The stomach is aligned nearly horizontally, with the duodenal bulb at the level of T11 to T12. The lesser and greater curvatures are demonstrated nearly on end, with the greater curvature being more anteriorly situated and the esophagogastric junction nearly on end (Figure 11-15).

Sthenic habitus: The stomach is aligned nearly vertically, with the duodenal bulb at the level of L1 to L2. The stomach is somewhat J-shaped, and its long axis is partially foreshortened. The lesser and greater curvatures, esophagogastric junction, pylorus, and duodenal bulb arc in partial profile (Figure 11-16).

Asthenic habitus: The stomach is aligned vertically, with the duodenal bulb at the level of L3 to L4. The stomach is J-shaped, and its long axis is demonstrated without foreshortening. The lesser and greater curvatures, esophagogastric junction, pylorus, and duodenal bulb are in profile (Figure 11-17).

- To obtain a PA stomach image, place the patient prone on the imaging table. Position the shoulders and pelvic ala at equal distances from the imaging table to prevent rotation, and draw the patient's arms away from the abdominal area to prevent them from being superimposed over the abdominal region (Figure 11-18).
- *Detecting abdominal rotation:* Rotation is effectively detected on a PA stomach image by comparing the distance from the pedicles to the spinous processes on both sides. The side demonstrating the greater distance from the pedicles to the spinous processes is the side positioned farther from the IR.

The pylorus is centered within the collimated field. The stomach and descending duodenum are included within the field.

- To position the pylorus in the center of the collimated field for the sthenic habitus, center a perpendicular central ray halfway between the vertebrae and left lateral rib border at a point approximately 1 to 2 inches (2.5 to 5 cm) above the lower rib margin. For the hypersthenic habitus, direct the central ray just to the left of the vertebrae at a level 2 inches (5 cm) superior to the sthenic habitus centering point. For the asthenic habitus, direct the central ray 2 inches inferior to the sthenic habitus centering point. Center the IR to the central ray.
- Open the longitudinally collimated field the full 14-inch (35-cm) IR length. Transverse collimation should be to the vertebrae and lateral rib border.

- An 11- × 14-inch (28- × 35-cm) IR placed lengthwise should be adequate to include all the required anatomical structures.

Posteroanterior Stomach and Duodenum Image Analysis

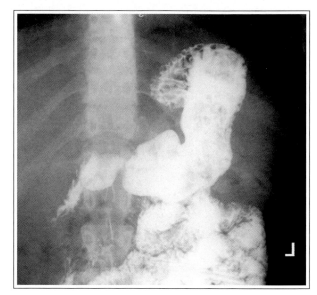

Image 5.

Analysis. The stomach demonstrates a blotchy appearance within the barium. The stomach contains residual food particles. The patient did not follow adequate preparation procedure.

Correction. The preparation procedure for the stomach includes NPO after midnight or for at least 8 hours before the examination and avoidance of gum and tobacco products before the procedure.

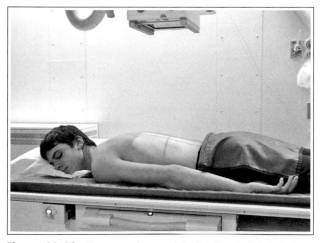

Figure 11-18. Proper patient positioning for posteroanterior stomach and duodenal image.

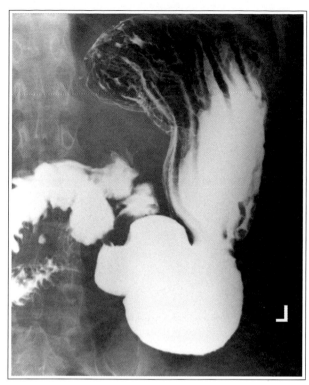

Image 6.

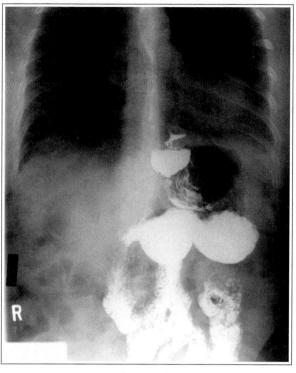

Image 7.

Analysis. The air-contrast fundus is overexposed, preventing demonstration of abnormalities. Either the mAs was too high or the AEC was positioned beneath the barium-filled body and pylorus.

Correction. Decrease the mAs enough to demonstrate the fundus, or manually set the mAs instead of using the AEC.

Analysis. The examination was obtained after full inspiration, compressing and foreshortening the stomach. Compare this image with the images obtained on expiration in Figures 11-3 and 11-16.

Correction. Expose the image on full, suspended expiration.

STOMACH AND DUODENUM: LATERAL PROJECTION (RIGHT LATERAL POSITION)

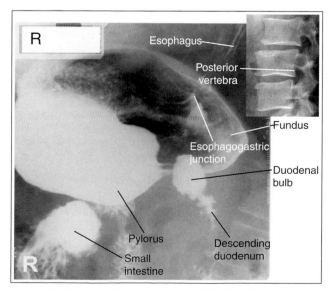

Figure 11-19. Hypersthenic right lateral spot stomach and duodenal image with accurate positioning.

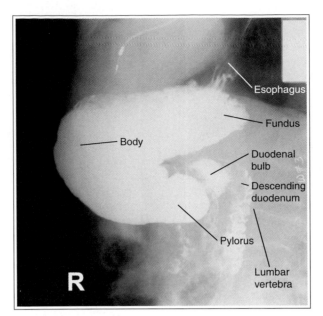

Figure 11-20. Sthenic right lateral stomach and duodenal image with accurate positioning.

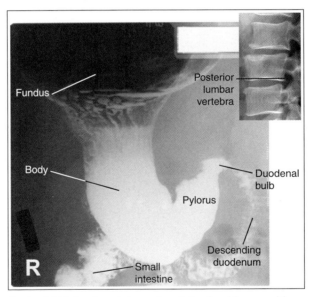

Figure 11-21. Asthenic right lateral spot stomach and duodenal image with accurate positioning.

Image Analysis

Contrast distribution: Air contrast is demonstrated in the fundus, and barium is visible in the pylorus, duodenum bulb, and descending duodenum.

An optimal right lateral stomach and duodenal image has been obtained when the thoracic and lumbar vertebrae demonstrate a lateral position, with the superimposed posterior surfaces of each vertebral body, when the stomach, duodenal bulb, and descending duodenum are anterior to the vertebrae, demonstrating

the retrogastric space, and when the correct aspect of the stomach, as defined by the body habitus, is in profile.

Hypersthenic habitus: The duodenal bulb and descending duodenum are in profile, and the long axis of the stomach demonstrates foreshortening with a closed lesser curvature (Figure 11-19).

Sthenic habitus: The duodenal bulb and descending duodenum are in profile, and the long axis of the stomach is partially foreshortened with a partially closed lesser curvature (Figure 11-20).

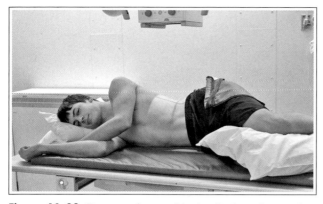

Figure 11-22. Proper patient positioning for lateral stomach and duodenal image.

Asthenic habitus: **The duodenal bulb and descending duodenum are in profile, the long axis of the stomach is demonstrated without foreshortening, and the lesser curvature is open (Figure 11-21).**

- To obtain a lateral stomach image, place the patient on the imaging table in a right lateral recumbent position. Flex the patient's knees and hips for support (Figure 11-22). To avoid rotation, align the shoulders, posterior ribs, and posterior pelvis perpendicular to the imaging table and IR. This is accomplished by resting your extended flat palm against each structure, individually, and then adjusting the patient's rotation until your hand is positioned perpendicular to the imaging table.

- *Detecting rotation:* Rotation can be detected on a lateral stomach and duodenal image by evaluating the superimposition of the right and left posterior surfaces of the vertebral bodies. On a nonrotated lateral stomach and duodenal image, these posterior surfaces are superimposed, appearing as one. On rotation, these posterior surfaces are not superimposed but are demonstrated one anterior to the other (see Image 8).

The pylorus is centered within the collimated field. The stomach and duodenal loop are included within the field.

- To place the pylorus in the center of the field, center a perpendicular central ray halfway between the midcoronal plane and anterior abdomen at the level of the inferior rib margin for the sthenic habitus. For the hypersthenic

habitus, direct the central ray at a level 2 inches (5 cm) superior to the sthenic habitus centering point. For the asthenic habitus, direct the central ray 2 inches inferior to the sthenic habitus centering point. Center the IR to the central ray.

- Open the longitudinally collimated field the full 14-inch (35-cm) IR length. Transverse collimation should be to the vertebrae and anterior abdomen border.

- An 11- × 14-inch (28- × 35-cm) IR placed lengthwise should be adequate to include all the required anatomical structures.

Lateral Stomach and Duodenum Image Analysis

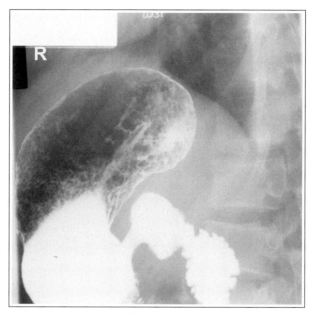

Image 8.

Analysis. The descending duodenum is partially superimposed over the duodenal bulb and vertebrae, and the posterior surfaces of the thoracic and lumbar vertebrae are not superimposed. The patient was not in a lateral position.

Correction. Align the shoulders, posterior ribs, and posterior pelvis perpendicular to the imaging table and IR.

STOMACH AND DUODENUM: ANTEROPOSTERIOR OBLIQUE PROJECTION (LEFT POSTERIOR OBLIQUE POSITION)

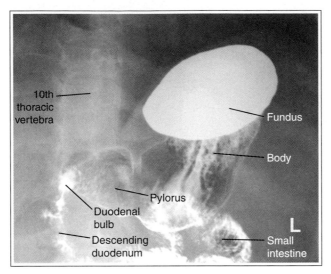

Figure 11-23. Hypersthenic left posterior oblique stomach and duodenal image with accurate positioning.

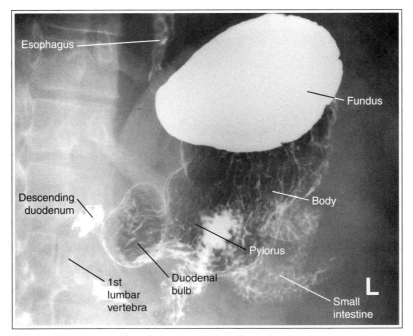

Figure 11-24. Sthenic left posterior oblique stomach and duodenal image with accurate positioning.

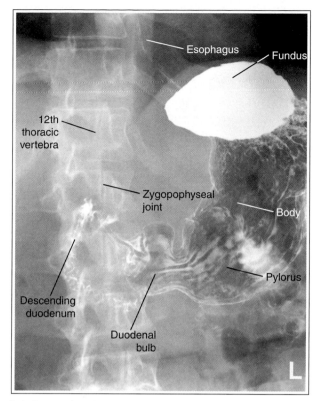

Figure 11-25. Asthenic left posterior oblique spot stomach and duodenal image with accurate positioning.

Image Analysis

Contrast distribution: Air-contrast is demonstrated in the pylorus, duodenal bulb, and descending duodenum, and barium is visible in the fundus.

An optimal AP oblique (left posterior oblique [LPO]) stomach and duodenal image has been obtained when the lumbar vertebrae demonstrate an oblique position with the degree of obliquity adequate for the body habitus and when the correct aspect of the stomach, as defined by the body habitus, is in profile.

Hypersthenic habitus: The patient has been rotated 60 degrees, as identified by the demonstration of the left lumbar zygapophyseal joints in the posterior third of the vertebral bodies. The duodenal bulb and descending duodenum are in profile, and the pylorus is superimposed over the vertebrae (Figure 11-23).

Sthenic habitus: The patient has been rotated 45 degrees, as identified by the demonstration of the left lumbar zygapophyseal joints at the midline of the vertebral bodies. The duodenal bulb and descending duodenum are in profile, and the vertebrae are demonstrated with little if any pyloric superimposition (Figure 11-24).

Asthenic Habitus: The patient has been rotated 30 degrees, as identified by the demonstration of the left lumbar zygapophyseal joints in the anterior third of the vertebral bodies. The duodenal bulb and descending duodenum are in profile, and the vertebrae are demonstrated with little if any pyloric superimposition (Figure 11-25).

- An AP oblique (LPO) stomach and duodenal image is obtained by placing the patient supine on the imaging table, then rotating the patient toward the left side until the midcoronal plane is at a 30- to 60-degree angle with the imaging table (Figure 11-26). The patient's right arm is drawn across the chest, the hand grasps the table edge, and the right knee is flexed for support. A radiolucent sponge positioned beneath the right surface may also help the patient maintain the LPO position. Rotate the patient with a hypersthenic habitus approximately 60 degrees and the patient with the asthenic habitus approximately 30 degrees.

The pylorus is centered within the collimated field. The stomach and duodenal loop are included within the field.

- To position the pylorus in the center of the collimated field, center a perpendicular central ray halfway between the vertebrae and left abdominal margin at a level

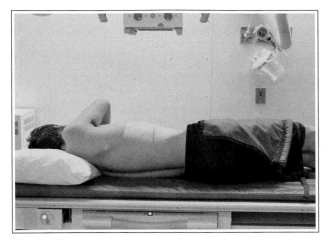

Figure 11-26. Proper patient positioning for left posterior oblique stomach and duodenal image.

midway between the xiphoid process and inferior rib margin for the sthenic habitus. Center the central ray at a level 2 inches (5 cm) superior to the sthenic habitus central ray centering for the hypersthenic habitus and 2 inches inferior for the asthenic habitus. Center the IR to the central ray.

- Open the longitudinally collimated field the full 14-inch (35-cm) IR length. Transverse collimation should be to the vertebrae and lateral rib border.
- An 11- × 14-inch (28- × 35-cm) IR placed lengthwise should be adequate to include all the required anatomical structures.

Posteroanterior Oblique Stomach and Duodenum Image Analysis

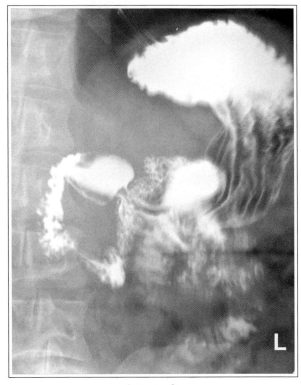

Image 9.

Analysis. The bony cortices are sharp, and the gastric and intestinal gases and barium are blurry. Peristaltic activity of the stomach and small intestine was occurring during the exposure.

Correction. Use a short exposure time.

STOMACH AND DUODENUM: ANTEROPOSTERIOR PROJECTION

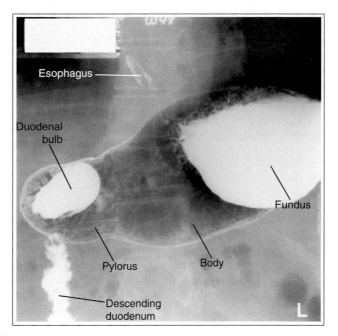

Figure 11-27. Hypersthenic anteroposterior spot stomach image with accurate positioning.

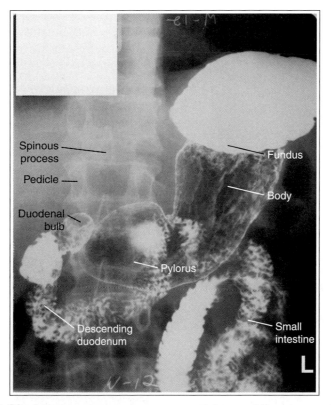

Figure 11-28. Sthenic anteroposterior spot stomach image with accurate positioning.

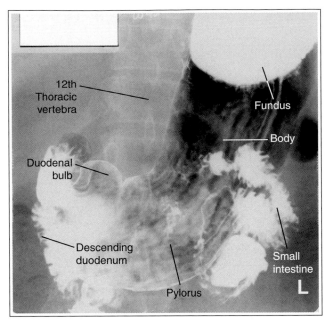

Figure 11-29. Asthenic anteroposterior spot stomach image with accurate positioning.

Image Analysis

Contrast distribution: **Air contrast is demonstrated in the pylorus, duodenal bulb, and descending duodenum, and barium is visible in the fundus.**

An optimal AP stomach image has been obtained when the spinous processes are aligned with the midline of the vertebral bodies, the distances from the pedicles to the spinous processes are the same on both sides, and the correct aspect of the stomach, as defined by the body habitus, is in profile.

Hypersthenic habitus: **The stomach is aligned nearly horizontally, with the duodenal bulb at the level of T11 to T12. The lesser and greater curvatures are demonstrated nearly on end, with the greater curvature being more anteriorly situated, and the esophagogastric junction is nearly on end (Figure 11-27).**

Sthenic habitus: **The stomach is aligned nearly vertically, with the duodenal bulb at the level of L1 to L2. The stomach is somewhat J-shaped, and its long axis is partially foreshortened. The lesser and greater curvatures, esophagogastric junction, pylorus, and duodenal bulb are in partial profile (Figure 11-28).**

Asthenic habitus: **The stomach is aligned vertically, with the duodenal bulb at the level of L3 to L4. The stomach is J-shaped, its long axis is demonstrated without foreshortening, and the lesser and greater curvatures, esophagogastric junction, pylorus, and duodenal bulb are demonstrated in profile (Figure 11-29).**

- To obtain an AP stomach and duodenal image, place the patient supine on the imaging table. Position the shoulders and ASISs at equal distances from the imaging table to prevent rotation, and draw the patient's arms away from the abdominal area to prevent them from being superimposed over the abdominal region (Figure 11-30).

- *Detecting abdominal rotation:* Rotation is effectively detected on an AP stomach and duodenal image by comparing the distance from the pedicles to the spinous processes on each side. The side demonstrating the greater distance from the pedicle to the spinous processes is the side positioned closer to the IR.

The pylorus is centered within the collimated field. The stomach and duodenal loop are included within the field.

- To position the pylorus in the center of the collimated field, center a perpendicular central ray halfway between the vertebrae and left abdominal margin at a level midway

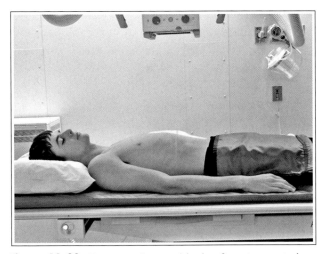

Figure 11-30. Proper patient positioning for anteroposterior stomach and duodenal image.

between the xiphoid process and inferior rib margin sthenic habitus. Center the central ray just medial to the left side of the vertebrae at a level 2 inches (5 cm) superior to the sthenic patient centering for the hypersthenic habitus and at a level 2 inches inferior for the asthenic habitus. Center the IR to the central ray.

- Open the longitudinally collimated field the full 14-inch (35-cm) IR length. Transverse collimation should be to the lateral rib border.
- An 11- × 14-inch (28- × 35-cm) IR placed lengthwise should be adequate to include all the required anatomical structures.

SMALL INTESTINE

SMALL INTESTINE: POSTEROANTERIOR PROJECTION

A marker indicating the amount of time that has elapsed since the patient ingested the contrast medium is included within the collimated field and is not superimposed over anatomical structures of interest.

- For studies of the small intestine, the patient drinks a large amount of barium, then the technologist obtains overhead images of the stomach and small intestine at timed intervals as peristalsis moves the contrast from the stomach through the small intestine to the cecum.

The timing begins when the patient ingests the contrast or as determined by the radiologist. Typically, the first prone overhead image is obtained at 15 minutes, then at 30 minutes, and then hourly until the barium is demonstrated in the cecum. The barium normally takes 2 to 3 hours to reach the cecum but may vary greatly from patient to patient. Each image in the timed series must contain a time marker to indicate the amount of time that has passed since the contrast was ingested.

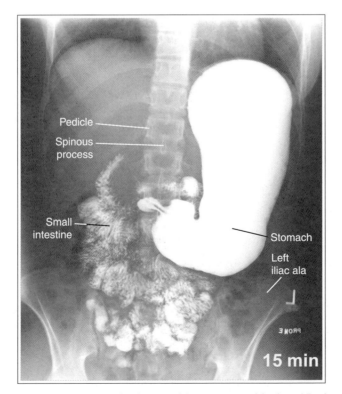

Figure 11-31. Posteroanterior small intestine image with accurate positioning; 15 minutes after ingestion.

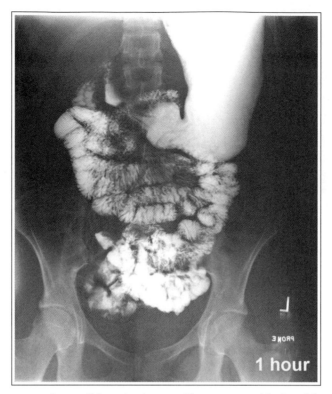

Figure 11-32. Posteroanterior small intestine image with accurate positioning; 1 hour after ingestion.

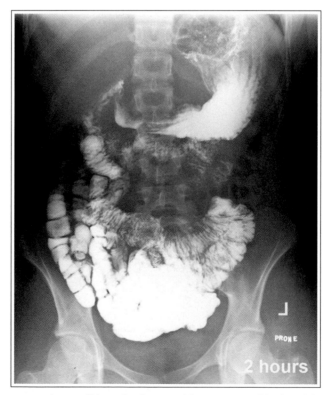

Figure 11-33. Posteroanterior small intestine image with accurate positioning; 2 hours after ingestion.

Image Analysis

The abdomen demonstrates a PA projection. The spinous processes are aligned with the midline of the vertebral bodies, the distances from the pedicles to the spinous processes is the same on both sides, and the iliac alae are symmetrical.

- To obtain a PA small intestine image, place the patient prone on the imaging table. Position the shoulders and ASISs at equal distances from the imaging table to prevent rotation, and draw the patient's arms away from the abdominal area to prevent them from being superimposed over the abdominal region (Figure 11-34). The prone position is chosen to demonstrate the small intestine because it will cause compression of the abdominal structures, increasing image quality.

- *Detecting abdominal rotation:* The upper and lower lumbar vertebrae can demonstrate rotation independently or simultaneously, depending on which section of the body is rotated. If the patient's thorax was rotated but the pelvis is not, the upper lumbar vertebrae and abdominal cavity demonstrate rotation. If the patient's pelvis was rotated but the thorax was not, the lower vertebrae and abdominal cavity demonstrate rotation. If the patient's thorax and pelvis were rotated simultaneously, the entire abdominal cavity demonstrates rotation. Rotation is effectively detected on a PA small intestine image by comparing the distances from the pedicles to the spinous processes on both sides and the symmetry of the iliac alae. The side demonstrating the greater distance from the pedicles to the spinous processes and the wider iliac ala is the side positioned farther from the IR.

The small intestine is centered within the collimated field. The stomach and proximal aspects of the small intestine are included within the field on images taken early in the series, and the small intestine and cecum are included on images taken later in the series.

- To include the stomach and small intestine on images obtained earlier in the series, use a perpendicular central ray with the midsagittal plane at a level 2 inches (5 cm) superior to the iliac crest. To include the small intestine and cecum on images obtained later in the series, direct the central ray to the midsagittal plane at the level of the iliac crest. Center the IR to the central ray (see Image 10).

- The longitudinal collimated field should remain fully open. Transversely collimate to within ½ inch (1.25 cm) of the patient's lateral skinline.

- *IR size and direction:* A 14- × 17-inch (35- × 43-cm) lengthwise IR should be adequate to include all the required anatomical structures on *sthenic* and *asthenic* patients, as long as the transverse abdominal measurement is less than 14 inches (35 cm).

  Use two 14- × 17-inch (35- × 43-cm) crosswise IRs on *hypersthenic* patients and on other patients who have a transverse abdominal measurement of 14 inches (35 cm) or greater, to include all the necessary anatomical structures. Take the first image with the central ray centered to the midsagittal plane at a level halfway between the symphysis pubis and ASIS. Position the bottom of the second IR so it includes 2 to 3 inches (5 to 7.5 cm) of the same transverse section of the peritoneal cavity imaged on the first image to ensure that no middle peritoneal information has been excluded. It may be necessary to obtain only the superiorly positioned image for the initially obtained image, because the barium may not travel to the inferiorly situated small bowel so soon in the procedure.

Anteroposterior Small Intestine Image Analysis

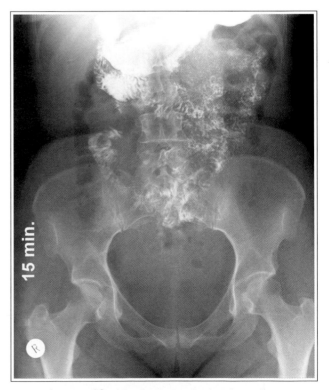

Image 10. 15-minute post-barium ingestion.

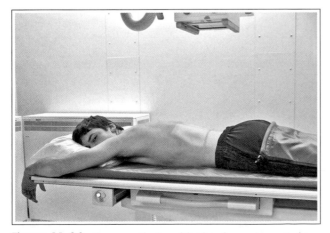

Figure 11-34. Proper patient positioning for posteroanterior small intestine image.

Analysis. Fifteen minutes after ingestion; the stomach and superior small intestine have not been included on the image. The central ray and IR were positioned too inferiorly.

Correction. Center the central ray 2 inches (5 cm) superior to the iliac crest. Center the IR to the central ray.

LARGE INTESTINE

The large intestine demonstrates adequate distention and mucosal covering. The lumina are distended without mucosal folds, the mucosal surface demonstrates a thin coating of barium, and barium pooling is limited to one third of the intestinal diameter.

- *Good double-contrast lower intestinal filling:* Good gaseous distention is demonstrated when the bowel lumina are distended, eliminating the mucosal folds and allowing all parts of the barium-coated mucosal lining of the colon and any small intraluminal lesions to be visualized.

  Good lower intestinal barium coating has been obtained when the surface positioned farther from the IR on recumbent images or superiorly on erect images, also called the *nondependent surface*, demonstrates a thin layer of barium coating the mucosal surface, and when the surface positioned closer to the IR on recumbent images or inferiorly on erect images, also called the *dependent (decubitus) surface*, demonstrates a thin layer of barium coating of the highest structures, with barium pooled in the lower crevices. The barium pools are used to wash away residual fecal material from the dependent

surface, coat the mucosal surface, and fill any depressed lesions as the patient is rotated. Ideally, barium should fill one third of the large intestine diameter; overfilling or underfilling may result in obscured lesions or inadequate intestinal washing, respectively. See Table 11-3 to determine where barium pooling will occur on a lower intestine image. Pooling will occur in the anterior surface on prone images, posterior surface on supine images, and inferiorly, between the mucosal folds, on erect images.

- *Poor double contrast:* Poor gaseous distention results in pockets of large barium pools, compacted intestinal segments with tight mucosal folds. Poor mucosal coating is demonstrated by thin, irregular or interrupted barium coating or excessive barium pooling. Poor coating may cause lesions to be easily missed. Although proper double-contrast filling is primarily the fluoroscopist's responsibility, the technologist's scope of practice may play a part in some of the causes for poor coating, such as using the wrong type of barium, improperly preparing the barium suspension, or performing poor lower intestinal preparation.

TABLE 11-3   Double-Contrast Filling of Large Intestinal Structures

Large Intestine	Supine Position	Prone Position
Cecum	Air	Barium
Ascending colon	Barium	Air
Ascending limb right colic (hepatic) flexure	Barium	Air
Descending limb right colic (hepatic) flexure	Barium	Air
Transverse colon	Air	Barium
Ascending limb left colic (splenic) flexure	Air	Barium
Descending limb left colic (splenic) flexure	Barium	Air
Descending colon	Barium	Air
Sigmoid colon	Air	Barium
Rectum	Barium	Air

LARGE INTESTINE: POSTEROANTERIOR OR ANTEROPOSTERIOR PROJECTION

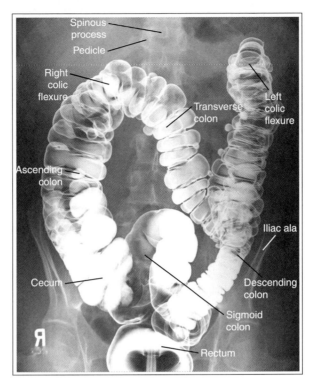

Figure 11-35. Posteroanterior large intestine image with accurate positioning.

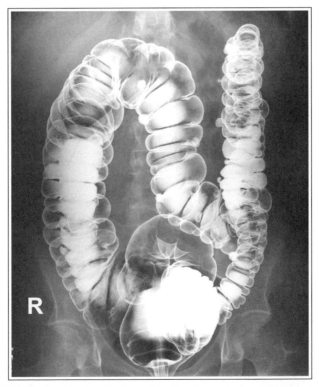

Figure 11-36. Anteroposterior large intestine image with accurate positioning.

Image Analysis

The abdomen image demonstrates a PA or AP projection. The spinous processes are aligned with the midline of the vertebral bodies, the distance from the pedicles to the spinous processes is the same on both sides, and the iliac ala are symmetrical. The ascending and descending limbs of the colic flexures demonstrate some degree of superimposition.

- To obtain a PA large intestine image, place the patient prone on the imaging table; to obtain an AP large intestine image, place the patient supine on the imaging table. Position the shoulders and ASISs at equal distances from the imaging table to prevent rotation, and draw the patient's arms away from the abdominal area to prevent them from being superimposed over the abdominal region (Figure 11-37).
- ***Detecting abdominal rotation:*** Rotation is effectively detected on a PA or AP lower intestine image by comparing the distances from the pedicles to the spinous processes on both sides, the symmetry of the iliac ala, and the superimposition of the colic flexures. *PA projection:* The side demonstrating the greater distance from the pedicles to the spinous processes, wider iliac ala, and colic flexure with greater ascending and descending limb superimposition is the side positioned farther from the IR (see Image 12). *AP projection:* The side demonstrating the greater distance from the pedicle to the spinous processes, wider iliac ala, and colic flexure with the greater ascending and descending limb superimposition is the side positioned closer to the IR.

  The beam divergence causes very different appearing iliac alae on an image that is obtained in a supine versus a prone position. Figure 11-38 demonstrates the iliac alae of a supine and prone abdomen; note that the iliac alae in an image obtained with the patient supine are wider than with the patient prone. This knowledge can be used to distinguish whether the image was taken with the patient in a supine or prone position, but the narrow iliac ala of the prone image should not be mistaken for narrowness caused by rotation.

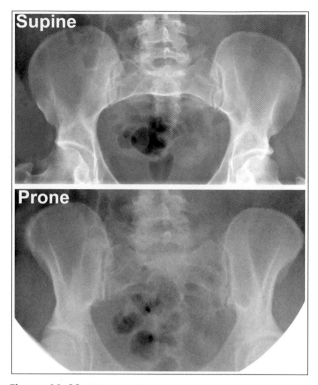

Figure 11-38. Iliac alae images of supine and prone patient.

The fourth lumbar vertebra is centered within the collimated field. The entire large intestine, including the left colic (splenic) flexure and rectum, is included within the field.

- To position the fourth lumbar vertebra in the center of the collimated field, center a perpendicular central ray with the patient's midsagittal plane at the level of the iliac crest. Center the IR to the central ray. The longitudinal collimated field should remain fully open. Transversely collimate to within ½ inch (0.6 cm) of the patient's lateral skinline.
- ***IR size and direction:*** A 14- × 17-inch (35- × 43-cm) lengthwise IR should be adequate to include all the required anatomical structures on *sthenic* and *asthenic* patients, as long as the transverse abdominal measurement is less than 14 inches (35 cm).

  Use two 14- × 17-inch (35- × 43-cm) crosswise IRs on *hypersthenic* patients and on other patients who have a transverse abdominal measurement of 14 inches (35 cm) or greater, to include all the necessary anatomical structures (Figure 11-39 and Image 13). Take the first image with the central ray centered to the midsagittal plane at a level halfway between the symphysis pubis and ASIS. Position the bottom of the second IR so it includes 2 to 3 inches (5 to 7.5 cm) of the same transverse section of the peritoneal cavity imaged on the first image to ensure that no middle peritoneal information has been excluded. The top of the IR should extend to the patient's xiphoid (which is at the level of the tenth thoracic vertebra) to make sure that the left colic (splenic) flexure is included.

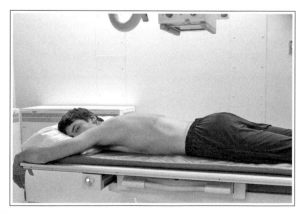

Figure 11-37. Proper patient positioning for posteroanterior large intestine image.

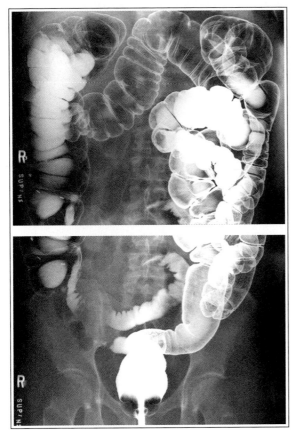

Figure 11-39. Proper patient positioning for posteroanterior large intestine images of hypersthenic patient.

Posteroanterior or Anteroposterior Large Intestine Image Analysis

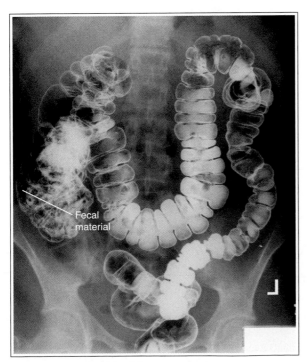

Image 11. PA projection.

Analysis. PA projection; remaining fecal material is visible in the cecum. Fecal material may obscure the mucosal surfaces and when barium coated may mimic polyps and small tumors.

Correction. Patient should follow large intestinal preparation procedure before examination.

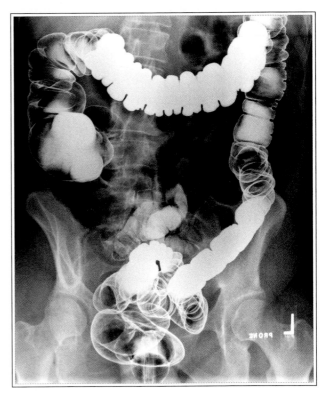

Image 12. PA projection.

Analysis. PA projection; the right iliac ala is narrow and the left wide, the distance from the right pedicles to the spinous processes is narrower than the same distance on the left side, and the left colic (splenic) flexure demonstrates greater ascending and descending limb superimposition. The patient was rotated toward the right side.

Correction. Rotate the patient toward the left side until the shoulders and iliac alae are at equal distances to the imaging table.

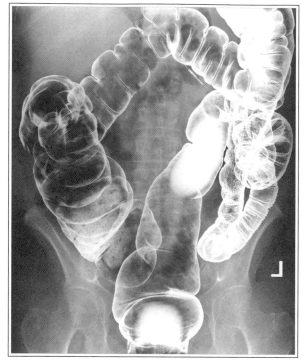

Image 13. PA projection.

Analysis. PA projection; the left colic (splenic) flexure and part of the transverse colon are not included on the image. The IR is not adequate to include the entire large intestine.

Correction. Use two crosswise IRs with 2 to 3 inches of overlap.

LARGE INTESTINE (RECTUM): LATERAL POSITION

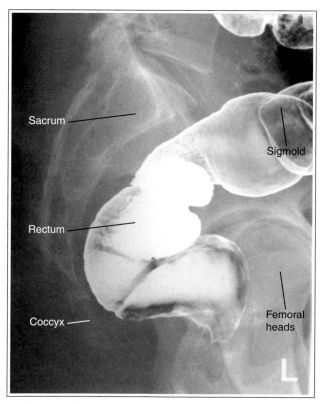

Figure 11-40. Lateral large intestine (rectum) image with accurate positioning.

Image Analysis

Scatter radiation is controlled.

- A grid and a lead sheet are placed on the imaging table at the edge of the posteriorly collimated field to reduce the amount of scatter radiation that reaches the IR, providing higher contrast and better visibility of recorded details.

The rectum is demonstrated in profile. The sacrum demonstrates a lateral position. The median sacral crest is demonstrated in profile, and the femoral heads are superimposed.

- To obtain a lateral sacral image, place the patient on the imaging table in a lateral recumbent position. Whether the patient is lying on the right or left side is not significant, although the left side positioning is easier for the technologist.

  Flex the patient's knees and hips for support, and position a pillow or sponge between the knees. The thickness of the pillow or sponge should be enough to prevent the side of the pelvis situated farther from the IR from rotating anteriorly, without being so thick as to cause this side to rotate posteriorly (Figure 11-41).

  To avoid rectal and vertebral rotation, align the shoulders, posterior ribs, and posterior pelvis perpendicular to the imaging table and IR. This is accomplished by resting your extended flat palm against each structure individually and adjusting the patient's rotation until your hand is positioned perpendicular to the imaging table.

- *Detecting rotation:* Rotation can be detected on a lateral rectum image by evaluating the degree of femoral head superimposition. On a nonrotated lateral rectal image, the femoral heads are directly superimposed. On rotation the femoral heads will move away from each other. When rotation has occurred, evaluate the placement of the femoral heads to determine the way in which the patient was rotated. The femoral head that demonstrates the greater magnification is the one situated farther from the IR (see Images 14 and 15).

The rectosigmoid region is at the center of the collimated field. The rectum, distal sigmoid, sacrum, and femoral heads are included within the field.

- To place the rectosigmoid region in the center of the field, center a perpendicular central ray to the midcoronal plane (between the ASIS and posterior sacrum) at the level of the ASIS. Center the IR to the central ray.
- Open the longitudinal and transverse collimation to the full IR field size.
- A 10- × 12-inch (24- × 30-cm) IR placed lengthwise should be adequate to include all the required anatomical structures.

Lateral Large Intestine (Rectum) Image Analysis

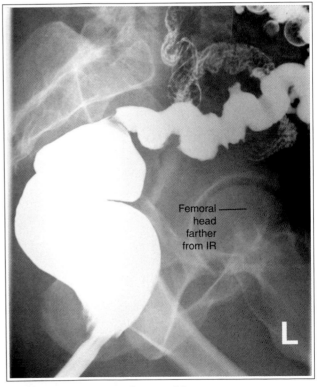

Image 14.

Analysis. A lateral position has not been obtained. The femoral heads are not superimposed; the right femoral head is rotated anterior to the left femoral head.

Correction. Rotate the right side of the patient posteriorly until the posterior pelvic wings are superimposed and aligned perpendicular to the imaging table.

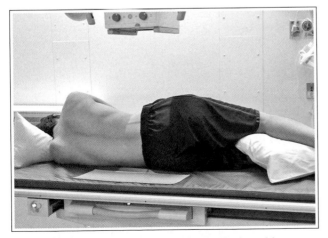

Figure 11-41. Proper patient positioning for lateral large intestine image.

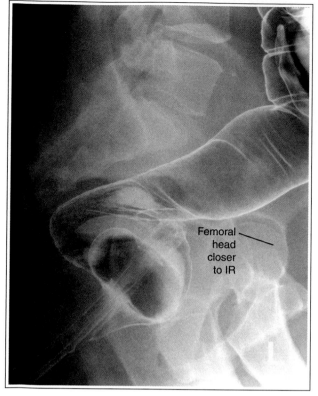

Image 15.

Analysis. A lateral position has not been obtained. The femoral heads are not superimposed; the right femoral head is rotated posterior to the left femoral head.

Correction. Rotate the right side of the patient anteriorly until the posterior pelvis wings are superimposed and aligned perpendicular to the imaging table.

LARGE INTESTINE: LATERAL DECUBITUS POSITION (ANTEROPOSTERIOR OR POSTEROANTERIOR PROJECTION)

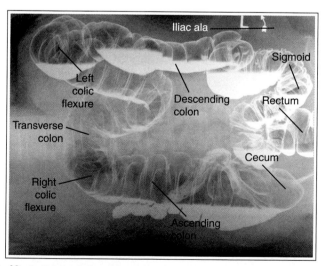

Figure 11-42. Left lateral decubitus large intestine image with accurate positioning.

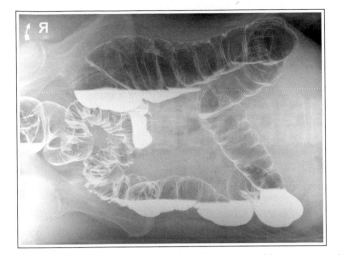

Figure 11-43. Right lateral decubitus large intestine image with accurate positioning.

Image Analysis

An arrow or word marker is present on the image, indicating the side of patient that was positioned up and away from the imaging table or cart.

- Place marker superiorly, away from anatomical structures of interest, and within the collimated field.

Density is uniform across abdomen structures.

- *Using a wedge-compensating filter:* When a decubitus large intestine image is obtained in a patient with *excessive abdominal soft tissue*, the soft tissue often drops toward the imaging table or cart. This movement results in a smaller AP measurement at the elevated side than at the side closer to the imaging table or cart. To compensate for this thickness difference, a wedge-compensating filter may be used. The wedge filter absorbs some of the x-ray photons before they reach the patient, thus decreasing the number of photons exposing the IR where the filter is located. The thick end of the wedge filter absorbs more photons than the thin end. When a wedge-compensating filter is used, attach it to the x-ray collimator head with the thick end positioned toward the patient's "up" side (thinnest part of abdomen) and the thin end toward the patient's "down" side (thickest part of abdomen). Then set a technique that will accurately expose the middle section of the abdomen. The wedge-compensating filter should absorb the needed photons to prevent overexposure of the thinner abdominal region. When the filter has been accurately positioned, image density is uniform throughout the abdominal structures. Positioning the filter too close to or too far away from the thickest part of the abdomen results in an overexposed or underexposed area on the image, respectively, and a line of density difference. If the compensating filter is inaccurately positioned,

a density variation line will appear, defining where the filter was and was not placed over the structures (Image 16).

The abdomen image demonstrates an AP projection. The spinous processes are aligned with the midline of the vertebral bodies, the distances from the pedicles to the spinous processes are the same on both sides, and the iliac alae are symmetrical. The ascending and descending limbs of the colic flexures demonstrate some degree of superimposition.

- Decubitus large intestine images are obtained by placing the patient in left and right lateral recumbent position on the imaging table or cart with the back or abdomen resting against a grid cassette or the upright IR holder. To avoid rotation, align the shoulders, the posterior ribs, and the posterior pelvis perpendicular to the imaging table or cart (Figure 11-44). Accomplish this alignment by resting an extended flat hand against each, respectively, and then adjusting the patient's rotation until the hand is positioned perpendicular to the imaging table or cart.

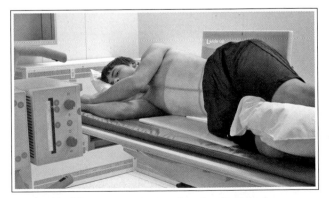

Figure 11-44. Proper patient positioning for lateral decubitus large intestine image.

Flex the patient's knees to support the patient's lateral position, although do not bring them to a 90-degree angle with the torso or they may be superimposed over the lateral aspect of the distal rectum (Image 17). It is most common for a patient to rotate the elevated thorax and iliac ala anteriorly. A pillow or other support placed between the patient's flexed knees may help to eliminate this forward rotation.

- *Detecting abdominal rotation:* Rotation is effectively detected on a PA or AP decubitus lower intestine image by comparing the distance from the pedicles to the spinous processes on each side, the symmetry of the iliac ala, and the superimposition of the colic flexures. *PA decubitus projection:* The side demonstrating the greater distance from the pedicles to the spinous processes, wider iliac ala, and colic flexure with greater ascending and descending limb superimposition is the side positioned farther from the IR (Image 18). *AP decubitus projection:* The side demonstrating the greater distance from the pedicle to the spinous processes, wider iliac ala, and colic flexure with greater ascending and descending limb superimposition is the side positioned closer to the IR (Image 19).

The abdominal field positioned against the imaging table or cart is demonstrated in its entirety and without artifact lines.

- Elevating the patient on a radiolucent sponge or on a hard surface such as a cardiac board positions the patient's abdomen above the IR's cassette border, preventing a part of the abdomen from being clipped, and prevents the abdomen from sinking into the table or cart pad. When the patient's body is allowed to sink into the cart pad, artifact lines are superimposed over the lateral abdominal field of the side that is down (Image 17).

The fourth lumbar vertebra is centered within the collimated field. The entire large intestine, including the left colic (splenic) flexure and rectum, is included within the field.

- To position the fourth lumbar vertebra in the center of the collimated field, center a perpendicular central ray with the patient's midsagittal plane at the level of the iliac crest. Center the IR to the central ray.
- The longitudinal collimated field should remain fully open. Transversely collimate to within ½ inch (1.25 cm) of the patient's lateral skinline.
- *IR size and direction:* A 14- × 17-inch (35- × 43-cm) lengthwise IR should be adequate to include all the required anatomical structures on *sthenic* and *asthenic* patients, as long as the transverse abdominal measurement is less than 14 inches (35 cm).
- Use two 14- × 17-inch (35- × 43-cm) crosswise IRs on *hypersthenic* patients and on other patients who have a transverse abdominal measurement of 14 inches (35 cm) or greater, to include all the necessary anatomical structures. Take the first image with the central

ray centered to the midsagittal plane at a level halfway between the symphysis pubis and ASIS. Position the bottom of the second IR so it includes 2 to 3 inches (5 to 7.5 cm) of the same transverse section of the peritoneal cavity imaged on the first image to ensure that no middle peritoneal information has been excluded. The top of the IR should extend to the patient's xiphoid (which is at the level of the tenth thoracic vertebra) to make sure that the left colic (splenic) flexure is included.

Lateral Decubitus Large Intestine Image Analysis

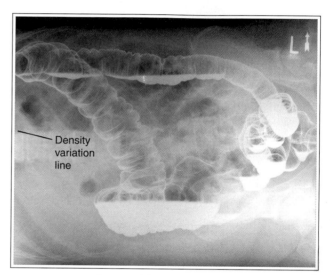

Image 16. AP projection.

Analysis. AP projection; the image density is not uniform across the abdomen. The right side of the abdomen is slightly underexposed, and the left side is slightly overexposed. Too much thickness of the compensating filter was positioned over the right side of the abdomen. A density difference line defines where the filter was and was not placed correctly over the abdomen.

Correction. Move the filter so less thickness is present over the right side of the abdomen.

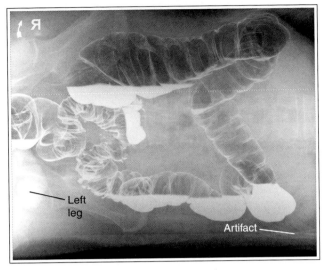

Image 17. PA projection.

Analysis. PA projection; artifact lines are superimposed over the left lateral abdominal region. The patient was not elevated on a radiolucent sponge. An underexposed area is present on the left side of the rectum. The patient's knee was bent to 90 degrees.

Correction. Elevate the patient on a radiolucent sponge or cardiac board to prevent the side of the abdomen from sinking into the table or cart pad. Decrease the amount of knee flexion.

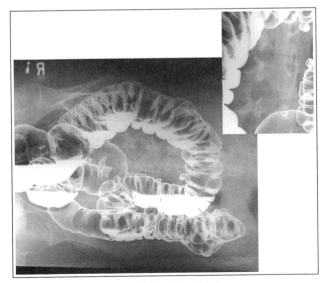

Image 18. PA projection.

Analysis. PA projection; the distance from the right pedicles to the spinous processes is less than the distance from the left pedicles to the spinous processes, the right iliac ala is narrower than the left, and the ascending and descending limbs of the left colic (splenic) flexure demonstrate increased superimposition. The left side of the patient was positioned closer to the IR than the right side.

Correction. Rotate the right side of the patient away from the IR until the shoulders and iliac ala are at equal distances to the IR.

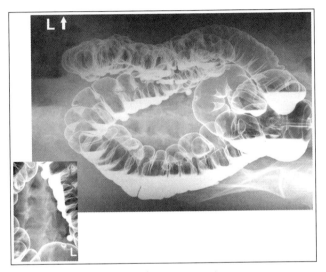

Image 19. AP projection.

Analysis. AP projection; the distance from the right pedicles to the spinous processes is less than the distance from the left pedicles to the spinous processes, the left iliac ala is wider than the right, and the left colic (splenic) flexure demonstrates increased superimposition. The left side of the patient was positioned closer to the IR than the right side.

Correction. Rotate the left side of the patient away from the IR until the shoulders and ASISs are at equal distances from the IR.

LARGE INTESTINE: POSTEROANTERIOR OBLIQUE PROJECTION (RIGHT ANTERIOR OBLIQUE POSITION)

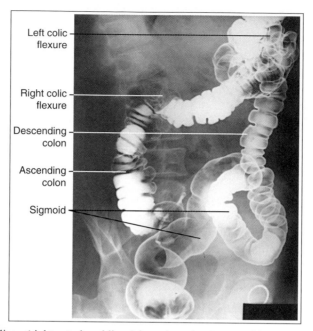

Figure 11-45. Posteroanterior oblique (right anterior oblique) large intestine image with accurate positioning. *(From Ballinger PW, Frank ED: Merrill's atlas of radiographic positions and radiologic procedures, vol 2, ed 10, p. 177.)*

Image Analysis

The ascending and descending limbs of the right colic (hepatic) flexure are demonstrated with decreased superimposition when compared with the PA projection, whereas the limbs of the left colic (splenic) flexure demonstrate increased superimposition and the rectosigmoid segments are demonstrated without transverse superimposition. The right iliac ala is narrow and the left is wide, and the distance from the right pedicles to the spinous processes is narrower than the distance from the left pedicles to the spinous processes.

- A PA oblique (RAO) large intestine image is obtained by positioning the patient prone on the imaging table and then rotating the torso toward the right side until the midcoronal plane is at a 35- to 45-degree angle with the imaging table. In the PA projection, the descending limb of the right colic (hepatic) flexure is superimposed over the ascending limb and the rectum is superimposed over the distal sigmoid. Rotating the patient toward the right side moves the ascending right colic limb from beneath the descending limb and the distal sigmoid from beneath the rectum (transversely), allowing better visualization of these structures. The left elbow and knee are partially flexed and are used to support the patient and maintain accurate obliquity (Figure 11-46).

  Detecting inadequate rotation on a PA oblique (RAO) image: Insufficient rotation of the colon is demonstrated on the PA oblique image when the ascending and descending limbs of the right colic flexure are superimposed

and the rectum is superimposed over the distal sigmoid (Image 20).

The midabdomen is at the center of the collimated field. The entire large intestine is included within the field.

- To place the midabdomen in the center of the field, center a perpendicular central ray approximately 1 to 2 inches (2.5 to 5 cm) to the left of the midsagittal plane at the level of the iliac crest. Center the IR to the central ray.
- The longitudinal collimated field should remain fully open. Transversely collimate to within ½ inch (1.25 cm) of the patient's lateral skinline.
- ***IR size and direction:*** A 14- × 17-inch (35- × 43-cm) IR placed lengthwise should be adequate to include all the required anatomical structures.

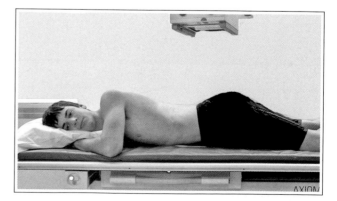

Figure 11-46. Proper patient positioning for posteroanterior oblique (right anterior oblique) large intestine image.

Posteroanterior Oblique (Right Anterior Oblique) Large Intestine Image Analysis

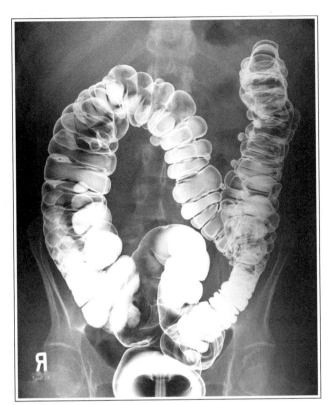

Image 20.

Analysis. The ascending and descending limbs of the right colic (hepatic) flexion and the rectum and distal sigmoid, respectively, demonstrate increased superimposition. The iliac ala are uniform in width. The patient was insufficiently rotated.

Correction. Rotate the patient toward the right side until the midsagittal plane is at a 35- to 45-degree angle with the IR.

LARGE INTESTINE: POSTEROANTERIOR OBLIQUE PROJECTION (LEFT ANTERIOR OBLIQUE POSITION)

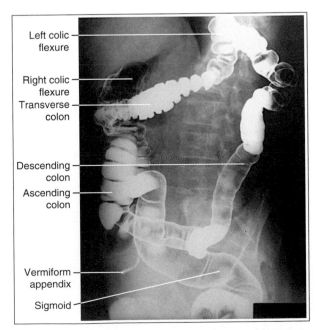

Figure 11-47. Posteroanterior oblique (left anterior oblique) large intestine image with accurate positioning. (*From Ballinger PW, Frank ED: Merrill's atlas of radiographic positions and radiologic procedures, vol 2, ed 10, p. 178*).

Image Analysis

The ascending and descending limbs of the left colic (splenic) flexure are demonstrated with decreased superimposition when compared with the PA projection, while the limbs of the right colic (hepatic) flexure demonstrate increased superimposition. The left iliac ala is narrow and the right is wide, and the distance from the left pedicles to the spinous processes is narrower than the distance from the right pedicles to the spinous processes.

- A PA oblique (LAO) large intestine image is obtained by positioning the patient prone on the imaging table and then rotating the torso toward the left side until the midcoronal plane is at a 35- to 45-degree angle with the imaging table. In the PA projection, the descending limb of the left colic (splenic) flexure is superimposed over the ascending limb, and the rectum is superimposed over the distal sigmoid. Rotating the patient toward the left side moves the descending left colic limb from beneath the ascending limb, allowing better visualization of these structures. The left elbow and knee are partially flexed and are used to support the patient and maintain accurate obliquity (Figure 11-48).

    Detecting inadequate rotation on a PA oblique (LAO) image: Insufficient rotation of the colon is demonstrated on the PA oblique image when the ascending and descending limbs of the left colic flexure are superimposed.

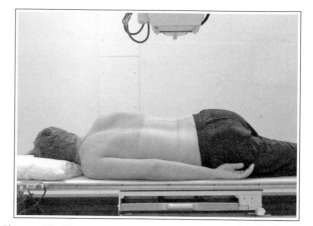

Figure 11-48. Proper patient positioning for posteroanterior oblique (left anterior oblique) large intestine image.

The midabdomen is at the center of the collimated field. The entire large intestine is included within the field.

- To place the midabdomen in the center of the field, center a perpendicular central ray approximately 1 to 2 inches (2.5 to 5 cm) to the right of the midsagittal plane at the level 1 to 2 inches (2.5 to 5 cm) superior to the iliac crest. Center the IR to the central ray.
- The longitudinal collimated field should remain fully open. Transversely collimate to within ½ inch (1.25 cm) of the patient's lateral skinline.
- ***IR size and direction:*** A 14- × 17-inch (35- × 43-cm) lengthwise IR placed lengthwise should be adequate to include all the required anatomical structures.

LARGE INTESTINE: POSTEROANTERIOR AXIAL OBLIQUE (RIGHT ANTERIOR OBLIQUE) OR POSTEROANTERIOR AXIAL PROJECTIONS (BUTTERFLY POSITIONS)

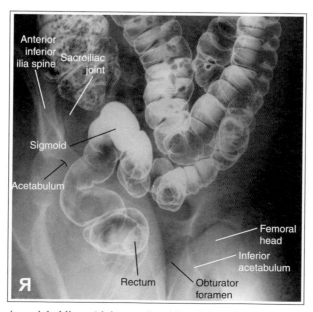

Figure 11-49. Posteroanterior axial oblique (right anterior oblique) large intestine image with accurate positioning.

Image Analysis

PA axial: **The pelvis is demonstrated without rotation: The iliac alae and obturator foramen are symmetrical.**

PA axial oblique (RAO): **The pelvis demonstrates adequate rotation when the rectosigmoid segments are demonstrated without transverse superimposition, the right sacroiliac (SI) joint is shown just medial to the ASIS, and the left obturator foramen is open.**

- *PA axial oblique (RAO):* A PA axial oblique (RAO) large intestine image is obtained by positioning the patient prone on the imaging table and then rotating the torso toward the right side until the midcoronal plane is at a 35- to 45-degree angle with the imaging table. In the PA projection the rectum is superimposed over the distal sigmoid, obscuring the rectosigmoid junction. Rotating the patient toward the right side moves the sigmoid from beneath the rectum (transversely), allowing better demonstration of this area. The left elbow and knee are partially flexed and are used to support the patient and maintain accurate obliquity (Figure 11-50).

    Detecting inadequate rotation on a PA axial oblique (RAO) image: Insufficient pelvic rotation of the rectosigmoid and pelvic area is demonstrated on the PA axial oblique image when the rectum is superimposed over the sigmoid colon, the right SI joint is too medial to the ASIS and the left obturator foramen is open. Too much pelvic rotation is demonstrated when the right SI joint is obscured and the left obturator foramen is closed (Images 21 and 22).

- *PA axial:* A PA axial large intestine image is obtained by positioning the patient prone on the imaging table with the legs extended. Position the shoulders and ASISs at equal distances from the imaging table to prevent rotation (Figure 11-51).

    Detecting rotation on a PA axial image: Rotation is effectively detected on a PA axial large intestine image by evaluating the symmetry of the iliac alae and obturator foramen. If the patient was rotated away from the

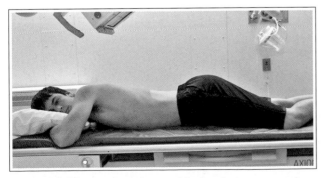

Figure 11-50. Proper patient positioning for posteroanterior axial oblique (right anterior oblique) large intestine image.

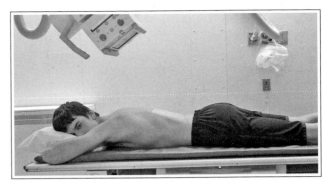

Figure 11-51. Proper patient positioning for posteroanterior axial large intestine image.

prone position, the iliac ala positioned farther from the IR will increase in width, the iliac ala positioned closer to the IR will narrow, the obturator foramina positioned farther from the IR will narrow, and the obturator foramina positioned closer to the IR will widen.

The rectosigmoid segment is demonstrated without inferosuperior superimposition, the pelvis demonstrates elongation, and the left inferior acetabulum is at the level of the distal rectum.

- The PA axial oblique (RAO) and PA axial projections of the large intestine are obtained to demonstrate the rectosigmoid area with less superimposition. To move the posteriorly situated rectum inferiorly and off the distal sigmoid, a 30- to 40-degree caudal angulation is used, decreasing rectosigmoid superimposition and better demonstrating the area. This angulation also elongates the pelvic structures.

- *Inadequate angulation:* When the rectosigmoid segment demonstrates inferosuperior overlap, the central ray angulation used was inadequate. If the inferior aspect of the left acetabulum is demonstrated superior to the distal rectum, the central ray was insufficient (Image 21). If the inferior aspect of the left acetabulum is demonstrated inferior to the distal rectum, the central ray angulation was too great (Image 22).

The rectosigmoid area is at the center of the collimated field. The rectum, sigmoid, and pelvic structures are included within the field.

- *PA axial projection:* To place the rectosigmoid area at the center of the collimated field, center the central ray to exit at the level of the ASIS and to the midsagittal plane.

- *PA axial oblique projection:* To place the rectosigmoid area in the center of the field, center the central ray to the exit at the ASIS and 2 inches (5 cm) to the left of the lumbar spinous processes. Center the IR to the central ray.

- An 11- × 14-inch (28- × 35-cm) or 14- × 17-inch (35- × 43-cm) IR placed lengthwise should be adequate to include all the required anatomical structures.

Posteroanterior Axial Oblique (Right Anterior Oblique) Large Intestine Image Analysis

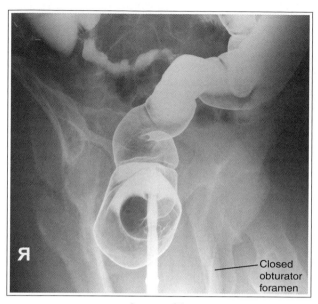

Image 21.

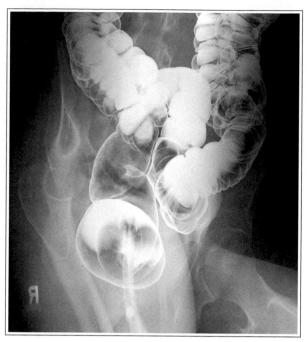

Image 22.

Analysis. The right SI joint is obscured, and the left obturator foramen is closed. The pelvis was rotated more than 45 degrees. The inferior aspect of the left acetabulum is demonstrated superior to the distal rectum. The central ray was insufficient.

Correction. Decrease pelvic rotation until the midcoronal plane is at a 30- to 45-degree angle with the imaging table, and increase the degree of central ray angulation.

Analysis. The right SI joint is obscured, and the left obturator foramen is closed. The pelvis was rotated more than 45 degrees. The inferior aspect of the left acetabulum is demonstrated inferior to the distal rectum. The central ray angulation was too great.

Correction. Decrease pelvic rotation until the midcoronal plane is at a 30- to 45-degree angle with the imaging table, and decrease the degree of central ray angulation.

Bibliography

Adler A, Carlton R: *Introduction to radiologic sciences and patient care,* ed 3, Philadelphia, 2003, Saunders.

Ballinger PW, Frank ED: *Merrill's atlas of radiographic positioning and radiologic procedures,* ed 10, St Louis, 2003, Mosby.

Bontrager K, Lampignano J: *Radiographic positioning and related anatomy,* ed 6, St Louis, 2005, Mosby.

Bushong SC: *Radiologic science for technologists,* ed 8, St Louis, 2004, Mosby.

Carroll, QB: *Fuchs's radiographic exposure and quality control,* ed 7, Springfield, Illinois, 2003, Charles C Thomas.

Ehrlich RA, McCloskey ED, Daly JA: *Patient care in radiography,* ed 6, St Louis, 2004, Mosby.

Eisenberg RL: *Gastrointestinal radiology: a pattern approach,* ed 4, Philadelphia, 2002, Lippincott Williams & Wilkins.

Fauber, TL: *Radiographic imaging and exposure,* ed 2, St Louis, 2004, Mosby.

Fraser RG, Colman N, Muller N, Pare P: *Synopsis of diseases of the chest,* ed 3, Philadelphia, 2005, Saunders.

Jeffrey RB, Ralls PW, Leung AN, Brant-Zawadzki M: *Emergency imaging,* Philadelphia, 1999, Lippincott Williams & Wilkins.

Levine MS, Rubesin SE, and Laufer I: *Double contrast gastrointestinal radiology,* ed 3, Philadelphia, 2000, Saunders.

Rogers LF: *Radiology of skeletal trauma,* ed 3, New York, 2002, Churchill Livingstone.

Shephard CT: *Radiographic image production and manipulation,* New York, 2003, McGraw-Hill.

Standring S: *Gray's anatomy: the anatomical basis of clinical practice,* ed 39, St Louis, 2004, Churchill Livingstone.

Statkiewicz MA, Visconti PJ, Ritenour ER: *Radiation protection in medical radiography,* ed 4, St Louis, 2002, Mosby.

Thornton A, Gyll C: *Children's fractures,* 2000, Baillière Tindall.

Tortora GJ, Derrickson BH: *Principles of anatomy and physiology,* ed 11, New York, 2005, Wiley.

Ward R, Blickman H: *Pediatric imaging,* St Louis, 2005, Mosby.

Williamson SL: *Primary pediatric radiology,* Philadelphia, 2002, Saunders.

Page numbers followed by f indicate figures; b, boxes.